Inherited Skin Disorders
The Genodermatoses

I dedicate this book to my patients and their families

John Harper

Inherited Skin Disorders
The Genodermatoses

Edited by

John Harper MD, FRCP

Consultant in Paediatric Dermatology
Great Ormond Street Hospital for Children
London, UK

Genetics Advisor

Marcus E. Pembrey MD, FRCP

Mothercare Professor of Paediatric Genetics
Mothercare Unit of Clinical Genetics and Fetal Medicine
Institute of Child Health
London, UK

Illustrative Editor

Simon Brown MSc, FIMI, FBIPP, FBPA

Director of Medical Illustration
Institute of Child Health
London, UK

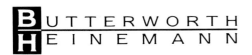
BUTTERWORTH
HEINEMANN

Butterworth-Heinemann Ltd
Linacre House, Jordan Hill, Oxford OX2 8DP
A division of Reed Educational & Professional Publishing Ltd

 A member of the Reed Elsevier plc group

OXFORD BOSTON JOHANNESBURG
MELBOURNE NEW DELHI SINGAPORE

First published 1996

British Library Cataloguing in Publication Data
Harper, John
    Inherited Skin Disorders: The Genodermatoses
    I. Title
    616.5042

ISBN 0 7506 1416 1

Composition by Genesis Typesetting, Rochester, Kent
Printed in Spain

Contents

Contributors

David J. Atherton MA, MB BChir, FRCP
Consultant and Senior Lecturer in Paediatric
  Dermatology
Great Ormond Street Hospital for Children
London, UK

Michael Baraitser FRCP
Consultant in Clinical Genetics
Great Ormond Street Hospital for Children
London, UK

Robert Baran
Centre for Diagnosis and Treatment of Nail Diseases
Cannes, France

Peter Beighton MD, PhD, FRCP, DCH
Professor of Human Genetics
University of Cape Town Medical School
South Africa

Stanley S. Bleehen
Formerly: Professor of Dermatology
Royal Hallamshire Hospital
Sheffield, UK

Graham B. Colver DM, FRCP
Consultant Dermatologist
Chesterfield Royal Hospital
Chesterfield, UK

Rodney P. R. Dawber MA, FRCP
Consultant Dermatologist and Clinical Senior
  Lecturer in Dermatology
Department of Dermatology
Churchill Hospital
Oxford, UK

Thierry Duvanel (Deceased)
Formerly: Chef de Clinique
Clinique de Dermatologie
Geneva University Hospital
Switzerland

R. A. J. Eady MD, BO, FRCP
Professor of Experimental Dermatopathology
Consultant Dermatologist
St John's Institute of Dermatology
St Thomas's Hospital
London, UK

Newton Freire-Maia
Doctor in Natural Sciences (Genetics)
Full Professor, Emeritus
Federal University of Parana
Brazil

David J. Gawkrodger MD, FRCP, FRCPE
Consultant Dermatologist and Honorary Clinical
  Lecturer
University of Sheffield
Royal Hallamshire Hospital
Sheffield, UK

Mary R. Judge MD, MRCP, DCH
Consultant Dermatologist
Bolton Royal Infirmary
Bolton, UK

Lennart Juhlin
Department of Dermatology
University Hospital
Uppsala, Sweden

Christine Kinnon PhD
Senior Lecturer in Molecular Immunology
Institute of Child Health
London, UK

Marc Lacour MD
University of Geneva
Switzerland

Muriel W. Lambert PhD
Professor of Medicine and Dermatology
UMD–New Jersey Medical School
Newark, New Jersey, USA

W. Clark Lambert MD, PhD
Professor of Pathology and Dermatology
UMD–New Jersey Medical School
Newark, New Jersey, USA

Gillian M. Murphy MD, FRCPI
Consultant Dermatologist and Lecturer in
   Dermatology
Beaumont and Mater Hospitals
Dublin, Ireland

D. G. Paige MA MRCP
Consultant Dermatologist
The Royal London Hospital
London, UK

Richard J. A. Penketh MBBS, BSc, MRCOG
Lecturer, Academic Department of Obstetrics and
   Gynaecology
University of Birmingham
Birmingham, UK

Marta Pinheiro
Doctor in Sciences (Biology)
Associate Professor
Federal University of Parana
Brazil

Linda G. Rabinowitz MD
Associate Professor of Dermatology and of
   Pediatrics
Medical College of Wisconsin
Milwaukee, Wisconsin, USA

Ramon Ruiz-Maldonado MD
Professor of Dermatology and Pediatric
   Dermatology
National Institute of Pediatrics
National University of Mexico
Mexico City, Mexico

Terence John Ryan DM, FRCP
Clinical Professor of Dermatology
Department of Dermatology
Churchill Hospital
Oxford, UK

Jean-Hilaire Saurat
Professor and Chairman
Department of Dermatology
Geneva University Hospital
Switzerland

Olivia M. V. Schofield MRCP (UK)
Department of Dermatology
Royal Infirmary of Edinburgh
Edinburgh, UK

Lourdes Tamayo MD
Head of the Department of Dermatology
National Institute of Pediatrics
National University of Mexico
Mexico City, Mexico

Lovell Robert Thomsett FRCVS, DVD
Formerly: Senior Lecturer in Veterinary Medicine
Royal Veterinary College
University of London
Consultant Veterinary Dermatologist
Watford, UK

Preface

The past decade has witnessed substantial advances in our understanding of the biological basis of many genetic skin diseases; one notable example being the molecular biology of keratins. For the most serious genetic skin diseases (such as epidermolysis bullosa and some forms of ichthyosis), this rapid expansion of knowledge will hopefully lead to routine earlier prenatal diagnosis using molecular genetic techniques on chorionic villus tissue and also the possibility, in the future, of specific treatments in the exciting new fields of preimplantation biology and gene therapy. This book aims to give insight into some of these newer aspects and their relevance to dermatological diseases.

JIH

Acknowledgements

I would like to thank the following for their major contributions: Professor Marcus Pembrey as genetics advisor; Simon Brown as illustrative editor; Rosemary Barton, my secretary; Anne Ashford as sub-editor and Cathie Staves as the development editor.

I also wish to thank the following for their helpful advice: Gareth Morgan, Howard Stevens and Professor Irene Leigh.

Finally I would like to acknowledge the support and help of my dear wife, Rowena.

Part One

Introduction

Chapter 1

Clinical perspectives in medical genetics

M. E. Pembrey

Introduction

Genetics is an integral part of modern medicine and clinicians have an important contribution to make in illuminating general aspects of human genetics as well as the pathogenesis of specific genetic disorders. This chapter is intended as a clinicians' guide to research strategies and the recent advances in our understanding of genetic mechanisms, illustrated where possible by the genodermatoses. A guiding principle in selecting topics to include has been the belief that physicians, indeed all those involved in clinical practice, have a responsibility not only to care for their patients, but also to learn from them. Research today underlies the improved diagnosis and treatment of tomorrow. In the absence of experiments to achieve desired matings or deliberately disrupt genes, advances in human genetics will always depend on a partnership between geneticists and clinicians. In medical genetics there has always been the possibility that a single family with a genetic disease, studied in depth, might clarify some genetic mechanism or provide a clue to the chromosomal location or nature of the causative mutation. Never before have there been so many opportunities to learn from the families we see with simply inherited disorders.

The revolutionary developments in our ability to map gene loci to particular chromosomal regions and ultimately to define genes, mutant or otherwise, in terms of their nucleotide base pair sequence, has opened the door to the definitive description of single gene disorders. There is now the real prospect that pathogenesis will be understood in molecular terms with the causal chain of events being traced from the genetic mutation, through the disruption of cell structure and function, to the signs and symptoms of the patient. Dermatologists have one great advantage: they have their organ of interest spread out before them, with a considerably greater prospect of obtaining tissue for histology than most specialists. Ready access to tissue will prove invaluable as it becomes commonplace to study tissue-specific expression of a gene by in situ hybridization, using a fluorescently labelled probe for the messenger RNA produced where the gene is active. Such a technique requires knowledge of a substantial part of the gene's nucleotide sequence, but the rate at which genes of interest are being characterized and sequenced is increasing all the time. The ability to view the whole skin also allows spatial variation in gene expression to be assessed. It is not surprising that it was in skin (actually, coat colour in mice) that Mary Lyon observed the functional genetic mosaicism in females, which in turn led her to propose her famous hypothesis of X inactivation.

As the fruits of the international Human Genome Project and related molecular genetic research come to be applied to medical genetics, it will be important to adopt a developmental perspective if we are to understand the patterns of damage as we see them in our patients. Why does one mutant gene produce overt effects only in skin, while a different mutant gene that produces similar skin lesions also affects certain internal organs? Questions like these will probably only be answerable when we know the role

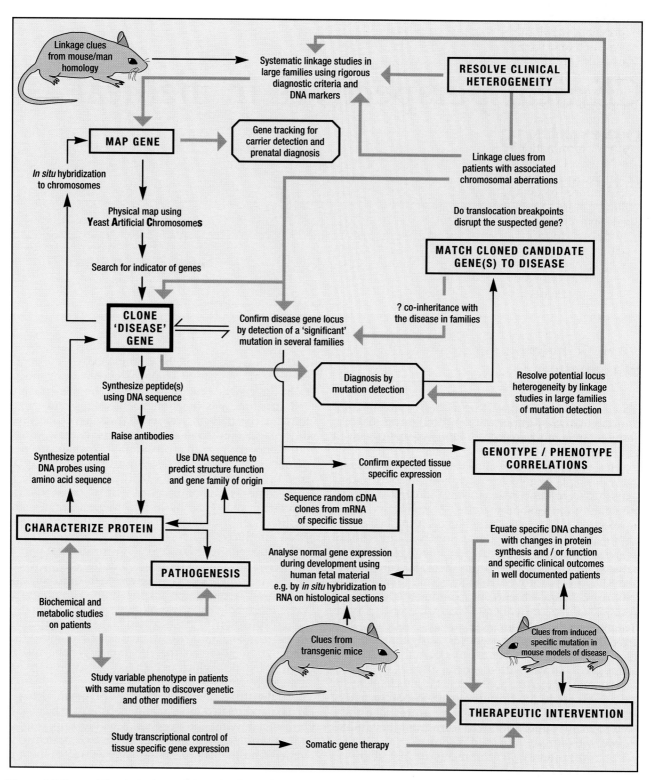

Figure 1.1 *Some of the strategies used in molecular medicine, centred on defining the mutant genes underlying disease. Note the need to integrate clinical and basic sciences*

of the normal gene during development. The need to perform studies on the developing fetus, to build up a sequential picture of the time and place of gene expression, highlights yet again the interdependence of research and clinical practice. While much may be learned from developmental studies in laboratory animals, in the end there will be a need to analyse human fetal material. There has been considerable progress in establishing ethical guidelines for research on material from aborted fetuses arising out of prenatal diagnosis for severe genetic disorders or as a result of termination of pregnancy for other reasons. As Figure 1.1 illustrates, most aspects of genetic research in the genodermatoses require the coordinated efforts of clinicians and geneticists, and none could be more forceful in encouraging these collaborations than the patients themselves and their families. The disease-specific patient organizations are usually keen to promote research and cooperate as fully as possible. With their help, the next decade should see major advances in our understanding of the pathogenesis of the genodermatoses described in this book.

Genetic heterogeneity and its resolution

The starting point of the clinician who deals with the genodermatoses is the patient and the patient's family; it is a matter of precise diagnosis to aid the choice of treatment, to guide prognosis and to allow appropriate genetic counselling. Accurate genetic counselling, particularly when accompanied by the offer of carrier detection or prenatal diagnosis, requires recognition of the problems that can arise from genetic heterogeneity, i.e. clinically similar disorders with different genetic causes. It is essential to distinguish *locus heterogeneity* from *allelic heterogeneity*, for they pose quite different problems in clinical practice.

Loci and alleles

The 50 000–100 000 human genes exist in a relatively fixed linear array along the 24 massive DNA molecules that are the key element of each of the 22 autosomes and the X or Y chromosome – the haploid genome of human gametes. The evolutionary importance of perfect alignment of homologous chromosomes at crossing over during meiosis and the success so far in establishing a linear map of human genes and other unique, but untranscribed, DNA sequences, indicate that the same genes on each of any pair of homologous chromosomes will be at exactly the same chromosomal location.

This particular position, together with the corresponding position on the homologous chromosome, constitute what is termed the *gene locus*. Alternative genes that can occupy the same locus are called *alleles*, and while many alleles (sometimes more than a hundred) may exist in a population, any one normal individual can, of course, have no more than two different alleles at a single locus. Where the alleles at an autosomal locus are the same, the individual is said to be *homozygous*. Where one allele is the normal, common or 'wild-type' allele and the other a mutant, the term *heterozygous* is used. An individual who has two different mutant alleles is called a *compound heterozygote*. This terminology works well in clinical genetics where one is dealing with harmful mutations and simple mendelian inheritance. Now that it is becoming possible to characterize the mutations in autosomal recessive disorders at the DNA sequence level, it turns out that many affected individuals are not homozygotes in the strictest sense (i.e. homo-allelic), but compound heterozygotes. Nevertheless, because both alleles are clinically significant mutants, the person has no normally functioning allele and is clinically affected. In Britain, about 60% of patients with cystic fibrosis are true homozygotes (e.g. a deletion of codon 508 of the *CFTR* gene on each chromosome 7), while the remainder are compound heterozygotes (e.g. delta 508 on one chromosome 7 and a point mutation at codon 551 on the other chromosome 7, or other combinations). In clinical genetics one needs to be able to describe the genotype in a meaningful way when it comes to DNA analysis, and so it is useful to use the term compound heterozygote for distinguishing these patients from healthy carriers or heterozygotes.

However, when dealing with highly polymorphic loci, with numerous normally functioning alleles (e.g. the HLA genes), the distinction between the terms heterozygote and compound heterozygote becomes meaningless and serves no purpose.

Allelic heterogeneity

Different mutations of the same gene can often produce different clinical outcomes – so different, indeed, that from the clinical point of view there would be little reason to suspect that the two diseases were due to mutations at the same gene locus. Sickle cell disease, with its vasculo-occlusive painful crises, presents a very different clinical picture from the transfusion dependence of beta-thalassaemia, yet both are due to mutations in the beta-globin gene. Sickle cell disease is unusual in that it always involves exactly the same mutation at codon 6 of the beta-globin gene, usually on both the chromosomes of the pair, although sickle/thalassaemia compound heterozygotes may present a very similar clinical picture. However, beta-thalassaemia is much more typical of genetic disease demonstrating considerable allelic heterogeneity, with over 60 different mutations capable of producing a very similar clinical picture. Such allelic heterogeneity is the rule rather than the exception with most genetic diseases. For example, within a year of cloning the human tyrosinase gene, located on chromosomal segment 11q14–21, eight different mutations causing oculocutaneous albinism type IA were defined[1]. The different classes of mutations and their effects on function are discussed later, but it is easy to imagine that any mutation that effectively knocks out gene expression will produce the same result, while two mutations that modify the protein product in very different ways could result in quite distinct phenotypes which are regarded clinically as different diseases.

From the practical point of view, allelic heterogeneity severely limits mutation detection by DNA analysis as a simple diagnostic tool. It is now technically easy to detect a *known* DNA sequence change in a gene, but if the result is negative, one is left uncertain as to whether there is another mutation within that gene, or whether it is the wrong gene locus altogether. There are increasingly powerful methods for detecting DNA sequence mismatches between the known normal sequence and the patient's gene, but this can be laborious for genes with huge coding regions. It may also be difficult to interpret any sequence differences that are discovered, because some amino acid changes in the gene product can be inconsequential polymorphisms. It is important to appreciate that inter-

preting DNA sequence changes, particularly those that change only one amino acid, often needs a substantial knowledge of the structure and function of the gene's protein product.

Locus heterogeneity

Locus heterogeneity refers to the same or similar clinical conditions being commonly due to mutations in genes at different gene loci, often on different chromosomes. This obviously causes difficulties when it comes to genetic counselling and predictive tests based on DNA analysis. There are many examples of disorders that can be inherited in either an X-linked or an autosomal fashion, and a good example is provided by chronic granulomatous disease. Figure 1.2 not only illustrates the different genes involved, but indicates one reason why locus heterogeneity so often arises. Many key biochemical functions depend on complexes assembled from more than one polypeptide chain, each encoded by a different gene. Mutations in any one of these genes can disrupt the function of the complex and produce a comparable disease. Chronic granulomatous disease represents a disease that is very well worked out at the biochemical level, but for many of the ill-understood disorders, locus heterogeneity poses

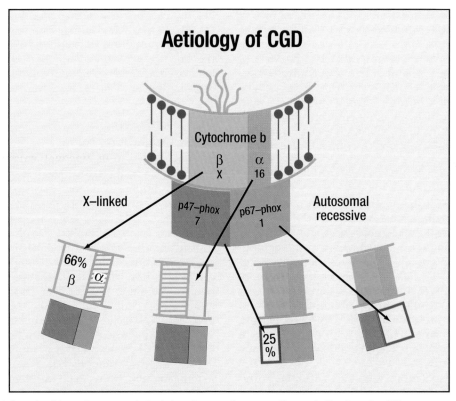

Figure 1.2 *The aetiology (and locus heterogeneity) of chronic granulomatous disease indicating the different gene products involved*

continuing problems in attempts to elucidate the genetics and, in turn, the pathogenesis. In tuberous sclerosis, for example, there is good evidence in some families that it is the result of a mutation on chromosome 9q, while most (perhaps all) others are due to mutation at a locus on chromosome 16p.

Locus heterogeneity compounds the problems of allelic variation when it comes to DNA analysis. Clearly the job is made more difficult when more than one gene has to be tested for mutations. Furthermore, there is not the fall-back strategy (as there is if the locus is known) of gene tracking for carrier or prenatal testing, a strategy that uses closely linked DNA markers and requires no knowledge of the precise mutation in that particular family.

Classification of genetic diseases

Some thought has to be given to how genetic diseases will be classified in the future, in view of the prospect of defining all single gene disorders at the DNA sequence level. There has to be a gradual convergence of the existing clinical classifications with the standardized listing of all monogenic disorders in McKusick's catalogue, *Mendelian Inheritance in Man* [2]. This catalogue has been adopted as the main clinical listing for the Human Genome Project and is increasingly arranged on a gene locus basis, so it does seem logical for the primary classification of monogenic disorders also to be by gene locus. The role of the clinician will be to compare similar diseases, known to arise as a result of mutations at two different loci, and to detect subtle differences in the clinical phenotype. These features will then serve as *clinical* guides as to which gene locus is mutant and where DNA analysis should be focused. It is likely that histological features will be an even better guide to which molecule is primarily involved in the pathogenesis of the disease and therefore which gene locus is mutant. Again, dermatology is well placed to move to this level of diagnostic precision.

While classification at the locus level will have to be incorporated into clinical definitions, it is insufficient by itself for clinical purposes. As indicated above, allelic heterogeneity can lead to two mutations in the same gene giving quite different diseases. Here progress will depend on studies of genotype and phenotype correlations. It should be noted that different mutations of the same gene locus can lead not only to different clinical manifestations but also to different patterns of *autosomal* inheritance. One mutation may only produce disease in the homozygous state (autosomal recessive inheritance), while another does so in the heterozygous state (autosomal dominant inheritance). It follows that just because two diseases are inherited in a different mendelian fashion, one should not necessarily assume that different gene loci are involved.

Chromosomal behaviour and patterns of inheritance

The basis of inheritance

The mendelian patterns of inheritance – autosomal dominant, autosomal recessive and X-linked – stem from a combination of the way chromosomes segregate at meiosis during gamete formation, and the nature of the mutation. Dominant or recessive inheritance is a question of reliance for adequate function on one or two active normal alleles, or how troublesome is the mutant gene product. The pedigree patterns and risks to offspring associated with different types of mendelian inheritance are well known and are discussed further in Chapter 20.

Human chromosomes function in pairs: a legacy of sexual reproduction. This in turn is an evolutionary device for maintaining a winning combination of genes in the face of mutations and ever-changing pathogens. Sexual reproduction requires a number of mechanisms to operate effectively at the level of the whole chromosome or at least substantial regions of it. First, homologous chromosomes have to segregate at meiosis. For this to be reliable there must first be pairing of homologues and probably also recombination (crossing-over to produce visible chiasmata) of chromatids of homologous chromosomes to assist correct disjunction. Errors such as non-disjunction result in the well-known, clinically important trisomies, as well as trisomic embryos that go on to be mosaics in which one line of cells is restored to normal by losing the extra chromosome. Rescued by the normal cell line, these embryos may develop the characteristic pigmentary and other disturbances of 'hypomelanosis of Ito'.

Secondly, recombination also has an important role in increasing the assortment of genes in the next generation; to be successful this requires near-perfect alignment of homologous chromosomes in meiosis. Errors can result in unequal crossing-over, giving deletions or duplications of genes or parts of genes. Perfect alignment of homologous chromosomes during meiosis is probably preceded by some initial trial pairings in which dispersed variable repeat DNA sequences (e.g. minisatellite DNA, of DNA 'fingerprinting' fame) seem to play a part. This 'junk' DNA may therefore have a useful purpose after all!

Thirdly, since chromosomes and their genes function in pairs, there are the problems of running a 'joint operation'. As yet very little is known about the extent or nature of 'cross-talk' between alleles, but there are reasons to believe this may exist. Until recently, identical alleles inherited from each parent were thought to be functionally equivalent, but now it is known that, at some loci, the *parental origin* of the allele influences its expression in the child. Some 'imprint' must be placed during parental gametogenesis to cause this differential allelic expression in the developing embryo. The nature of this genomic imprinting is still to be elucidated, but seems to involve a silencing of one of the alleles, and has some parallels with the phenomenon of X inactivation. This brings us to the fourth aspect of chromosomal behaviour, gene dosage compensation between the unequal sex chromosomes.

X Inactivation

There are very few genes on the Y chromosome for the simple reason that half the humans in the world could not benefit from any genes located there! Genes that are Y-linked are likely to be primarily involved in male sex determination (like the testis determining factor gene, *SRY*) or spermatogenesis. The X and Y chromosomes do, however, pair during meiosis, with synapsis occurring between homologous DNA sequences on the tip of the short arm of the X and the short arm of the Y. This pairing region is called the pseudoautosomal region, because there is at least one obligatory crossing-over during meiosis, and therefore genes here segregate just as they do on the autosomes. Appropriately these genes escape X inactivation; both sexes have the same gene dosage.

For the remainder of the X-linked genes, most have no counterpart on the Y, and so females would have twice the dose of gene product that males do, unless one or other of the alleles were 'silenced'. In fact, inactivation of one or other of the alleles does occur with most genes, just as Lyon proposed in 1961. The inactivation process operates essentially at the whole chromosome level, so in females any one cell has either one or the other X chromosome inactivated (to become the late replicating X, which is the Barr body during interphase). Females are therefore mosaics with respect to X-linked genes, with about half their cells functionally dependent on the paternal X, and the others operating with the maternal X. This random X inactivation process is of no consequence if the woman carries no X-linked mutation, but the extent to which the process deviates from 50:50 can be critical if she does. Unfavourable X inactivation is the most likely cause of a female heterozygote suffering more marked clinical manifestations of an X-linked disease than usual, whereas favourable X inactivation will result in no detectable signs of the disorder. There is an interesting clinical result in those rare instances when a balanced X/autosome reciprocal chromosomal translocation disrupts a critical gene on the X. In this situation the normal X is inactivated and the cells are therefore reliant on the translocated X which lacks expression of the disrupted gene. The woman is functionally the same as an affected male and suffers to the same extent. It is likely that this distortion of random X inactivation stems from the selective loss of those cells in which the translocated X is the inactive one. The inactivation process may spread to the attached length of autosome to fatally silence gene expression there. Alternatively, the part of the translocated X without the inactivation centre cannot inactivate as it should, and the cell's function is compromised. One always has to remember that in the patient we see only the end result of the long cell proliferation process of embryological development. These X/autosome translocations provide valuable clues to the location of X-linked disease loci and have provided the initial mapping information for many genes, including those involved in anhidrotic ectodermal dysplasia and Hunter's syndrome.

How X inactivation happens is not really known. It spreads from an inactivation centre located at Xq12 and a candidate for the key gene located there has been cloned[3]. This gene, *XIST*, is only expressed when on the *inactive* X. What is known is that some alleles on the active and inactive X can be distinguished by their pattern of DNA methylation. Many of the cytosines of DNA are methylated and variation in this is connected in a complicated way with the switching on and off of many genes (not just on the X chromosome) during cellular differentiation.

DNA methylation

The long-term silencing of genes, which underpins differentiation and the inactivation of one or other of the two X chromosomes in female cells (X inactivation), is probably consolidated by shifts in DNA packing that serve to limit the access of RNA polymerase, the enzyme responsible for gene transcription. A key challenge for any such mechanism for maintaining differentiation is how to cope with successive cell divisions, since DNA replication is likely to disrupt protein–DNA binding. Here the methylation of DNA seems to play an important role in mammals (but not in lower animals). The selective methylation of DNA appears to be essential for mammalian development, and the pattern of methylation can be preserved during DNA replication and cell division. In general there is preferential methylation of the cytosine of CpG dinucleotides and these have an interesting distribution within the genome. They tend to cluster, in what are called CpG islands, in the promoter region (usually upstream) of housekeeping genes where they are *not* methylated, and in a low-density fashion in relation to tissue-specific genes where their methylation plays a part, via methyl-CpG-binding proteins, in appropriate gene expression.

Uniparental disomy and genomic imprinting

It was noted earlier that trisomic embryos may lose a chromosome and revert to the correct number. This process can result in the embryo having two copies of a chromosome from one parent and none from the other, a condition called uniparental disomy. This is of clinical significance if that chromosome carries a gene locus that is subject to genomic imprinting, because the person can lack the necessary contribution from one parent. For example, the gene whose failure causes Prader–Willi syndrome is located on chromosome 15 and is subject to imprinting. Only the allele transmitted by the father is active, the one from the mother being 'silenced' by the imprint picked up during oogenesis. About 25% of patients with Prader–Willi syndrome have uniparental maternal disomy with no chromosome 15 from the father. The remainder have a paternal deletion of the critical 15q12 region. In either case the patient has no transcriptionally active gene, i.e. no paternally derived allele.

Mosaics

The assumption that all our cells have the same genes depends on the faithful replication and segregation of the chromosomes during mitosis as the embryo grows. Errors do, of course, occur and the effects are often visible in the skin. Many of the trivial circumscribed lesions on the skin, e.g. depigmented patches, are probably due to somatic mutations either at the DNA level or involving whole chromosomes. It is also likely that genes may become 'silenced' by the sort of factors involved in imprinting (epigenetic factors) in some somatic cells during life.

When the mosaicism arises early in development the abnormal cell line may be widely distributed throughout the tissues causing malfunction in several organs. An important example here is the group of disorders subsumed under the term 'hypomelanosis of Ito' (HI) (Chapter 13). The relationship between pigmentary dyplasias, genetic mosaicism and HI has been the subject of discussion[4]. In the minority of cases of HI, chromosomal mosaicism can be demonstrated by a combination of blood and skin fibroblast karyotyping. If one were able to take multiple biopsies, no doubt the proportion of HI patients showing chromosomal or genetic mosaicism (demonstrable by DNA fingerprinting) would be much greater. In keeping with the chromosomal mosaic pathogenesis is the wide variety of associated malformations and the sporadic nature of the disorder. With respect to the latter point, the assumption must be that it is the normal cell line that rescues the embryo from lethality (or an established trisomic phenotype), and therefore any offspring inheriting the abnormal genotype from a mosaic parent would not be viable. In theory, such affected offspring could themselves become mosaic by losing the additional chromosome, but such 'transmission' of mosaicism from one generation to the next must be rare. Happle[5] proposed that sporadic disorders where cutaneous lesions tend to follow the lines of Blaschko, such as the McCune–Albright, Schimmelpenning–Feuerstein–Mims (linear sebaceous naevus) and Proteus syndromes, might be due to lethal mutations that can only exist in a mosaic

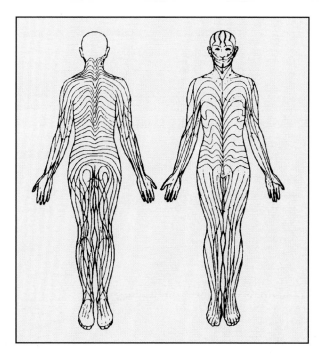

Figure 1.3 *Blaschko's lines as illustrated in his 1901 article, 'A system of lines on the surface of the human body which the linear naevi and dermatoses follow'*

state, which in turn explains the patchy distribution of lesions along Blaschko's lines (Figure 1.3). However, the transmission of probable Proteus syndrome from father to son[6] is difficult to explain using Happle's hypothesis.

The nature of Blaschko's lines is itself unclear. They are thought to reflect the dorsoventral outgrowth of two functionally different populations of cells during early embryogenesis. It is proposed that the two different population of cells can be generated by either random X inactivation in a female carrying an X-linked mutation (e.g. as incontinentia pigmenti), or mosaicism. How the presence of two different cell lines leads to the pigmentary disturbances is not known, but presumably stems from altered developmental signals concerned with melanocyte migration.

Genes and the disruption of gene function by mutation

Organization and function of genes

The term 'gene' is used to describe a DNA sequence that is transcribed into RNA. Genes fall into three main functional types: those that encode an enzyme or structural protein; those that encode a DNA-binding protein involved in the regulation of other genes; and

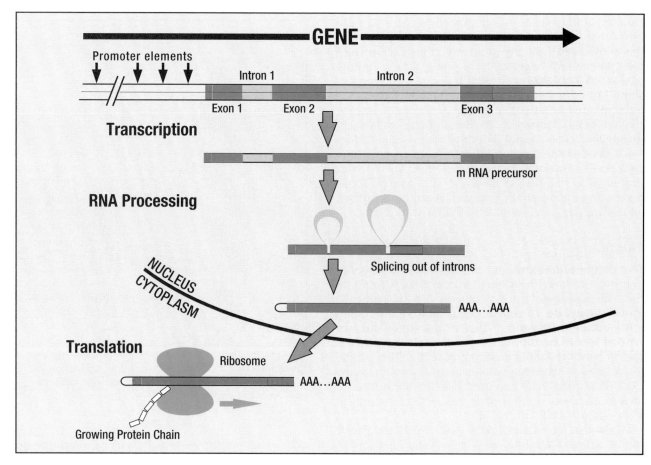

Figure 1.4 *Outline of a gene*

those where the gene product is RNA rather than protein, such as the ribosomal genes. Although most genes are present only once per haploid genome, the genes for some abundant essential products (e.g. histones, ribosomal RNAs or transfer RNAs) are present many times within the genome and are often clustered together. Figure 1.4 illustrates the general features of a gene. The coding regions (exons) for the amino acids of the protein gene product are separated by intervening sequences (introns), which although transcribed initially into RNA, are spliced out before the definitive messenger RNA (mRNA) leaves the nucleus. In general, the introns are very much larger in total than the exons; for example the neurofibromatosis 1 gene (*NF1*) on chromosome 17 is about 300 000 base pairs (bp) in total length, although the mRNA is 13 000 bp long. Why exons or coding regions are split up by introns, often many introns, is not obvious. There are likely to have been some evolutionary gains from this arrangement in that coding regions for particular protein domains could more easily be shuffled around to generate new combinations. With

some genes there is differential splicing of the initial RNA transcript in the nucleus, with different combinations of exons being put together to produce different mRNAs, and therefore different proteins, in different tissues. For example, the primary RNA transcript from the alpha-tropomyosin gene is spliced into nine different mRNAs depending on the cell type.

One surprise has been the discovery of genes within genes. Three small genes, *OMGP* (encoding an oligodendrocyte myelin glycoprotein), *EV12B* and *EV12A* (encoding transmembrane proteins), are located within a large intron of the *NF1* gene. They are oriented in the opposite direction to *NF1*, i.e. they are transcribed from the other DNA strand.

Functionally, it would be wrong to think of a gene as just the exons and introns – the bit that is transcribed. The transcription of the gene is critically dependent on specific DNA sequences in the promoter region 'upstream' (the terms 5' and 3', based on the orientation of the transcribed RNA, are given to the upstream and downstream directions respectively whether referring to RNA or DNA). These 5' sequences are DNA-binding sites for transcription factors, proteins concerned with the initiation and regulation of transcription of the gene by RNA polymerase. The increased transcription of genes in response to steroid hormones, for example, is mediated through specific DNA sequences (usually 5') that are binding sites for the hormone receptor/hormone complex. Some of the sequences concerned with the modulation of transcription, so-called enhancer elements, can be thousands of base pairs away from the gene they influence.

Gene families

Many genes are part of a family of genes with similar functions and DNA sequence. Once one gene has been sequenced, it is usually fairly easy to exploit sequence homology to clone the other members of the family. The different members of the family may be clustered together along the same chromosomal region or dispersed throughout the genome. For example, there are a large number of alpha-keratins falling into two main groups, type I and type II. The genes for several type I keratins, including keratin 14, are clustered on chromosomal region 17q12–21, while those for type II keratins, including keratin 5, are clustered at 12q11–13. In addition to functional genes, a gene family may contain pseudogenes, evolutionary relics of duplicated gene sequences that have accumulated mutations and are no longer functional. The keratin type I cluster on 17q12–21 contains two keratin 14 pseudogenes, for example. Pseudogenes can complicate DNA analysis and can sometimes contribute to mutation by predisposing to unequal crossing-over (see below). The gene family 'likeness' can be exploited in research aimed at matching a cloned gene to a genetic disease. If a mutation cannot be found in a particular 'candidate' gene from patient DNA, then it is worth considering other genes of the same family, for they are likely to serve a similar function and a mutation within them might produce a similar disease.

In choosing prospective candidate genes to test for mutations causing a particular disease, the role of the different genes in normal development and differentiation needs to be borne in mind. This approach to matching candidate genes and diseases is well illustrated by early research into epidermolysis bullosa simplex (EBS). In the basal cell layer, keratins 5 and 14 are the main constituents of the keratin filaments, but as these cells stratify and differentiate so the keratin 5 and 14 genes are downregulated, and the transcription of other keratin gene pairs is increased in a tissue-specific way. Keratins 1 and 10 predominate in differentiating skin, keratins 4 and 13 in oesophageal cells and keratins 3 and 12 in corneal cells. With keratins 5 and 14 being equally necessary

for the assembly of the keratin filaments of the cytoskeleton of the basal cells and thereby the integrity of the epithelium, it was possible that one or other (or both) of these genes could be involved in EBS. In fact, after clues from a transgenic mouse model discussed below, it was found that two unrelated EBS patients with the Dowling–Meara type of disease each had a (different) mutation changing an arginine at residue 125 within the helical rod domain of the keratin 14 molecule[7]. Subsequently, Lane et al[8] found a keratin 5 mutation converting a glutamine to glycine at the end of the helical rod domain in a large family, also with Dowling–Meara EBS. A mutation of the keratin 14 gene, changing a leucine to a proline at residue 384, has been found in a large kindred with Koebner EBS[9], while a Weber–Cockayne EBS mutation in one family has been shown to co-inherit with the type II keratin cluster on chromosome 12, thereby implicating the keratin 5 gene. Thus there is strong evidence that these three major forms of EBS are due to mutations in either the keratin 5 or 14 gene.

Much basic work had already been done on the genetics and cellular biology of the keratins before mutations in EBS were sought. Sometimes DNA sequence homology can identify a related gene, which although poorly understood can still be a sensible candidate for a disease-related gene. Recently, one type of retinitis pigmentosa (RP) was shown to be due to mutation in the peripherin gene on chromosome 6. A peripherin-like gene (*ROM1*) was identified on chromosome 11 on account of its sequence homology to the peripherin gene. It too appears to have a developmental and structural role in the rod photoreceptor and therefore became a prime candidate for the gene involved in some forms of RP. It was not long before a putative mutation causing RP was found.

Types of mutation

From the clinical standpoint, a relatively simplistic idea of how genes work will allow the disruptive effect of most mutations to be understood in principle. As indicated in Figure 1.4, the primary RNA transcript includes both the coding regions (exons) and the intervening sequences (introns). The introns have to be spliced out to produce the mature messenger RNA (mRNA), which can then leave the nucleus with the full coding sequence as one contiguous length of RNA. Nearly all exon/intron boundaries have a specific nucleotide sequence that facilitates the precise recognition and action of the splicing machinery. Introns usually begin with GU(AAGU) and end with (C)AG. The RNA also has to have a poly(A) tail added to its 3' end and a CAP complex added to the 5' end to ensure RNA stability and normal function. At the 3' end of most genes there is a sequence motif that is transcribed into

AAUAAA in the corresponding RNA where it acts as the polyadenylation signal. Once in the cytoplasm, the mRNA is translated at the ribosomes, amino acids being added to the nascent polypeptide chain in accordance with the RNA three-base codons, until a Stop codon is reached.

The transcription of a gene is dependent on the assembly of a multiprotein transcription complex that includes RNA polymerase at the appropriate position upstream (5′) to the gene sequence to be transcribed into RNA. This is turn requires the presence of certain sequence motifs, such as the TATAA motif often found about 25–30 bp 5′ to the start of transcription. Other sequences commonly found further upstream of genes include CCAAT and GGGCG. As noted earlier, there are also enhancer sequences that can be found in various positions in relation to the gene that they influence. These play a role in the modulation of gene activity during development, differentiation and metabolism. Other genes, developmental genes for example, encode DNA-binding proteins that bind to these specific enhancer sequences which may be connected to several genes. In this manner, a DNA-binding protein and the gene encoding it can orchestrate the coordinated expression of many other genes. The DNA-binding proteins include one of several characteristic types of domain (the 'zinc finger' for example) that represent the actual DNA-binding site. Mutations in these domains can sometimes have quite specific but complex phenotypic effects. The Wilms' tumour-related gene on chromosome segment 11p13, the *WT1* gene, provides an example. The *WT1* gene encodes a DNA-binding protein that is normally involved in renal and urogenital development. A mutation at nucleotide position 1180 which changes an arginine to tryptophan in one of the zinc finger DNA-binding domains produces the Denys–Drash syndrome, in which there is a characteristic glomerulonephritis, male pseudohermaphroditism and a predisposition to Wilms' tumour.

Clearly much has to be elucidated before it will be easy to appreciate the full chain of events between some mutations and the phenotypic changes they produce, particularly if the effect is mediated through transcriptional modification of the expression of other genes. One of the lessons coming from the rapid advances in mammalian developmental genetics, is that the tissue-specific phenotypic effects of a mutation in a developmental gene are not merely a reflection of the tissue-specific expression of the normal gene, but a reflection of the ability of some but not all tissues to compensate for the loss of the normal function of that gene.

However, for many mutations the phenotypic effects are much more direct and can be simply classified into mutations that have their effect by making a functionally different protein, and those mutations that result in a reduction or absence of the gene product.

Changes in the structure of the protein gene product

Amino acid substitution or mis-sense mutation

The amino acid substitution or mis-sense mutation is the simplest of mutations, usually caused by a single nucleotide base change that alters the codon. The impact this has on the function of the protein depends on how critical that particular amino acid is. The triple helix domain of all collagens has a glycine every third residue, because this small amino acid packs neatly into the centre of the helix. Substitution of any larger amino acid tends to disrupt the helix and allow overhydroxylation, etc. Mis-sense mutations have been found at codons 382, 383 and 373 of the tyrosinase gene in individuals with type IA oculocutaneous albinism[10]. All these mutations involve the location of the proposed copper B region of tyrosinase and probably inhibit the catalytic function of the enzyme.

Loss or addition of one or a few codons

Provided the reading frame for translation of the RNA into polypeptide is preserved, a slightly modified protein can be produced, despite the loss or addition of a few codons. The most famous codon deletion is the 508 deletion in the *CFTR* gene – the most common mutation in cystic fibrosis.

Exon skipping

Exon skipping can arise when there is a mutation that alters the recognition of the splice sites by the exon/intron splicing machinery.

Unequal crossing-over to produce a hybrid protein

Unequal crossing-over arises when homologous chromosomes misalign at meiosis, and is discussed below.

Truncated or novel peptides at the C-terminus

A single base change towards the end of the translated region of a gene can sometimes create a Stop codon, which leads to a slightly truncated protein being produced. Alternatively, the base change may remove the normal Stop codon, converting it to a codon for an amino acid. This results in a novel, additional string of peptides until another Stop codon is reached. A deletion or addition of one or two bases (or any number of bases that is not a multiple of three) generates a shift in the reading frame. If this occurs close to the end of the gene, again a partially functional protein with a truncated or novel C-terminus can be produced.

Deletion within the gene

Provided the reading frame is maintained intact, small to large deletions within the gene can often result in a partially functional protein. The best-known example is Becker's muscular dystrophy, where some huge in-frame deletions of the dystrophin gene result in relatively minor effects on muscle function. One of the first Waardenburg's type I mutations found in the *PAX3* gene was an in-frame 18 bp deletion in the central region of exon 2[11].

Changes in the amount of protein gene product

Deletion

Deletion of the whole of a gene results in the absence of gene product. The phenotype in such a situation is a guide to what will happen with the many other types of mutation (considered below) that result in a 'knock out' of the gene. Interestingly, there are many situations in autosomal dominant disorders where the complete absence of a gene product from one allele is less troublesome than an altered protein that can act as a 'spanner in the works'. This phenomenon goes by several different names, such as protein suicide, included/excluded mutants or dominant negative effect, but in essence it is a case of a faulty gene product being more trouble than it is worth when it comes to assembling multimeric proteins. It is better to do without and use an unconventional but correctly formed protein as a partner.

RNA that cannot be processed properly

As mentioned above, the intron/exon boundaries have highly conserved DNA sequences, and mutations within one of these sequences can prevent the splicing out of an intron, which, of course, cannot code for protein. Depending on the exact base change, only abnormally spliced mRNA may be produced, or there may be a combination of abnormal and normal mRNA. In the latter case the result will be a reduced amount of normal gene product. Another type of mutation which can produce a reduced amount of normal mRNA is a change in the polyadenylation site, so that the mRNA is somewhat unstable.

Premature Stop codons and frame-shift mutations

When a Stop codon is generated by a base change in a codon relatively early in the gene sequence, then the severely truncated protein produced at translation is generally useless. It is either unstable or missing a crucial functional domain. As indicated earlier, the deletion of one or two bases leads to a shift in the reading frame, generating a novel amino acid sequence from that point onwards. More often than not this frame shift results in a Stop codon within a short distance, so the protein in such mutations is usually severely truncated as well as having an inappropriate amino acid sequence.

Impaired transcription

Mutations in the special sequences upstream needed for the efficient assembly of various transcription factors and RNA polymerase usually result in a reduced level of gene product. As discussed below, the full mutation in the fragile-X mental retardation syndrome, where there is a marked expansion of a CGG repeat within the 5' region of the *FMR1* gene, is associated with widespread local DNA methylation, and it seems that it is this that blocks transcription of the gene.

Mutational mechanisms

As more mutations underlying human diseases are described, so some of the more common mutational mechanisms have been revealed. Some DNA sequences are more liable to mutation than others.

The dinucleotide CpG is a mutational hot spot, and is under-represented in the genome just because of this propensity to mutate. The C is often methylated and deamination tends to result in a CG to TG or a CG to CA substitution. Such mutations are estimated to account for about a third of all single base pair substitutions causing human disease[12]. By way of illustration, Spritz et al[13] described a mis-sense mutation (CG to CA) at codon 383 (previously numbered 365) in the tyrosinase gene causing oculo-cutaneous albinism (OCA) type IA.

Oetting et al[10] noted that a Japanese frame-shift mutation (a single cytosine insertion within a run of four cytosines) reported in two unrelated type IA OCA patients by Tomita et al[14] occurs within a repetitive base sequence, as do two of the three frame-shift mutations they reported causing type IA OCA (each a single bp deletion within a string of five guanidines). Such potential Z-DNA forming sequences are regarded as frame-shift mutation hot spots[15]. Interestingly, the 18 bp deletion within the *PAX3* gene causing Waardenburg's syndrome, mentioned earlier, occurred between two directly repeated GGCCC sequences in exon 2.

The recent discoveries of the mutational events underlying the fragile-X syndrome[16] and myotonic dystrophy[17] broaden the concept of mutational instability dramatically. Here a normal string of up to 50 CGGs in the *FMR1* gene increases to 70–200 in number to become the asymptomatic premutation in incipient fragile-X families. Passage of this premutation through oogenesis can result in a massive, variable amplification of the CGG repeat, associated methylation of neighbouring DNA and loss of *FMR1* gene transcription, giving the full fragile-X phenotype. A similar progressive amplification of a CTG repeat in the myotonic dystrophy gene correlates with the increasing severity of the disease as it is transmitted from one generation to the next (a phenomenon called anticipation). Here the progression of the mutation is not dependent on just female transmission, as it is in fragile-X syndrome.

The last common mutational event worthy of comment is unequal crossing-over. If homologous chromosomes misalign during pairing at meiosis and then recombination takes place in the normal way, one chromatid ends up with a deletion and one with a corresponding duplication, while the two uninvolved chromatids are normal. This is a very common cause of deletional mutations, such as those that remove the steroid sulphatase gene in the great majority of patients with X-linked ichthyosis. A prerequisite for unequal crossing-over is the existence of local repeated homologous or near-homologous DNA sequences, for it is in these situations that misalignment due to 'mistaken identity' can occur (much like partnership errors in square-dancing with many sets of identical twins!). The repeated sequences can be duplicated active genes, neighbouring inactive pseudogenes or dispersed non-coding repeat sequences such as the 300 bp Alu repeat.

The Alu repeat, of which there are some 300 000–500 000 copies in the human genome, also plays a role in one of the more intriguing but rarer forms of mutation. Although not a proper gene as such, most – if not all – Alu sequences are transcribed into RNA. The presence of a poly(A) tail at the 3' end of the genomic Alu repeats suggests that they have integrated at new genomic positions through an RNA intermediate. A recently described de novo mutation in the *NF1* gene, causing neurofibromatosis 1, has turned out to be just such a spontaneous genomic integration. An Alu repeat had 'jumped' into the intron between exons 5 and 6! This caused skipping of exon 6 in the mRNA, and the splicing of exon 5 to exon 7 resulted in a frame shift which in turn generated a premature Stop codon such that the NF1 protein (normally 2818 amino acids long) would be missing 771 amino acids from the C-terminus[18].

Closing the gap between chromosomal abnormalities and mendelian disorders

So far we have only considered mutations affecting a single locus, but mutations may involve a few or many loci. Some of the past distinction between mendelian disorders and structural (as opposed to numerical) chromosomal abnormalities was largely a reflection of the limitations of the methods employed for genetic analysis. With better cytogenetic resolution including fluorescent in situ hybridization (FISH)

Table 1.1 *Selected autosomal microdeletion syndromes*

Disorder	Chromosomal region
Alagille syndrome	20p11.23–12.1
Angelman syndrome	15q11–13
DiGeorge's syndrome (velocardiofacial)	22q11.2
Langer–Giedion syndrome	8q24.1
Miller–Dieker syndrome (isolated lissencephaly)	17p13.3
Prader–Willi syndrome	15q11–13
Smith–Magenis syndrome	17?
Rubinstein–Taybi syndrome	16p13.3
WAGR syndrome	11p13

discussed below, for defining microdeletions, duplications and other rearrangements, plus more extensive DNA sequences and better physical maps linking up neighbouring genes, the 'no-man's land' of genome analysis from 50 kilobases to 5 megabases is beginning to yield its secrets. The mutation causing Charcot–Marie–Tooth disease (hereditary motor and sensory neuropathy, type I) is a duplication of some 2 mb at 17p11.2, and there is a growing list of microdeletion syndromes (Table 1.1). For the most part, disorders due to autosomal, multilocus mutations are transmitted (when the severity of their effect does permit childbearing) as autosomal dominant disorders.

Contiguous gene disorders

A syndrome due to a deletion that extends to remove more than one gene is called a contiguous gene disorder or contiguous deletion syndrome, with the combination of features being a reflection of the number and function of genes knocked out. Thus there are two main ways of disrupting the function of multiple genes to give a multifeature disorder; a contiguous gene deletion or a mutation in a developmental gene that is a transcription factor for several other genes further down the developmental pathway. A good example of both causes of a multisystem disorder comes from the work on the *WTI* gene on chromosome 11p13. We have already noted that a point mutation in this zinc finger transcription factor gene can cause the Denys–Drash syndrome of male pseudohermaphroditism, glomerulonephritis and a predisposition to Wilms' tumour. If a microdeletion knocks out both the *WT1* gene and the aniridia gene (*AN2*) that is located about 5 kb distant, you get the WAGR contiguous gene disorder of predisposition to Wilms' tumour, aniridia, genital abnormalities, and growth and mental retardation (if the deletion is relatively large). A list of X-linked contiguous deletion syndromes is given in Table 1.2. A well-established

Table 1.2 *X-linked contiguous deletion syndromes*

Disorder	Chromosomal region
X-linked ichthyosis	Xp22.3
Kallmann's syndrome	
Chondrodysplasia punctata	
Mental retardation	
Short stature	
Ocular albinism	
Duchenne's muscular dystrophy	Xp21
Chronic granulomatous disease	
McLeod phenotype	
Retinitis pigmentosa	
Mental retardation	
Glycerol kinase deficiency	
Adrenal hypoplasia	
Alland's eye disease	
Choroideraemia	Xq21
Deafness (with gusher at surgery)	
Mental retardation	

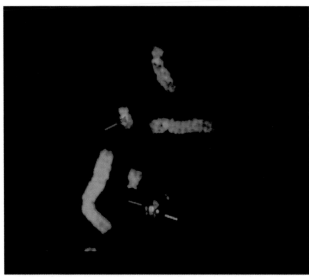

Figure 1.5 *A microdeletion at 22q11.2 demonstrated by fluorescent in situ hybridization (FISH) in a case of DiGeorge's (velocardiofacial) syndrome. A control probe (red) gives a signal on both chromosomes 22, while a probe from the deleted region (yellow) is present on only one. Double signals are usually seen because at metaphase the chromosomes have divided into two chromatids (courtesy of Dr Peter Scambler)*

'set' of contiguous gene disorders involve the steroid sulphatase locus (Xp22.3), deletion of which causes X-linked ichthyosis[19]. In fact, over 90% of the mutations causing X-linked ichthyosis are deletions. Deletions of different sizes and location within Xp22.3 give varying combinations of the following six diseases: X-linked ichthyosis, Kallmann's syndrome (hypogonadotrophic hypogonadism and anosmia), chondrodyplasia punctata, ocular albinism, mental retardation and short stature. Like the deletions of just the steroid sulphatase gene, the high rate of deletions in this area appears to be due to abnormal pairing and unequal crossing-over between low copy number repeat elements in the region. A number of cases are due to abnormal exchanges between Xp22.3 and Yq11 (which carries homologous sequences) that give rise to terminal deletions of the distal Xp region. It is becoming increasingly important to be able to investigate mendelian disorders with high-resolution cytogenetic methods, particularly those that employ DNA probes.

Fluorescent in situ hybridization

It is now possible to hybridize fluorescently labelled DNA probes directly to regular metaphase spreads of chromosomes and see where they 'light up'. This technique goes by the acronym FISH, and can be used in two ways. By using a mixture of many probes specific for a particular chromosome, the whole of both chromosomes of the pair can be 'painted' with a specific fluorochrome. Other chromosomes can be painted with fluorochromes giving different colours. Chromosome painting is very helpful for revealing the chromosomal origin of fragments attached to other chromosomes or lying free. It also helps to resolve the nature of complex translocations, important in general clinical genetics as well as in cancer cytogenetics. An alternative approach is the use of a gene-specific or marker-specific probe to determine its rough location on the chromosome and its relationship to other sequences. Not only is this a very powerful way to map newly cloned cDNAs, but it can be used in clinical practice to look for the deletion or relocation of known genes, or parts of large genes. Figure 1.5 shows this technique used to detect a microdeletion at 22q11.2 in a patient with DiGeorge's syndrome.

DNA analysis

Mutation detection and the polymerase chain reaction

Mutation detection will eventually become the mainstay of the diagnosis of all mendelian disorders, whichever clinical specialist is involved, and also contribute significantly to the diagnostic work-up of most cancers and many other multifactorial diseases such as eczema. If the past is anything to go by, it will take some time before clinicians appreciate that diagnostic classification by mutation, although not the whole story, will be the best starting point from which to consider prognosis, patient treatment and care, and counselling to the family. The next few years will see the development of large-scale, automated mutation detection methods. Clinical acumen will, in part, be judged by the ability to predict at which gene locus the mutation will be found. This revolution in the diagnosis of genetic disease stems from the development of the polymerase chain reaction (PCR). This is a technique for replicating in vitro a known target section of DNA from the patient's total DNA, thereby simplifying analysis. Like virtually all genetic engineering techniques, PCR exploits the pairing of DNA strands with complementary sequences and naturally occurring enzymes, in this case a thermally stable DNA polymerase. The steps in the reaction are as follows:

1. Oligonucleotide primers, about 20 nucleotides long, are synthesized in the laboratory such that one is complementary to one DNA strand at one end of the desired target sequence, while the other is complementary to the sequence of the other DNA strand at the other end of the target section of DNA.
2. Heating the patient's total DNA causes the two strands of the DNA double helix to separate and allows the primers to have access to the sequences at either end of the target DNA.
3. Cooling the DNA causes the primers to hybridize to the ends of the target DNA strands to form short, double-stranded lengths of DNA that will be recognized by the DNA polymerase enzyme. Because of the short lengths involved, this primer pairing occurs ahead of full restoration of double-stranded DNA.
4. Warming the DNA in the presence of DNA polymerase and a supply of nucleotides causes this enzyme to start replicating the single-stranded DNA from the point where the primers have hybridized. In this way each target DNA sequence is doubled.
5. Repeating steps 2–4 in the presence of thermally stable DNA polymerase and enough nucleotides and primer will lead to an exponential increase in copies of the target DNA sequence. Each newly synthesized strand will act as a template for primer hybridization in the next round of DNA replication.

It can be seen from the above that the design of the primers, the temperature settings and the time spent at each temperature are key aspects of successful amplification by PCR. This reaction allows clinical molecular geneticists to generate millions of copies of the target DNA sequence of interest in a matter of hours. The quantity of PCR product can be so great that it can be visualized directly after simple staining with ethidium bromide, for example, and so mutation detection becomes a matter of detection of PCR products that differ in size or presence, depending on the existence or not of a specific mutation in the initial DNA. The simplest system is illustrated (Figure 1.6) by detection of the three-nucleotide deletion at codon 508 of the *CFTR* gene – the most common mutation in cystic fibrosis. Primers either side of codon 508 generate a 50 bp PCR product from a normal gene, but a 47 bp product from a mutant gene. Other mutation detection strategies have one of the primers hybridizing to the precise site of the mutation. If the mutant sequence is present, PCR amplification takes place and a product will be detected, but not if the sequence is normal. The result is confirmed by a second test using a different primer set that works with the normal sequence but not the mutant one. These and some other systems detect *known* mutations. Searching for unknown single nucleotide mutations in the exons and exon/intron boundaries of specific genes requires other approaches that can indicate the existence of some sequence difference from normal. The precise nature of the change can then be established by DNA sequencing.

Knowing the mutation in a particular patient is important both for immediate advice to the patient

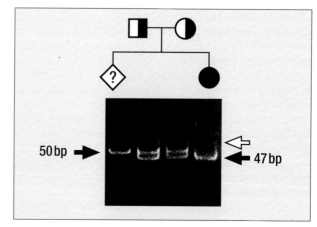

Figure 1.6 *Pedigree showing a girl with cystic fibrosis, her carrier parents, and a fetus undergoing prenatal diagnosis. Below each individual in the pedigree is the DNA track showing the normal 50 base pair DNA fragment and/or the 47 base pair fragment, due to deletion of codon 508. The open arrow shows a faint band in the heterozygotes due to a pairing between the 50 bp and 47 bp DNA strands (heteroduplex) which travels more slowly in the polyacrylamide gel. The fragments are generated by the polymerase chain reaction using primers that flank codon 508 and are just stained with ethidium bromide (from Pembrey ME. Impact of molecular biology on clinical genetics. In: Basic Cell and Molecular Biology. British Medical Association, London, 1992; 20)*

and for the eventual elucidation of the pathogenesis of the disorder.

While rapid technical progress in mutation detection can be expected, there are still many situations where families wish to have genetic predictions made even though mutation detection has not proved possible. Much can be offered if the gene locus involved, or the chromosomal region, is known. Mapping disease gene loci (Figure 1.7) is not only the first step in positional cloning strategies, but also allows genetic prediction by gene tracking provided there is no significant unresolved locus heterogeneity.

Gene mapping and tracking

There has been phenomenal progress in gene mapping techniques in the last few years, with thousands of DNA 'markers' being defined that cover all the chromosomes. These greatly facilitate linkage studies within large families affected by a mendelian disease. In essence, linkage analysis simply asks the question whether each DNA marker co-inherits with the disease more often than expected by chance. The statistical test of this is expressed as a log of the odds (LOD) score for a specified recombination fraction, theta (i.e. a specified genetic distance between disease locus and marker). With uncomplicated inheritance a LOD score of 3 or greater is accepted as evidence of linkage, while a LOD score of –2 excludes linkage at that theta. The closer the marker (of known chromosomal location) is to the unknown disease locus, the less likely it is to be separated by recombination between the two chromosomes when they pair at meiosis, and the more likely that the disease and a particular marker allele will travel together through the generations. The traditional DNA marker is a restriction fragment length polymorphism (RFLP) analysed by Southern blotting of restricted (digested) DNA, with the fragments detected by a radioactive probe. An RFLP is a common variation in DNA sequence (usually of no genetic significance) that removes or creates a cutting site for a particular restriction enzyme or alters the distance between two sites, such that on digestion different-sized DNA fragments are generated by the two homologous chromosomes. The parent has to be heterozygous for the RFLP as well as at the disease locus in order to obtain linkage information, so there has been a constant search for highly polymorphic markers where nearly everyone is heterozygous. There has also been a move to the quicker PCR-based methods of analysis, exploiting an abundant class of DNA sequence polymorphisms, dinucleotide (CA) or tetranucleotide repeats.

Gene tracking is the term given to the use of a known linkage between a marker and a disease locus to predict the genotype at the disease locus in a particular family member, such as in asymptomatic carrier testing or prenatal diagnosis. The marker is often a DNA polymorphism within the disease gene locus itself. Gene tracking is widely used in clinical DNA analysis services to assist genetic counselling and provide the option of early prenatal diagnosis where mutation detection is not feasible. There are several limitations to gene tracking. Distinguishing the two homologous chromosomes in key family members is one requirement, and the new markers have gone some way to overcoming this limitation in the application of gene tracking. Another limitation is the need to obtain blood or other samples for DNA extraction from other family members. A third limitation of gene tracking is the difficulty that arises when the stated father turns out not to be the biological father. Finally, even when using a polymorphism within the disease gene itself as a marker, there is the small chance that a recombination between the marker and the mutation will result in a wrong prediction. Set against these limitations when compared to mutation detection is the huge advantage of gene tracking being entirely independent of the particular type of mutation in that family. All that is required is to know which gene locus is involved, i.e. not to be faced with unresolved locus heterogeneity.

Linkage studies are just the first step in positional cloning of a disease gene. The next step is to create a physical map that incorporates the linked DNA markers. Rapid progress is occurring in this field as well. At the time of writing, all the DNA (bar some blocks of repetitive DNA) from each of the smallest human chromosomes, the Y and 21, has already been cloned as fragments into yeast artificial chromosomes (YACs) and ordered with respect to each other to create a vast 'contig' of overlapping DNA fragments stretching from one end of the chromosome to the other. This will greatly facilitate positional cloning of genes on these chromosomes.

Mouse models

The next chapter considers the genodermatoses that occur in the domestic and farm animals of veterinary practice. This section considers the laboratory mouse, which is playing an increasingly important complementary role in medical genetics. The discovery that there is considerable evolutionary conservation of the DNA sequence within important genes between the mouse and human (mouse/man homology) means that once a mouse gene is cloned, its human equivalent is usually detectable using a probe to the mouse sequence, and vice versa. Comparative gene mapping is also enhanced by the fact that there is

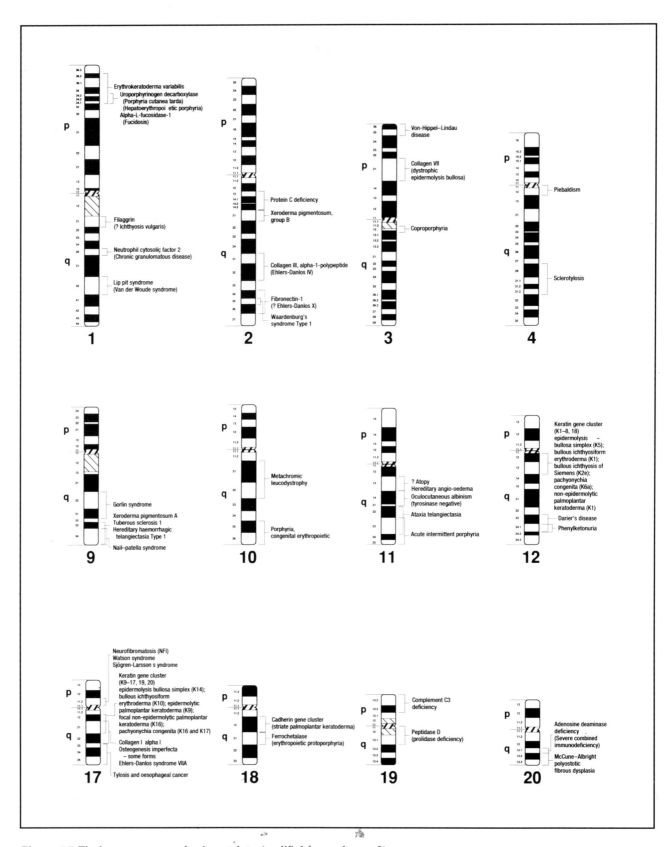

Figure 1.7 *The human gene map for dermatology (modified from reference 2)*

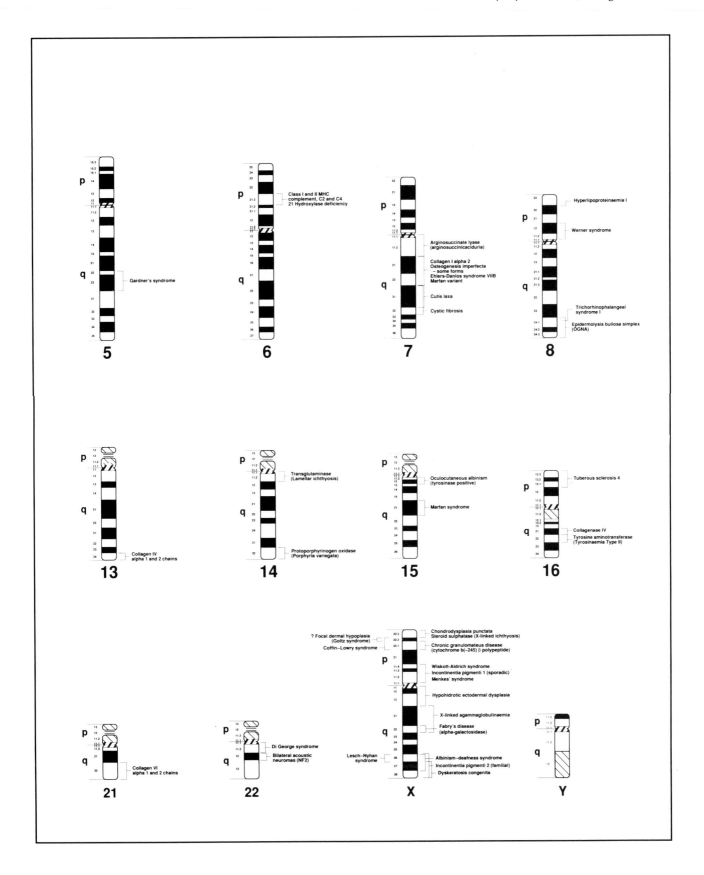

chromosomal region homology between mouse and human, with many large linkage groups of gene loci being the same in the two species despite large-scale rearrangements of the chromosomes themselves during evolution.

There is an internationally organized mouse genome project akin to the human endeavour, and a systematic listing of genetic variants and strains of laboratory mouse[20]. As mentioned at the beginning of this chapter, the clinician deals with many patients who represent 'experiments of nature', and where genetic disorders are concerned, attempts to match a particular disorder or phenotype with its causative change in DNA sequence. One has to look to the laboratory mouse and other animals if one wants to resolve genetic heterogeneity by selective breeding, analyse tissue gene expression throughout development or deliberately change the DNA to see what phenotype emerges. It can be important to develop mouse models of human diseases, such as cystic fibrosis, by site-directed mutagenesis to study pathogenetic mechanisms and develop new treatments. There are several types of mouse model, which include the following:

1. The naturally occurring mutant, which is usually mapped by traditional linkage studies to a mouse chromosomal region, which in turn might suggest a human chromosomal region through knowledge of homology.
2. Mutant phenotypes that arise as a result of disruption of an existing gene during experimental insertion of a transgene, where the transgene DNA sequence provides a tag on the location of the disrupted gene.
3. The precise 'knock out' or mutation of the wild-type gene by some form of targeted mutagenesis, which usually exploits homologous recombination technology in embryonic stem cells.

It has already been noted how it was a transgenic mouse model that alerted investigators to the likelihood that mutations in the basal cell keratin genes could cause epidermolysis bullosa simplex. However, spontaneously arising mouse mutants have recently proved to be extremely useful in identifying the mutations underlying Waardenburg's syndrome type I, piebaldism and at least one form of tyrosinase-positive albinism.

Genetic linkage studies in large families with Waardenburg's syndrome type I (following up a clue from a patient with a chromosomal deletion) mapped the mutation to the q37 region of chromosome 2. A naturally occurring mutation in mouse, called Splotch because of its depigmented patches, was shown to be due to a mutation in the developmental gene, *Pax3*. The *Pax* family of developmental genes are so-called because they all have a DNA motif termed 'paired'. *Pax3* also has a homeodomain. The *Pax3* gene maps to that part of mouse chromosome 1 which is known to be homologous to human chromosome region 2q37. Thus the human *PAX3* gene (capitals are used for the human gene) became a prime 'candidate' gene for Waardenburg's syndrome type 1. Mutations were duly found in some patients[11]. Interestingly, one such mutation was an 18 bp deletion of a highly conserved (and therefore functionally important) 'paired' domain region of the gene and yet the clinical disorder was not particularly severe. To date there is no correlation with the type and location of mutation and the severity of the deafness, and interestingly the Splotch mice heterozygotes do not appear to have any ear abnormalities.

The story behind identifying the mutant gene in piebaldism is similar. It was noted that there was a similar mouse mutant 'dominant white spotting' (W), which also had defects in haematopoiesis and germline development. This mouse phenotype was eventually shown to be due to mutations in the c-*kit* proto-oncogene, which encodes the tyrosine kinase cell-surface receptor for the mast/stem cell growth factor. The human c-*kit* gene was known to map to chromosome region 4q12 and interstitial deletions of this region had been found in some patients with piebaldism, so c-*kit* became a prime 'candidate' gene in which to search for mutations. They were duly found in at least four unrelated families with piebaldism[21,22].

It was interest in the relative lack of pigmentation in some individuals with Prader–Willi or Angelman's syndrome that initially focused attention on chromosome region 15q12–13, the location of the microdeletions found in these disorders. However, it was the mapping of tyrosinase-positive type II albinism locus to 15q12 by traditional linkage studies[23] that strengthened the likelihood that this locus was homologous with the pink-eyed dilute locus p in mouse. The p locus was known to be on mouse chromosome 7 in a linkage group homologous to human 15q11–13. A combined mouse/human study cloned a cDNA from a gene that revealed mutations in both the mouse mutants and patients with type II oculocutaneous albinism[24].

The power of combining mouse and human studies is clear from these three examples, as is the value of the occasional patient with a chromosomal abnormality in providing the first mapping clue. It has to be remembered that partial cDNA sequences of thousands of 'random' human genes are being generated each year. They are being classified into known gene families, which in turn can hint at their function. That is a lot of genes to be matched with 'candidate' diseases! Knowledge of the naturally occurring mouse phenotypes[20,25] and genetically engineered mouse models is likely to contribute to the genetic analysis, and thereafter elucidation of the pathogenesis, of a number of the genodermatoses that are the subject of this book.

References

1 Giebel LB, Strunk KM, Spritz RA. Organization and nucleotide sequence of the human tyrosinase gene and a truncated tyrosinase pseudogene. *Genomics* 1991; **9**: 435–45.

2 McKusick VA, *Mendelian Inheritance in Man*. 11th ed. Johns Hopkins University Press. Baltimore, 1994. 11th ed.

3 Brown CJ, Ballabio A, Rupert JL et al., A gene from the region of the human X inactivation centre is expressed exclusively from the inactive X chromosome. *Nature* 1991; **349**: 38–44.

4 Flannery D. Pigmentary dysplasias, hypomelanosis of Ito, and genetic mosaicism. *Am J Med Genet*, 1990; **35**: 18–21.

5. Happle R. Cutaneous manifestations of lethal genes. *Hum Genet* 1986; **72**: 280.

6 Goodship J, Redfearn A, Milligan D, Gardner-Medwin D, Burn J. Transmission of Proteus syndrome from father to son? *J Med Genet* 1991; **28**: 781–5.

7 Coulombe PA, Hutton ME, Letai A et al. Point mutations in human keratin 14 genes of epidermolysis bullosa simplex patients: genetic and functional analyses. *Cell* 1991; **66**: 1301–11.

8 Lane EB, Rugg EL, Navsaria H et al. A mutation in the conserved helix termination peptide of keratin 5 in hereditary skin blistering. *Nature* 1992; **356**: 244–6.

9 Bonifas J, Rothman AL, Epstein E. Linkage of epidermolysis bullosa simplex to probes in the region of keratin gene clusters on chromosomes 12q and 17q. *J Invest Dermatol* 1991; **96**: 550a.

10 Oetting WS, Mentink MM, Summers CG et al. Three different frameshift mutations of the tyrosinase gene in type 1A oculocutaneous albinism. *Am J Hum Genet* 1991; **49**: 199–206.

11 Tassabehji M, Read AP, Newton VE et al. Waardenburg's syndrome patients have mutations in the human homologue of the *Pax-3* paired box gene. *Nature* 1992; **355**: 635–6.

12 Cooper DN, Krawczak M. The mutational spectrum of single base-pair substitutions causing human genetic disease: patterns and predictions. *Hum Genet* 1990; **85**: 55–74.

13 Spritz RA, Strunk KM, Giebel LB, King RA. Detection of mutations in the tyrosinase gene in a patient with type IA oculocutaneous albinism. *New Engl J Med* 1990; **322**: 1724–7.

14 Tomita Y, Takeda A, Okinaga S, Tagami H, Shibahara S. Human oculocutaneous albinism caused by single base insertion in the tyrosinase gene. *Biochem Biophys Res Commun* 1989; **164**: 990–6.

15 Fuchs RPP, Freund A-M, Bichara M. Potential Z forming DNA sequences are frameshift mutation hot spots. In: Friedberg EC, Hanawalt PC, eds. *Mechanisms and Consequences of DNA Damage Processing*. Alan R. Liss, New York, 1988; 33–42.

16 Fu Y-H, Kuhl DPA, Pizzuti A et al. Variation of the CGG repeat at the fragile X site results in genetic instability: resolution of the Sherman paradox. *Cell* 1991; **67**: 1–20.

17 Buxton J, Shelbourne P, Davies J et al. Detection of an unstable fragment of DNA specific to individuals with myotonic dystrophy. *Nature* 1992; **355**: 547–8.

18 Wallace MR, Andersen LB, Saulino AM et al. A *de novo* *Alu* insertion results in neurofibromatosis type 1. *Nature* 1991; **353**: 864–6.

19 Ballabio A, Andria G. Deletions and translocations involving the distal short arm of the human X chromosome: review and hypotheses. *Hum Mol Genet* 1992; **1**: 221–7.

20 Lyon MF, Searle AG, eds. *Genetic Variants and Strains of the Laboratory Mouse*. 2nd ed. International Committee on Standardized Genetic Nomenclature for Mice. Oxford University Press, 1989.

21 Giebel LB, Spritz RA. Mutation of the *c-kit* (mast/stem cell growth factor receptor) proto-oncogene in human piebaldism. *Proc Natl Acad Sci USA* 1991; **88**: 8696–9.

22 Spritz RA, Giebel LB, Holmes SA. Dominant negative and loss of function mutations of the *c-kit* (mast/stem cell growth factor receptor) proto-oncogene in human piebaldism. *Am J Hum Genet* 1992; **50**: 261–9.

23 Ramsey M, Colman M-A, Stevens G et al. The tyrosinase-positive oculocutaneous albinism locus maps to chromosome 15q11.2–q12. *Am J Hum Genet* 1992; **51**: 879–84.

24 Rinchik EM, Bultman SJ, Horsthemke B et al. A gene for the mouse pink-eyed dilution locus and for human type II oculocutaneous albinism. *Nature* 1993; **361**: 72–6.

25 Winter RM. Malformation syndromes: a review of mouse/human homology. *J Med Genet* 1988; **25**: 480–7.

Chapter 2

Naturally occurring genetic skin diseases in animals

L. R. Thomsett

Knowledge of genetics as it applies to animals living in the wild is scant. Long-term observation of wild animal family groups presents many difficulties, even without the consideration of any danger involved.

The chance appearance of a genetic abnormality, the result of the normal process of reproduction to replenish and maintain herd or group numbers, is unlikely to establish a defect and lead to its perpetuation. The outcome of such an event would be the ultimate rejection of the affected animal by the family group. A similar situation is seen where sick or injured members of the group are eventually abandoned to fend for themselves, where they readily become the prey of natural predators.

Where an animal is affected with a disability that prevents it being at one with its environment, unable to nourish itself or to protect itself against predators, its chances of survival are meagre.

The domesticated species – cattle, sheep, goats, pigs and to a limited extent the horse (i.e. livestock reared for food, hide or wool production) – are complemented by the competitive and companion animal group – horses (non-farm breeds), dogs, cats and a variety of small animals which are kept as pets.

Genetic disease is rare in domestic animals. Should it occur, once recognized its perpetuation is unlikely, since in well-managed breeding establishments and farms any affected animals would be culled and appropriate changes made in the breeding programme; while any animals that were retained would be prevented from breeding by sterilization.

Table 2.1 lists those genetic skin disorders recognized to occur in domestic animals.

A further group comprises a number of species, some of specialized breeding, classified as laboratory animals, e.g. rat, mouse, guinea-pig, rabbit and hamster, together with certain of the monkeys.

Clinical manifestations of genodermatoses in animals

Pituitary dwarfism

The German shepherd dog, one of the most popular breeds of dog, is reported as having the highest incidence of pituitary dwarfism, although it does occur in other breeds from time to time; its mode of inheritance is as an autosomal recessive trait.

Clinical signs develop at 2–3 months of age, prior to which time all littermates are physically comparable.

Coat development is poor and hair length shorter than normal, with the woolly puppy coat retained. Primary hairs do not develop other than on the face, distal limbs, head and tail, and the animal fails to grow.

A bilateral symmetrical alopecia subsequently develops on the neck and upper thighs. The skin becomes thin, scaly and inelastic and the hair follicles become plugged with comedones. Skin hyperpigmentation increases progressively until the whole becomes densely melanic. Genital development varies from normal to severe hypogonadism.

Behavioural disorders in the form of aggression are common in pituitary dwarfs.

Table 2.1 *Congenital and hereditary skin disorders of domestic animals*

Disorder	Species affected
Acral mutilation and analgesia	Dog
Albinism	Sheep (especially Icelandic), dog (Dobermann pinscher, Rottweiler)
Black hair follicular dysplasia	Dog (spaniel)
Bovine erythropoietic porphyria	Cattle
Chédiak–Higashi syndrome	Cattle (Hereford, Angus), cat (Blue Persian), mink, white tiger
Colour mutant alopecia	Dog (Dobermann pinscher, Irish setter, dachshund, Great Dane)
Congenital hyperbilirubinaemia and photosensitivity	Sheep
Congenital myxoedema	Dog (Shar-pei)
Curly coat	Cattle, pig, horse, cat
Cutaneous asthenia	Cattle, sheep, pig, horse, dog, cat, rabbit, mink
Cyclic haematopoiesis	Dog (grey collie syndrome)
Dermatosis vegetans	Pig
Dermoid sinus (neutral tube defect)	Dog (Rhodesian ridgeback)
Epidermolysis bullosa	Cattle, sheep
Epitheliogenesis imperfecta	Cattle, horse, pig, sheep, dog, cat
Familial acantholysis	Cattle
Familial canine dermatomyositis	Dog (collie, Shetland sheepdog)
Hereditary multifocal cystadenocarcinomas and nodular dermatofibrosis	Dog (German shepherd)
Hereditary zinc deficiency	Cattle
Hypertrichosis	Cattle, pig, sheep
Hypothyroidism	Cattle (Afrikander), merino sheep, goat (Saanen–dwarf)
Hypotrichosis	Cattle, pig, sheep, horse, goat, cat (Siamese, Sphinx)
Ichthyosis	Cattle, pig, dog
Idiopathic seborrhoea	Dog (cocker spaniel)
Kinky hair syndrome (Menkes' disease)	Mouse
Lentiginosis profusa	Dog
Lethal acrodermatitis	Dog (bull terrier)
Lethal white foal disease	Horse
Lupus erythematosus	Dog, cat, horse
Marfan's syndrome	Cattle
Pattern baldness	Dog, monkey
Piebaldism	Dog (sheepdog)
Pili torti	Cat
Pituitary dwarfism	Dog (German shepherd)
Primary lymphoedema	Cattle, dog
Pustular psoriasiform dermatitis	Pig

Life expectation is less than for others of the breed, death commonly occurring between 3 and 8 years of age.

Hypothyroidism

Hypothyroidism occurs in cattle (Afrikander), merino sheep and Saanen–dwarf cross-bred goats. It is char-

acterized by poor coat quality and density, as well as length. The skin is thickened and myxoedematous.

Congenital myxoedema of the Shar-pei dog

The sharpei is a breed notable for its excessive skin folds which are present from birth[1]. To date, in dogs dermal mucinosis associated with excessive skin folding is unique to the Shar-pei breed.

Many years of breeding in China have resulted in the establishment of the genetic defect characterized by the abnormal synthesis of dermal glycosamino-glycans.

The Shar-pei breed, established in the USA for over 20 years, has now become established in the UK.

Reference

1 Dunstan RW, Rosser EJ. Congenital myxoedema of the Shar Pei dog. Newly recognised and emerging geno-dermatoses in domestic animals. *Curr Prob Dermatol* 1987; **17**: 216–35.

Cutaneous asthenia

Synonyms: *Dermatosparaxis, cutis laxa, Ehlers-Danlos syndrome*

Cutaneous asthenia (known as Ehlers–Donlos syndrome in humans) has been reviewed by Minor et al[1].

Cattle – both pedigree and crossbred cattle have been shown to be affected by skin fragility, coupled with both hyperextensibility of skin and joints.

Sheep – pedigree and crossbred sheep of a number of breeds have been affected similarly with loose hyperextensible skin which was readily torn with minor trauma.

In both sheep and cattle the disorder is usually fatal; its mode of inheritance is lethal autosomal recessive.

Pig, horse – similar conditions, varying in severity, have been described in the pig and horse; although in the latter lesions tend to be localized to the back and thorax. The outcome is not fatal.

Dog, cat, mink – skin hyperelasticity is well-recognized in these species (Figure 2.1), and varying

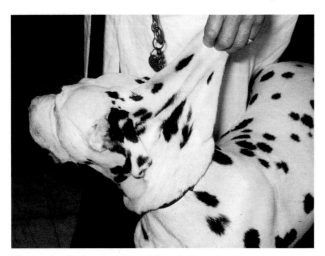

Figure 2.1 *Dalmatian dog with cutis laxa*

degrees of hyperextensibility and fragility are seen. Spontaneous tearing and tearing under minor trauma are commonly recorded clinical signs. Dominant cutaneous asthenia is found in dogs, cats and mink where inheritance is as a simple autosomal trait.

Recessive cutaneous asthenia has recently been described in the cat.

Harvey et al[2] described a condition in *rabbits* similar to the Ehlers–Danlos syndrome.

Hegreberg and Counts[3] summarized the expression of cutaneous asthenia (Ehlers–Danlos syndrome) in animals and humans as shown in Table 2.2.

References

1 Minor RR, Wootton, Joyce AM, Prockop DJ, Patterson DF. Genetic disease of connective tissues in animals. *Curr Probl Dermatol.* 1987; **17**: 199–215.
2 Harvey RG, Brown PJ, Young RD, Whitbread TJ. A connective tissue defect in two rabbits similar to the Ehlers-Danlos syndrome. *Vet Record* 1990; **120**: 351.
3 Hegreberg GA, Counts DF. Ehlers-Danlos syndrome. In: Andrews EJ, et al, (eds.) *Spontaneous Animal Models of Human Disease.* American College of Laboratory Medicine Series, vol. II. New York, Academic Press, 1979; 36–9.

Epitheliogenesis imperfecta

Congenital inherited discontinuities of Squamous epithelia of skin and oral mucous, membranes occur occasionally in calves and piglets, are rare in foals and, lambs and very rare in puppies and kittens[1]. Epitheliogenesis imperfecta has been recorded in several breeds of cattle, in which it is characterized by the absence of epithelium on the limbs and areas of the head – cheeks, pinnae, muzzle and nostrils, with involvement of the oral cavity (tongue and hard palate). Hoof deformity has also been recorded, as have developmental anomalies involving the jaws, teeth, anus and other organs.

In the horse lesions are more commonly found involving the limbs and head. Selmanowitz[2] compared certain features of this disease, as it is seen in cattle and pigs, to a congenital ectodermal defect, focal dermal hypoplasia and a form of epidermolysis bullosa in humans. The inheritance of this disorder is autosomal recessive.

References

1 Jubb KVF, Kennedy PC, Palmer N. *rainology of domestic Animals*, vol. I. *Congenital and Hereditary Diseases of Skin.* 4th ed. Academic Press, New York; 1993. 553.
2 Selmanowitz VJ. Ectodermal dysplasias including epitheliogenesis imperfecta, ichthyoses and follicular/glandular anomalies. In: Andrews EJ et al, eds. *Spontaneous Animal Models of Human Disease.* American College of Laboratory Animal Medicine Series vol. II. Academic Press, New York, 1979; 3–10.

Table 2.2 *Human and animal expression of Ehlers–Danlos syndrome*

	Inheritance	Clinical expression
Types I–III Human, dog, cat, mink	Autosomal dominant	Type I – skin fragility, hyperextensibility, bruising Type II – less severe form of type I Type III – excess joint mobility, minimal skin involvement
Type IV Human	Autosomal recessive	Rupture of large blood vessels, bowel. Thin, easily bruised skin. Deficient synthesis of type III collagen
Type V Human, mouse	Sex-linked recessive	Hyperextensibility of the skin, fragility and hyperextensibility of joints. Short stature
Type VI Human	Autosomal recessive	Some skin and joint hyperextensibility. Severe spinal curvature. Retinal detachment
Type VII Human, cattle, sheep	Autosomal recessive	Severe joint laxity, dislocation, short stature, moderate skin changes

Dermoid sinus, neural tube defect, dermoid cyst

In the dog the condition is a developmental defect whereby there is a perpetuation of the connection between the skin and the neural tube. In its most severe form the clinical manifestation is of a tube of skin extending to the spinal canal connecting with the dura mater. When mildly expressed there is only a small saccular indentation of the skin[1].

Keratinous follicular debris, secretions of skin glands and shed hair accumulate within the tube, which becomes dilated and cystic with subsequent inflammation.

Any infection which develops in the severe form may extend to the neural canal causing meningitis.

The most commonly affected breed is the Rhodesian ridgeback, in which the lesion occurs along the dorsal midline of the cervical region.

Although incompletely determined, the mode of inheritance is considered to be autosomal recessive.

Reference

1 Thomson RE, ed. *Special Veterinary Pathology. Cogenital and Hereditary Conditions.* BC Decker, Toronto, 1988; 10.

Primary lymphoedema

Primary lymphoedema is associated with developmental anomalies in lymph nodes and lymphatics and has been shown to occur as an autosomal recessive trait in cattle and as an autosomal dominant with variable expressivity in dogs.

In cattle, the condition affects the Ayrshire breed in particular and is present at birth. Severely affected calves are anasarcous and die, while those less severely affected, although showing oedema of the head and distal extremities, may survive.

Canine lymphoedema is seen in several breeds of dog and, as in cattle, occurs in early life – commonly within 3 months of birth. The oedema affects the hind-limbs more often than the fore limbs, although other areas of the body may also be involved.

In both cattle and dogs the skin exhibits the characteristic pitting oedema response on pressure.

Patterson[1] described the features of the disease as it affected the offspring of 100 dogs and stressed the great variation in clinical characteristics. Severely affected animals showed the subcutaneous tissues of the whole body to be involved, and most succumbed to the disease. Those less affected showed pitting oedema of the hind-limbs at birth or up to 3 months old, after which stage of development the condition resolved and affected puppies were no different from normal puppies of comparable age.

It has been suggested that studies of these animals may provide, embryologically, an understanding of the development of the lymphatic system.

Reference

Patterson DF. Hereditary lymphoedema. *Comp Pathol Bull* 1971; **3**: 2.

Hypotrichosis

Hypotrichosis has been seen in many species and breeds of domesticated animals, particularly in the dog and certain breeds of cattle.

The clinical manifestation of hypotrichosis is commonly seen as a generalized disorder, but on occasion the pattern of hairlessness may be regional. Scott[1] and Selmanowitz[2] have discussed the heritability and clinical signs in cattle.

Clinically recognized forms of hypotrichosis in animals are described below.

Hypotrichosis in cattle

Lethal hypotrichosis

Lethal hypotrichosis is an autosomal recessive disorder occuring in cattle, especially the Holstein-Friesian breed. Hair is present only on the muzzle, eyelids, ears, tail and pasterns. Calves die soon after birth. Histologically the anomaly is of follicular and apocrine duct dysplasia.

Semi-hairlessness

Semi-hairlessness is a non-lethal, autosomal recessive condition of cattle. The animals have a thin coat of short, curly hair of fine texture, becoming coarser and more wiry with age. Hair tends to be longer on the legs than elsewhere. The skin is wrinkled and scaly. Developmental retardation and temperamental aberration also occur in some calves. Histologically the hypotrichosis is associated with a follicular dysplasia.

Hypotrichosis and anodontia

A lethal sex-linked recessive disorder has been recorded particularly in crossbred male Maine–Anjou–Normandy cattle. Hairless and toothless at birth, the calves have been seen eventually to develop a fine coat and partial dentition, but survive no longer than 6 months. Anatomical abnormalities of the tongue, genitalia and horns are also a clinical feature. Histologically, follicular and apocrine duct dysplasia with abnormal dermal vascularization has been demonstrated in this syndrome, which is considered to be similar to human hypohidrotic ectodermal dysplasia.

Viable hypotrichosis

Viable hypotrichosis is an autosomal recessive disorder seen in Guernsey, Jersey and Holstein cattle. Calves are born virtually hairless except for hairs present on the ears, eyelids, legs and tail. A certain amount of hair may subsequently develop. Histologically the abnormality has been shown to be a follicular and apocrine gland hypoplasia.

Streaked hypotrichosis

Streaked hypotrichosis is a sex-linked dominant condition lethal for males. Female Holstein–Friesian cattle show vertical streaks of alopecia over the hips, legs and sides. The syndrome is thought to be similar to human focal dermal hypoplasia.

Tardive hypotrichosis

Thought to be sex-linked recessive, tardive hypotrichosis is seen in Friesian cattle. Female calves are apparently normal until 6 months of age, from which time they suffer a progressive hair loss commencing on the face and neck, extending towards the tail and down the legs. Histologically there is a follicular keratosis. The syndrome in cattle has some similarity to tardive cystic atrichia in humans.

'Baldy' calf syndrome

This autosomal recessive disorder is lethal for homozygous males. Affected calves are normal at birth but do not survive more than 8 months, having shown a noticeable deterioration from 1–2 months of age. A progressive hair loss with scaly, wrinkled skin develops over the neck, shoulders, axillae, stifle, hocks, elbows and periocular regions. Curling of the ear tips is also a clinical feature.

Hypotrichosis of polled and horned Hereford cattle (USA)

Hypotrichosis in these cattle is an autosomal dominant condition, characterized by generalized hypotrichosis from birth with thin skin, poor-quality curly hair with follicular hypoplasia and hoof abnormalities.

Hypotrichosis of polled Dorset sheep and German and Mexican hairless pigs

The disorder is similar to that seen in cattle.

Hypotrichosis in small animals

In small domestic animals there are a number of genetically associated hypotrichotic conditions. Some of these occur as spontaneous abnormalities, others have been perpetuated by breeders who accept and cultivate the hairlessness as the major characteristic of the breed.

Hypotrichosis of cats

Hypotrichosis, although rare, occurs in cats as an autosomal recessive trait. Affected animals become alopecic within 2 weeks of birth. Hair growth has in some cases been seen up to 10 weeks of age, after which time total hair loss becomes established.

Feline alopecia universalis of the Sphinx and Siamese breeds of cat is a naturally occurring total alopecia caused by a genetic mutation. In affected cats the follicular dysplasia is manifested as an absence of primary hairs with limiited regional distribution of secondary follicles. The epidermis is thicker than normal for the species and breed. In normality the sebaceous and apocrine glands open into the upper portion of the hair follicle; in Sphinx cats these open directly onto the surface of the skin.

Hypotrichosis of dogs

Canine alopecic breeds vary considerably in the degree of abnormality which is clinically expressed. The Chihuahua and Mexican hairless (particularly the former) are quite well coated, whereas others such as the Chinese crested dog are virtually devoid of hair, except for a crest of hair on the top of the head.

Congenital alopecia in dogs occurs sporadically in litters of puppies of many breeds in both pedigree and non-pedigree matings. The author investigated a congenitally hypotrichotic whippet showing partial absence of hair similar to that described by Selmanowitz et al[3]. Since that report, litters of crossbred smooth-coated terrier puppies (Jack Russell) have been investigated by the author. These showed bilaterally symmetrical areas of total alopecia involving the temporal region of the head, ears, lumbosacral region, axillae, abdomen, groin and posterior aspect of the thighs (Figure 2.2). The remaining haired areas of the head, body and limbs were covered in coarse guard hairs. Affected puppies were all males, all of which showed genital hypoplasia. Histological examination of hairless skin of the affected males showed total absence of hair follicles and skin glands.

Congenital hypotrichosis universalis of beagles was reported by Dunstan and Rosser[4]. It is characterized by virtualy total hairlessness, apart from small numbers of primary hairs. There was only a fine, almost invisible stubble of hairs, each of which protruded slightly from the follicular opening. The dogs did, however, have whiskers. Histologically the feature was of follicular atrophy with most follicles in telogen arrest. Although the mode of inheritance is not known, it appears that should any two affected animals be mated, then all their offspring manifest the abnormality. It was suggested by the authors that since the feature of the condition is atrophy of primary follicles to the point where they only produce small hair shafts, there is some similarity to male pattern alopecia of humans.

Pattern baldness in domestic animals

A condition not commonly encountered in domestic animals, pattern baldness is recognized as an inherited alopecia of the dachshund breed of dog; occurring in both males and females, it is not strictly analogous to human pattern baldness. In dogs it commences at maturity, approximately 1 year of age. Males show bilateral symmetrical hair loss on the pinnae which becomes total by the age of 8–9 years. Females show alopecia of the ventrum[5]. Many types of pattern baldness occur in dogs in which the underlying cause is found to be an endocrinopathy; the clinical features referable to the skin being bilaterally symmetrical hair loss of the trunk and proximal limbs with sparing of the distal limbs, tip of tail, head and ears. Histologically the condition is characterized by orthokeratotic hyperkeratosis, telogen arrest and plugging of hair follicles with keratinous masses.

A condition more akin to pattern baldness of man has been described by Uno[6] in stump-tailed macaques. Eighteen adults over 6 years old showed advanced baldness of the frontal region. In animals 3–5 years old the hair in the early bald areas was shorter and thinner as well as less pigmented than elsewhere on the head. In well-established cases the normal hair of the adolescent was replaced by short, thin hair over the whole of the balding area. In the absence of any demonstrable pathological change the baldness appeared to be due to a diminution in the size of hair follicles, thus producing small, fine hairs rather than terminal hairs.

References

1 Scott DW. *Large Animal Dermatology*. WB Saunders, Philadelphia, 1988; 334–7.
2 Selmanowitz VJ. Ectodermal dysplasias in cattle. Analogues in man. *Br J Dermatol* 1970; **84**: 258.
3 Selmanowitz VJ, Kramer KM, Orentreich N. Congenital ectodermal defect in miniature poodles. *J Hered* 1970; **61**: 196–9.
4 Dunstan RW, Rosser JR Jr. Newly recognised and emerging genodermatoses in domestic animals. *Curr Probl Dermatol* 1987; **17**: 216–35.
5 Muller GH, Kirk RW, Scott Danny W. *Small Animal Dermatology*. 4th ed. WB Saunders, Philadelphia, 1989.

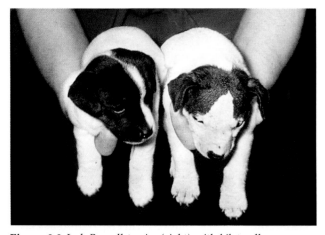

Figure 2.2 *Jack Russell terrier (right) with bilaterally symmetrical alopecia sex-linked to the male*

6 Uno H. Baldness. Model No. 212. In: Capen C et al, eds. *Handbook – Animal Models of Human Disease*. Armed Forces Institute of Pathology, Washington, DC, 1981.

Colour mutant alopecia

Colour mutant alopecia is a hereditary ectodermal defect seen in its most typical form in the Dobermann pinscher breed of dog, in which it is referred to as 'blue Dobermann' syndrome. It is also recognized in other breeds, e.g. Irish setter, dachshund and Great Dane[1,2].

Clinically the condition is a progressive deterioration in coat density and quality with concurrent scaliness of the skin which develops from birth and involves only those areas of the animal carrying the blue coat colouration; areas carrying normal tan coat hair remain unaffected. Coat changes are accompanied by histologically demonstrable abnormalities of the hairs. Such hairs as are present contain abnormal massive deposits of melanin which contribute to cortical fragility and fracture of the hair shafts.

In addition to the hair dystrophy the hair follicles become dilated with keratinous debris, subsequently developing pustular lesions of secondary pyoderma[3,4].

The mode of inheritance of this defect has, as yet, not been determined.

References

1 Foil CS. Comparative genodermatoses. *Clin Dermatol* 1985; **3**: 175.
2 Carlotti DN. Canine hereditary Blackhair follicular dysplasia and colour mutant alopecia. Clinical and histopathological aspects. In: Von Tscharner C, Halliwell REW, eds. *Advances in Veterinary Dermatology*, vol. I. Baillière Tindall, London, 1990; 43–6.
3 Prieur DJ, Fittschen C, Collier LL. Blue Dobermann syndrome of dogs: a deleterious macromelanosomal trait. *Fed Proc* 1984; **43** (3): 603.
4 Dunstan RW, Rosser EJ. Colour mutant alopecia in dogs. Newly recognised and emerging genodermatoses in domestic animals. *Curr Probl Dermatol* 1987; **17**: 229–31.

Black hair follicle dysplasia

Black hair follicle dysplasia occurs in dogs having particoloured coats made up of black and white or brown and white patches. The areas of white hair are normal from birth, but those composed of black or brown hair show a variety of abnormalities. Such hair is shortened, stubby, lacks lustre and is accompanied by a scaliness of the skin. The condition has been seen in crossbreds as well as in a small number of pedigree breeds.

The author has seen a less severe form of the disease in black-and-white cocker spaniels and brown-and-white springer spaniels. In these the hair in the white patches is normal and the black or brown body coat is of poor quality, fine and woolly as well as lacking in lustre.

Although the mode of inheritance of the condition is unclear, it is thought to be an autosomal dominant trait.

Similar black-and-white hair dystrophies have been seen in horses, the aetiology of which is unclear.

Hypertrichosis

Hirsutism is a rare occurrence in animals and is more likely to be the result of endocrinopathy than of genetic origin.

In sheep, Border disease, a combination of togavirus infection and genetic disorder, results in lambs having a long birthcoat and accompanying neurological signs, for which the term 'hairy shakers' has been coined.

The dystrophic change is due to an enlargement of the primary hair follicles resulting in the production of very large wool fibres[1].

Reference

1 Darbyshire MB, Barlow RM. Experiments in Border disease IX. The pathogenesis of the skin lesion. *J Comp Path* 1976; **86**: 557–70.

Pili torti

A condition resembling human pili torti has been seen in a litter of domestic short-haired cats[1]. The litter of eight (five females and three males) were born of a sibling mating. All were normal at birth. One female died within 5 days; the remaining kittens showed a rapidly developing alopecia at 10 days of age. When 18 days old, only one kitten retained a good hair coat; in the affected kittens hair was readily epilated. All the kittens were apparently mentally alert and there was no evidence of deafness.

In addition to the abnormal coat there were inflammatory ocular lesions, a mild pedal dermatitis and paronychia. By day 26, a further kitten had died and four were destroyed on humane grounds.

Microscopic examination of hair showed a uniform rotation about the long axis of 360 degrees in a clockwise manner. The follicle dystrophy showed as a marked hyperkeratosis with dense whorls of keratin; some follicles were cystic and in some follicular curvature could be seen.

The condition was considered comparable to the autosomal dominant condition as seen in humans.

Reference

1 Geary MR, Baker KP. The occurrence of pili torti in a litter of kittens in England. *J Small Animal Pract* 1986; **27** (2): 85–8.

Curly coat

Curling abnormalities of hair as part of a lethal skin defect have been recorded in Japanese black cattle[1]. Alopecia developed within a week and extended over several areas of the body. The hair present was short, bristly and kinked at birth; the skin was found to be excessively thick and hung in folds around the animals' neck. Corneal opacity was also seen, with subsequent purulent ocular infection. Affected animals only survived for up to a month. The follicular abnormality was seen to be a diminution in follicle numbers with an increase in the number of abnormally large sweat glands. Inheritance was autosomal recessive.

Scott[2] listed the breeds of cattle showing abnormal coat curliness, the inheritance in the Ayrshire breed being autosomal dominant and in Swedish cattle autosomal recessive. In horses, curly coat has been shown to be autosomal recessive in the Percheron breed, as well as in some American breeds of horse.

References

1 Hamana K. Congenital lethal skin defects in Japanese cattle. *Proceedings of the 14th World Congress on Diseases of Cattle.* Dublin, 1986; 181–5.
2 Scott DW. *Large Animal Dermatology.* WB Saunders, Philadelphia, 1988.

Kinky hair syndrome of mice (Menkes' disease)

Prins and Van den Hamer[1] described a disease of laboratory mice in which the brindled mutation homozygous male is characterized by depigmented white fur, curled whiskers and wavy pelage.

Most of the affected mice die at 14–21 days of life. The cause of death is a severe copper deficiency due to inactivity of copper-containing enzymes.

Reference

Prins HW, Van den Hamer CJA. Menkes disease. Model No. 244. In: Capen CC et al, eds. *Handbook – Animal Models of Human Disease.* Armed Forces Institute of Pathology, Washington, DC, 1982.

Albinism

In domestic animals the true albino is rare, although it has been described in Icelandic sheep[1,2].

A variety of manifestations of partial hypopigmentation are, however, recognized across the species, e.g. hypopigmentation of the lips and nose is considered to be a congenital disorder of Dobermann pinschers, Rottweilers and certain other breeds of dog[3].

Canine cyclic haematopoiesis (grey collie syndrome)

Canine cyclic haematopoiesis is a lethal autosomal recessive condition affecting puppies born with pale, depigmented noses and silver-grey coat colour in contradistinction to the normal sable colouration of this breed.

Within 2–3 months after birth affected puppies show poor growth and development with concurrent illness having a variety of clinical signs, i.e. fever, diarrhoea, enlarged lymph nodes.

Accompanying these signs is alternating neutropenia and neutrophilia, and non-regenerative anaemia. Puppies do not usually survive over the age of 6 months, certainly no longer than 2 years.

Chediak–Higashi syndrome

Padgett[4] reviewed this pigmentation anomaly which is recognized as partial oculocutaneous albinism of Hereford cattle, and Cole[5] described similar symptoms in Angus cattle which was confirmed as a simple autosomal recessive trait following the results of breeding trials.

The condition in cats – Persian cats with yellow eyes and blue smoke hair colour – is described by Holzworth[6], and it is similarly seen in Aleutian mink and white tigers. In the cat the condition is manifested as the abnormal deposition of greatly enlarged melanin granules within the hairs as well as abnormal granules in a number of other cell types.

Owing to other cellular abnormalities the affected animals are more susceptible to infection and suffer from spontaneous haemorrhages.

Tyrosinase deficiency in the chow-chow dog

Depigmentation, changes seen in puppies with this syndrome[7] are associated with the hair and in particular with the characteristic blue-black tongue of this breed. The colour of the tongue changes to pink, accompanied by whitening of parts of the hair shafts, spontaneous remission of which is recorded within 2–4 months.

Lethal white foal disease

Two forms of inheritance are described – autosomal dominant and autosomal recessive. Scott[8] summarized the autosomal dominant trait as 'non-viable embryos in the homozygous state'.

In the autosomal recessive form, foals born to the mating of two horses of the Overo paint breed show albinism and congenital defects of the intestinal tract[9].

Albinism in humans

In comparison with animals in which there are few manifestations of albinism, six forms of human oculocutaneous albinism are recognized: tyrosinase negative albino, tyrosinase positive albino, yellow type albino, Chediak–Higashi syndrome, Hermansky–Pudlak syndrome and Cross's syndrome.

In some patients albinism is linked with congenital deafness; in animals this feature occurs only in white piebald cats and Dalmatian dogs in whom deafness is well recognized.

References

1 Adalsteinsson S. Depressed fertility in Icelandic sheep caused by a single colour gene. *Ann Géne Sélect Anim* 1975; **7** (4): 445–7.
2 Adalsteinsson S. Albinism in Icelandic sheep. *J Hered* 1977; **68** (6): 347–9.
3 Schaible RH. Introduction to hypopigmentation. In: Andrews EJ et al, eds. *Spontaneous Animal Models of Human Disease.* American College of Laboratory Medicine Series, vol. II. New York, Academic Press, 1979; 11.
4 Padgett GA, Holland JM, Davis WC, Henson JB. The Chediak–Higashi syndrome: a comparative review. *Curr Top Pathol* 1970; **51**: 175–94.
5 Cole DE. Oculo-cutaneous hypopigmentation of Angus cattle. *Dissert Abs Int* 1985; **45** (10): 3128.
6 Holzworth J. Diseases of the cat. *Medicine and Surgery*, vol. I. WB Saunders, Philadelphia, 1987; 625–8.
7 Engstrom D. Tyrosinase deficiency in the Chow Chow. In: Kirk RW, ed. *Current Veterinary Therapy II.* WB Saunders, Philadelphia, 1966.
8 Scott DW. *Large Animal Dermatology.* WB Saunders, Philadelphia, 1988.
9 Jones WE. The overo white foal syndrome. *J Eq Med Surg* 1979; **3**: 54–6.

Piebaldism

Piebaldism is an autosomal dominant condition characterized by the congenital absence of pigment cells in the white areas of the skin. Piebald colouration is present in many domestic species.

Ichthyosis

Ichthyosis (Figure 2.3 and 2.4) is a rare hereditary disease which has been reported in dogs, cats, cattle and pigs[1], as well as It is characterized by the accumulation of masses of scales on the surface of the skin due to increased corneocyte cohesion. It is suggested that this is associated with abnormal lipid metabolism during the production of intercellular cement substances[3].

In cattle a severe form of autosomal recessive ichthyosis occasionally occurs. The disease is present at birth, the fetus being covered in hyperkeratotic plate-like scales divided by intraepidermal fissures. Affected animals survive but a very short period of time. Hair is mostly absent. When present it may grow in variable density in a furrowed pattern. The stratum

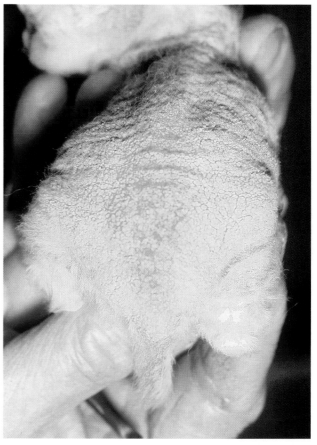

Figure 2.3 *Kitten with ichthyosis*

corneum of the surface epidermis shows orthokeratotic hyperkeratosis, as does the lining of the ducts of the skin glands.

In dogs, ichthyosis appears to simulate lamellar ichthyosis as an autosomal recessive trait. The clinical picture in the dog is of masses of grey scale and keratinous projections from the skin. Large amounts

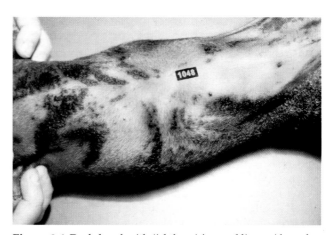

Figure 2.4 *Dachshund with 'ichthyosis' resembling epidermal naevi and the lines of Blaschko*

of debris are shed. The foot pads are affected by accumulations of masses of keratin at the pad periphery.

References

1 Baker JR, Ward WR. Ichthyosis in domestic animals: a review of the literature and a case report. *Br Vet J* 1985; **141**: 1–8.
2 Jubb KVF, Kennedy PC, Palmer N. *Pathology of Domestic Animals*, vol. I. 4th ed. Academic Press, New York, 1993; 554–5.
3 Dunstan RW, Rosser EJ Jr. Newly recognised and emerging genodermatoses of animals. *Curr Probl Dermatol* 1987; **17**: 217–18.

Lentiginosis profusa

Lesions of lentigo are not uncommon in the dog and take the form of multiple intensely black macules, particularly on the ventral surfaces of the body. Other areas of the body and the limbs may, however, also be affected. The lesions are discrete, sharply circumscribed and only occasionally raised above the level of the surrounding skin. Their presence causes no inconvenience or discomfort to the patient, only concern to the owner.

Histologically, there is no epidermal abnormality in the early stage of development and only mild thickening, acanthosis and hyperkeratosis with dense hypermelanosis once the lesion is fully developed.

The author has seen the condition particularly in breeds which are naturally hyperpigmented in certain areas of the skin, e.g. the miniature schnauzer. The pug, in which the hereditary form of lentiginosis profusa has been described by Briggs[1], is similarly hyperpigmented. This is autosomal dominant.

Reference

1 Briggs OM. Lentiginosis profusa in the pug: three case reports. *J Small Animal Pract* 1985; **26**: 675–80.

Familial acantholysis

Jolly et al[1] described familial acantholysis, an autosomal recessive condition, in Aberdeen Angus calves in New Zealand. The disease was present at birth or developed within 2 weeks and was invariably fatal. Lesions of hoof separation, ulceration and erosion of the epithelium covering areas of the limbs subject to pressure or rubbing as well as ulceration and erosion of the oral cavity.

Although in many respects this disease is similar to epidermolysis bullosa of sheep, the two conditions differ in the pathogenesis of lesions. In the calf the disorder is an acantholysis with separation between the prickle cells and the basal layer.

Reference

1 Jolly RD, Alley MR, O'Hara PJ. Familial acantholysis of Angus calves. *Vet Pathol* 1973; **10**: 473–83.

Epidermolysis bullosa

Epidermolysis bullosa is a complex of hereditary bullous diseases whose cardinal signs are spontaneous blistering or blisters induced by trauma. An autosomal recessive condition resembling the dystrophic form of human epidermolysis bullosa has been described in Swiss sheep in which sporadic hereditary bullous skin disease occurred in newborn lambs[1]. Lesions were found to occur from birth and took the form of blisters in and around the mouth and on the coronary bands.

A similar condition occurs in newborn Suffolk and South Dorset Down breeds of sheep in New Zealand.

Dystrophic epidermolysis bullosa has been described in the cat[2]. Lesions were seen on the gums, tongue, palate and Oropharynx with ulceration and crusting of the metacorpal, metatarsal and digital pads as well as paronychia.

Bassett[3,4] described epidermolysis bullosa in cattle in Ireland, in which calves showed growth retardation and abnormal susceptibility to skin damage by minor trauma, shown histologically as dermoepidermal separation.

References

1 Ehrensperger F, Hauser B, Wild P. Epidermolysis in lambs. *Tierarztl Umsch* 1987; **42** (9): 677–98.
2 White SD, Dunstan RW, Olivry T et al. Dystrophic (dermolytic) epidermolysis bullosa in a cat. *Vet Dermatol* 1993; **4** (2): 91–5.
3 Bassett H. Bovine epidermolysis, an inherited disease of cattle. *Proceedings of the 14th World Congress on Diseases of Cattle*. Dublin, 1986; 75–80.
4 Bassett H. A congenital bovine epidermolysis resembling epidermolysis bullosa simplex of man. *Vet Record* 1987; **121** (1): 8–11.

Canine familial dermatomyositis

Canine familial dermatomyositis was first documented in detail by Hargis et al[1,2] and is presumed autosomal dominant with variable expressivion. It occurs particularly in dogs of the collie and Shetland sheepdog breeds and of crosses of these breeds. Although there is an established breed predilection, no sex predilection has been recorded.

Kunkle et al[3] described three forms of the disease: (i) where affected puppies outgrow the disease and show no further signs; (ii) where the appearance of lesions decreases in frequency until by 1 year of age the dog is free of the condition except for residual scarring; and (iii) recurrent episodes of lesions throughout life.

Clinical signs show marked variation and may appear as early as 7–11 weeks of age, but more commonly between the third and sixth month. Lesions in the form of pustules, vesicles and ulcers, some of which show spontaneous regression, are seen on the face, lips, ears and nose, progressively involving other areas such as the paws, tip of tail and skin over the stifle region. Lesions vary in their persistence, some being indolent and persisting for 6–8 months. The resulting scarring and alopecia may be permanent.

Myositis is variable in its manifestation. Severely affected animals show clinical signs of muscle involvement resulting in temporal and masseter atrophy, in some cases to the degree that eating and swallowing are impaired. Poor physical development with generalized muscle atrophy also occurs.

Histopathological examination of early skin lesions shows pustules or subepidermal vesicles; vacuolar degeneration of basal cells with both superficial and deep perivascular dermatitis is seen. Late cases show hyperkeratosis, epidermal hyperplasia, dermal fibrosis and follicular atrophy. Hydropic degeneration of basal cells and the formation of colloid bodies are seen in association with intrabasal or subepidermal clefts and vesicles[4].

References

1 Hargis AM, Haupt KH, Hegreberg GA, Prieur DJ, Moore MP. Familial canine dermatomyositis. Initial characterisation of the cutaneous and muscular lesions. *Am J Pathol* 1984; **116**: 234–44.
2 Hargis AM, Haupt KH, Prieur DJ, Moore MP. Familial canine dermatomyositis. *Am J Pathol* 1985; **120**: 323–5.
3 Kunkle GA, Gross TL, Fadok V. Dermatomyositis in Collie dogs. *Compend Cont Educ Pract Vet* 1985; **7**: 185–92.
4 Gross TL, Kunkle GA. The cutaneous histology of dermatomyositis in Collie dogs. *Vet Pathol* 1987; **24**: 11–15.

Dermatosis vegetans

Dermatosis vegetans is a genetically transmitted skin and respiratory tract disorder which has been seen widely throughout Europe as well as in Canada. Its mode of inheritance is autosomal recessive. Initially seen as a disease of Landrace pigs[1], it has been shown to be a semilethal hereditary disorder characterized by a maculopapular dermatitis in erythematous symmetric patterns. The skin lesions are often present at birth and are found particularly on the ventral abdomen and medial thighs. The erythematous eruption when fully developed becomes covered in a dark-brown papillomatous crust. Exudative lesions on the coronary band of the claws also show accumulations of brown material and the claw itself becomes ridged and deformed.

Symptoms of respiratory distress develop concurrently with the skin lesions and are shown to be associated with giant cell pneumonia.

Progressive deterioration in the condition of affected pigs is terminated in most cases by death in 6 weeks. Animals that survive remain stunted. Skin lesions histologically demonstrate an intraepidermal pustular dermatitis with epidermal microabscesses containing eosinophils and neutrophils in the early stage of the disease. Older lesions show a hyperplastic superficial perivascular dermatitis with multinucleate giant cells. Lung lesions are those of a giant cell interstitial pneumonia[2].

Reference

1 Done JT, Loosemoore RM, Saunders CN. Dermatosis vegetans in pigs. *Vet Record* 1967; **80**: 292–7.
2 Evensen O, Bratberg B. An ultrastructural and cytochemical study of the pulmonary lesions and multinucleate giant cells in porcine dermatosis vegetans. *Acta Pathol Microbiol Immunol Scand* 1992; **100**: 515–22.

Pustular psoriasiform dermatitis of swine

Pustular psoriasiform dermatitis[1] is a skin disease, thought to be genetic, of young pigs (more commonly of white breeds), which occurs spontaneously in the 12–18 month age group, with no sex predilection. Rarely associated with any systemic illness, it is seen as asymmetrical papular eruptions, not unlike those of dermatosis vegetans, having a raised erythematous border and central area of bran-like scale and crust.

The pattern of lesions is often bizarre, coalescent arciform or serpiginous over the ventral body with extension to involve the lateral and dorsal aspects as well as the medial thighs. Pruritus is absent and lesions heal spontaneously in 3–10 weeks.

Histologically the initial lesions are of intraepidermal pustules containing eosinophils and neutrophils with parakeratosis. Once established, the histological picture is of a superficial perivascular dermatitis and psoriasiform epidermal hypoplasia.

The human disease equivalent is considered to be familial annular erythema or familial pustular psoriasis.

Reference

1 Scott DW. Porcine juvenile pustular psoriasiform dermatitis. In: *Large Animal Dermatology*. WB Saunders, Philadelphia, 1988; 351–2.

Systemic lupus erythematosus

In domestic animals Systemic lupus erythematosus is rare; it occurs in dogs and cats and very rarely in horses. It is included in the group of genodermatoses because of the genetic predilection shown in what is a disease of multifactorial aetiology[1]. No age or sex predilection has been shown in the dog and cat, although two breeds of dog, the Shetland sheepdog and German shepherd dog, appear to be predisposed.

Clinical signs in the dog are varied: fever, anaemia, polyarthritis, skin disease, oral ulceration and proteinuria as well as a variety of other signs affecting the cardiovascular, nervous, respiratory and lymphatic systems and some large viscera.

In the cat, fever, anaemia, skin infection and glomerulonephritis are some of the signs of what is a somewhat bizarre disease.

Diagnosis is difficult. The antinuclear antibody titre is the most reliable confirmatory test available, which is up to 90% positive when active disease is present. Skin lesions vary greatly, and may be generalized and involve particularly the face, ears and distal extremities. Skin histology is very variable and may be nondiagnostic. The most common lesion is an interface dermatitis. Hydropic lichenoid change involving the hair follicle outer root sheath, subepidermal vacuolar alteration and myxoedema are described[2]. Direct immunofluorescence testing has shown variable, equivocal results.

References

1 Hubert B, Teichner M, Fournel C, Monier JC. Spontaneous familial systemic lupus erythematosus in a canine breeding colony. *J Comp Pathol* 1988; **98** (1): 81–9.
2 Scott DW, Walton DK, Manning TO, Smith CA, Lewis RM. Canine lupus erythematosus II. Systemic lupus erythematosus. *J Am Animal Hosp Assoc* 1983; **19**: 481–8.

Bovine erythropoietic porphyria

Jorgensen and with[1] reviewed the hereditary porphyrias in animals other than humans, and Scott[2] discussed the role of porphyrias in the causation of photodermatitis.

A number of breeds of cattle have been reported as being affected by bovine erythropoietic porphyria, e.g. Hereford, Shorthorn, Holstein and Danish Red, and the disorder is known throughout the world. The cardinal signs are discolouration of the teeth, bones and most soft tissues due to the accumulation of uroporphyrin I and coproporphyrin.

Clinically, animals with porphyria are anaemic owing to haemolysis with consequent high levels of porphyrins accumulating in the blood and skin, predisposing to photosensitiation, pale mucous membranes and discolouration of the teeth (pink tooth) to a pink or dark-brown colour. Urine on standing turns dark red or reddish-brown in sunlight, or may be dark when voided. Photodermatitis is the major clinical sign and affects the non-pigmented or lightly pigmented most-exposed areas of skin; it follows the pattern of white to black pigmentation absolutely.

Diagnosis is on clinical grounds together with Wood's light red or orange fluorescence of teeth and urine in positive cases. The determination of raised levels of porphyrins in blood and urine and also the results of skin biopsy examination are further confirmation. Inheritance is autosomal recessive.

References

1 Jorgensen SK, With TK. Congenital porphyria in animals other than man. In: Rook AJ, Walton GS, eds. *Comparative Physiology and Pathology of Skin*. Blackwell, Oxford, 1965; 317–31.
2 Scott DW. Environmental diseases. In: *Large Animal Dermatology*. WB Saunders, Philadelphia, 1988; 81–3.

Congenital hyperbilirubinaemia and photosensitivity

Congenital hyperbilirubinaemia and photosensitivity is a disorder that has been reported to affect specifically Southdown lambs in New Zealand[1].

Reference

1 Clare NT. Photosensitising diseases in New Zealand *IV*. The photosensitising agent in Southdown photosensitivity. *NZ J Sci Technol* 1945; **27A**: 23–31.

Hepatic pigmentation with photosensitivity

A form of hepatogenous light sensitization has been recorded in sheep, which has some similarity to Dubin–Johnson syndrome in humans[1].

Reference

1 Cornelius CE, Osburn BI. Hepatic pigmentation with photosensitivity. A syndrome in Corriedale sheep resembling Dubin–Johnson syndrome in man. *J Am Vet Med Assoc* 1965; **146**: 709–13.

Lethal acrodermatitis in bull terriers

Lethal acrodermatitis in bull terriers[1,2] is an autosomal recessive condition with similarities to human acrodermatitis enteropathica. Puppies are weak at birth with pale pigmentation. Exudative lesions develop around the body orifices accompanied by nail dystrophy. Behavioural changes occur at weaning onwards with marked aggressive behaviour. Affected pups die by the age of 15 months.

References

1 Jezyk PF, Haskins ME, Mackay-Smith WE, Patterson DF. Lethal acrodermatitis in bull terriers. *J Am Vet Med Assoc* 1986; **188**: 833–9.
2 Smits B, Croft DL, Abrans-Ogg ACB. Lethal acrodermatitis in bull terriers: a problem of defective zinc metabolism. *Vet Dermatol* 1991; **2** (2): 91–6.

Hereditary zinc deficiency (parakeratosis)

A less severe disease of cattle, similar to that seen in the bull terriers, is hereditary zinc deficiency or parakeratosis[1,2]. at birth and develop exudative skin lesions with scale, crust and hair loss on the face, distal limbs and mucocutaneous junctions. Other general clinical signs are seen affecting the respiratory and alimentary tracts (diarrhoea). Skin biopsy shows parakeratosis, hyperkeratosis with a superficial perivascular dermatitis.

A genetic defect in some breeds of dog, e.g. malamutes, in which there is decreased capability for zinc absorption, also gives rise to similar skin lesions.

References

1 Dyson DA. Inherited parakeratosis in Friesian calves. *Vet Record* 1986; **119** 635.
2 Weisman K, Flagstad T. Hereditary zinc deficiency (Adema disease) in cattle, an animal parallel to acrodermatitis enteropathica. *Acta Dermatovenereol* 1976; **56**: 151.
3 Jubb KVF, Kennedy PC, Palmer N. *Pathology of Domestic Animals*, vol. I. 4th ed. Academic Press, New York, 1993; 553–5.

Acral mutilation and analgesia syndrome

Acral mutilation and analgesia syndrome is an autosomal recessive condition affecting certain breeds of dog, in particular German shorthaired pointers and English pointers[1]. There is a degenerative neuropathy with lesions at the level of the primary sensory neuron. Clinical signs are first seen in puppies on reaching 3–5 months of age. No sex predilection has been demonstrated.

Affected puppies show habitual biting and licking of the paws in response to loss of temperature and pain responses in the affected feet; occasionally the legs and trunk may be similarly affected. Hind-limbs are more severely affected than the fore-limbs. Consequent upon the changes there is swelling of the toes and feet with paronychia and self-amputation of the toes.

Reference

1 Cummings JF, de Lahunta A, Winn SS. Acral mutilation and nociceptive loss in English pointer dogs. *Acta Neuropathol* 1981; **53** (2): 119–27.

Idiopathic seborrhoea of cocker spaniels

Idiopathic seborrhoea of cocker spaniels[1,2] is a disease exclusive to spaniels which does not become apparent until 2–3 years of age.

Clinically the condition is characterized by a greasy coat, ceruminous otitis, compacted yellow scale and crust-forming keratinous plaques. This form of seborrhoea is accompanied by marked skin malodour. Moderate to mild pruritus may also be seen. The syndrome is in some respects similar to human seborrhoeic dermatitis.

There is an increased epidermal turnover of 10–11 days compared with the normal of 21–24 days. Histologically, the change in the skin is seen as orthokeratosis and parakeratosis with 'basket-weave' laminated masses of keratin, and follicular dilatation with keratinous plugging. There are areas of epidermal spongiosis and a superficial perivascular dermatitis.

References

1 Dunstan RW, Rosser EJ Jr. Newly recognised and emerging genodermatoses in animals. Idiopathic seborrhoeic dermatitis of spaniel dogs. *Curr Probl Dermatol* 1987; **17**: 219–20.
2 Muller GH, Kirk RW, Scott DW. *Small Animal Dermatology*. 4th ed. WB Saunders, philadelphia; 1989; 727.

Hereditary multifocal renal cystadenocarcinomas and nodular dermatofibrosis in the German shepherd dog

An autosomal dominant syndrome characterized by multifocal renal tumours and lesions of dermatofibrosis was described by Lium and Moe in 1985[1]. The condition was investigated in 43 German shepherd dogs. Kidney lesions were multiple solid and cystic tumours with metastases in 43% of affected animals. Ten of 11 affected bitches had multiple uterine leiomyomas. Skin lesions were composed of dense collagen fibres.

Reference

1 Lium B, Moe L. Hereditary multifocal cystadenocarcinomas and nodular fibrosis in the German Shepherd dog: microscopical and hishopathologic changes. *Vet Pathol* 1985; **22** (5): 447–55.

The relevance of animal genodermatoses to human disease

From this review of domestic animal genodermatoses it can be seen that there is a vast amount of knowledge to be gained by observation of these species (Table 2.3). The observation of disease in animals provides essential information relevant to the understanding of human disease and offers opportunities for both natural and experimental matings which can never be used as investigational aids in humans.

While the animal kingdom can contribute much information on the genetic disorders, whether of skin or other systems or organs, it has always to be

Table 2.3 *Animal models of human genodermatoses, spontaneous and experimental; a partially tapped resource*

Animal condition	*Relevant human condition*
Albino and beige mice	Albinism
Anodontia and macroglossia – cattle	Ectodermal dysplasia
Atrichia, tardive symmetrical – cattle, hairless mouse	Tardive cystic atrichia
Canine and equine immune-mediated thrombocytopenic purpura	Immune-mediated thrombocytopenia, autoimmune thrombocytopenia
Canine familial dermatomyositis	Human genetically controlled immune-mediated diseases, dermatomyositis
Congenitally athymic mouse, rat, guinea-pig	Thymic aplasia,
Congenital ectodermal defect, sex-linked – dog	Sex-linked hypohidrotic ectodermal dysplasia
Congenital ichthyosis – cattle, mouse	Recessive ichthyoses and ichthyosis congenita
Congenital lymphoedema – dog	Lymphatic abnormalities
Congenital myxoedema – dog	Scleromyxoedema
Cutaneous asthenia (Ehlers–Danlos syndrome and variants)	
EDS I–III – dog, cat, mink	EDS I–III
EDS V – mouse	EDS V
EDS VII – cattle, sheep, cat	EDS VII
Epidermolysis bullosa – cattle, sheep, cat	Dystrophic recessive epidermolysis bullosa
Epitheliogenesis imperfecta – cattle, foal, pig, dog	Congenital ectodermal defect, focal dermal hypoplasia, aplasia cutis, epidermolysis bullosa
Familial acantholysis – cattle	Hailey–Hailey disease
Follicular glandular dysplasia – cattle	Ectodermal dysplasia
Genetic mast cell deficiency – mouse	Study of mast cell function; comparative studies of normal and abnormal mast cell populations
Hypotrichosis and anodontia – cattle	Ectodermal dysplasia
Idiopathic thrombocytopenia	Idiopathic thrombocytopenic purpura; investigation of basic immune mechanism involved in thrombocytopenia
Kinky hair syndrome (Menkes' disease) – mouse	Menkes' disease; investigation of copper metabolism
Lentiginosis profusa – dog	Lentiginosis
Marfan's syndrome – cattle	Marfan's syndrome
Melanoma – Sinclair swine	Melanoma
Melanosis – grey horse	Factors affecting abnormal growth of melanocytes; study of melanocytic activity and melanin transfer
Merle dog (Shetland sheepdog, mouse)	Piebaldism
Near-total hairlessness of newborn – cattle	Aplasia of hair follicles, follicular hypoplasia
Pattern baldness – chimpanzee	Male pattern baldness
Pili torti – cat	Pili torti
Pustular psoriasiform dermatitis – pig	Human psoriatic disease
Seborrhoeic disease – dog	Seborrhoea
Streaked hairlessness – female cattle	Focal dermal hypoplasia
Woolly semi-hairlessness – cattle	Pili torti
X-linked sparse fur mutation – mouse	Type II X-linked ornithine transcarboxylase deficiency

remembered that human and animal diseases are never directly comparable in all respects in either aetiology or effect.

Some conditions have been fully or partially reproduced experimentally in laboratory animal species, the advantage of these being the ease and speed with which new generations can be bred. However, the laboratory animal species are phylogenetically further from humans than are companion animals. A further advantage of non-laboratory species of animals is that they are more likely to show the heterogeneity of response to causal factors that is characteristic of the human[1].

Similarly, in respect of the genodermatoses of domestic animal species, their occurrence and study as spontaneous disorders has the advantage over experimentally induced disease in that they arise under natural circumstances where interactions between a variety of causal factors, both genetic and environmental, may occur[2].

References

1 Calabrese EJ. Animal extrapolation and the challenge of human heterogeneity. *J Pharmaceut Sci* 1986; **75**: 1041–6.
2 Thrusfield M. Companion animal epidemiology, its contribution to human medicine. *Acta Vet Scand* 1989; **84** (suppl.): 57–65.

Further reading

Davidson MK, Lindsey JR, Davis JK. Requirements and selection of an animal model. *Israel J Med Sci* 1987; **23**: 551–5.

Foil C. Comparative genodermatoses. *Clin Dermatol.* 1985; **3**: 175–83.
Freeman DJ, Hegreberg GA. Congenital skin diseases. *Probl Vet Med* 1990; **2** (3): 523–47.
Frenkel JK. Choice of animal models for the study of disease processes in man. *Fed Proc* 1969; **28**: 160–1.
Hoskins JD, Taboada J. Congenital defects of the dog. *Comp Cont Educ Pract Vet* 1992; **14** (7): 873–97.
Jubb KVF, Kennedy PC, Palmer N. *Pathology of Domestic Animals*, vol. I. 4th ed. Academic Press, New York, 1993; 553–79.
Kirk RW (ed). A catalogue of congenital and hereditary disorders of dogs (by breed). In: *Current Veterinary Therapy IX*. WB Saunders, Philadelphia, 1986; 1281–5.
Muller GH, Kirk RW, Scott DW. *Small Animal Dermatology*. 4th ed. WB Saunders, Philadelphia, 1989.
Patterson DF, Haskins ME, Jezyk PF. Models of human genetic disease in domestic animals. In: Harris H, Hirschhorn K, eds. *Advances in Human Genetics*. Plenum, New York, 1982; 263–339.
Scott DW. *Large Animal Dermatology*. WB Saunders, Philadelphia, 1988.
White SD. Congenital and genetic skin disease. *Tijdschr Diergeneesk* 1993; **118** (suppl.): 53–7.

Acknowledgements

I wish to acknowledge with gratitude the assistance of Professor John E. Harkness, College of Veterinary Medicine, Mississippi State University, in the preparation of this contribution, the forbearance of the editor Dr John Harper, and Mrs Rosemary Barton for typing the manuscript.

Chapter 3

The skin before birth

O. M. V. Schofield and R. A. J. Eady

Introduction

The embryological development of human skin has been accurately documented using the techniques of light microscopy, and transmission and scanning electron microscopy [1–3]. Studies have been performed on samples of presumed normal pregnancies that have been terminated. The estimated gestational age (EGA) is vital to the study of skin throughout pregnancy and is assessed by maternal menstrual dates, ultrasound measurements and direct fetal measurements such as heel–toe and crown–rump lengths. The histological atlas of developing skin is useful, but chronologically an oversimplification as it excludes the important regional variation which is also apparent in immunohistochemical[4,5] and biochemical[6,7] studies of developing skin.

A knowledge of the morphological development of human skin is important for many reasons. It establishes the normal sequence of events in skin development and allows an improved understanding of the normal anatomy and physiology of the skin; a chronological standard enables any developmental abnormality or delay to be identified; most importantly it provides a template to investigate developmental genetics of the skin.

The control mechanisms involved in developing skin are far from clear. All the cells have the same genetic composition and both the nucleus and the cytoplasm are essential for determining cellular differentiation. In other tissues nucleoproteins and hormones have been identified as the mediators of differentiation. At the molecular level both histone and non-histone chromosomal proteins and chalones are implicated in gene control, and the repression and derepression of individual genes govern cellular differentiation. Developing skin is a useful organ to investigate these phenomena, because they are naturally occurring processes throughout gestation.

Until the gene defects in certain genodermatoses are identified, thereby enabling prenatal diagnosis to be made using chorionic villus sampling, fetal skin sampling remains an important method of antenatal diagnosis in a number of skin diseases. A thorough knowledge of normal fetal skin development allows a comparison to be made and in many conditions a knowledge of regional variation is vital.

An understanding of the normal morphological characteristics of developing skin provides an insight into the normal physiological properties of skin and its various and varying functions. The subject is complex, because the skin of the developing human in a fluid environment acts as a protective and possibly nutritive organ, becoming an immunologically competent and protective organ after birth.

This chapter describes the changes seen in the skin in early embryogenesis, through the embryonic–fetal transition to the second and then third trimester. Understanding the normal anatomy and functions during this final trimester enables better clinical care of the preterm infant. The periderm, immigrant cells and the development of skin adnexa are described. Finally, the similarities between fetal skin and fetal membranes, and the potential uses of this genetically identical tissue, are discussed.

Early embryology (up to 30 days)

Skin is derived from two germ layers: the ectoderm, including the neural crest, which gives rise to the epidermal component, and the mesoderm, which is the source of the dermis. By the end of the third week after fertilization, that is at the time of the first missed menstrual period, the embryo consists of a trilaminar embryonic disc (Figure 3.1) and the embryonic ectoderm, mesoderm and endoderm can be individually identified[8]. The embryonic ectoderm and mesoderm are continuous peripherally with the amnion. The ectoderm gives rise to surface ectoderm which in turn comprises epidermis, hair, nails, cutaneous and mammary glands, enamel of teeth (Table 3.1) and the neuroectoderm, which is the source of melanocytes. The paraxial portion of the mesoderm gives rise to the dermis. By 4 weeks EGA, skin consists of two layers: the single-layered epidermis overlying a watery mesenchyme.

Epidermis

The single layer of epidermal cells (less than 10 μm in thickness) consists of loosely integrated keratinocytes, joined apically by desmosomes. Morphologically, both dark and light keratinocytes are recognized[1]. The basal boundary is reinforced by a horizontal layer of fine filaments lying beneath the plasma membrane, and this layer decreases as hemidesmosomes form.

Table 3.1

Surface ectoderm	*Neuroectoderm*
Epidermis, hair, nails	Neural crest: cranial
Cutaneous and mammary	and sensory ganglia
glands	and nerves, medulla of
Anterior pituitary gland	the adrenal gland,
Enamel of teeth	pigment cells
Inner ear	Neural tube: central
Lens of the eye	nervous system, retina,
	pineal body, posterior
	pituitary gland

By 28 days the epidermis is two-layered, consisting of the basal cell layer and the periderm[9]. The basal cells and the periderm cells can be distinguished morphologically by the presence of microvilli on the amniotic surface of the periderm cells[10,11].

Dermoepidermal junction

The basement membrane is flat with a recognizable lamina lucida and lamina densa. By 5 weeks, fine filaments extend from the basal cells across the lamina lucida, and extend from the lamina densa to a proximal network of 25 nm in depth[12].

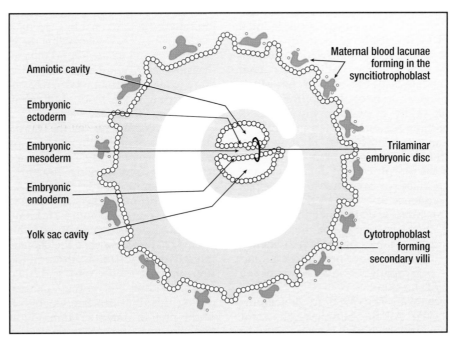

Figure 3.1 *At week 3 of gestation, the conceptus is embedded in the uterine wall, surrounded by cytotrophoblast which is beginning to form the placenta. The embryo consists of a trilaminar disc, and the ectoderm can be seen to be in direct continuation with the future amniotic cavity and reflected amnion*

Dermis

There is no distinction at this stage between the dermis and subcutis. The dermis consists of a network of stellate mesenchymal cells, with poorly developed organelles, which join with one another through junctions on cellular processes. The matrix secreted is a watery gel containing periodic acid–Schiff (PAS) positive material, rich in sugar and sparse in fibrils[13].

The second month (30–60 days): embryonic skin

Epidermis

The epidermis is present as a two-layered epithelium consisting of the basal cell layer covered by the periderm cells (Figure 3.2). Both these cell types contain large amounts of glycogen and are rapidly dividing[14]. They are attached by desmosomes[9]. The basal and periderm cells express keratins of low molecular weight (Table 3.2) – 40 kDa (keratin 19), 52.5 kDa (keratin 8), indicative of a simple epithelium, and 50 kDa (keratin 14), characteristic of basal cells[6]. In addition the periderm cells express a 45 kDa keratin (keratin 18) that is peculiar to normal simple epithelium. These keratin filaments are visible ultrastructurally as a filamentous network in the

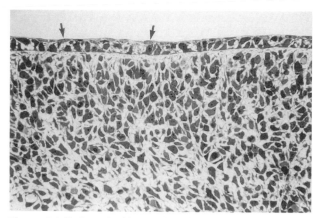

Figure 3.2 *Embryonic skin consists of a two-layered epithelium, the basal cell layer covered by the flatter periderm (arrowed)*

basal cells and bundles of filaments in association with the desmosomes[1]. Filaggrin is not present at this stage. The epidermal lipid content is mostly phospholipids and free sterol, indicating that the plasma membrane is the main contributor[7].

Dermoepidermal junction

Laminin 1[15] and type IV collagen are identifiable immunohistochemically (Table 3.3) at 6 weeks EGA at the basement membrane. There is a regional

Table 3.2 *Keratin expression throughout gestation*

		Keratin composition
Embryonic skin	Periderm	Simple (8, 18, 19)
	Basal cells	Proliferative (16) Basal cell (5, 14)
Stratification	Periderm	Simple Proliferative (16)
	Intermediate cells	Simple (8) Proliferative (1, 6) Cornifying (10)
	Basal cells	Simple (8) Basal Proliferative
Follicular keratinization	Follicles	Cornifying (1, 10) Simple (7, 8)

Cytokeratin 9, which pairs with 1, is site-specific and found in the palms and soles late in development [5]

Table 3.3 *Development of the basement membrane zone*

	Embryonic		Fetal						
	1	2	3	4	5	6	7	8	9
Lamina lucida and densa	×								
Hemidesmosomes			×						
Anchoring fibrils			×						
Antigens									
Laminin 1		×							
Type IV collagen		×							
Type V collagen			×						
Type VII collagen			×						
Bullous pemphigoid Ag*		×							
Laminin 5		×							
19 DEJ-1		×							

*Determined using patient's sera, possibly recognizing both 230 kDa and 180 kDa antigens.

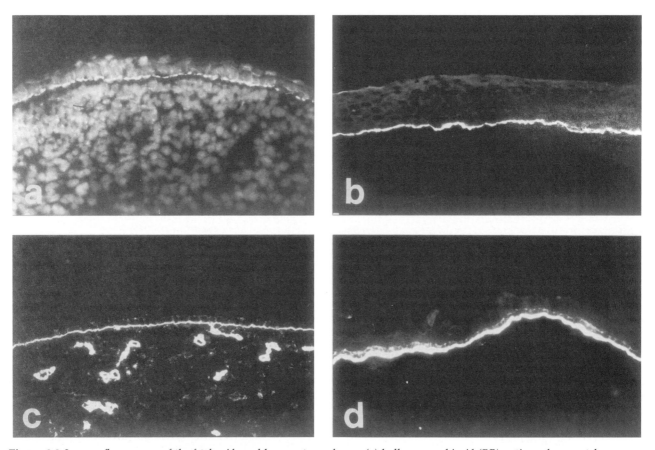

Figure 3.3 *Immunofluorescence of the fetal epidermal basement membrane: (a) bullous pemphigoid (BP) antigen shows patchy staining at 8 weeks estimated gestational age (EGA) (counterstained with propidium iodide); (b) BP antigen shows bright staining by 15 weeks EGA; (c) type IV collagen at 11 weeks EGA; and (d) type VII collagen at 13 weeks EGA. The staining within the basal cells represents the epidermal contribution of type VII collagen seen at this early gestational age*

differential expression of bullous pemphigoid antigen, being present in the palms and soles at 9 weeks EGA but not on the trunk until later in gestation (Figure 3.3) [4, 16, 17].

Dermis

The dermis is twice as thick as the epidermis and continues to be cellular[13]. It shows a regional variation and is cellular and dense over bony areas, but on the trunk it is more loosely organized with widely separated cells. The dermal matrix is rich in hyaluronic acid and contains collagen types I, III, IV and V, i.e. an increased amount of collagen in the extracellular matrix; collagenase is also present[18].

Computer reconstructions with light and electron microscopy have identified endothelial cells as early as 45 days EGA, and by 40–45 days vessels are seen to lie in a single plane parallel to the epidermis and the dermal/subcutis interface[19]. Nerve growth patterns precede angiogenesis.

At this early stage the skin is thicker on distal extremities, particularly overlying bone. There is no appendageal formation, but volar pads (mounds of mesenchyme) are beginning to form.

The third month: embryonic–fetal transition

The third month of the first trimester represents an important transition point in the development of the human fetus. The skin undergoes a series of changes which render it compositionally very similar to adult skin although it remains morphologically different.

Epidermis

At 60–65 days EGA the basal cells start to proliferate and form an intermediate cell layer (Figure 3.4). The intermediate cells are like adult cells in their keratin composition, possessing differentiation-specific keratins of high molecular weight, types 1 (67 kDa) and 10 (56.5 kDa), long before cornification is apparent histologically[20]. The basal and periderm cells continue to express simple keratins (Figure 3.5). Cell surface changes occur with this onset of stratification: desmosomes are present in increasing numbers, and the pemphigus antigen is first expressed[4,17].

Glycolipid and glycoprotein blood groups are identified. The cell surface carbohydrates, including *n*-acetyl lactosamine, are the same as in the embryo[21]. The basal cells now contain less glycogen than the intermediate or periderm cells and their dividing capacity is the same as in the adult. The

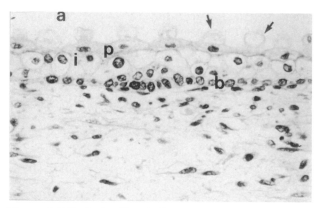

Figure 3.4 *The fetal epidermis during month 3 develops an intermediate cell layer (i). The periderm cells (p) are now supporting large blebs (arrowed) protruding into the amniotic cavity (a); (b) is the basal cell layer*

epidermal thickness increases from less than 10 μm to 66 μm[22].

Dermoepidermal junction

At the basal surface of the basal cells, bullous pemphigoid antigen, laminin 5, and 19 DEJ-1 are expressed and hemidesmosomes increase in number[23]; punctate type VII collagen expression is seen as anchoring fibrils begin to be formed (Figure 3.6)[12,24]. The dermoepidermal junction is irregular.

Dermis

During this embryonic–fetal transition period, the dermis changes from a relatively cellular structure to a more fibrous matrix[13]. This change is accompanied by an alteration in the cells from an undifferentiated mesenchymal phenotype to a more fibroblastic one,

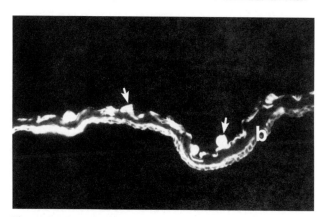

Figure 3.5 *Immunofluorescence micrograph showing expression of keratin 19 at 13 weeks' gestation in the basal cells (b) and periderm cells (arrowed) only*

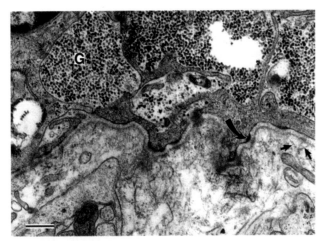

Figure 3.6 *Electron micrograph of the fetal epidermal basement membrane at 18 weeks EGA. The basal cells are full of glycogen (G). Both hemidesmosomes (curved arrow) and anchoring fibrils (straight arrows) are present (scale bar 0.5 μm)*

although no new gene products are produced at this stage. Cell orientation conforms to different patterns. Firstly, some cells are concentrated along the basement membrane in association with the collagen fibrils. In the deeper portion of the dermis, now identifiable as the reticular dermis, the fibroblasts are elongated and oriented horizontally. Microfibrils of the elastic fibre system are present. The thickness of the dermis remains constant but there is an increase in fibrous collagen accumulation. Types I (70%), III (20%) and V collagens are present[18]. Type III collagen has an important role in establishing dermal architecture, and both types III and V outline the vessels[18,25]. At this stage a deep reticular vascular plexus is present; smaller vessels are found throughout the dermis up to the epidermal basement membrane accompanied by unmyelinated nerve fibres[26]. Nerves consist of fibre bundles rather than individual fibres, surrounded by a Schwann cell process.

Periderm

The periderm is a specialized epithelium that is peculiar to fetal skin[11]. It is present at 4 weeks EGA as the most superficial layer of the epidermis in direct contact with the amniotic cavity, and invests the fetus until the end of the second trimester. Its cycle of development has been divided into stages (Figure 3.7)[11]. Its origin is unknown, but it is thought to arise either from the basal cells[27] or as an extension of amnion[28] over the embryo. The similarities between periderm and amnion are evidenced by common antigen expression on the cell surface as recognized by Peri-1[28] and GB1[29] (Figure 3.8). In addition these two tissues express

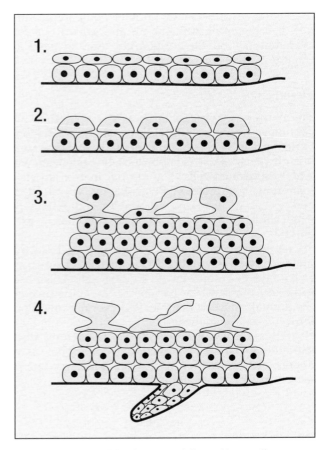

Figure 3.7 *Stages of development of the periderm cells: (1) 35–55 days: the periderm cells are flat and simple, overlying the basal epidermal cells; (2) 55–75 days: the periderm cells become more dome-shaped; (3) 65–120 days: the cells develop blebs which become increasingly complex, extending into the amniotic cavity; (4) 110–160 days: with the onset of interfollicular cornification the periderm cells are shed into the amniotic cavity. Modified from Holbrook KA, and Odland GF. The fine structure of developing human epidermis* J Invest Dermatol 1975; 65: 16–38.

similar keratins. The periderm cell progresses from a flattened squamous cell (Figure 3.7) to a simple bleb-forming cell which increases in complexity with microvilli formation, intracellular vesicles and cellular indentations. Finally, the capacity of the periderm cell to divide diminishes, its glycogen content falls and the periderm regresses at the time of interfollicular keratinization of the epidermis, i.e. at the end of the second trimester. The cells are then shed into the amniotic fluid which at that time changes from a serum dialysate to a solution containing the products of fetal renal excretion[30].

The function of this epithelium is not clear. Its changing ultrastructural characteristics and data in vitro suggest that it may have a secretory or absorptive role, and it acts as a protective layer for the fetus.

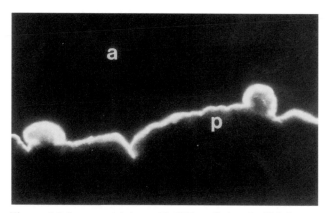

Figure 3.8 *Immunostaining with GB1 outlining the bleb formation of the periderm cell; a, amniotic cavity; p, periderm cell*

Melanocytes, Langerhans and Merkel cells

During the second month of gestation, immigrant cells are identifiable. Langerhans cells[31] are recognized by positive ATPase and HLA-DR reactivity by 45 days, but are still CD1 negative. By about 90 days EGA, HLA-DR+ and CD1+ cells are present in a constant ratio. It is not clear if this is due to an influx of HLA-DR+/CD1+ cells coincident with the onset of a functional fetal bone marrow, or to phenotypic changes within the epidermal cells involving de novo synthesis of the epitopes reacting with the OKT6+ antibody. A regional difference is seen, as Langerhans' cells are numerous in the palms and soles until 12 weeks EGA and then decline in numbers. Elsewhere on the body there is a gradual increase in the number of Langerhans' cells after 16 weeks' gestation[32]. Melanocytes migrate from the neural crest to the skin crossing the basement membrane. Fibronectin may be important in this process via integrin receptors[33].

By month 2, melanocytes can be identified by immunohistochemical means between the basal and periderm cells, with dendritic processes extending to the basement membrane. They express a melanoma-associated antigen, HMB45[34,35]. Histologically, melanocytes have smaller, more darkly stained nuclei than keratinocytes[36]. Ultrastructurally, by month 3, melanocytes have premelanosomes in the cytoplasm and show some degree of melanization[37]. At this stage melanocytes are present in relatively high numbers (mean value 1050 cells per mm^2) They increase in density to 2300 per mm^2 during the early second trimester and then decline to a density of 800 per mm^2, which is in the range for a newborn.

Transplantation models of fetal skin grafted onto nude mice suggest that Merkel cells arise in situ from the epidermal cells. By the third month of gestation, Merkel cells can be ultrastructurally identified on the palms and soles[38]. At 15 weeks EGA, Merkel cells have been identified in the dermis expressing nerve growth factor receptors; at the same time cutaneous nerves start to form the subepidermal nerve plexus

and it is hypothesized that Merkel cells have an inductive influence on these nerves[39]. Merkel cells have been demonstrated in association with sweat glands and bulbous hair pegs[40].

The second trimester (12–24 weeks)

Epidermis

During the second trimester there is increased stratification of the epidermis (Figure 3.9), the development of epidermal appendages and the onset of cornification. Keratinization (terminal differentiation) starts in the hair follicles and proceeds in a cephalocaudal direction[41]. There is an increased coordinated expression of keratins 1 (67 kDa) and 10 (56.5 kDa) which are markers of keratinizing epithelia. There is a regional difference in the expression of lipids[7]. In the epidermis, an increase in the content of sterol, wax ester and triglyceride occurs in the more cephalad specimens, but in the legs the profile is more

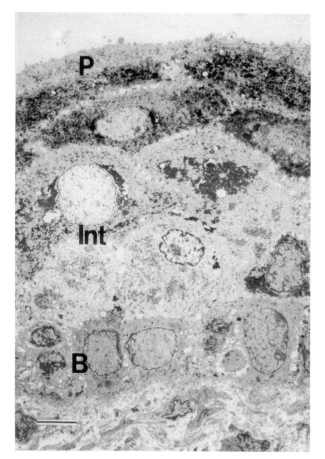

Figure 3.9 *Electron micrograph of fetal skin at 18 weeks' gestation showing stratification into several layers including basal (B) and intermediate (Int). The periderm (P) is still present (scale bar 1 μm)*

like earlier fetal skin. This expression correlates with the appearance of lipid in the sebaceous glands and with follicular keratinization. Sterol esters are thought to represent a marker of fetal cornification. Carbohydrate changes occur, possibly playing a role in cell recognition, cell differentiation and morphogenesis[21].

Dermoepidermal junction

Hemidesmosomes and anchoring fibrils are well developed. Bullous pemphigoid antigen is present in all sites by 17 weeks EGA and its expression is fully linear by 23 weeks EGA. The basement membrane surrounds the developing adnexae (Figure 3.10).

Dermis

The dermis is a fibrous matrix that is five times as thick as the epidermis. The papillary region contains finer collagen fibrils and a higher density of cells compared with the reticular region. Immunohistochemical techniques show that the distribution of types I and III collagen remains constant throughout the dermis. The amount of type III collagen in the fetal dermis at this stage is about 30–60% of total skin collagen, whereas in the adult it is only 10–20%. At 15–18 weeks EGA the ratio of $\alpha1(I)$ to $\alpha1(III)$ collagen mRNA is 0.8[25], which correlates well with the protein levels, suggesting that the control is mainly at the transcriptional level and degradation does not play a large part. Type II collagen has been detected in fetal scalp skin at 17–23 weeks EGA[42]. Type V collagen is present within the epidermis, in the basal cells, periderm and diffusely in the suprabasal layers[18]. Together with type III collagen it surrounds the dermal blood vessels. Light and electron microscopy demonstrate a continuing maturation of the vascular system in the dermis. At 100 days, Weibel–Palade bodies (ultrastructural markers of the endothe-

lial cell) which contain factor VIII-related antigen are seen[26]. The venular basement membrane is multilaminated, but not as complex as in the adult. Elastic fibres are now formed, appearing first in the reticular dermis and 3–4 weeks later in the papillary dermis. Between 13 weeks and 19 weeks EGA the production of elastin by fibroblasts increases by 7–14 times, reaching neonatal levels. Messenger RNA levels are similarly increased 6–15 times by 19 weeks[43].

During this trimester, after 100 days, adipocytes are present in the subcutaneous tissues.

The third trimester (from 24 weeks)

The third trimester constitutes a period of growth and reorganization[3].

Epidermis

From 24 weeks to 40 weeks EGA the epidermis becomes more stratified. The stratum corneum is only a few cell layers thick at the beginning of the third trimester, but by the time of birth it has thickened considerably. Appendages are by now fully developed (see below).

Dermoepidermal junction

The dermoepidermal junction becomes more irregular and continues to mature with an increasing number of hemidesmosomes and anchoring fibrils.

Dermis

The dermis remains thin but contains all the components of the adult dermis. Its expansion continues after birth (see below). Blood vessels are now in an adult pattern[44].

In view of the difficult ethical and technical problems involved in examining skin during this period of development, far fewer chronological data are available. Premature skin has been studied and the dermis in particular is found to increase its bulk and maturation after birth. An examination of preterm infants from 24 weeks gestation reveals that the maturity of the skin accelerates outside the womb, and within 2 weeks post partum – regardless of the gestational age at birth – the skin is histologically similar to that of a normal term infant[45]. This finding holds important implications for clinical management[46]. Thus, the initial fragile skin with poor temperature control, increased fluid loss and high absorbing capacity of the preterm infant will resolve over the first 2 weeks of life. The increased transcutaneous permeability may have therapeutic potential for fluid delivery; however, drug absorption is potentially toxic.

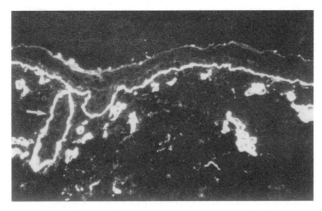

Figure 3.10 *Immunofluorescence micrograph showing laminin at 14 weeks EGA at the dermoepidermal junction extending around developing hair follicles and blood vessels (arrowed)*

Table 3.4 *Ontogeny of skin appendages*

					Months of gestation				
	Embryonic					*Fetal*			
	1	2	3	4	5	6	7	8	9
Hair									
germ			×						
peg				×					
Exposed hair					×				
Nail					×				
Sebaceous gland					×				
Apocrine gland						×			
Eccrine gland						×			

Epidermal appendages

The development of the epidermal appendages is summarized in Table 3.4.

Hair follicles

Month 3 (pregerm)

The development of hair follicles[47] starts at about 75–80 days' gestation with the development of primary follicles on the face and scalp. Focal aggregations of basal cells (pregerms) are matched by aggregated mesenchymal cells within the adjacent dermis which give rise to the dermal papilla. Initially melanocytes are present in the same proportions as in the epidermis. Intermediate cells crowd together above the follicle primordium (Figure 3.11). At the end of the third month, hair follicles project at an angle into the upper and mid-depth regions of the dermis but show no further differentiation.

Month 4

Hair follicle development continues in a cephalocaudal direction during month 4. There are regional differences depending on the underlying tissues. Follicles are growing obliquely, thus determining a caudal direction for the erupted hair. Two or three cell layers of mesenchymal cells surround the hair peg and secrete the connective tissue that becomes the fibrous root sheath.

Month 5 (bulbar hair peg)

Collections of cell 'bulges' appear from the posterior surface of the follicle along its length (Figure 3.12). The

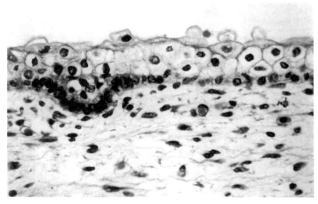

Figure 3.11 *Hair follicle development: during the third month of gestation, the pregerms develop with a focal aggregation of intermediate and basal cells as the first indication of hair follicle development*

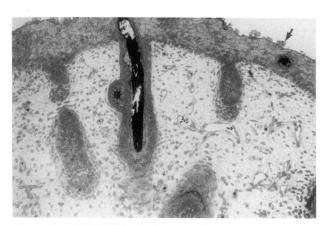

Figure 3.12 *Hair follicle development: during the second trimester the hair follicle develops 'bulges' (starred) which give rise to the apocrine glands, sebaceous glands and arrector pili muscles. Periderm is still present (arrowed)*

most inferior 'bulge' usually forms the attachment for the arrector pili muscle. The middle 'bulge' gives rise to the sebaceous gland (see later), and the most superficial 'bulge', in certain areas, forms the apocrine gland. As these appendages are forming, an intra-epidermal pathway for the passage of hair is organized.

Follicular keratinization is starting at this stage. The hair cone is the projection from the matrix that differentiates into five dissimilar products that form the hair and inner root sheath.

Month 6

Melanocytes concentrate in the peripheral layer of the outer root sheath of the infundibulum, lower bulb and pigment matrix. Development of hair follows excavation of the hair canal. Squamous cells of the inner root sheath cuticle form within the layers of Huxley and Henle as the cuticle and cortex of a fetal (lanugo) hair keratinize. Lanugo hairs lack a medulla. Fully formed hairs lie within the epidermal canal until they are released by erosion of the roof of the canal[48]. Hairs are released on the eyebrows and forehead at 16 weeks EGA and by 18 weeks on the scalp.

Sebaceous glands

With the onset of the 'bulge' formation during the fifth month, the differentiation of the primordial cells into sebum-producing cells proceeds rapidly. There are three main layers to the gland: in the centre are cells with large cytoplasmic vacuoles containing lipid[49]; surrounding these cells is a layer of cells containing glycogen, admixed with melanocytes and Langerhans' cells; and the most superficial cell layer of the gland consists of immature, glycogen-rich cells. The duct of the sebaceous gland is formed at the site of origin from the follicle, by degeneration of the central cells and keratinization of the surrounding cells[1].

Eccrine sweat glands

During the third month of gestation, undulations of the basal cell layer of the epidermis of the palms and soles give rise to the sweat gland primordia[50,51]. Cords of outer columnar (basal) and inner rounded (intermediate) cells develop and extend into the dermis. At 16 weeks EGA, the secretory coil forms and by 22 weeks both secretory and myoepithelial cells can be recognized. The duct and secretory coil become patent by separation of the cells, and the intra-epidermal portion becomes patent by fusion of intracellular vesicles. This process occurs on the rest of the body during month 5.

Apocrine glands

At 6 months EGA the most superficial bulge on the hair follicle gives rise to the apocrine gland[52]. Like eccrine glands, these glands have two-layered secretory and ductal portions, but they extend deep into the subcutaneous fat. The lumen is formed by the same process as in the eccrine gland. It is thought that apocrine glands develop all over the body but regress in all areas except the areolae, axillae, scalp, eyelids, external auditory meati, umbilicus and anogenital areas[52].

Nails

Between 8 weeks and 10 weeks EGA, the nail primordia form[53]. The primary nail field, a smooth, shiny, rectangular surface delineated by continuous shallow grooves, is present at 10 weeks. The nail bed lies underneath the primary nail field. The nail fold consists of both dorsal and ventral epithelial cell layers and gives rise to the nail itself. The dorsal nail plate starts keratinizing at 11 weeks EGA. By 14 weeks both the nail bed and the dorsal and ventral matrix primordia are contributing to nail formation. The nail is covered by periderm which eventually degenerates. By month 5, nail formation is complete; the nail consists of two layers. By 32 weeks, the nail reaches the tip of the finger, and by 36 weeks the tip of the toe. At term, three distinct layers to the nail plate are seen: the superficial layer arising from the dorsal nail fold; the middle layer from the ventral nail fold; and finally the ventral portion from the distal two-thirds of the nail bed.

Controlling factors in developing skin and cutaneous appendages

The control of fetal skin and appendage formation is complex and, although much investigated, is largely unknown. There are two levels of organization in fetal skin development that require control: the development of single specialized structures, and their specific pattern arrangements. The main control mechanisms which may have important actions on the gene expression of the individual cells have been studied:

1. Epithelial–mesenchymal interactions.
2. Extracellular matrix proteins.
3. Growth factors.
4. Homeobox genes.

Epithelial–mesenchymal interactions

It is now well recognized that both epidermis and dermis play interacting roles in development control[54]. This has been studied mainly in chick embryos by recombination experiments. The embryonic dermis is essential to maintain a proliferative epidermis which is region-specific. In appendage formation, reptilian scales, avian feathers and mammalian hair have been studied. The morphology and pattern of mammalian hair formation require controlling influences from both epidermis and dermis which are correct for both site and age. For example, an interplay of controlling factors allows the dermis to determine a site-specific expression of keratins, once primed by the epidermis. It has been suggested that *HOX* genes, while being expressed in murine skin in a similar fashion to keratin genes, may be in part responsible for these inductive dermal signals[55].

Extracellular matrix proteins

The substances (known as morphogens) that exert the controlling mechanisms seen in the epidermal–dermal interactions are not well understood, but appear numerous. Collagen fibrils in different arrays have been implicated as a morphogenetic message. Laminin has been implicated in epidermal and neuronal guidance; while fibronectin, although diffusely distributed, is implicated in the migration of the neural crest cells. Tenascin, an extracellular matrix glycoprotein, has been proposed as the modulator of appendage formation and neural crest migration[56,57] and is considered to be a marker for epithelial–mesenchymal interactions[58]. In gut and teeth, the epithelium is thought to produce a soluble factor that induces tenascin production by the underlying mesenchyme. This in turn allows mesenchymal condensation. Integrins may play a role in tissue organization during skin embryogenesis[59]. Embryonic and fetal keratinocytes express the adhesion molecule E-cadherin, but only the embryonic epidermal keratinocytes express the neural crest adhesion molecule, N-CAM. The P-cadherin molecule has been implicated in eccrine gland development[60]. More recently, a mesenchymal protein, epimorphin, has been found to be important in hair follicle formation[61]. However, the exact role of tenascin is unclear[62].

Growth factors

Many peptides have now been identified with stimulatory effects on epithelial and mesenchymal cells. These humoral regulators include peptide hormones such as chalones, and growth factors such as epidermal and fibroblast growth factors. Chalones have been shown to maintain controlled proliferation and stratification of basal epidermal cells. Epidermal growth factor receptor (EGF-R), which is also recognized by transforming growth factor alpha, has been systematically examined during development[63], and in the first trimester is found on the basal cells of the epidermis. During stratification, it appeared to be membrane-bound on the basal and intermediate cells,

as well as involving (to a lesser extent) some of the dermal mesenchymal cells. At the site of hair follicle formation, EGF-R appears to be lacking in the basal cells, but by the stage of the bulbous hair peg, it has expressed in the cells of the outer root sheath, the matrix region of the hair bulb and the sebaceous gland. Epidermal growth factor is known to delay the development of the first coat of hair follicles in mice and can cause abnormal growth patterns of wool in sheep. In adult skin, EGF-R is only found in the basal and spinous cell layers of the epidermis. The more extensive expression in fetal skin suggests its importance in human skin development, and in particular, the first indication of a difference in the basal cells destined to become appendages.

Homeobox genes

One of the main controlling factors that determine the complex three-dimensional network of the skin seems likely to be the homeobox genes[64]. Homeobox genes have been intensively studied in the fruit fly, *Drosophila melanogaster*, and have been described in diverse species, from nematodes to mammals. One of the major groups of homeobox genes are *HOX* genes. In vertebrates there are 38 *HOX* genes organized into four clusters on separate chromosomes. They all contain a 180 homeodomain, and are expressed in spatial and temporal patterns during murine embryogenesis[65]. From the fruit fly studies it seems likely that they encode transcription factors which control effector genes for the organization of three-dimensional structure.

In human fetal skin, *HOX* genes have been found as early as 6 weeks EGA. Cultured human fetal melanocytes express several members of *HOX* A and C families. In the developing chick, homeobox genes *MsX-1* and *MsX-2* are specifically associated with developing skin appendages[66].

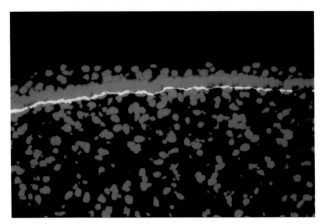

Figure 3.13 *Type VII collagen at the basement membrane of cord amnion at 19 weeks EGA, counterstained with propidium iodide*

Amnion and fetal skin: similarities and potential uses

Amnion develops in close proximity to fetal skin and has an identical genotype. It is antigenically similar to fetal skin especially at the basement membrane zone, but displays a more pluripotential phenotype within the epithelium and mesenchyme. Amnion is abundantly available and is a valuable tissue for the examination of individual antigens, fetal membrane function and possibly the control mechanisms regulating gene expression. Morphologically there are three main types of amnion[10]: cord amnion with a stratified squamous epithelium, reflected amnion with a simple cuboidal epithelium and placental amnion with a columnar epithelium. The underlying fetal mesenchyme is composed of a reticular layer and a cellular layer.

The similarities between amnion and skin have been demonstrated principally by immunohistochemical techniques using reflected amnion. Antigen expression is almost invariably synchronous, for example at the basement membrane zone where antigens such as laminin 1, types IV and VII collagen (Figure 3.13) and laminin 5 are present in both tissues in the first trimester. In addition, identical characteristic abnormalities are found at the basement membrane zone in the inherited condition of epidermolysis bullosa[67]. This is further supported by similar ultrastructural changes in both tissues in this condition, which has led to the suggestion that amnion could potentially be sampled in place of fetal skin in prenatal diagnosis[68].

Pemphigus and bullous pemphigoid antigens are also expressed in amniotic epithelium and basement membrane respectively[69].

The fetal mesenchymal cells and amniotic epithelium both express keratins and vimentin[70], suggesting a multipotential state. This fetal membrane might therefore be useful for examining the profound inductive influences that the mesenchyme appears to exert over epithelial differentiation.

Conclusion

The complexity of developing skin is just beginning to be revealed. Systematic morphological examination shows well-ordered developmental stages in all the layers of the skin from the early embryo to the infant. The regional variation of specialized areas such as the scalp, face, eyelids and plantar and palmar surfaces can now be individually studied in vivo following the successful transplantation of fetal skin to a nude mouse[71] and fetal skin culture in vitro[58]. The finding of both antigenic and biochemical 'markers of differentiation' in the first trimester fetus suggests, however, that skin does not develop in a progressively more complex fashion but is highly mature very early in gestation. Molecular biology is providing a means to an even greater understanding of development, and further studies are needed to address gene control including the inductive signals and regional differences among skin cell populations.

References

1 Breathnach A. *An Atlas of the Ultrastructure of Human Skin*. Churchill, London, 1971.
2 Hashimoto K, Gross B, DiBella AR, Lever W. The ultrastructure of the skin of human embryo. *J Invest Dermatol* 1966; **47**: 317–35.
3 Holbrook KA, Hoff MS. Structure of the developing human and embryonic and fetal skin. *Sem Dermatol* 1981; **3**: 185–202.
4 Lane AT, Helm KF, Goldsmith LW, Identification of bullous pemphigoid, pemphigus, laminin, and anchoring fibril antigens in human fetal skin. *J Invest Dermatol* 1985; **84**: 27–30.
5 Moll I, Heid H, Franke W, Moll R. Distribution of a special subset of keratinocytes characterized by the expression of cytokeratin 9 in adult and fetal human epidermis of various body sites. *Differentiation* 1987; **33**: 254–65.
6 Dale B, Holbrook KA, Kimball JR, Hoff M, Sun T-T. Expression of epidermal keratins and filaggrin during human fetal skin development. *J Cell Biol* 1985; **101**: 1257–69.
7 Williams ML, Hincenbergs M, Holbrook KA, Skin lipid content during early fetal development *J Invest Dermatol* 1988; **91**: 263–8.
8 Moore KL. *The Developing Human*. 2nd ed. WB Saunders, Philadelphia, 1977.
9 Breathnach AS, Robins J. Ultrastructural features of epidermis of a 14 mm (6 weeks) human embryo. *Br J Dermatol* 1969; **81**: 504–16.
10 Bourne G. *The Human Amnion and Chorion*. Lloyd-Luke, London, 1962.
11 Holbrook KA, Odland GF. The fine structure of developing human epidermis: light, scanning and transmission electron microscopy of the periderm. *J Invest Dermatol* 1975; **65**: 16–38.
12 Smith LT, Sakai LY, Burgeson RE, Holbrook KA. Ontogeny of structural components at the dermal-epidermal junction in human embryonic and fetal skin: the appearance of anchoring fibrils and type VII collagen. *J Invest Dermatol* 1988; **90**: 480–5.
13 Smith LT, Holbrook KA. Embryogenesis of the dermis in human skin. *Pediatr Dermatol* 1986; **3**: 271–80.
14 Bickenbach JR, Holbrook KA. Label-retaining cells in human embryonic and fetal epidermis. *J Invest Dermatol* 1987; **88**: 42–6.
15 Burgeson RE, Chiquet M, Deutzmann R et al. A new nomenclature for the laminins. *Matrix Biol* 1994; **14**: 209–11.
16 Fine J-D, Smith LT, Holbrook KA, Katz SI. The appearance of four basement membrane zone antigens in developing human fetal skin. *J Invest Dermatol* 1984; **83**: 66–9.

17 Muller HK, Kalnins R, Sutherland RC. Ontogeny of pemphigus and bullous pemphigoid antigens in human skin. *Br J Dermatol* 1973; **88**: 443–6.

18 Smith LT, Holbrook KA, Madri JA. Collagen types I, III and V in human embryonic and fetal skin. *Am J Anat* 1986; **175**: 507–21.

19 Johnson CL, Holbrook KA. Development of human embryonic and fetal dermal vasculature. *J Invest Dermatol* 1989; **93** (suppl.): 10–17.

20 Holbrook KA, Dale BA, Smith LT et al. Markers of adult skin expressed in the skin of the first trimester fetus. *Curr Probl Derm* 1987; **16**: 94–108.

21 Dabelsteen E, Holbrook K, Clausen H, Hakomori S. Cell surface carbohydrate changes during embryonic and fetal skin development. *J Invest Dermatol* 1986; **87**: 81–5.

22 Foster CA, Bertram JF, Holbrook KA. Morphometric and statistical analyses describing the in utero growth of human epidermis. *Anat Rec* 1988; **222**: 201–6.

23 Riddle CV. Development of hemidesmosomes: an intra-membranous view. *Anat Embryol* 1986; **174**: 153–60.

24 Paller A, Queen L, Woodley DT et al. Organ specific, phylogenetic and ontogenetic distribution of the epi-dermolysis bullosa acquisita antigen. *J Invest Dermatol* 1986; **86**: 376–9.

25 Sandberg M, Makela JK, Multimaki P, Vourio T, Vuorio E. Construction of a human proα1(III) collagen cDNA clone and localisation of type III collagen expression in human fetal tissues. *Matrix* 1989; **9**: 82–91.

26 Tonnesen MG, Jenkins D, Siegal SL et al. Expression of fibronectin, laminin and factor VIII related antigen during development of the human cutaneous micro-vasculature. *J Invest Dermatol* 1985; **85**: 564–8.

27 Holbrook KA. Human epidermal embryogenesis. *Int J Dermatol* 1979; **18**: 329–56.

28 Lane AT, Negi M, Goldsmith LA. Human periderm: a monoclonal antibody marker. *Curr Probl Dermatol* 1987; **16**: 83–93.

29 Schofield OMV, McDonald JN, Fredj-Reygrobellet D et al. Common antigen expression between human periderm and other tissues identified by GB1-monoclonal anti-body. *Arch Dermatol Res* 1990; **282**: 143–8.

30 Lind TG, Parkin FM, Cheyne C. Biochemical and cytological changes in fluid amnii with advancing gestation. *J Obstet Gynaecol Br Commonw* 1968; **76**: 693.

31 Foster CA, Holbrook KA, Farr A. Ontogeny of Langer-hans cells in human embryonic and fetal skin: expression of HLA-DR and OKT6 determinants. *J Invest Dermatol* 1986; **86**: 240–3.

32 Fujita M, Furukawa F, Horiguchi Y et al. Regional development of Langerhans cells and formation of Birbeck granules in human embryonic and fetal skin. *J Invest Dermatol* 1991; **97**: 65–72.

33 Scott G, Ryan DH, McCarthy JB. Molecular mechanisms of human melanocyte attachment to fibronectin. *J Invest Dermatol* 1992; **99**: 787–94.

34 Smoller BR, McNutt NS, Hsu A. HMB-45 recognises stimulated melanocytes. *J Cutan Pathol* 1989; **16**: 49–53.

35 Holbrook KA, Underwood RA, Vogel AM, Gown AM, Kimball JR. The appearance, density and distribution of melanocytes in human embryonic and fetal skin revealed by the antimelanoma antigen, HMB 45. *Anat Embryol* 1989; **180**: 443–5.

36 Mishima Y, Widlan S. Embryonic development of mela-nocytes in human hair and epidermis. *J Invest Dermatol* 1966; **46**: 263–77.

37 Breathnach AS, Wyllie L. Electron microscopy of melano-cytes and Langerhans cells in human fetal epidermis at fourteen weeks. *J Invest Dermatol* 1964; **42**: 389–94.

38 Moll I, Lane AT, Franke W, Moll R. Intraepidermal formation of Merkel cells in xenografts of human fetal skin. *J Invest Dermatol* 1990; **94**: 359–64.

39 Narisawa Y, Hashimoto K, Nihei Y, Pietruk T. Biological significance of dermal Merkel cells in the development of nerves in human fetal skin. *J Histochem Cytochem* 1992; **40** (1): 65–71.

40 Kim D-K, Holbrook KA. The appearance, density and distribution of Merkel cells in human embryonic and fetal skin: their relation to sweat gland and hair follicle development. *J Invest Dermatol* 1995; **104**: 411–16.

41 Holbrook KA, Odland GF. Regional development of the human epidermis in the first trimester embryo and the second trimester fetus (age related to the timing of amniocentesis and fetal biopsy). *J Invest Dermatol* 1980; **80**: 161–8.

42 Azumo N, Izumi T, Tajima S et al. Expression of Type II collagen at the middle stages of chick embryonic and human fetal skin development. *J Invest Dermatol* 1994; **102**: 958–62.

43 Sephel GC, Buckley A, Davidson JM. Developmental initiation of elastin gene expression by human fetal skin fibroblasts. *J Invest Dermatol* 1987; **88**: 732–5.

44 Ryan TJ. Structure, pattern and shape of blood vessels of the skin. In: Jarrett N, ed. *The Physiology and Pathophysiol-ogy of the Skin.* Academic Press, New York, 1973; 577–651.

45 Evans NJ, Rutter N. Development of the epidermis in the newborn. *Biol Neonate* 1986; **49**: 73–80.

46 Lane AT. Development and care of the premature infant's skin. *Pediatr Dermatol* 1987; **4**: 1–5.

47 Pinkus H. Embryology of hair. In: Montagna W, Ellis RA, eds. *Hair Growth.* Academic Press, New York, 1958; 1–32.

48 Holbrook KA, Odland GF. Structure of the human fetal hair canal and initial hair eruption. *J Invest Dermatol* 1978; **71**: 385–90.

49 Fujita H, Asagami C, Murota S, Murozumi S. Ultra-structural study of embryonic sebaceous cells, especially of their droplet formation. *Acta Derm Venereol* 1972; **52**: 99–155.

50 Hashimoto K, Bernard G, Gross MD, Lever WF. Ultra-structure of the skin of human embryos. I: The intra-epidermal eccrine sweat duct. *J Invest Dermatol* 1966; **45**: 139–151.

51 Hashimoto K, Bernard G, Gross MD, Lever WF. Ultra-structure of the skin of human embryos. II: The forma-tion of the intradermal portion of the eccrine sweat gland and of the secretory segment during the first half of embryonic life. *J Invest Dermatol* 1966; **46**: 513–29.

52 Serri F, Montagna W, Mescon H. Studies of the skin of the fetus and the child II. *J Invest Dermatol* 1962; **39**: 199–217.

53 Zaias N. Embryology of the human nail. *Arch Dermatol* 1963; **87**: 37–53.

54 Sengel P. Epidermal-dermal interactions during forma-tion of skin and cutaneous appendages. In: Lowell A, ed. *Biochemistry and Physiology of the Skin,* vol. 1. Oxford University Press, 1983; 102–131.

55 Byrne C, Tainsky M, Fuchs E. Programming gene expression in developing epidermis. *Development* 1994; **120**: 2369–83.

56 Chiquet-Ehrismann R, Mackie E, Pearson C, Sakakura T. Tenascin: an extracellular matrix protein involved in tissue interactions during fetal development and oncogenesis. *Cell* 1986; **47**: 131–9.

57 Mackie E, Tucker RP, Halfter W, Chiquet-Ehrismann R, Epperlain HH. The distribution of tenascin coincides with pathways of neural crest cell migration. *Development* 1988; **102**: 237–50.

58 Holbrook KA, Smith LT, Kaplan ED et al. Expression of morphogens during human follicle development in vivo and a model for studying follicle morphogenesis in vitro. *J Invest Dermatol* 1993; **101**: 39–49S.

59 Hertle MD, Adams JC, Watt FM, Integrin expression during human epidermal development in vivo and in vitro. *Development* 1991; **112**: 193–206.

60 Fujita M, Furukawa F, Fujii K et al. Expression of cadherin cell adhesion molecules during human skin development: morphogenesis on epidermis, hair follicles and eccrine sweat ducts. *Arch Dermatol Res* 1992; **284**: 159–66.

61 Hirai Y, Takebe K, Takashina M, Kobyashi S, Takeishi M. Epimorphin, a mesenchymal protein essential for epithelial morphogenesis. *Cell* 1992; **69**: 471–81.

62 Lightner VA. Tenascin; does it play a role in epidermal morphogenesis and homeostasis? *J Invest Dermatol* 1994; **102**: 273–7.

63 Nanney LB, Stoscheck CM, King LE, Underwood RA, Holbrook KA. Immunolocalisation of epidermal growth factor receptors in normal developing human skin. *J Invest Dermatol* 1990; **94**: 742–8.

64 Scott GA, Goldsmith LA. Homeobox genes and skin development: a review. *J Invest Dermatol* 1993; **101**: 3–8.

65 Mathews CHE, Datmer K, Lawrence HJ, Largman C. Expression of the HOX 2.2 homeobox gene in murine embryonic epidermis. *Differentiation* 1993; **52**: 177–84.

66 Noveen A, Jiang T-X, Ting-Berreth SA, Chuong C-M. Homeobox genes MsX-1 and MsX-2 are associated with induction and growth of skin appendages. *J Invest Dermatol* 1995; **104**: 711–19.

67 Eady RAJ, Heagerty AHM, Kennedy AR et al. Lethal junctional epidermolysis bullosa: a disorder of hemidesmosome formation, but not bullous pemphigoid antigen. *J Invest Dermatol* 1986; **87**: 144 (abstract).

68 Hausser I, Anton-Lamprecht I. Prenatal diagnosis of genodermatoses by ultrastructural diagnostic markers in extraembryonic tissues: defective hemidesmosomes in amnion epithelium of fetuses affected with epidermolysis bullosa Herlitz type. *Hum Genet* 1990; **85**: 367–75.

69 Robinson HN, Anhalt GJ, Patel HP et al. Pemphigus and pemphigoid antigens are expressed in human amnion epithelium. *J Invest Dermatol*; 1984; **83**: 234–7.

70 Regauer S, Franke WW, Vartanen I. Intermediate filament cytoskeleton of amnion epithelium and cultured amnion epithelial cells: expression of epidermal cytokeratins in cells of a simple epithelium. *J Cell Biol* 1985; **100**: 997–1009.

71 Lane A, Scott GA, Day KH. Development of human fetal skin transplanted to the nude mouse. *J Invest Dermatol* 1989; **93**: 787–91.

Part Two

Specific Disease Groups

Chapter 4

Epidermolysis bullosa

D. J. Atherton

Introduction

Epidermolysis bullosa is the term used to describe a number of genetically determined disorders, whose principal characteristic is the exceptional ease with which the skin and/or mucosae will blister as a response to mechanical trauma.

Some object to the use of the term for diseases that fulfil the above criteria but do not feature true epidermolysis, i.e. lysis of keratinocytes, and would prefer to call these conditions 'hereditary mechano-bullous diseases', rather than epidermolysis bullosa. However, the term epidermolysis bullosa is used in the wider sense in this chapter.

There are three broad categories of epidermolysis bullosa: epidermolysis bullosa simplex, dystrophic epidermolysis bullosa and junctional epidermolysis bullosa (Table 4.1) (Figure 4.1). Within each of these categories, there are several subtypes which are clinically (and probably genetically) distinct[1,2].

Table 4.1 *Categories of epidermolysis bullosa*

Epidermolysis bullosa simplex
   Generalized (Koebner type)
   Localized to the hands and feet
     (Weber–Cockayne type)
   Herpetiformis (Dowling–Meara type)
Dystrophic epidermolysis bullosa
Junctional epidermolysis bullosa

References

1 Fine J-D, Bauer EA, Briggaman RA, Carter DM et al. Revised clinical and laboratory criteria for subtypes of inherited epidermolysis bullosa. *J Am Acad Dermatol* 1991; **24**: 119–35.
2 Priestley G, Tidman M, Weiss J, Eady R, eds. *Epidermolysis Bullosa: A Comprehensive Review of Classification, Management and Laboratory Studies*. DEBRA, Crowthorne, 1990.

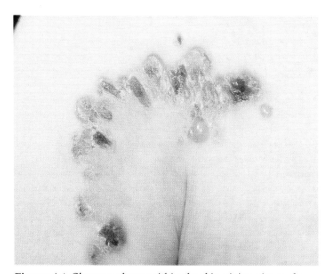

Figure 4.1 *Cleavage planes within the skin giving rise to the different types of epidermolysis bullosa*

Epidermolysis bullosa simplex

Definition

Epidermolysis bullosa simplex comprises a group of inherited disorders characterized by mechanically induced blistering occurring within the epidermis itself as a result of keratinocyte lysis. Because of the characteristic level of cleavage, epidermolysis bullosa simplex is sometimes termed 'epidermolytic' epidermolysis bullosa.

There are several established variants, of which the following are the most important:

1. Generalized epidermolysis bullosa simplex (Koebner type).
2. Epidermolysis bullosa simplex localized to the hands and feet (Weber–Cockayne type).
3. Epidermolysis bullosa simplex herpetiformis (Dowling–Meara type).

Clinical features

Generalized epidermolysis bullosa simplex (Koebner type)

Generalized epidermolysis bullosa simplex tends to have an early onset, either during the perinatal period or during the first few months of life. It is not infrequently already present at birth. Rubbing of the skin tends to be the main provocative factor. The blistering tendency is much more apparent in warm weather, to the extent that some patients' problems are more or less confined to the summer months.

In the perinatal period, blistering and erosions occur at sites determined by trauma during delivery and by handling in the nursery. Lesions heal quickly without scarring. Thereafter, the rate of new blister formation tends to slow down, with new lesions only appearing at sites of continuing friction, particularly in the napkin area.

Oral lesions do occur, but tend not to be prominent, and only rarely interfere with feeding. Nail involvement is unusual, and when nails are occasionally shed following subungual blistering, they generally regrow without dystrophy.

As the child starts to crawl, lesions may occur on the knees, feet, elbows and hands. With the onset of walking, the principal problem localizes to the feet and ankles, with the hands being the next most frequently affected site. In adults, it is rare for lesions to occur elsewhere, though blisters can be provoked at any site under appropriate provocation. Rubbing of the feet by footwear is generally the major problem that patients face.

Though it is sometimes implied that epidermolysis bullosa simplex is a relatively trivial disease, some patients experience significant disability, mainly because of difficulty in walking. Some individuals may only be able to walk one or two hundred metres on a summer day before painful blistering occurs. Other patients may have problems with manual tasks, and may find it impossible to use hand tools for more than very brief periods.

Blisters tend to be small, up to about 2 cm in diameter, and, despite their relatively superficial localization, they are generally tense, and may even be haemorrhagic. A particular feature of epidermolysis bullosa simplex is a halo of erythema around blisters, a characteristic which is generally lacking in other types of epidermolysis bullosa in the absence of secondary infection. Nevertheless, secondary infection appears particularly common in this type of epidermolysis bullosa. Though the blisters will heal rapidly in the absence of such secondary infection, the frequent recurrence of the provocative trauma at affected sites tends to cause new blisters to occur underneath and at the margins of ones that are in the process of healing. A degree of hyperkeratosis often marks the site of recurrent blistering.

Epidermolysis bullosa simplex localized to the hands and feet (Weber–Cockayne type)

The localized variant of epidermolysis bullosa simplex tends to have its onset rather later in childhood, not infrequently in adolescence or even in early adult life. Those who have this condition often do not consider themselves to have a medical problem, merely an exaggeration of the normal tendency to blister during or after hard walking or running, or after intensive use of the hands. Their blistering tendency may not become apparent until they are required to undertake unusual activity, for example a forced march in the army.

Areas of the body other than the hands and feet are not affected, nor are the nails or the mouth. The blisters are tense and occur at the same sites on the hands and feet as in the generalized type of epidermolysis bullosa simplex. Likewise, secondary infection is perhaps the principal complication of the disorder. In the absence of such infection, the blisters heal fairly rapidly without blistering.

Epidermolysis bullosa simplex herpetiformis (Dowling–Meara type)

Epidermolysis bullosa simplex herpetiformis or Dowling–Meara type (Figures 4.1 and 4.2) is a less common but increasingly recognized form of epidermolysis bullosa simplex [1–3]. Clinically, it generally causes widespread blistering, which is relatively easily provoked, with an onset in early infancy. Blistering may be severe during the neonatal period, and some babies have died. Blisters are perhaps more often haemorrhagic than in other forms of epidermolysis bullosa simplex, and milia may be a feature for a few weeks after blisters have healed. It is important to be aware that milia are not pathognomonic of dystrophic forms

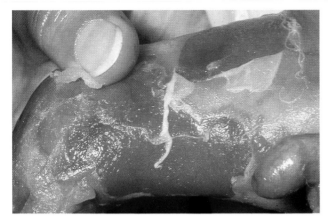

Figure 4.2 *Extensive skin loss in a baby with Dowling–Meara epidermolysis bullosa simplex*

of epidermolysis bullosa, and that they may occur, albeit rather transiently, in all the other forms, but perhaps particularly in epidermolysis bullosa simplex herpetiformis.

The hands and feet are the sites of predilection, and blisters in these sites are identical to those seen in other forms of epidermolysis bullosa simplex. However, blisters frequently occur at other sites on the face, trunk and limbs, and tend to be disposed in groups on an erythematous background; hence the term 'herpetiformis'. However, these groups are perhaps more often annular or arcuate than truly herpetiform. The neck is particularly commonly affected, perhaps due to friction related to clothing, though in this condition groups of blisters may appear with remarkably little provocation. High environmental temperatures seem not to be of great importance in reducing the threshold for blistering. Like other types of epidermolysis bullosa simplex, secondary infection is very common, perhaps more of a problem in this than any other form of epidermolysis bullosa. Mild oral involvement may occur. The nails may be lost, but generally regrow without the development of dystrophic changes. A few patients ultimately develop thickening of nails that have been lost frequently, associated with a degree of subungual hyperkeratosis.

Perhaps the most characteristic clinical feature of epidermolysis bullosa herpetiformis is the frequent development in later childhood of increasing degrees of rather verrucous palmoplantar keratoderma. This is usually focal at first, becoming more diffuse with time.

Pathology

The technique of taking biopsies in epidermolysis bullosa is of the greatest importance if the procedure is to provide useful tissue for the pathologist. The biopsy should be taken from clinically unaffected skin. Disruption of the skin should be induced by rubbing the area to be biopsied with a finger or an india-rubber

for about a minute. There should follow a delay of 5–10 minutes, after which the biopsy should be taken. In the author's unit, the shave technique is found to provide the best-quality material, because artefact is minimal, fixation is rapid, orientation is easier and healing is good.

Epidermolysis bullosa simplex is characterized at the pathological level by true 'epidermolysis', i.e. intracellular keratinocyte lysis. In all forms, this lysis occurs in the basal keratinocytes. Pathologically, epidermolysis bullosa simplex of the generalized and localized types cannot currently be distinguished. On the other hand, epidermolysis bullosa simplex herpetiformis shows the distinctive ultrastructural feature of tonofibril clumping occurring within basal keratinocytes prior to their lysis. It has been demonstrated that these tonofilament clumps contain the basal keratins 5 and 14[4].

Prenatal diagnosis of epidermolysis bullosa simplex is discussed in Chapter 21.

Genetics

These disorders are inherited as autosomal dominant traits in the vast majority of cases. There have been a few reports of autosomal recessive inheritance of epidermolysis bullosa simplex [5–7], including a form which was frequently lethal[6], and one in which some affected individuals also demonstrated neuromuscular abnormalities[7].

In both the generalized and the localized forms of epidermolysis bullosa simplex, patients almost always have extensive family histories of the condition, and the occurrence of sporadic cases is relatively unusual. As is generally the case with dominantly inherited diseases, severity may vary considerably between affected members of a single family. The majority of cases of epidermolysis bullosa simplex herpetiformis have to date been sporadic, but where other family members have been affected, inheritance has been autosomal dominant.

It was initially shown that the genetic defect in one family with localized epidermolysis bullosa simplex was on chromosome 12, in a region known to code for keratin 5, and the defect in another family with generalized epidermolysis bullosa simplex was localized to chromosome 17, in a region known to code for keratin 14[8]. It was more or less simultaneously demonstrated that 2 patients with epidermolysis bullosa simplex herpetiformis had point mutations in the keratin 14 gene[9], and that the tonofilament clumps seen ultrastructurally in this condition contain keratins 5 and 14[4]. It has now been substantiated that the three main forms of epidermolysis bullosa simplex result from mutations in the genes encoding keratins 5 and 14 expressed in basal keratinocytes, and that the differing clinical severity of these disorders reflects the resulting degree of disturbance of keratin filament assembly[10].

Differential diagnosis

The only time at which differential diagnosis may present some difficulty is in the neonatal period. This problem is discussed below in the section on dystrophic epidermolysis bullosa.

Treatment

In generalized and localized epidermolysis bullosa simplex, the long family association with the disease, combined with an awareness both of the provoking influences and the limitations of available therapy, make it fairly unusual for patients to seek medical assistance. When they do, the most useful contribution the clinician can make is to provide advice about suitable footwear and general care of the feet, and about genetic aspects.

Fresh blisters should be drained after puncture with a sterile disposable needle, as they tend to extend if left alone. The blister roof should be left in situ. It is often useful to bathe blistered feet and hands in warm water containing potassium permanganate at a dilution of about 1:8000. The ideal dressing for erosions and blisters in patients with epidermolysis bullosa simplex has yet to be invented, and none of the currently available products seems to fit these patients' requirements exactly. Patients and their parents generally make up their own minds about the dressing materials that most suit their own needs, and the dermatologist's job is really to ensure, firstly, that patients are properly informed about the range of different types of dressing available, and, secondly, that they are able to secure a supply of their chosen dressings as economically as possible.

Because of the frequent occurrence of secondary bacterial infection, patients often like to use topical antimicrobial applications. However, there is no ideal topical antimicrobial agent to protect these patients from secondary bacterial infections, and the regular use of any particular preparation tends to be associated with the development of bacterial resistance to the antimicrobial employed. At Great Ormond Street Hospital the practice is to concentrate on physical cleansing and the use of potassium permanganate soaks as described above. If anything is to be applied to individual lesions, an antiseptic is preferred to an antibiotic, and of those preparations that are currently available, the following seem most suitable: 1.5% hydrogen peroxide cream (Hioxyl, made by Quinoderm, UK), 10% povidone-iodine aqueous solution or ointment (Betadine, Seton, UK), 0.5% cetrimide cream (Cetavlex, Zeneca Pharma, UK) and 1% silver sulphadiazine cream (Flamazine, Smith & Nephew, UK).

It is important to provide children with epidermolysis bullosa simplex with footwear which allows them the maximum mobility while providing the best possible protection for their feet. Many children can wear 'off the peg' shoes if these incorporate appropriate design features. Ideally, these shoes are made of very soft leather, with the minimum number of internal seams. There should be plenty of room for the toes, in both the horizontal and vertical planes. Both the uppers and the insock should be made of permeable leather, in order to keep the foot as cool and dry as possible, and the inside of the sole should have a shape which is as anatomically appropriate as possible. Few 'off the peg' shoes fulfil these criteria, other than certain lines of Elephanten shoes (UK agents: Intershoe Ltd, Stockton on Tees) which have been found to be more or less ideal.

Socks should be absorbent and should therefore contain a high proportion of cotton. They should also provide additional cushioning; the towelling type of sport sock is ideal. It is sometimes useful for the patient to wear two pairs of socks as this helps to reduce friction.

A small proportion of babies and young children with generalized epidermolysis bullosa simplex, and a larger proportion with epidermolysis bullosa simplex herpetiformis, may be very fragile, and they will need protective measures as described for dystrophic epidermolysis bullosa (see below). Fortunately, however, this fragility generally reduces over a period of a few years. In children with epidermolysis bullosa simplex herpetiformis it seems to be important to check that clothing does not have rough internal seams, and that it fits loosely, especially at the neck, wrists and ankles.

References

1 Anton-Lamprecht I, Schnyder UW. Epidermolysis bullosa herpetiformis Dowling–Meara: report of a case and pathomorphogenesis. *Dermatologica* 1982; **164**: 221–35.
2 Hachem-Zadeh S, Rappersberger K, Livshin R, Konrad K. Epidermolysis bullosa herpetiformis Dowling–Meara in a large family. *J Am Acad Dermatol* 1988; **18**: 702–6.
3 Buchbinder LH, Lucky AW, Ballard E et al. Severe infantile epidermolysis bullosa simplex Dowling–Meara type. *Arch Dermatol* 1986; **122**: 190–8.
4 Ishida-Yamamoto A, McGrath J, Chapman SJ et al. Epidermolysis bullosa simplex (Dowling–Meara type) is a genetic disease characterized by an abnormal keratin-filament network involving keratins K5 and K14. *J Invest Dermatol* 1991; **97**: 959–68.
5 Fine J-D, Johnson L, Wright T, Horiguchi Y. Epidermolysis bullosa simplex: identification of a kindred with autosomal recessive transmission of the Weber–Cockayne variety. *Pediatr Dermatol* 1989; **6**: 1–5.
6 Salih MAM, Lake BD, ElHag MA, Atherton DJ. Lethal epidermolytic epidermolysis bullosa: a new autosomal recessive type of epidermolysis bullosa. *Br J Dermatol* 1985; **113**: 135–43.
7 Fine J-D, Stenn J, Johnson L, Wright T et al. Autosomal recessive epidermolysis bullosa simplex. *Arch Dermatol* 1989; **125**: 931–8.
8 Bonifas J, Rothman AL, Epstein EH. Epidermolysis bullosa simplex: evidence in two families for keratin gene abnormalities. *Science* 1991; **254**: 1202.

9 Coulombe PA, Hutton ME, Letai A et al. Point mutations in human keratin 14 genes of epidermolysis bullosa simplex patients: genetic and functional analyses. *Cell* 1991; **66**: 1301–11.

10 Coulombe PA, Hutton E, Vassar R, Fuchs E. A function for keratins and a common thread among different types of epidermolysis bullosa simplex diseases. *J Cell Biol* 1991; **115**: 1661–74.

Dystrophic epidermolysis bullosa

Definition

Dystrophic epidermolysis bullosa is the name given to a group of inherited disorders characterized by mechanically induced blistering occurring immediately below the lamina densa of the basement membrane zone.

Because of the characteristic level of cleavage, dystrophic epidermolysis bullosa is sometimes termed 'dermolytic' epidermolysis bullosa. These disorders derive the name 'dystrophic' from the tendency of the blisters to heal with atrophic scarring.

There are several clinical variants, but these have not been precisely separated on genetic or biochemical grounds, and their status is therefore still unclear[1]. It is often possible to distinguish an autosomal dominant or recessive pattern of inheritance in individual families, but there may be considerable overlap of clinical features between the two.

Clinical features

The clinical hallmark of this group of disorders is the tendency for blistered areas to heal with the appearance of milia and with atrophic scarring (Figures 4.3–4.6). However, as discussed above, milia are not confined to dystrophic epidermolysis bullosa, though they do tend to be more prominent and longer-lasting in dystrophic epidermolysis bullosa. Furthermore, scarring is often not apparent after a particular area of

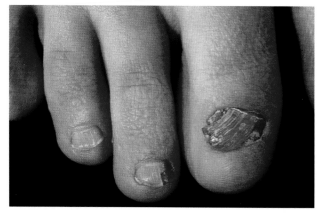

Figure 4.4 *Dominant dystrophic epidermolysis bullosa with typical nail dystrophy*

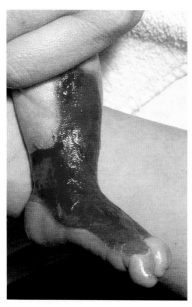

Figure 4.5 *Localized absence of skin at birth in a child with dystrophic epidermolysis bullosa*

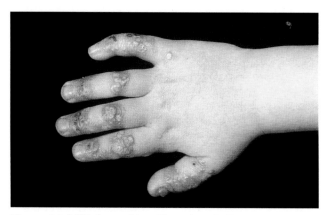

Figure 4.3 *Mild dystrophic epidermolysis bullosa*

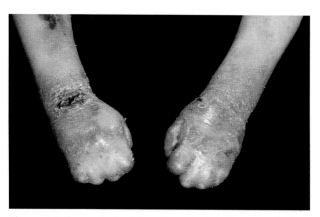

Figure 4.6 *Severe dystrophic epidermolysis bullosa: acquired syndactyly*

skin has only blistered once, but becomes progressively more apparent the more often blistering occurs.

Clinically, dystrophic epidermolysis bullosa varies from being an extremely disabling disease at one end of the spectrum, to a trivial disease at the other. While it is asserted that a wide variety of distinct subtypes of dystrophic epidermolysis bullosa can be separately identified, it is the writer's view that an obsession with precise categorization of the individual case is generally unnecessary. It is all too easy for an academic preoccupation with classification to distract from the more urgent and important matter of providing care and advice to patient and family. In the individual case it is sufficient for the purpose of clinical management to establish that the patient has a dystrophic form of epidermolysis bullosa. Beyond this the most important issue is whether the patient's disease has been transmitted as an autosomal dominant or recessive trait, for the purposes of genetic counselling and prenatal diagnosis.

Blistering in dystrophic epidermolysis bullosa tends to be provoked predominantly by knocks and blows to the skin, rather than by rubbing as in epidermolysis bullosa simplex. Blisters in dystrophic epidermolysis bullosa therefore occur most frequently at skin sites where this type of trauma is common, such as the dorsa of the hands and feet, and the elbows and knees. However, persistent rubbing of the skin also predisposes to blistering, especially rubbing by clothing and bedding such as occurs around the neck, the waist, groin, hips and the lumbosacral area.

The blisters may vary considerably in size, and some patients may develop blisters that exceed 10 cm in diameter. The blisters tend to be rather flaccid, and are filled with either clear or bloodstained fluid. Healing is generally fairly rapid. Crops of milia are common following initial re-epithelialization, but where an area is not subject to further blistering, the milia cease to appear after a few months. Scarring is unusual following a single episode of blistering in a particular area, and generally only follows recurrent blistering. Blistering is much more easily provoked in areas that have previously been blistered, particularly when scarring has occurred. Healing areas tend to itch, and when the patient scratches, further blistering is likely to follow. This can establish a cycle of blistering, itching and reblistering, the situation being made ever worse by the increasing ease with which reblistering occurs.

In the great majority of cases, blisters – or more often erosions – are present at or very shortly after birth (Figure 4.5). Commonly, an extensive eroded area is present at birth on one or both lower legs, usually on the dorsum and lateral aspect of the foot and the shin. This type of lesion almost certainly evolves in utero as a result of the fetus rubbing its legs together. In the absence of other lesions suggestive of epidermolysis bullosa, this type of lesion may mis-takenly be regarded as cutis aplasia congenita[2]. These areas usually heal fairly rapidly, though the resulting scarring frequently leads to some deformity of the foot, particularly to upward displacement of the great toe.

In all types of epidermolysis bullosa, new blisters develop less frequently with increasing age. It is unclear whether this is because of a genuinely decreased tendency of the skin to blister or is simply a reflection of more effective avoidance of trauma by older patients. However, in the case of patients afflicted by severe dystrophic epidermolysis bullosa, this gradual improvement is counterbalanced by the steadily increasing fragility of skin that has been repeatedly ulcerated in the past, and is now atrophic and as delicate as tissue paper. Whereas previously ulcerated areas would usually heal rapidly, these atrophic areas may now break down so frequently that they never seem to heal. The neck, axillae, elbows, hands, hips, knees and ankles seem to be among the most troublesome sites from this point of view.

Cutaneous scarring in dystrophic epidermolysis bullosa may lead to a variety of complications, particularly to joint contractures, and to fusion of the fingers and toes. Progressive hand deformity is common in patients who blister readily. When digital fusion is going to develop, the earliest signs that this is happening can usually be detected within the first year of life. By this age also, some idea of the likely speed of progression of the process can usually be gained. The process of fusion seems to occur insidiously in the apices of the interdigital spaces, where careful examination will generally reveal small fissures. Occasionally, accidental trauma will lead to denudation of skin on the apposing aspects of more than one finger. If the fingers are apposed during healing, they may become fused acutely. Good hand function may be retained despite marked digital fusion, so long as apposition of index finger and thumb is retained. More disabling is the development of flexion contraction of the hand, due to fibrosis of the skin on the palmar aspects of the fingers and hand.

Subungual blisters are common, and are generally followed by partial or complete separation of the nail plate. The nail will usually regrow normally after this has occurred on one or two occasions, but repeated nail loss will lead to the development first of nail dystrophy and then of permanent nail loss. In the very mildest cases of dystrophic epidermolysis bullosa, nail dystrophy may be an important diagnostic aid, particularly dystrophy of the great toenails.

Blistering of the oral, pharyngeal and oesophageal mucosa is common in dystrophic epidermolysis bullosa, and may lead to a number of problems, of which the most important are:

1. Pain, leading to reduced nutritional intake.
2. Progressive contraction of the mouth.
3. Progressive fixation of the tongue.

4. Dental caries caused by oral infection and impaired dental hygiene due to (2) and (3) above.
5. Oesophageal dysmotility and strictures.

Dysphagia is a common complication of dystrophic epidermolysis bullosa, particularly of the recessive types, though it is certainly not restricted to them. There may be little correlation between the severity of the skin disease and the severity of dysphagia in the individual patient. Many factors contribute to dysphagia in these patients, and although great emphasis has been given to the oesophageal strictures that may develop, these are certainly not the only cause of the dysphagia. Important contributions are made by oral problems, especially by submucous fibrosis in the oral cavity, contraction of the oral and pharyngeal openings, and by fixation of the tongue. In addition, the teeth are often very poor and many may have been extracted. Extremely painful erosions are frequently present in the mouth and pharynx. Combinations of these problems cause patients great difficulties in chewing and swallowing normal food. Eating is often painful, slow and exhausting, so that only relatively small quantities of food can be coped with at any meal.

Anal fissuring is also common, and leads to faecal retention, faecal soiling, and eventually to constipation. The tendency to constipation is aggravated by a low dietary fibre intake. It seems probable that these patients' tendency to take food in frequent small quantities, rather than in discrete meals of reasonable size, leads to a degree of disordered intestinal peristalsis, which will tend to aggravate the constipation still further.

Conjunctival bullae are not infrequent in patients with severe dystrophic epidermolysis bullosa, and lead to conjunctival ulceration and painful corneal erosions. These may result in conjunctival and corneal scarring, and thus threaten vision in the longer term, both directly and by interfering with tear film stability and tear production.

A few boys will develop phimosis, and children of either sex may very occasionally develop strictures of the urethral meatus, resulting in urinary retention.

Anaemia is a problem in most patients with severe dystrophic epidermolysis bullosa. Investigations demonstrate haematological features both of iron deficiency and of decreased red cell iron utilization ('anaemia of chronic disease'). The iron deficiency probably reflects both chronic blood loss from skin, mouth, oesophagus and anal canal, and poor iron intake.

Patients with dystrophic epidermolysis bullosa frequently have nutritional problems, which may be serious in the more severely affected. Most prominent among these are:

1. Poor nutritional intake, mainly due to oral, pharyngeal and oesophageal disease and to anorexia secondary to constipation.

2. Loss of nutrients due to seepage of serum and blood through the skin and mucosae.
3. Increased nutritional requirements for healing.

Children with more severe dystrophic epidermolysis bullosa tend to grow poorly. A decrease in linear growth velocity is usually preceded by a decrease in weight gain, implying that the growth effect is secondary to inadequate nutrition. Anaemia probably also makes a significant contribution, and as discussed above, is not entirely of nutritional origin.

The most sinister late complication of dystrophic epidermolysis bullosa is the tendency for epitheliomas, predominantly squamous cell carcinomas, to develop in recurrently ulcerated areas[3]. Such tumours appear to cause the death of substantial numbers of patients from the second decade onwards. Patients may be unaware of this danger and may therefore fail to bring such lesions to medical attention in good time. It is of the greatest importance that all patients with dystrophic epidermolysis bullosa be fully aware of this risk, and of the need to report any unusual skin lesion, particularly lumps, nodules or ulcers that seem particularly unwilling to heal.

The literature suggests that various subtypes of dystrophic epidermolysis bullosa can be distinguished clinically, e.g. a 'transient' type ('transient bullous dermolysis of the newborn'), an 'inverse' type, a 'pretibial' type and Bart's syndrome (congenital absence of skin)[1]. In the author's view, there is too much clinical overlap between these alleged subtypes, and there is little to suggest that such a segregation is helpful from the patients' point of view.

Pathology

At the pathological level, dystrophic epidermolysis bullosa appears to reflect abnormalities in the attachment of the basement membrane to the underlying dermis, and particularly by reduced numbers or absence of anchoring fibrils[4]. These anchoring fibrils have been shown largely to comprise type VII collagen[5]. Ultrastructural abnormalities of the anchoring fibrils are not necessarily visible in autosomal dominant forms of dystrophic epidermolysis bullosa.

The monoclonal antibody LH7:2 binds to the basement membrane zone in normal skin, but not in severe recessive dystrophic epidermolysis bullosa. It is now clear that this antibody binds to type VII collagen. Binding is weak but generally present in milder recessive dystrophic epidermolysis bullosa, but is normal in dominant dystrophic epidermolysis bullosa[6]. This suggests that recessive dystrophic epidermolysis bullosa may be a heterogeneous disorder. While it appears that type VII collagen is absent from the skin in the most severe form of recessive dystrophic epidermolysis bullosa, functional abnormalities of type VII collagen are perhaps more likely to be responsible for other forms of dystrophic epidermolysis bullosa. Support for this concept is provided by the demonstration of linkage of dominant dystrophic epidermolysis bullosa to the collagen VII gene[7]. The finding of intracellular type VII collagen in the epidermis of some patients with dystrophic epidermolysis bullosa has suggested that its absence at the dermoepidermal junction may reflect an abnormality of its secretion into the extracellular compartment[8].

Genetics

As with epidermolysis bullosa simplex, there is a wide variation in the severity of the dystrophic epidermolysis bullosa in different patients. At its least severe, dystrophic epidermolysis bullosa can allow an almost normal quality and length of life, while at its most severe, it may cause major handicap and a brief, painful lifetime.

Dystrophic epidermolysis bullosa may be inherited as an autosomal dominant or an autosomal recessive trait. In general, it tends to be most severe when inheritance is recessive, and mildest when inheritance is dominant, but there are many exceptions to this generalization, and the mildest cases of recessive dystrophic epidermolysis bullosa have less severe disease than the worst cases of dominant dystrophic epidermolysis bullosa. In the great majority of cases of dominant dystrophic epidermolysis bullosa there is a clear family history, suggesting a low rate of new mutations. Most sporadic cases of dystrophic epidermolysis bullosa seem to be of recessive type, even where clinically mild. Unfortunately, the LH7:2 monoclonal antibody appears to be of limited value in distinguishing dominant and recessive dystrophic epidermolysis bullosa, a distinction that is not possible by electron microscopy alone.

Both recessive and dominant forms of dystrophic epidermolysis bullosa result from mutations in the type VII collagen gene (COL7A1) on chromosome 3p21. Clinical variants such as the Bart's syndrome[9] and pretibial epidermolysis bullosa[10] have also been linked to the COL7A1 locus.

Prenatal diagnosis of dystrophic epidermolysis bullosa is discussed in Chapter 21.

Differential diagnosis

Differential diagnosis in epidermolysis bullosa is normally only a problem during the neonatal period. Conditions that require consideration at this time include 'sucking' blisters, congenital herpes simplex, cutis aplasia, incontinentia pigmenti, focal dermal hypoplasia, bullous ichthyosiform erythroderma, transplacental herpes gestationis and pemphigus vulgaris, miliaria crystallina, staphylococcal scalded skin and congenital acrokeratotic poikiloderma.

During the neonatal period, attempts to distinguish the various types of epidermolysis bullosa clinically are unwise. The later appearance of milia is indicative of dystrophic epidermolysis bullosa, though small numbers of milia can undoubtedly be seen from time to time in non-dystrophic types.

Early diagnostic biopsy is helpful, but considerable skill is required in interpretation of results.

Treatment

Skin care

Skin care in patients with epidermolysis bullosa must incorporate the twin objectives of protection against trauma and provision of optimal conditions for rapid healing of blisters and erosions. A third objective, relevant in the older patient, is surveillance for epidermal neoplasia.

The skin of neonates with epidermolysis bullosa may be extraordinarily sensitive, even to 'normal' handling. Infants are often seen with erosions on each side of the trunk as a result of being picked up. Sometimes there are five lesions on each side, one for each of the nurse's fingers. Therefore, special handling techniques must be used in the nursing of these infants.

At Great Ormond Street Hospital, babies with epidermolysis bullosa are nursed on a piece of foam 2.5 cm thick, measuring about 90 cm × 90 cm, which is covered by a silk sheet. Using this arrangement, the baby can be held without direct contact, making it possible to feed, comfort and move the baby about safely (Figure 4.7).

Dressings are changed twice daily (Figure 4.8). New blisters are punctured with a sterile disposable needle and drained as they will often extend if left alone. The blister roof is left in situ. The baby is dried with a hair drier, after which eroded areas should, if necessary, be gently cleaned with cotton-wool balls soaked with sterile normal saline. Vaseline gauze (Sherwood, Davis and Geck, UK) is then applied to eroded and blistered areas. If eroded areas are obviously infected, stabilized hydrogen peroxide cream (Hioxyl, made by Quinoderm, UK) is spread on to the Vaseline gauze on the side that will come into direct contact with the skin. Great caution must be exercised in the choice of topical antibacterial agents for these children because of the very real danger of induction of bacterial resistance, and because of the danger of toxicity that may follow the systemic absorption which is inevitable when a topical agent is applied to de-epithelialized areas under more or less occlusive dressings. The use of topical antimicrobial agents should not be routine. Vaseline gauze is an extremely fine paraffin gauze, superior to standard paraffin gauze because of its greatly reduced thread diameter and mesh size. This gauze is also available in a ribbon form, which is useful for weaving between fingers and toes. Over the

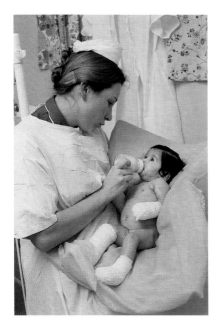

Figure 4.7 *Special care must be taken in handling babies with severe epidermolysis bullosa*

Vaseline gauze is applied a layer of Melolin roll (Smith & Nephew, UK); this comprises wadding, with a non-adherent film applied to the underside. This is now secured by a suitable conforming bandage, e.g. J-Fast (Johnson & Johnson, UK), and/or a tubular stretch bandage such as Tubifast (Seton, UK).

Such dressings will generally not adhere to eroded areas, and their use is associated with a good rate of re-epithelialization, probably reflecting both their occlusive and protective properties. They are, however, not used solely to encourage healing of blistered areas; they are used for protection in any area, whether affected or not at the time, that may be liable

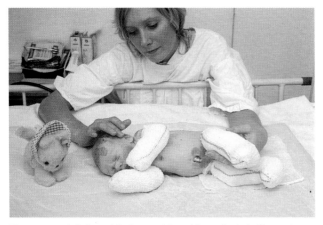

Figure 4.8 *A baby with dystrophic epidermolysis bullosa after the dressings have been applied*

to blistering. The department is now using another dressing, Mepitel (Molynycke, Luton, UK) applied directly to the skin, which has the advantage that it can be left in place for up to 7 days.

Babies with epidermolysis bullosa should not be nursed completely naked. Such babies are usually uncomfortable, irritable and restless; they therefore tend to do themselves considerable harm, for example by rubbing their legs together, and their lesions heal relatively slowly. These dressings described above are almost always used on the arms and legs, and often on the trunk also. Babies wearing such dressings are usually more comfortable and are shielded from external mechanical trauma, particularly self-induced trauma. Parents are encouraged to learn the technique and use it after they take the baby home.

Over the months that follow birth, it becomes decreasingly appropriate to employ the type of dressing described above. The danger of self-inflicted trauma decreases as the need for mobility and play gradually increases. However, as the child becomes more mobile, the risk of external trauma from falls and knocks initially increases. As the child slowly learns to become more careful, so the amount of mechanical trauma again diminishes. Sadly, toddlers are notoriously careless, and certain sites tend to become recurrently blistered. The sites that are at special risk in the toddler are the elbows, wrists, hands, knees, shins, ankles and feet. Many parents elect to use protective dressings to cushion these sites. An appropriate technique is to use Melolin roll next to the skin, over which is applied J-Fast, then Tubifast, over the area to be protected.

Different patients use a great variety of topical agents, most of which are antimicrobial in their effects. Secondary bacterial infection is a constant problem in blistered and eroded areas, and it frequently delays healing. There is still no ideal topical antimicrobial agent to protect the patient from the secondary bacterial infections that tend to be such a major problem. Of those preparations that are currently available, the following seem most suitable: 1.5% hydrogen peroxide cream (Hioxyl, Quinoderm, UK), 10% povidone-iodine aqueous solution or ointment (Betadine, Seton, UK), 0.5% cetrimide cream (Cetavlex, Zeneca Pharma, UK) and 1% silver sulphadiazine cream (Flamazine, Smith & Nephew, UK). Antibiotics of value in the systemic treatment of serious infections should not be used topically to treat chronic dermatoses such as epidermolysis bullosa, nor should important topical antibiotics, especially mupirocin (Bactroban, Smith Kline and Beecham, UK), because the selection of resistant bacteria is virtually inevitable; indeed, one of the first reports of mupirocin-resistant *Staphylococcus aureus* related to a patient with epidermolysis bullosa.

Clearly, avoidance of trauma is an important facet of treatment of these children. It is extremely difficult, however, for parents to find the right balance between what could be regarded as appropriate avoidance of trauma and overprotection of the developing child. Children with epidermolysis bullosa should be brought up as normally as possible, in order to maximize their physical, manipulative and social skills. They gradually learn to take extra care themselves, and to avoid situations in which trauma is likely to occur. Older children with epidermolysis bullosa learn to stand back when other children scuffle. However, during the toddler phase, they tend to be rather careless, and will benefit from constant vigilance on the part of those who are caring for them. In order to give them the best chance of taking part in normal activities, the emphasis should be on the provision of protective dressings and clothing, rather than on the avoidance of all remotely physical activities. It is particularly important to provide children suffering from epidermolysis bullosa with footwear that allows them maximum mobility while providing the best possible protection for their feet. Socks should be absorbent and should therefore contain a high proportion of cotton; they should also provide additional cushioning – the towelling type of sport sock is ideal. Other clothing needs to be chosen carefully. Before purchase, all items should be inspected to check that they do not have rough internal seams, and that they fit loosely, especially at the neck, wrists and ankles.

Systemic therapy

Over the years a number of systemic agents have been reported to have beneficial effects in dystrophic epidermolysis bullosa; the principal claim for such agents has been accelerated healing. Early ultrastructural studies of recessive dystrophic epidermolysis bullosa suggested that collagen breakdown in the papillary dermis might contribute to the development of blisters. The subsequent observation that skin fibroblasts cultured from patients appeared to synthesize increased amounts of collagenase appeared consistent with such a hypothesis, and provided the rationale for the therapeutic use of phenytoin, as this agent appeared able to reduce this collagenase production in vitro. The successful use of oral phenytoin in patients with this disease has been reported; however, more recent studies have not supported a major therapeutic role for this agent, and it is no longer used in most centres.

Following the demonstration that retinoids are able to inhibit collagenase activity in vitro, there was interest in their possible therapeutic value in recessive dystrophic epidermolysis bullosa. However, these drugs have not to date turned out to be helpful in practice.

High-dose oral corticosteroids were at one time widely used for the control of blistering in severe dystrophic epidermolysis bullosa, often as a long-term therapy. However, in the author's view, the morbidity associated with oral corticosteroid therapy, particularly in the very young, far outweighs its benefits, and at the Great Ormond Street Hospital this approach has not been used for several years. In the author's experience, the mortality of severe epidermolysis bullosa in the neonate is now less than it was when such treatment was in vogue.

Patients with recessive dystrophic epidermolysis bullosa who have restorative hand surgery appear to do no better if they are given oral corticosteroids during the months after surgery, and it remains to be shown that this form of treatment is beneficial overall to those with severe dysphagia.

Over the years there has been interest in the possible value of vitamin E as a treatment for dystrophic epidermolysis bullosa, but little objective evidence of benefit.

Prevention and treatment of complications

Digital fusion and contracture. Corrective surgery should be undertaken as soon as the function of the hand is significantly impaired. Only one hand should be operated upon at a time. The surgical procedure involves firstly separating the fused digits, and then releasing any contractures as completely as possible. Split-skin grafts are then sewn into place in the resulting defects along the separated surfaces and on the palmar aspect of previously flexed joints. Where the hand is almost completely encased, the whole extremity may be more conveniently 'degloved' before proceeding to separate the fingers completely and release the contractures.

Kirschner wires are not used routinely, but they can be useful to maintain extension during the immediate postoperative period. It is, however, of great importance to splint the hand in a flat position (Figure 4.9), with all joints extended as fully as possible over a

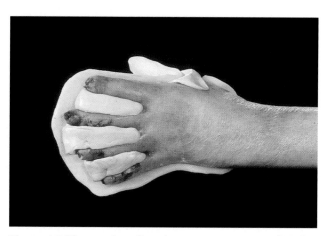

Figure 4.9 *The use of a splint after surgery to prevent digital fusion and contracture*

volar plaster-of-Paris slab. The dressings are changed under general anaesthesia at 2 and 3 weeks.

In the past, impressions were taken of the hand at the second dressing change to enable technicians to make accurately fitting acrylic gloves to act as longer-term splints. The aim of such splints is to retard recurrence of the fusion and contractures. These gloves are traditionally made in two halves, a palm and a dorsum, to enable them to be taken on and off easily. After surgery, children are requested initially to wear the splints continuously for 3 months, then for decreasing periods during the day, until after 6 months they need wear them only at night. Thermoplastic splints are now being evaluated; they are much easier to make, and can be altered or remade as required by the physiotherapist.

Unfortunately, these operations often need to be repeated from time to time. It may be necessary to relieve similar flexion contractures at other joints, especially in the feet, and at the knees and hips.

It is perhaps surprising that skin autografts can be so easily and successfully undertaken in patients with dystrophic epidermolysis bullosa. Attempts to grow therapeutically useful autologous keratinocyte sheets in vitro from patients with dystrophic epidermolysis bullosa have been frustrated by the tendency of the cells to separate from one another in culture. However, sheets of cultured allogeneic keratinocytes may prove valuable in the surgical treatment of dystrophic epidermolysis bullosa.

Physiotherapy and early splintage may help to delay the development of these deformities, and allow surgical treatment to be postponed. In the author's view, children and adults with dystrophic epidermolysis bullosa should maintain activity levels that are as high as are reasonably possible. Sadly, they are sometimes mistakenly immobilized by well-meaning parents or doctors, and this merely serves to accelerate the progression of their disability.

Dysphagia. Babies who are bottle-fed require the softest available teats (generally those designed for premature infants). The opening can be enlarged by use of a hot needle to make feeding easier. Some babies find it easier to take milk from a spoon than from a bottle.

For children with severe dystrophic epidermolysis bullosa it may be wise to liquidize solid foods from the start. This probably helps reduce mucosal trauma, as well as providing food that can be more easily eaten when swallowing difficulties are already established.

Many children with severe dystrophic epidermolysis bullosa experience periods when they cannot eat at all, either because of pain in the mouth or throat, or because of obstruction in the pharynx or oesophagus. If they are also unable to drink, it may be necessary to give fluid intravenously. A short admission for intravenous fluid administration allows the affected part to 'rest', and seems to accelerate recovery. Nasogastric feeding can be used to provide longer periods of rest.

Where swallowing difficulties occur, particularly when oesophageal strictures have developed, it is often assumed that the situation will inevitably worsen progressively. This may not be the case, at least in childhood. Dysphagia is prominent in the 3–7 year age group, but often becomes less of a problem as the child grows. For this reason, any question of highly invasive surgery, such as oesophageal replacement, should be delayed until every chance of spontaneous improvement has passed.

Oesophageal strictures that seriously reduce the patient's nutritional intake over long periods may require surgical dilation. However, difficulties arise where there is more than one stricture, or where there is an atonic segment proximal to a stricture. Solitary strictures respond well to dilation, though further dilations will generally be required. The balloon technique appears to be superior to traditional bougienage.

Oesophageal replacement may need to be considered in patients who require extremely frequent dilation, or when dilation is not possible. However, this situation only arises very rarely, and should not be considered before puberty. At least in children, the author prefers to bypass the oesophagus by use of gastrostomy feeding.

Anaesthesia. Despite the delicacy of the oral and pharyngeal mucosa, and anxieties about acute laryngeal obstruction if blistering of the larynx were to occur following intubation, general anaesthesia has proved to be fairly straightforward in patients with epidermolysis bullosa, if certain precautions are taken.

All those involved in handling these children before, during and after surgery must be made aware of the extreme vulnerability of their skin. Patients must be moved about with great care. Trolleys and operating table should be well padded so that pressure on the skin is kept to a minimum. No-one should lean on the patient during the operation. Plenty of non-adherent soft gauze padding such as Melolin roll should separate blood pressure cuffs and tourniquets from the skin. Sticky tapes and other adhesive materials, such as those used to attach electrocardiograph electrodes, must be avoided as the skin will come away when they are removed; elasticated netting, conforming bandages, and sutures if necessary, should be substituted. Heart rate is probably best monitored by the use of pulse oximetry. The corneas should be protected with simple eye ointment.

General anaesthesia is to be preferred to extensive local anaesthesia, because the latter may cause blistering. Access to the mouth may be poor due to an inadequate oral aperture, but this can be improved, often dramatically, by physiotherapy, using a variety of mouth-opening exercises.

To avoid undue facial manipulation, intubation is generally preferable, and an uncuffed tracheal tube should be selected, a size smaller than one would normally use. The tracheal tube and laryngoscope blade should be well lubricated. The tube should be fixed using ribbon gauze. Where the tube touches the lips or skin, Vaseline gauze should be interposed. Occasionally, limitation of mouth opening or dental problems may make intubation difficult; in such cases, and for short procedures, inhalational anaesthesia can be maintained by means of a face mask, which should have a soft air cushion separated from the skin by Vaseline gauze. Vaseline gauze should also be placed against the patient's skin where the underside of the jaw is held by the anaesthetist. Oropharyngeal airways should not be used.

The author is unaware of any reported cases in which laryngeal or tracheal obstruction has occurred following intubation in patients with dystrophic epidermolysis bullosa, or in the smaller number of patients with junctional epidermolysis bullosa who have required surgery.

Anaemia. Where there is evidence of iron deficiency, oral iron supplements should be given; liquid preparations tend to be most appropriate. Iron therapy alone will be ineffective where 'anaemia of chronic disease' is prominent, and in this situation blood transfusion may be necessary. It has been the author's policy not to transfuse unless the anaemia is causing significant symptoms or handicap; in these relatively immobile individuals, transfusion is therefore rarely necessary until haemoglobin levels fall below 7 G/dL. It must be borne in mind that iron overload may become a problem if transfusions are given more often than every 6–8 weeks over prolonged periods. Every effort should be made to improve the patient's general condition, with particular attention to nutrition and to care of the skin, as these measures may reduce the frequency at which transfusion is required.

Constipation. The management of constipation comprises firstly softening residual faecal material with softeners such as docusate sodium (Dioctyl Paediatric Syrup, Schwarz Pharma Ltd, UK), then emptying any accumulated faecal load by careful use of phosphate or sodium citrate enemas, or sodium picosulphate (Picolax, Ferring Pharma Ltd, UK) by mouth. The prior application of topical local anaesthetic makes the procedure much less unpleasant for the patient. It is then worth while to encourage daily defecation by the regular oral administration of senna; it may be necessary to do this for a period of a few months. The senna dose should then be progressively reduced.

In the longer term, it is important to prevent the recurrence of constipation by increasing the dietary fibre content or by the administration of bulk-forming agents, such as methylcellulose. In many cases, it is also necessary to give a faecal softening agent such as lactulose which has the additional benefit of increasing bulk. The routine administration of liquid paraffin is contraindicated because of the real risk of its entry into the respiratory tract in these patients.

A beneficial effect has been observed in constipated children with epidermolysis bullosa from the daily administration of a fibre-containing liquid nutritional supplement (Enrich, Abbott Laboratories Ltd, UK). This appears to be more acceptable than other sources of fibre, either dietary or pharmaceutical, and can be given easily to children who are being fed by nasogastric tube or via a gastrostomy.

If constipation persists despite these measures, and where anal pain on attempted defecation is marked, it may be worth considering an anal stretch under general anaesthesia.

Nutrition. Overcoming the combination of nutritional problems presented by these patients is exceedingly difficult. Some patients with dysphagia find it helpful to have their food liquidized, but others never accept this, unless they have been fed nothing else from infancy. Apart from making it easier for the patient to eat, liquidizing the diet may help prevent further damage to the pharynx and oesophagus, and may reduce the frequency of episodes of acute dysphagia. However, liquidizing food usually involves increasing its fluid content and therefore its bulk, which often results in a diminished total food intake. If water or gravy is used for this purpose, the nutrient value of the food will be reduced. This effect can be minimized by the use of milk, soup or flavoured white sauce. The process may make food blander and less appetizing, so that ingenuity is required to ensure that all meals do not taste the same. Liquidized food retains most of its fibre content; this is removed by sieving, which should therefore be avoided.

Many patients' diets are heavily dependent upon milk. This should not be discouraged, but such a diet may be far from complete from a nutritional point of view, tending to be low in iron and fibre, for example. High-fibre foods should be encouraged where practical, but they tend to have a lower energy content, and usually require more effort to eat than foods with a low fibre content.

The addition of glucose polymers such as Caloreen (Clinitec Nutrition Ltd, UK) or fat emulsions such as Calogen (Scientific Hospital Supplies, UK) is not routinely recommended. While these may increase energy intake, they will not improve overall nutrition. However, they are useful in certain circumstances, e.g. to supplement infant formula, or where protein intake intake from other foods is already high.

Though sucrose provides a highly effective means of increasing the patient's energy intake, high-sucrose foods such as chocolate are best restricted to mealtimes, to minimize their harmful effect on the teeth.

In the author's experience, the best approach is to inform parents and patients of the nutritional properties of different foods, and to encourage them to focus on those that provide nutrition in its most concentrated and best-balanced form. The aim is a well-balanced diet with a higher than normal content of protein, vitamins and minerals. The emphasis is on foods of soft, manageable consistency, with an attractive appearance and flavour.

Patients should be encouraged to take their food in discrete meals, rather than small quantities continuously throughout the day. This encourages a regular bowel habit, and reduces the risk of dental caries. However, many children with epidermolysis bullosa will be unable to eat enough at only three meals, mainly because they find the process of eating both painful and tiring. A system of three or four main meals per day, plus two or three snacks, will often be more appropriate. It is often a good idea to put a limit on the time allowed for each meal or snack, to prevent one meal from overlapping with the next.

The first 2 years of life are probably critical to the nutritional status of children with epidermolysis bullosa, and great efforts need to be directed towards improving nutrition during this period. It seems possible that children who show signs of dysphagia from early life should not be encouraged to move on to solid foods at all, but should be maintained on a liquidized diet throughout their life.

Since few patients do succeed in achieving even a normal nutritional intake, multinutrient supplements are frequently required. There are many palatable preparations available in liquid or powder form. Some, such as Complan (Heinz HJ. Co. Ltd, UK) and Build-Up (Nestlé, UK), are only available by purchase from a pharmacy or supermarket. Others, such as Fresubin (Fresenius, UK), Enrich (Abbott Laboratories Ltd, UK) and Fortisip (Cow & Gate, UK), are available in the UK on prescription from a general practitioner.

Vitamin and mineral supplements are frequently advisable, but care must be taken not to give excessive amounts which may be harmful. Children taking multinutrient supplements may already be receiving adequate amounts of vitamins and minerals. When appropriate, the patient may be given a complete vitamin supplement such as Ketovite (Paines & Byrne, UK), a liquid iron supplement such as Sytron (Link Pharm Ltd, UK) or one in the form of granules that can be dispersed in food, such as Feospan (Evans Medical Ltd, UK), and a zinc supplement such as Z Span (Goldshield Pharm Ltd, UK), which also takes the form of granules that can be dispersed in food. A fluoride supplement such as En-De-Kay (Stafford-Miller, UK) may be advisable depending on the fluoridation level of local water supplies.

Teeth. While the teeth are usually structurally normal in dystrophic epidermolysis bullosa, they are prone to severe caries due to several factors, including chronic intraoral infection and gum disease, a high sucrose intake and the absence of the normal physical cleansing effect of food owing to the diet being more or less liquid. The situation is made worse in severe dystrophic epidermolysis bullosa by the loss of the gingivobuccal sulci, causing residual food to remain applied to the buccal surfaces of the teeth for long periods, and by the loss of the normal cleansing of the teeth because of fixation and shrinkage of the tongue.

Appropriate dental care includes improvements in the diet, improved cleaning of the teeth, the regular use of an antiseptic mouthwash after meals to clean away as much of the residual food as possible, and oral fluoride supplements in areas where it is not adequately present in tap water.

In dystrophic epidermolysis bullosa, a conservative approach to dental therapy should be adopted, rather than wholesale extraction as has been recommended elsewhere. Those who propose this approach argue that the patients do not require teeth as their diet is more or less liquid. However, the possession of teeth is helpful in giving the patients a more normal facial appearance, since these patients will not tolerate dentures. Furthermore, shrinkage of the mouth appears to be accelerated by dental extractions. Undoubtedly, extraction is sometimes the only practical option for severely carious teeth because of the difficulty of doing conservative dental work through these patients' very restricted oral opening. Where extraction is necessary, healing is rapid.

Eyes. The use of lubricants such as simple eye ointment BP (10% liquid paraffin, wool fat 10%, in yellow soft paraffin) is valuable when patients have bullae. Topical corticosteroids without preservative may be indicated in the acute phase of ulceration, but their use should not be prolonged unless it is possible to monitor intraocular pressure.

References

1 Fine J-D, Bauer EA, Briggaman RA, Carter DM et al. Revised clinical and laboratory criteria for subtypes of inherited epidermolysis bullosa. *J Am Acad Dermatol* 1991; **24**: 119–35.

2 Bart BJ, Gorlin RJ, Anderson DE, Lynch FW. Congenital absence of skin and associated abnormalities resembling epidermolysis bullosa. *Arch Dermatol* 1966; **93**: 296–304.

3 Tidman MJ, Atherton DJ, Eady RAJ. Squamous carcinoma as a complication of dystrophic epidermolysis bullosa. *J Roy Soc Med* 1984; **77**(suppl. 4): 37–9.

4 Tidman HJ, Eady RAJ. Evaluation of anchoring fibrils and other components of the dermal-epidermal junction in dystrophic epidermolysis bullosa by a quantitative

ultrastructural technique. *J Invest Dermatol* 1985; **84**: 374–7.

5 Sakai LY, Keene DR, Morris NP, Burgeson RE. Type VII collagen is a major structural component of anchoring fibrils. *J Cell Biol* 1986; **103**: 1577–86.

6 Heagerty AHM, Kennedy AR, Leigh IM, Purkis PE, Eady RAJ. Identification of an epidermal basement membrane defect in recessive forms of dystrophic epidermolysis bullosa by LH 7:2 monoclonal antibody: use in diagnosis. *Br J Dermatol* 1986; **115**: 125–31.

7 Ryynanen M, Knowlton RG, Parente MG et al. Human type VII collagen: genetic linkage of the gene (COL7A1) on chromosome 3 to dominant dystrophic epidermolysis bullosa. *Am J Hum Genet* 1991; **49**: 797–803.

8 Phillips RJ, Harper JI, Lake BD. Intraepidermal collagen type VII in dystrophic epidermolysis bullosa: report of five new cases. *Br J Dermatol* 1992; **126**: 222–30.

9 Zelickson B, Matsumura K, Kist D, Epstein EH, Bart BJ. Bart's syndrome: ultrastructure and genetic linkage. *Arch Dermatol* 1995; **131**: 663–8.

10 Christiano AM, Lee JYY, Chen WJ et al. Pretibial epidermolysis bullosa: genetic linkage to COL7A1 and identification of a glycine-to-cysteine substitution in the triple-helical domain of type VII collagen. *Hum Mol Genet* 1995; **9**(4): 1579–83.

Junctional epidermolysis bullosa

Definition

Junctional epidermolysis bullosa is a group of inherited disorders characterized by mechanically induced blistering occurring within the lamina densa of the basement membrane zone.

Previously, junctional epidermolysis bullosa was more usually known as epidermolysis bullosa 'letalis'. However, although junctional epidermolysis bullosa is undoubtedly more likely than other categories of epidermolysis bullosa to result in death in infancy, some children do survive a number of years, and a few patients will survive into adult life, occasionally with relatively little handicap. Because of these survivors, the term epidermolysis bullosa 'letalis' is usually now avoided. Although not yet adequately differentiated, it seems clear that there are several distinct varieties of junctional epidermolysis bullosa. From the clinician's point of view it is currently practical to consider there to be three broad groups of patients:

1. Those who die within approximately 2 years after birth (Herlitz type junctional epidermolysis bullosa).
2. Those who survive into adult life ('benign' junctional epidermolysis bullosa).
3. Those whose disease takes a course which is intermediate between these two extremes, terminating in death in childhood, after the end of the second year.

These distinctions are to some extent arbitrary, and there is likely to be considerable overlap.

Clinical features

Herlitz type junctional epidermolysis bullosa

In the great majority of cases, blistering is present at birth or develops within the first few days of life. Despite the likelihood of an early lethal outcome, the initial lesions may be deceptively mild. It is always a mistake to try to guess the type of epidermolysis bullosa or the prognosis on clinical grounds alone in the neonate, as there is little correlation between initial severity and outcome, either in terms of life expectancy or ultimate degree of handicap.

In the infant, the sites of blistering are essentially the same as in other types of epidermolysis bullosa. Subungual and mucosal blisters are equally typical and frequent in junctional epidermolysis bullosa as they are in dystrophic epidermolysis bullosa. Initially, healing is rapid, and milia are not infrequent, though they are not as persistent as they are in dystrophic epidermolysis bullosa. Scarring is not a prominent feature as it is in dystrophic epidermolysis bullosa, but slightly atrophic areas are a not infrequent sequel to previous blistering. In the absence of profound scar formation, digital fusion and hand and foot deformity do not occur, nor do oral submucous fibrosis, or pharyngeal and oesophageal strictures.

As time passes, healing tends to become more and more sluggish, and by the second year of life, where the child survives, the disease is often typified by the development of more or less extensive areas of non-healing ulceration. These are perhaps most characteristically seen around the mouth and nose (Figure 4.10). Chronic paronychia with nail loss is another highly

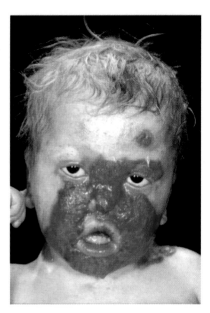

Figure 4.10 *Junctional epidermolysis bullosa*

characteristic feature, which leads to a 'drumstick' appearance of the tips of the fingers and toes. The development of excessive granulation tissue in non-healing areas is a peculiarity of junctional epidermolysis bullosa, and is perhaps most obvious in association with smaller ulcerations.

Congenital pyloric stricture occurs in a small but significant number of infants with junctional epidermolysis bullosa, though it remains unclear whether this reflects genetic linkage of genes for junctional epidermolysis bullosa and pyloric atresia, the different manifestations of a single gene, or merely a tendency for junctional epidermolysis bullosa to cause damage to the pyloric area in utero[1].

The disease is serious because of its tendency to affect the larynx. Many babies with junctional epidermolysis bullosa become hoarse very early in life; indeed the appearance of this symptom seems to be one of the few reliable features that allow a clinical distinction to be made between junctional and dystrophic epidermolysis bullosa in the first weeks of life. Hoarseness is usually followed by recurrent bouts of stridor, each of which carries a serious risk of fatal asphyxiation. This laryngeal disease is probably the principal cause of death in junctional epidermolysis bullosa.

Another distinctive feature of 'lethal' junctional epidermolysis bullosa is the early appearance of profound failure to thrive. The development of this complication of the disease has ominous significance for the infant as it tends to fail to respond to all attempts at correction, including the use of nasogastric hyperalimentation.

As in severe dystrophic epidermolysis bullosa, a degree of anaemia is common. In some cases this is severe. As in dystrophic epidermolysis bullosa, the pattern is a mixture of iron deficiency anaemia and 'anaemia of chronic disease'.

As in dystrophic epidermolysis bullosa, anal fissuring, faecal retention and constipation are common.

Rapid dental degeneration is the rule. Dental enamel hypoplasia appears to be common in junctional epidermolysis bullosa, and the resulting development of caries is accelerated by the dietary preference of affected children for foods and drinks with a high sucrose content.

Ocular disease similar to that described in dystrophic epidermolysis bullosa may occur.

Urethral and ureteral strictures have also been observed in patients with junctional epidermolysis bullosa, almost certainly secondary to direct involvement of the urethral and bladder epithelia by the disease. Interestingly, genitourinary involvement has been more prominent in those children who also had congenital pyloric strictures.

Benign type junctional epidermolysis bullosa

The early clinical course of individuals with the benign type of junctional epidermolysis bullosa seems to be similar to that of children with lethal junctional epidermolysis bullosa[2], although the development of excessive granulation tissue, growth failure and anaemia seems to be less prominent. The patient survives through early childhood, with a gradually decreasing tendency to develop new blisters. Non-healing areas may remain a lifelong problem for such patients.

Areas of previous blistering show a variable degree of atrophy, and both nail dystrophy and scarring alopecia are prominent sequelae of previous blistering and ulceration.

Distinction of the 'lethal' and 'benign' types of junctional epidermolysis bullosa is complicated by the reported death in early infancy of some of the siblings of patients with the clinically 'benign' type[2].

Pathology

In junctional epidermolysis bullosa, separation of the epithelium occurs between the lamina densa of the basement membrane and the basal keratinocytes, i.e. through the lamina lucida. Hemidesmosomes are believed to have a role in bonding these two structures. A reduction in the numbers of ultrastructurally visible hemidesmosomes, which are also usually structurally abnormal, is generally present in children with the Herlitz type of junctional epidermolysis bullosa, and in a proportion of those with non-Herlitz junctional epidermolysis bullosa[3]. However, these structures may be present in normal numbers and with apparently normal morphology in a small proportion of children with Herlitz type junctional epidermolysis bullosa, and in greater numbers in those with more benign forms of the disease.

In junctional epidermolysis bullosa, reduced basement membrane zone binding of a monoclonal antibody, GB3, has been demonstrated[4].

It has emerged that though GB3 antibody does not label the basement membrane zone in Herlitz junctional epidermolysis bullosa, it may do so in individuals with more benign variants of junctional epidermolysis bullosa and may therefore have some prognostic value. It has now been shown that GB3 binds to laminin 5, a constituent of the anchoring filaments that are a component of the hemidesmosome complex.

Exactly what is happening pathologically in the larynx is uncertain, but blistering on the edges of the cords is probably followed by the development of granulations, and eventually by squamous metaplasia and the resulting development of mucous retention cysts[5].

The pathological basis for the profound failure to thrive observed in many babies remains unclear, though involvement of the gastrointestinal tract with resulting malabsorption and/or protein loss might play a part.

Genetics

All types of junctional epidermolysis bullosa are transmitted as autosomal recessive traits. The different phenotypes of junctional epidermolysis bullosa are caused by mutations: in the genes *LAMA3*, *LAMB3* and *LAMC2* encoding for laminin 5[6]; in the gene for the integrin β4 subunit associated with junctional epidermolysis bullosa and pyloric atresia[7] and in the gene for bullous pemphigoid antigen (*BPAG2*) in a patient with generalized atrophic benign epidermolysis bullosa[8].

Differential diagnosis

The only point at which differential diagnosis may present some difficulty is in the neonatal period. This problem is discussed above under dystrophic epidermolysis bullosa.

Treatment

As for other forms of epidermolysis bullosa, specific treatment is not available, and there is no evidence that patients benefit from the administration of any systemic therapy other than nutritional supplements.

General skin care, and the management of complications such as constipation, malnutrition, ocular disease and anaemia, are essentially the same as in the case of dystrophic epidermolysis bullosa.

Patients with junctional epidermolysis bullosa usually tolerate a less liquid diet and, because there is much less mucosal scarring, the teeth are more accessible to the dentist. A normal conservative approach to dental treatment is therefore both more necessary and feasible.

Autologous epidermal grafts have been successfully used for the treatment of chronic facial ulceration in junctional epidermolysis bullosa[9]. These lesions have been treated in a child with junctional epidermolysis bullosa using keratinocyte allografts grown from healthy donors. Perhaps the major problem in treating lesions of this type is to prevent traumatization of the grafts once they have been positioned; this can be done by the use of a suitable 'helmet', particularly at night.

In the author's unit, humidification of inspired air has been found to be valuable in babies with subacute stridor. The onset of acute laryngeal obstruction in these cases is possibly more likely to reflect the development of granulations on the vocal cords than intact blisters, and more intense stridor is therefore treated by inhalation of nebulized racemic adrenaline (racepinephrine) 0.5 ml in 2 ml normal saline (Vaponephrin, limited supplies available from Fisons Pharmaceuticals, Loughborough, UK, for named patients) and corticosteroids, such as beclomethasone dipropionate 100 µg (Becotide suspension, Allen & Hanburys, Greenford, UK), both as often as 2-hourly.

Although it would be helpful to know the precise cause of the obstruction, laryngoscopy is not routinely undertaken because this would require the clinician to be prepared if necessary both to intubate the patient in emergency, and to undertake tracheostomy later. Tracheostomies have been found to be too difficult to maintain in babies with junctional epidermolysis bullosa because of the ulceration that occurs at the insertion of the tube and along the line of the ties used to hold it in place. Therefore, because of the increased morbidity associated with this procedure, it is never undertaken.

The recent advances in molecular genetics for both dystrophic and junctional epidermolysis bullosa have provided the basis for DNA-based prenatal diagnosis during the first trimester of gestation, and sets the stage for the application of gene therapy to these devastating skin diseases in the future.

References

1 Hayashi AH, Galliani CA, Gillis DA. Congenital pyloric atresia and junctional epidermolysis bullosa: a report of long-term survival and a review of the literature. *J Pediatr Surg* 1991; **26**: 1341–5.

2 Paller AS, Fine J-D, Kaplan S, Pearson RW. The generalised atrophic benign form of junctional epidermolysis bullosa. *Arch Dermatol* 1986; **12**: 704–10.

3 Tidman MJ, Eady RAJ. Hemidesmosome heterogeneity in junctional epidermolysis bullosa revealed by morphometric analysis. *J Invest Dermatol* 1986; **86**: 51–6.

4 Heagerty AHM, Kennedy AR, Eady RAJ et al. GB3 monoclonal antibody for diagnosis of junctional epidermolysis bullosa. *Lancet* 1986; **1**: 860.

5 Davies H, Atherton DJ. Acute laryngeal obstruction in junctional epidermolysis bullosa. *Pediatr Dermatol* 1987; **4**: 98–101.

6 Kivirikko S et al. A homozygous nonsense mutation in the alpha 3 chain gene of laminin 5 (LAMA3) in lethal (Herlitz) junctional epidermolysis bullosa. *Hum Mol Genet* 1995; **4**: 959–62.

7 Vidal F et al. Mutations in the gene for the integrin β4 subunit are associated with junctional epidermolysis bullosa and pyloric atresia. *Nature Genet* 1995; **10**: 229–34.

8 McGrath JA, Gatalica B, Christiano AM et al. Mutations in the bullous pemphigoid antigen (BPAG2), a hemidesmosomal transmembrane collagen (COL17A1), in generalized atrophic benign epidermolysis bullosa. *Nature Genet* 1995; **11**: 83–6.

Chapter 5

The ichthyoses

M. R. Judge and J. I. Harper

Introduction

The term 'ichthyosis' describes dry, rough skin with persistent visible scaling, which may resemble fish scales (Greek *ichthys*, fish). The condition results from a disorder of keratinization or cornification, associated with abnormal epidermal differentiation and desquamation. The histopathological changes in ichthyosis are most obvious in the stratum corneum of the epidermis, but some cases show changes in the granular and basal layers. Inflammatory ichthyoses are associated with a cellular infiltrate in the dermis.

The hereditary ichthyoses are a large and heterogeneous group of disorders comprising primary ichthyotic diseases and a number of multisystem ichthyosiform syndromes (Table 5.1). They range from the barely noticeable scaling of mild ichthyosis vulgaris to florid scaling and erythroderma in non-bullous ichthyosiform erythroderma. Blistering occurs in bullous ichthyosis, and harlequin ichthyosis is often lethal.

The more severe recessive forms of ichthyosis may present as a collodion baby at birth. The majority of these develop non-bullous ichthyosiform erythroderma or lamellar ichthyosis. Rarely trichothiodystrophy, neutral lipid storage disease, Conradi–Hünermann syndrome or Gaucher's disease ensues[1]. However, 10% of collodion babies subsequently have a good outlook, with only mild, dry, scaly skin or limited areas of hyperkeratosis[2] (Figure 5.1).

The treatment of mild ichthyosis includes the application of emollients and keratolytic agents. For the more severe forms the retinoid drug etretinate has revolutionized the lives of many affected children[3]

and has improved the survival of the harlequin fetus. Etretinate (Tigason) has now been superseded by its major active metabolite, acitretin (Neotigason), which has a shorter half-life of 50–60 hours compared with 120 days for etretinate[4].

References

1 Lui K, Commens C, Choong R, Jaworski R. Collodion babies with Gauchers disease. *Arch Dis Child* 1988; **63**: 854–6.
2 Frenk E. Spontaneously healing collodion baby: a light and electron microscopical study. *Acta Derm Venereol* 1981; **61**: 168–71.
3 Paige DG, Judge MR, Shaw DG, Atherton DJ, Harper JI. Bone changes and their significance in children with ichthyosis on longterm etretinate therapy. *Br J Dermatol* 1992; **127**: 387–91.
4 Pilkington T, Brogden RN. Acitretin. A review of its pharmacology and therapeutic use. *Drugs* 1992; **43** (4): 597–627.

Ichthyosis vulgaris

Definition

Ichthyosis vulgaris (IV) is the most common of the hereditary ichthyoses, with an incidence of approximately 1 in 250 people[1]. It may be mild, clearing completely in the summer months, or severe enough to be a troublesome problem year-round. There is an association with atopy in up to 50% of individuals[2].

Table 5.1 *The ichthyoses*

Ichthyosis vulgaris
X-linked ichthyosis
Non-bullous ichthyosiform erythroderma
Lamellar ichthyosis
Bullous ichthyosiform erythroderma
Ichthyosis hystrix
Harlequin ichthyosis
Netherton's syndrome
Sjögren–Larsson syndrome
Refsum's disease
Keratitis–ichthyosis–deafness (KID) syndrome
Trichothiodystrophies (IBIDS, PIBIDS, Tay's
    syndrome)
Conradi-Hünermann syndrome
Neutral–lipid storage disease (Chanarin–Dorfman
    syndrome)
Other ichthyotic disorders
    CHILD syndrome
    Multiple sulphatase deficiency
    Ichthyosis follicularis with alopecia and
    photophobia (IFAP)
    Familial peeling skin syndrome
Isolated genetic disorders with ichthyosis
    Ichthyosis associated with renal disease
    Congenital ichthyosis with neural deafness
    Ichthyosis associated with other neurological
    disorders
    Ichthyosis and skeletal defects
    Ichthyosis with immune defects
    Miscellaneous

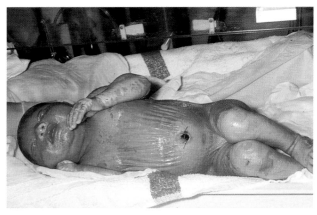

Figure 5.1 *Collodion baby born within a tight membrane which was shed within the first weeks of life. Although collodion membrane may precede the development of severe recessive ichthyosis, this girl now has only residual mildly dry, scaly skin*

Clinical features

The skin may be dry and scaly from the neonatal period, but more usually scaling is obvious from 2 months onwards and it may be delayed until childhood. The scale is white, small, light and flaky, and is most pronounced on the extensor surfaces of the arms and lower legs, characteristically sparing the flexural creases. The trunk, especially the abdominal wall, is often mildly affected. Facial scaling and involvement of the pinnae are sometimes seen. The palms and soles are usually free of scale but palmoplantar hyperlinearity, a reflection of mild hyperkeratosis, is a feature of IV patients, whether they have coexistent eczema or not. It may also be seen in patients with atopic eczema alone[3,4].

Symptoms of IV are few and limited to complaints of dryness and roughness of the skin. In isolated IV pruritus is not a problem, but in patients who also have eczema, flexural lichenification and pruritus with excoriation are additional features. Ichthyosis vulgaris shows a marked seasonal variation in most patients, improving in warm and sunny weather, probably as a result of ambient humidity. Many sufferers report a gradual improvement in adolescence, though a small number actually worsen with age.

Pathology

Histological examination of affected skin shows a mild hyperkeratosis and, usually, a diminished or absent granular layer in the epidermis. Electron microscopy reveals scanty and fragmented keratohyalin granules in the granular cells, whereas the keratin filaments appear normal.

Biochemical studies indicated that, in affected skin only, uptake of radiolabelled histidine by the granular layer was reduced[5]. Histidine is important in the synthesis of profilaggrin, a major component of the keratohyalin granule and necessary for keratin filament assembly. Cultured keratinocytes from affected skin in IV patients failed to react to monoclonal antibody to filaggrin, and electron microscopy showed an absence of keratohyalin granules[6]. Filaggrin synthesis is indeed reduced but keratin filaments are formed and, to date, it is not known what role this defect in epidermal protein metabolism plays in the pathogenesis of the ichthyosis. Amino acid breakdown products of filaggrin have the ability to retain water in the outer stratum corneum, and their deficiency may contribute to the scaling. No consistent lipid abnormality has yet been found in IV, although total ceramide content is reduced in the stratum corneum in atopic eczema[7].

Genetics

Ichthyosis vulgaris is an autosomal dominant disorder with variable penetrance such that disease severity can vary between generations and affected siblings. Atopic eczema in many families also follows an autosomal dominant pattern, although its expression may be polygenic. When both conditions are combined it is likely that gene linkage or contiguous gene defects are responsible.

References

1 Wells RS, Kerr CB. Clinical features of autosomal dominant and sex-linked ichthyosis in an English population. *Br Med J* 1966; **1**: 947–50.
2 Kuokkanen K. Ichthyosis vulgaris: a clinical and histopathological study of patients and their close relatives in the autosomal dominant and sex-linked forms of the disease. *Acta Derm Venereol* 1969; **49** (suppl. 62): 1–4.
3 Uehara M, Hayashi S. Hyperlinear palms. *Arch Dermatol* 1981; **117**: 490–1.
4 Mevorah B, Marazzi A, Frenk E. The prevalence of accentuated palmoplantar markings and keratosis pilaris in atopic dermatitis, autosomal dominant ichthyosis and control dermatological patients. *Br J Dermatol* 1985; **112**: 679–85.
5 Dale BA, Sybert VP, Holbrook KA. Ichthyosis vulgaris: identification of a defect in the synthesis of filaggrin correlated with an absence of keratohyaline granules. *J Invest Dermatol* 1984; **19**: 191–4.
6 Fleckman P, Holbrook KA, Dale BA, Sybert VP. Keratinocytes cultured from subjects with ichthyosis vulgaris are phenotypically abnormal. *J Invest Dermatol* 1987; **88**: 640–5.
7 Imokawa G, Abe A, Jin K et al. Decreased levels of ceramides in stratum corneum of atopic dermatitis: an aetiologic factor in atopic dry skin? *J Invest Dermatol* 1991; **96**: 523–6.

X-linked ichthyosis

Definition

Wells and Kerr[1] differentiated X-linked ichthyosis (XLI) from ichthyosis vulgaris in 1966, and the former condition is now recognized to be associated with steroid sulphatase deficiency. Of clinical significance is the association of XLI with important extracutaneous manifestations and with potential perinatal complications.

Clinical features

In the UK, the incidence of XLI is approximately 1 in 6000[1]. Only males manifest the ichthyosis, while carrier females are generally asymptomatic. The disorder has a worldwide distribution.

In many cases scaling is evident within the first 2 weeks of life, although parents may describe it as 'redness' and 'peeling' at this stage and may not become aware of persistent scaling until some months later. In a significant number (10 out of 25 patients in a personal series), a history of delayed onset of scaling from the age of 3 months to 5 years of age was elicited.

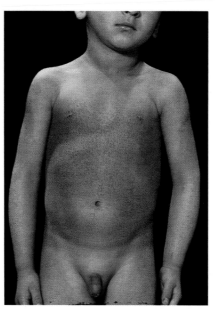

Figure 5.2 *X-linked ichthyosis in a boy with prominent dark scaling*

However, a prospective study of 21 patients in Denmark revealed onset of light flaky scaling before 1 month with more typical scale by 6 months in all but 2 children[2]. The scaling of XLI increases throughout childhood, often spreading up from the lower legs to the trunk. It stabilizes in the teenage years with little subsequent change. In most patients scaling improves markedly in the summer months.

Scaling in XLI is most prominent on the extensor surfaces of the upper arms, the outer thighs and around the lower legs. The scale is medium to large, polygonal, adherent, dull and usually light-brown in colour. The posterior and lateral neck, upper and lateral abdominal wall and preauricular facial skin are often affected (Figure 5.2). In more severe cases, the face, scalp, axillae, flexor aspects of the limbs and dorsal surfaces of hands and feet may be involved, but the palms and soles are spared.

Extracutaneous features

An increased incidence of testicular maldescent, cryptorchidism, abnormalities of sperm count or motility and testicular cancer have been reported in patients with XLI[3]. Inguinal hernias are often noted.

Rarely, XLI is associated with hypogonadotropic hypogonadism, anosmia and a variety of neurological defects, including nystagmus and mirror movements of the hands and feet, which together constitute Kallmann's syndrome. These associations are presumed to arise because of variable large deletions of the short arm of the X chromosome. Rud's syndrome was said to comprise X-linked ichthyosis, obesity, hypogonadism and mental retardation with a variety of other features in some reported cases. However, its existence as a separate entity is in doubt, and the associated features can (in some instances at least) be ascribed to complications of a difficult labour or to a hypogonadotrophic state.

Corneal opacities, detected with the slit-lamp microscope, occur in up to 50% of patients and in 24% of female carriers, but are apparently of no functional significance. They were thought to be due to deposits on the posterior surface of Descemet's membrane, but a recent study raised the possibility of a physicochemical effect of cholesterol sulphate on the cornea[4]. An increased incidence of apparently unassociated congenital defects was noted by the authors in a group of XLI patients, including skeletal dysplasia with spangled hair in one patient.

Perinatal manifestations of steroid sulphatase deficiency

It was noted in the 1970s that low maternal urinary oestriol excretion in the third trimester of pregnancy was not invariably associated with intrauterine growth retardation. The male offspring were often healthy and well-developed, and when followed they developed ichthyosis. Some had suffered perinatal complications as a result of a difficult, prolonged labour[5]. The underlying defect, placental steroid sulphatase deficiency, was identified, and coincidentally steroid sulphatase deficiency was noted in boys with XLI. Jobsis linked the two conditions in 1976[6].

In the authors' group of 25 XLI patients, 8 were born after labours exceeding 8 hours and in 2 cases labour continued for 36 hours or more. Two had suffered neurological damage, apparently as a result of problems in delivery.

Pathology

Biopsy of affected skin in XLI shows an expanded stratum corneum without parakeratosis or acanthosis. The granular cell layer is usually normal but may be mildly thickened or even (rarely) absent, which makes histologic differentiation from ichthyosis vulgaris difficult. The keratohyalin granules are normal on electron microscopy in contrast to ichthyosis vulgaris but desmosomes are more persistent than normal[7]. Kinetic studies have shown normal rates of cell turnover.

Biochemical basis of XLI

Steroid sulphatase deficiency was identified in 1976 as the cause both of placental sulphatase deficiency and X-linked ichthyosis[5]. In fact fibroblasts, leucocytes, lymphocytes, hair root epithelium, nail matrix and amniocytes can all be assayed and reveal the enzyme deficiency.

Steroid or cholesterol sulphatase is an isomer of aryl sulphatase C and one of a large group of microsomal enzymes responsible for hydrolysing sulphate groups from, in this case, cholesterol sulphate. However, the sulphated forms of other steroid sex hormones such as pregnenolone, 17-hydroxyprogesterone, progesterone, dehydroepiandrosterone and 5-androsterone are also increased. Testosterone sulphate is reduced but testosterone levels are normal, as its synthesis can be mediated by a desaturase enzyme system. Pituitary gonadotrophins and prolactin are normal. The altered sex hormone profile may in part explain the abnormal testicular development in some XLI patients.

Pathogenesis of scaling

Evidence of a direct causal link between elevated cholesterol sulphate levels and scaling is accumulating. Topical application of cholesterol sulphate in the hairless mouse induced a reversible retention ichthyosis and a threefold increase in stratum corneum thickness after 1 week. The scaling cleared within 3 days of stopping the treatment and did not occur if other sulphated substrates of the enzyme were applied. Topical cholesterol prevented this effect and also temporarily reduced the scaling of XLI but not of other ichthyoses. Many cholesterol-lowering drugs have caused ichthyosis as a side-effect[8].

Lipid analysis of normal epidermis shows a gradual decline in the cholesterol sulphate content from a level of 6% in the granular layer to 3% in the stratum corneum. A concomitant rise in cholesterol which triggers lipid bilayer disintegration reflects the increasing activity of steroid sulphatase, which reaches its maximum concentration in the inner stratum corneum membranes. In XLI steroid sulphatase is absent in all layers of the epidermis and cholesterol sulphate content ranges from 12% to 30% in stratum corneum lipids.

Calorimetric studies have identified a failure of the normal liquid–crystalline transition phase in the stratum corneum intercellular lipids in XLI, presumably due to the polar subgroups of cholesterol sulphate[9]. This provides strong evidence for the central role played by abnormal lipid metabolism in the induction of scaling in certain ichthyoses.

Investigation

Increased serum cholesterol sulphate in patients with XLI can be detected on a serum lipoprotein electrophoresis strip[10]. Cholesterol sulphate carries a stronger electronegative charge than cholesterol, resulting in an increased mobility of the beta low-density lipoprotein fraction towards the anode. This simple screening test requires an experienced eye to detect the often subtle change. A more specific diagnostic test is assay of steroid sulphatase activity in leucocytes or skin fibroblasts, which is available in selected research centres. Serum cholesterol levels are normal in XLI as the main cholesterol biosynthetic enzyme, hydroxymethylglutamyl-CoA reductase, is unaffected.

Carrier detection

Corneal stromal deposits have been detected on slit-lamp examination in a proportion of carriers, and it has been claimed that carriers have an increased incidence of xerosis and mild scaling.

Lipoprotein electrophoresis is normal in obligatory female carriers. It has been reported that steroid sulphatase levels in leucocytes, fibroblasts or hair roots are higher in normal females than in normal males because the Lyon effect (inactivation of one X chromosome in normal female cells) does not apply to the steroid sulphatase gene. This should be of help in detecting female carriers of the XLI gene since they would be expected to have 50% of the steroid sulphatase values of non-carrier females. Lykkesfeldt reported that 30 of 31 carriers had a leucocyte steroid sulphatase level below the 2.5 percentile of normal females, indicating gene heterozygosity[11]. In practice, partial X inactivation seems to occur, and other studies have yielded enzyme values in the range 40–86% in different tissues in known carriers. Leucocyte steroid sulphatase assay, using oestrone sulphate as substrate, is probably the most reliable biochemical test for heterozygote detection, but is by no means always clear-cut.

Some authorities prefer visual assessment of stained hair roots to detect steroid sulphatase. Each hair root represents a clonal proliferation of an epithelial cell which either stains positively where there is partial or no inactivation, or negatively where inactivation of the normal X chromosome has occurred with absence of steroid sulphatase expression in that clone.

Bonifas reported on the success of Southern blot hybridization of leucocyte DNA in diagnosing suspected carriers[12]. This provides an accurate measure of the 50% gene dosage of steroid sulphatase in carriers, but is applicable only in the 90% of XLI families who have a complete deletion of the steroid sulphatase gene.

Genetics

The linkage of XLI and the Xg red blood cell marker in the 1960s was an early example of chromosome localization by tracking linked traits in family studies[13]. The rare association of XLI with a variety of congenital defects such as stunted growth, hypogonadism and loss of olfaction has enabled mapping of the relevant genes on the short arm of the X chromosome.

Gene mapping in families with X to Y translocations helped to place the steroid sulphatase gene at the distal tip (Xp) of the short arm of the X chromosome at the Xp22.3 locus[14]. It is close to the pseudoautosomal region of the X chromosome and contiguous with the genes that regulate olfaction. A partial deletion of the distal short arm of the X chromosome has been noted in patients with related disorders such as Kallmann's syndrome and chondrodysplasia punctata.

The absence of immunoreactive steroid sulphatase in the great majority of XLI patients implies a gene defect and this is borne out by the absence of lymphocyte DNA hybridization to steroid sulphatase cDNA probes[15]. Southern blot analysis of genomic DNA shows absence of steroid sulphatase gene common core sequences in 89% of XLI patients from 45 families, and a large deletion of up to 2 megabases was calculated in studies using a range of DNA probes. There is considerable genetic heterogeneity between XLI families with often sizeable DNA loss detected by flow cytometry (up to 3.4%)[16] in some and in other cases evidence of X–Y translocations[17].

Isolated X-linked ichthyosis is generally a mild disease, though cosmetically troublesome, and few families would in retrospect have been interested in prenatal diagnosis. However, placental steroid sulphatase deficiency is a risk factor in affected pregnancies and highlights the importance of identifying carrier females in affected families so that they can be forewarned of possible perinatal complications. The rare associated syndromes such as Kallmann's syndrome are more significant and in these families genetic counselling, heterozygote detection and (if requested) prenatal diagnosis – maternal urinary oestriol levels or chorionic villus sampling for steroid sulphatase assay – are indicated[18].

References

1 Wells RS, Kerr CB. Clinical features of autosomal dominant and sex-linked ichthyosis in an English population. *Br Med Journal* 1966; **1**: 947–50.

2 Hyer H, Lykkesfeldt G, Ibsen HH, Brandrup F. Ichthyosis of steroid sulphatase deficiency. Clinical study of 76 cases. *Dermatologica* 1986; **172**: 184–90.

3 Lykkesfeldt G, Lykkesfeldt AE, Hoyer H, Skakkebaek NE. Steroid sulphatase deficiency associated with testis cancer. *Lancet* 1983; **ii**: 1456.

4 Costagliola C, Fabbrocini G, Illiano GM, Scibelli G, Delfino M. Ocular findings in X-linked ichthyosis: a survey of 38 cases. *Ophthalmologica* 1991; **202**: 152–5.

5 Traupe H, Happle R. Clinical spectrum of steroid sulphatase deficiency: X-linked ichthyosis, birth complications and cryptorchidism. *Eur J Pediatr* 1983; **140**: 19–21.

6 Jobsis AC, van Duuren CY, van de Vries GP et al. Trophoblast sulphatase deficiency associated with X-chromosomal ichthyosis. *Ned Tijdschr Geneeskd* 1976; **120**: 1980.

7 Anton-Lamprecht I, Hofbauer M. Ultrastructural distinction of autosomal dominant ichthyosis vulgaris and X-linked recessive ichthyosis. *Hum Genet* 1972; **15**: 261–4.

8 Winklemann RK, Perry HO, Achor RWP et al. Cutaneous syndromes produced as side effects of triparanol therapy. *Arch Dermatol* 1963; **87**: 372–7.

9 Elias PM, Williams ML, Maloney ME et al. Stratum corneum lipids in disorders of cornification: steroid sulphatase and cholesterol sulphate in normal desquamation and the pathogenesis of recessive X-linked ichthyosis. *J Clin Invest* 1984; **74**: 1414–21.

10 Epstein EH, Krauss RM, Schackleton CHL. X-linked ichthyosis: increased blood cholesterol sulfate and electrophoretic mobility of low density lipoprotein. *Science* 1981; **214**: 659–60.

11 Lykkesfeldt G, Lykkesfeldt AE. Carrier identification in steroid sulphatase deficiency and recessive X-linked ichthyosis. *Acta Derm Venereol* 1986; **66**: 134–8.

12 Bonifas JM, Epstein EH. Detection of carriers for X-linked ichthyosis by Southern blot analysis and identification of one family with a de novo mutation. *J Invest Dermatol* 1990; **95**: 16–19.

13 Adam A, Ziprkowski L, Feinstein A et al. Linkage relations of X-borne ichthyosis to the Xg blood group. *Ann Hum Genet* 1969; **32**: 323–32.

14 Tiepolo L, Zuffardi O, Fraccaro M et al. Assignment by deletion mapping of the steroid sulphatase X-linked ichthyosis locus to Xp 223. *Hum Genet* 1980; **54**: 205–6.

15 Yen PH, Allen E, Marsh B et al. Cloning and expression of steroid sulphatase cDNA and frequent occurrence of deletions in STS deficiency: implications for X-Y interchange. *Cell* 1987; **49**: 443–54.

16 Cooke A, Gillard EF, Yates JRW et al. X-chromosome deletions detectable by flow cytometry in some patients with steroid sulphatase deficiency (X-linked ichthyosis). *Hum Genet* 1988; **79**: 49–52.

17 Ballabio A, Carrozzo R, Parenti G et al. Molecular heterogeneity of steroid sulphatase deficiency. *Genomics* 1989; **4** (1): 36–40.

18 Paige DG, Emilion GG, Bouloux PMG, Harper JI. A clinical and genetic study of X-linked ichthyosis and contiguous gene defects. *Br J Dermatol* 1994; **131**: 622–9.

Non-bullous ichthyosiform erythroderma

Definition

Non-bullous ichthyosiform erythroderma (NBIE) is a usually severe inflammatory ichthyosis, with an incidence of approximately 1 in 300 000. It occurs in all races, especially in groups where consanguineous marriage is common.

Clinical features

In over 90% of cases, NBIE presents at birth as a collodion baby, with a yellow, glistening membrane resembling sausage skin, which envelops the neonate; it produces ectropion and sometimes lip eversion and nasal obstruction. The membrane soon dries and cracks. The small number in whom this is not a recorded feature are erythrodermic from birth and

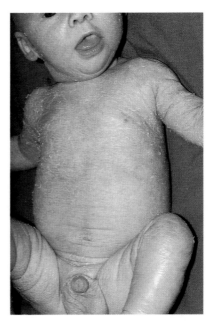

Figure 5.3 *Non-bullous ichthyosiform erythroderma*

some are significantly premature. Shedding of the collodion membrane within the first few weeks of life reveals persistent, generalized scaly erythroderma (Figure 5.3). Presentation as a collodion baby may precede other rarer forms of ichthyosis[1].

Erythroderma generally lessens in childhood. Scaling can affect all areas including the scalp, ears, face, flexures, palms and soles. The scales of NBIE are white or grey, light, superficial and semiadherent. They appear feathery on the face, arms and trunk, but may be lamellar or plate-like on the lower legs. Scaling may be cyclical with build-up and shedding over periods of 2–4 weeks. Palmoplantar hyperkeratosis occurs in 70% of patients; if severe, it can cause recurrent painful fissures, digital contractures and loss of pulp volume. Scalp involvement often causes tinea amiantacea, and may lead to patchy cicatricial alopecia.

Ectropion improves during infancy but may persist into adult life and, if untreated, carries the risk of exposure keratitis and blindness[2]. The loss of eyebrows and lashes in severe cases accentuates the ocular problem. Hypoplasia of the nasal and aural cartilages may occur as a result of compression and scarring, and the resultant deformity increases the cosmetic burden on these patients.

A mild nail dystrophy consisting of ridging, subungual hyperkeratosis or hypoplasia occurs in up to 50% of patients, but hair, teeth and mucosal surfaces are normal. Nail growth and skin healing are rapid. In most patients sweating is compromised and markedly reduced from infancy onwards; care is needed to avoid hyperpyrexia during intercurrent illness, leisure pursuits or in hot climates. Sweat gland function may partially recover in adolescence and has been observed in patients treated with retinoids. Pruritus is often a feature of NBIE.

Less severely affected patients may present with either an intertrigo-like pattern or scant, light scale and mild palmar hyperkeratosis. Subtle facial tautness and accentuated skin lines may persist into childhood.

Many affected children are of short stature but most catch up with a delayed growth spurt in adolescence. The disorder may limit a child's ability to take part in sports, but if encouraged, most of these children enjoy swimming and less vigorous activities. Psychological problems often arise at school because of insensitive comments and reactions of others. However, in general children with NBIE seem to cope remarkably well with their disability and academically achieve on a par with their peers. Career advice and continuing support assist young adults in adjusting to the occupational and social problems arising from the chronic skin disease.

Pathology

Light microscopy of skin sections reveals a variable hyperkeratosis, mild parakeratosis and acanthosis with a normal or reduced granular layer. There is usually a mild lymphocytic infiltrate and prominent blood vessels may be present in the dermis. Periodic, acid–schiff (PAS) staining of frozen sections shows characteristic staining of cell membranes in the stratum corneum and granular layer and in the basement membrane[3]; PAS bonds with glycoconjugates in cell membranes and staining is absent in normal skin and in other ichthyoses, with the possible exception of Netherton's syndrome.

Electron microscopy may show increased mitotic activity, slightly reduced levels of keratohyalin and tonofilaments, and lipid vacuolation in the stratum corneum. German and Swedish groups have defined subtypes 1–5 of 'ichthyosis congenita' based on skin ultrastructural findings, but these subtypes do not correlate closely to recognized clinical phenotypes and their use in specific diagnosis is, thus far, limited [4–6].

Kinetic studies, using labelled thymidine, confirm an increased epidermal turnover rate in NBIE similar to the 7-day cycle of psoriasis and in contrast to the normal epidermal kinetics of lamellar ichthyosis[7].

Biochemical studies

Williams and Elias reported that lipid analysis of untreated skin scale from patients with NBIE consistently yielded an excess of the saturated hydrocarbon group, *n*-alkanes[8]. These accounted for up to 25% of total scale lipids compared to an average of 5% in normal skin scale and 7% in patients with lamellar ichthyosis. Topical application of alkanes to normal epidermis induced scaling, erythema and increased epidermal turnover rate. However, alkanes are breakdown products of petroleum chemicals and are prevalent in the environment and in petroleum-containing emollients. Carbon-dating of skin alkanes revealed a half-life of 30 000 years or more, indicating that they could not have been synthesized in the epidermis[9]. This finding led to the suggestion that skin alkanes are merely contaminants and of no significance in the pathogenesis of ichthyosis. Work in the authors' unit has shown that although alkane levels were raised in certain hereditary ichthyoses, this measurement was neither sensitive nor specific for any one type[10].

Stratum corneum enzyme studies highlight differences between NBIE and other autosomal recessive ichthyoses. In NBIE scale, the lamellar body enzyme beta-glucosidase was reduced while butyrase levels were maintained[11].

Genetics

Classical NBIE is an autosomal recessive condition but there has been one report of a similar condition occurring in a mother and 2 of her children[12]. In the authors' group of 25 NBIE patients, 5 had affected siblings, and a sixth, an Indian child from a consanguineous family, had 2 affected cousins with similar mild NBIE. In all, 7 patients (of whom 3 were Caucasian) were the offspring of consanguineous parents.

In consanguineous families genetic counselling is straightforward and prenatal diagnosis can be discussed with parents of severely affected cases. However, in the absence of a positive family history, a risk of further affected children of 1 in 4 for each child is given, and affected individuals will not have affected children although half of their offspring may be carriers. The proband may, however, represent a sporadic mutation with no adverse implications for subsequent pregnancies, and the possibility of dominant transmission must be borne in mind[12].

Prenatal diagnosis by fetal skin biopsy at 20–22 weeks is far from satisfactory for two reasons. Phenotypic heterogeneity can exist between members of the same family so that the severity of disease in the proband may not reflect that of the affected fetus; and secondly, prenatal second-trimester skin biopsy to detect premature keratinization is not always reliable[13]. Specific ultrastructural or biochemical changes in a proband may be used in the future to improve the sensitivity of prenatal testing, but these features are not sensitive enough at present.

References

1 Larregue M, Ottavy N, Bressieux JM, Lorette J. Bébé collodion: trente-deux nouvelles observations. *Ann Derm Venereol* 1986; **113**: 773–85.

2 Murdoch ME, Judge MR, Dowd P. Non-bullous ichthyosiform erythroderma: response to etretinate therapy. *Br J Dermatol* 1991; **125**: 62–4.

3 Williams ML, Elias PM. Heterogeneity in autosomal recessive ichthyosis. *Arch Dermatol* 1985; **121**: 477–88.

4 Hazell M, Marks R. Clinical, histologic and cell kinetic discriminants between lamellar ichthyosis and non-bullous congenital ichthyosiform erythroderma. *Arch Dermatol* 1985; **121**: 489–93.

5 Arnold ML, Anton-Lamprecht I. Problems in prenatal diagnosis of the ichthyosis congenita group. *Hum Genet* 1985; **71**: 301–11.

6 Niemi KM, Kanerva L, Kuokanen K. Recessive ichthyosis congenita, type 2. *Arch Dermatol Res* 1991; **283**: 211–18.

7 Arnold ML, Anton-Lamprecht I, Melz-Rothfuss B, Hart-schuh W. Ichthyosis congenita, type 3. *Arch Dermatol Res* 1988; **280**: 268–78.

8 Williams ML Elias PM. Elevated n-alkanes in congenital ichthyosiform erythroderma: phenotypic differentiation of two types of autosomal recessive ichthyosis. *J Clin Invest* 1984; **74**: 296–300.

9 Bortz JT, Wertz PW, Downing DT. The origin of alkanes found in human skin surface lipids. *J Invest Dermatol* 1989; **93**: 723–7.

10 Judge MR, Morse-Fisher N, Manku M, Harper JI. Quantification of n-alkanes in stratum corneum in the hereditary ichthyoses. *Br J Dermatol* 1992; **127**: 91–6.

11 Bergers M, Traupe H, Mier PD, Steijlen P, Happle R. Enzymatic distinction between two subgroups of autosomal recessive lamellar ichthyosis. *J Invest Dermatol* 1990; **4**: 407–12.

12 Rossmann–Ringdahl I, Anton-Lamprecht I, Swanbeck G. A mother and two children with non-bullous congenital ichthyosiform erythroderma. *Arch Dermatol* 1986; **122**: 559–64.

13 Holbrook KA, Dale BA, Williams ML et al. The expression of congenital ichthyosiform erythroderma in second trimester fetuses of the same family: morphologic and biochemical studies. *J Invest Dermatol* 1988; **91**: 521–31.

Lamellar ichthyosis

Definition

Lamellar ichthyosis (LI) is the less common of the two major autosomal recessive ichthyoses, with an incidence of approximately 1 in 600 000. It is generally a severe ichthyosis but, as with NBIE, mild forms do occur. The term 'lamellar ichthyosis' means different things to different people. In the early twentieth century lamellar ichthyosis implied any congenital ichthyosis excluding harlequin fetus. Then it was applied to the dry (non-bullous) type of congenital ichthyosiform erythroderma, and by the 1960s was also being used to describe the collodion baby. Many still use the term for all autosomal recessive ichthyoses, qualifying it by the prefixes 'erythrodermic' (ELI) or 'non-erythrodermic' (NELI), which correspond to the NBIE and LI categories recognized in the UK[1]. Citing evidence of clinical, histological and

biochemical heterogeneity in autosomal recessive ichthyosis, Williams and Elias supported the case for separating it into two distinct entities, congenital ichthyosiform erythroderma (CIE) and LI[2].

Traupe et al have described an autosomal dominant pattern of inheritance of LI (ADLI)[3].

Clinical features

At birth most affected infants present as collodion babies and after shedding show a less intense erythroderma than infants with NBIE, an important and persistent distinguishing feature. Scaling occurs within the first month of life and may affect the whole skin surface or localize to the scalp, abdomen and lower legs.

The scale in LI is usually plate-like, large, pigmented and firmly adherent (Figure 5.4). In severely affected individuals, focal intermittent shedding causes deep and painful fissures, especially around flexures and on the palms and soles. Limitation of joint movement and flexion contractures due to constriction bands and scarring may result.

Additional features in some patients are palmoplantar keratoderma, scarring alopecia, ectropion and hypoplastic aural and nasal cartilages. As in NBIE, hair, teeth and mucous membranes are not affected, and growth and intellectual ability are normal. Extracutaneous manifestations have not been reported. Severe forms of LI seldom improve with age, and psychological problems due to cosmetic effects and limited mobility can lead to isolation, depression and poor school performance.

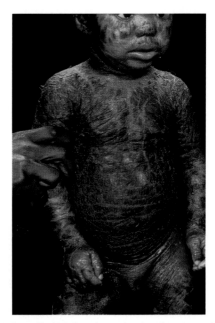

Figure 5.4 *Lamellar ichthyosis: severe involvement with large, plate-like scales*

Milder forms of LI occur[4]; in the authors' group of 4 affected children, all of whom were collodion babies, 2 fitted into this category, while the third was moderately and the fourth severely affected. In mild cases, typical large, brown, adherent scale was present on the lower legs, upper arms and, in one, on the forehead and lateral trunk. Fine, white, branny scales occurred on the flexures and neck. The patients were hypohidrotic, had normal palms and soles and their condition tended to improve in summer months. One had cycles of scale building up over 3 weeks before spontaneously shedding.

Erythroderma is absent or mild in LI. Pruritus rarely occurs and sweating is impaired. Ectropion may persist when the face is affected.

Autosomal dominant lamellar ichthyosis

Traupe et al outlined the clinical, ultrastructural and biochemical features of an ichthyosis that clinically resembled LI but showed an autosomal dominant transmission in 4 members, 2 male and 2 female, through three generations of a German family[3]. These patients had non-erythrodermic, lamellar-type, generalized scaling from birth, palmoplantar hyperkeratosis, and lichenification of the dorsal hands and feet and at the major flexures. They did not have a collodion membrane at birth and pruritus was a problem in one child, though none had signs of atopy. Other autosomal dominant ichthyoses were ruled out by ultrastructural examination of skin biopsies, and the light microscopical features were similar to those of classical LI.

Since then, reports of a similar disorder in separate families have appeared, though in these cases a collodion baby phenotype and subsequent mild erythroderma were notable features[5,6]. In Larregue's series of collodion babies, 10% were said to have developed ADLI but the disease phenotype was not clearly defined.

Pathology

Light microscopy of the skin in LI shows variable parakeratosis and massive orthohyperkeratosis with a stratum corneum thickness at least twice that of NBIE. The granular layer appears normal or increased and the remainder of the epidermis may be of normal thickness. Generally, epidermal structure resembles that of palmar or plantar skin, but there may be mild papillomatosis, extension and blunting of rete ridges and dilatation of dermal capillaries reminiscent of psoriasis.

Special histochemical stains, PAS, lectin binding for glycoconjugates and free-sterol localization, showed a staining pattern similar to that of normal skin[2]. On the other hand faint PAS positivity in the stratum corneum was noted by Traupe[1].

Electron microscopy features in LI are variable and do not match the recognized clinical variants. Niemi reported finding prominent cholesterol clefts and crystals in the stratum corneum, lipid droplets in corneocytes and thin or absent corneocyte envelopes in 7 kindred, at least some of whom had typical LI[7]. Arnold and Anton-Lamprecht's group examined skin biopsies from 9 patients with a reticulated form of recessive ichthyosis with features of both NBIE and LI[8]. They found cytoplasmic vacuoles, elongated membrane structures and abnormal vesicles within lamellar bodies and suggested that defective lipid metabolism caused the scaling disorder.

Kinetic studies surprisingly revealed a normal transit time in contrast to the hyperproliferative epidermis of NBIE and psoriasis, and LI is classified as a retention ichthyosis[9].

Biochemical studies

Scale lipid analysis in classical severe LI by the Williams group showed a mild but significant rise in levels of sphingolipids (ceramides) and free sterols, a pattern similar to that of normal palmoplantar skin[2]. Alkanes were normal.

Lipid analysis of plantar scale from 2 patients with autosomal dominant LI revealed increased levels of free fatty acids, triglycerides, sterol esters and alkanes. In contrast to classical LI, levels of free sterols and ceramides were reduced[10].

Genetics

Classical LI is an autosomal recessive disorder and the same principles apply in the counselling of families as outlined for NBIE. The disorder has been shown to be associated with a defect in keratinocyte transglutaminase (TGK) activity[11] and mapped to chromosome 14q11[12].

Because of the existence of apparent autosomal dominant LI, examination of any relative with skin disease is indicated and the implications of dominant transmission should be borne in mind.

References

1 Traupe H. *The Ichthyoses: A guide to Clinical Diagnosis, Genetic Counselling and Therapy.* Springer, Heidelberg, 1989.

2 Williams ML, Elias PM. Heterogeneity in autosomal recessive ichthyosis. *Arch Dermatol* 1985; **121**: 477–88.

3 Traupe H, Kolde G, Happle R. Autosomal dominant lamellar ichthyosis: a new skin disorder. *Clin Genet* 1984; **26**: 457–61.

4 Arnold ML, Anton-Lamprecht I, Melz-Rothfuss B, Hartschuh W. Ichthyosis congenita, type 3. *Arch Dermatol Res* 1988; **280**: 268–78.

5 Larregue M, Ottavy N, Bressieux JM, Lorette J. Bébé collodion; trente-deux nouvelles observations. *Ann Derm Venereol* 1986; **113**: 773–85.

6 Toribio J, Redondo VF, Peteiro C, Zulaica A, Fabeiro JM. Autosomal dominant lamellar ichthyosis. *Clin Genet* 1986; **30**: 122–6.

7 Niemi KM, Kanerva L, Kuokanen K. Recessive ichthyosis congenita, type 2. *Arch Dermatol Res* 1991; **283**: 211–18.

8 Arnold ML, Anton-Lamprecht I, Melz-Rothfuss B, Hartschuh W. Ichthyosis congenita, type 3. *Arch Dermatol Res* 1988; **280**: 268–78.

9 Hazell M, Marks R. Clinical, histologic and cell kinetic discriminants between lamellar ichthyosis and nonbullous congenital ichthyosiform erythroderma. *Arch Dermatol* 1985; **121**: 489–93.

10 Melnik B, Kuster W, Hollman J, Plewig G, Traupe H. Autosomal dominant lamellar ichthyosis exhibits abnormal scale lipid pattern. *Clinical Genet* 1989; **35**: 152–6.

11 Huber M, Rettler I, Bernasconi K et al. Mutations of keratinocyte transglutaminase in lamellar ichthyosis. *Science* 1995; **267**: 525–6.

12 Russell LJ, DiGiovanna JJ, Rogers GR et al. Mutations in the gene for transglutaminase 1 in autosomal recessive lamellar ichthyosis. *Nature Genet* 1995; **9**: 279–83.

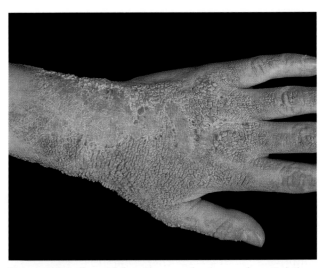

Figure 5.5 *Bullous ichthyosiform erythroderma: characteristic erosions and thickened scaling*

Bullous ichthyosiform erythroderma

Synonym: *Epidermolytic hyperkeratosis*

Definition

Bullous ichthyosiform erythroderma (BIE) is a disorder of keratinization which is associated in younger patients with blistering. More than half of those affected do not have a family history of the disease and are thought to represent new mutations. The incidence is said to be less than 1 in 100 000, though it is likely that some mild cases are not recognized. A characteristic histological picture of hyperkeratosis with lytic changes in the epidermis characterizes this condition, and in many countries BIE is known as 'epidermolytic hyperkeratosis' (EHK).

Clinical features

Apart from a mild generalized erythroderma the skin may appear normal immediately after birth. More usually fragility with often extensive flaccid blisters and peeling are apparent within the first few hours of life. Even normal delivery and subsequent handling may lead to widespread areas of denuded skin on the limbs and trunk. Frequent misdiagnoses at this stage include staphylococcal scalded skin syndrome and epidermolysis bullosa. However, the baby is generally apyrexial and well, and if focal hyperkeratosis is not already present to suggest BIE, a skin biopsy will readily establish the diagnosis.

In the past many of these infants developed severe infection, dehydration and malnutrition and death was common, but with intensive neonatal care their prognosis has greatly improved. The superficial erosions heal rapidly without scarring and with good nursing care these babies should thrive. Widespread blistering ceases in the first few months of life but localized blisters at sites of trauma (especially the nappy area) or skin infection continue into childhood. Erythroderma fades in infancy while the characteristic grey, waxy scale progresses.

Increasing hyperkeratosis is obvious from early childhood and is most prominent in the flexures (wrists, cubital and popliteal fossae, axillae), scalp, anterior neck, abdominal wall and infragluteal folds (Figure 5.5). At these sites, yellow-brown, waxy and ridged scale builds up, sometimes forming spiny outgrowths. Chunks of scale may dislodge leaving raw, tender erosions where scale slowly accumulates again. Colonization by bacteria and yeasts causes a distinctive and embarrassing body odour in children as well as adults and it responds only partially to prolonged antimicrobial or antiseptic therapy. Repeated infections with pustulation and cellulitis are a troublesome complication in childhood and may necessitate long-term or cyclical antibiotics. The central face is generally spared but scalp involvement can be severe and cause patchy alopecia. Some develop more generalized scaling with brown, semiadherent scale on the limbs and trunk (notably around the areolae), which, along with the tendency to blistering and infections, improves in adolescence.

Palmoplantar hyperkeratosis develops in many patients with BIE and occasionally results in recurrent painful fissures, contractures and sclerodactyly with functional disturbance. This feature does not relate to disease severity as 8 of 24 BIE patients seen in the authors' department had normal palms and soles, although 6 of these 8 had moderate to severe skin disease. Nail dystrophy is rare in BIE though increased curvature may result from periungual infection or pulp atrophy.

Growth retardation occurs in severely affected children though many catch up in adolescence. In the authors' group varus deformity of the feet, necessitating surgical correction, occurred in 2 patients with BIE-associated plantar keratoderma.

Severely affected patients with skin fragility, painful fissures, recurrent infections, contractures, unsightly scale and body odour suffer significant physical and psychological morbidity. However, against the odds, the majority lead a relatively normal life. Some mildly affected individuals have only transient blistering in infancy with focal hyperkeratosis thereafter.

Evolution of BIE is variable but in common with other autosomal dominant skin disorders it tends to improve with age. Spontaneous blistering diminishes in childhood and virtually disappears by adolescence. Infections, which often start in the moist flexures, can still trigger focal blisters and pustulation. Scaling and flexural hyperkeratosis may persist except for slight seasonal variation. Severely affected patients have a persistent mild background erythema which is most noticeable on eroded patches.

Three severely affected adult patients in the authors' group of 24 had mental retardation, mild in 1 patient and moderate in 2. Two had suffered perinatal complications associated with fits. All had attended special schools and achieved a reasonable level of employment and independence, though one had difficulty keeping his job owing to complaints about his body odour.

Bullous ichthyosis of Siemens

A mild variant of BIE was described by Siemens in 1937 in a large Dutch kindred[1] and recently the concept was revived by Traupe[2]. The features of bullous ichthyosis of Siemens are delayed onset, episodes of blistering (after minor trauma or associated with infection) persisting into adult life and focal patchy 'moulting' of scale which Siemens called *'Mauserung'*. Erythroderma does not occur in these patients, and blistering is more problematic in the summer months.

In the authors' group of 24 BIE patients, 4 had the Siemens variant. Their blisters were episodic and superficial, often becoming pustular before crusting and peeling. In 1 child the correct diagnosis was made only after he presented with widespread bullous impetigo superimposed on mild hyperkeratosis which had been attributed to eczema. Blistering rarely occurred in the 2 adults but hyperkeratosis was mild, grey in colour and limited to the flexures with scattered patches elsewhere. Scaling was usually mild and between attacks there were few clues. Body odour was not a problem and the palms and soles, nails and scalp were normal. The 3 patients who had skin biopsies showed the changes of typical EHK.

Naevoid BIE

There have been several reports of individuals with a linear, focal or naevoid hyperkeratosis, showing histological features of epidermolytic hyperkeratosis, who have had a child with classical generalized BIE [3–5]. The limited disease expression in the parent, which sometimes presented with atypical lesions distributed in Blaschko's lines, was suggestive of a spontaneous somatic mutation at an early stage in embryonic life. This resulted in some skin clones being affected while others remained unaffected (mosaicism). Germ cell lines were also involved in those who passed the trait on to their offspring, with the result that the child had universal involvement.

Two such mother-child pairs have been seen at Great Ormond Street Hospital. Each of the mothers had asymmetric hyperkeratotic scaling or papules which had been diagnosed in one as a systematized epidermal naevus and in the other as Darier's disease. The correct diagnosis was made following repeat skin biopsy, only after the babies were born with unequivocal BIE. In one reported case, the parental lesion was an insignificant comedonal naevus on the neck which histologically showed epidermolytic hyperkeratosis[4]. It is therefore important to biopsy congenital naevoid or focal warty lesions and, in the presence of epidermolytic hyperkeratosis, to counsel the individual accordingly.

Pathology

Skin biopsy shows marked epidermal acanthosis and hyperkeratosis. In the cells of the prominent granular layer and in the upper spinous layers there are perinuclear vacuoles and large, clumped keratohyalin granules. Intercellular and intracellular clefts may form, and in a blister lesion cytolysis is seen in the spinous and granular layers. These are the hallmarks of 'epidermolytic hyperkeratosis', but in mild forms of the disease these changes may be subtle. The basal keratinocytes are normal.

Electron microscopy reveals clumped keratin filaments dispersed around the keratinocyte nucleus[6]. Desmosomes are disrupted to a variable degree and clefts appear between keratinocytes. However, this histological picture is not unique to BIE and it may be seen occasionally in diverse conditions such as solitary acanthoma, overlying a dermatofibroma, in the walls of epidermal cysts and even in normal oral mucosa[7]. It occurs in some epidermal naevi (possibly mosaic forms of EHK) and in Vorner's type palmoplantar keratoderma without ichthyosis[8].

Molecular biology

The aggregation of tonofilaments in the suprabasal layers of the epidermis and adnexa in BIE suggests a defect in keratins 1 and/or 10 which are distributed in this pattern in normal skin. Immunoelectron microscopy, using keratin monoclonal antibodies, confirmed that the aggregated tonofilaments expressed keratins 1 and 10, whereas non-aggregated filaments were composed of keratins 5 and 14[9]. Linkage of EHK to the keratin gene cluster on chromosome 12 has been reported. Transgenic mice with a K10 gene mutation have an EHK phenotype, and point mutation of K1/K10 genes in EHK have been found[10,11].

Tonofilament aggregation also occurs in the Dowling–Meara variant of epidermolysis bullosa simplex (see Chapter 4) which is also characterized by recurrent blistering and palmoplantar keratoderma. The ultrastructural defect in this condition appears predominantly in basal keratinocytes which normally express keratins K5 and K14. Indeed, the tonofilament clumps in Dowling–Meara EB are strongly labelled with the K5 and K14 monoclonal antibodies, suggesting a distinctive molecular pathogenesis for each of these two bullous disorders[12].

In ichthyosis bullosa of Siemens, a mutation in keratin K2e, has been described in two unrelated British families[13].

Biochemical findings

The finding of an elevated alpha-mannosidase level in one case of apparent BIE suggested a possible cutaneous lysosomal abnormality[14]. Another group reported elevated serum beta-glucuronidase levels in a kindred with an autosomal dominant keratoderma and ichthyosiform dermatoses[15]. In other BIE patients, a raised filaggrin content in the epidermis, similar to that seen in ichthyosis vulgaris, has been identified[16].

Scale lipid analysis in the authors' department has shown a modest elevation of total ceramide content in BIE scale, the significance of which is unknown.

Genetics

At least half of cases of BIE have no family history of the disease and are presumed to represent new mutations. However, in the light of the genetic mosaicism that may occur, both parents of a BIE child should be carefully examined for focal keratotic lesions. In the absence of parental EHK, any further siblings should not be at risk, but the patient will transmit the condition in an autosomal dominant fashion to any offspring.

The accepted wisdom has been that BIE breeds true within a family, but this may be misguided. A mildly affected parent may have a severely affected child, either because the parent's condition has improved with age or because parent has a focal or naevoid epidermolytic hyperkeratotic lesion due to genetic mosaicism. If genetically mosaic parents have germ cell involvement they run the same 50% risk of each of their children being affected, except that in such an instance the child will have generalized disease which may be both unexpected and severe.

Rarely the reverse can happen, with an attenuated form of BIE appearing in the next generation. This occurred in one family in the authors' experience. A mother who had been severely affected as a child had four children, three of whom were moderately affected and the fourth had only transient blistering in infancy followed by focal hystrix-like scaling. Genetic counselling for BIE sufferers is by no means easy.

Prenatal diagnosis is carried out at around 20 weeks of gestation by identifying the characteristic ultrastructural changes on fetal skin biopsy using ultrasound guidance[16]. Tonofilament clumping occurs during the second trimester, and precedes the formation of keratohyalin granules and stratum corneum[17]. It should soon be possible to apply recently developed immunohistochemical techniques to identify specific defects in keratins 1 or 10 earlier in gestation.

References

1 Siemens HW. Dichtung und Wahrheit über die 'Ichthyosis bullosa', mit Bemerkungen zur Systematik der Epidermolysen. *Arch Dermatol Syphilol* 1937; **175**: 590–680.
2 Traupe H, Kolde G, Hamm H, Happle R. Ichthyosis bullosa of Siemens: a unique type of epidermolytic hyperkeratosis. *J Am Acad Dermatol* 1986; **14**: 1000–5.
3 Barker LP, Sachs W. Bullous congenital ichthyosiform erythroderma. *Arch Dermatol Syphilol* 1953; **67**: 443–55.
4 Lookingbill DP, Ladda RL, Cohen C. Generalized epidermolytic hyperkeratosis in the child of a parent with nevus comedonicus. *Arch Dermatol* 1984; **120**: 223–6.
5 Nazzaro V, Ermacora E, Santucci B, Caputo R. Epidermolytic hyperkeratosis: generalized form in children from parents with systematized linear form. *Br J Dermatol* 1990; **122**: 417–22.
6 Anton-Lamprecht I, Schnyder UW. Ultrastructure of inborn errors of keratinization, VI. Inherited ichthyoses – a model system for heterogeneities in keratinization disturbances. *Arch Dermatol Forsch* 1974; **250**: 207–27.
7 Ackerman AB. Histopathologic concept of epidermolytic hyperkeratosis. *Arch Dermatol* 1970; **102**: 253–9.
8 Hamm H, Happle R, Butterfass T, Traupe H. Epidermolytic palmoplantar of Vorner: is it the most frequent type of palmoplantar keratoderma? *Dermatologica* 1988; **177**: 138–45.
9 Ishida-Yamamoto A, McGrath JA, Judge MR et al. Selective involvement of keratin 1 and 10 in the cytoskeletal abnormality of epidermolytic hyperkeratosis. *J Invest Dermatol* 1992; **99**: 19–26.
10 Fuchs E. Genetic skin disorders of keratin. *J. Invest Dermatol* 1992; **99**: 671–4.
11 Irwin McLean WH, Eady RAJ, Dopping-Hepenstal PJC et al. Mutations in the rod 1A domain of keratins 1 and 10 in bullous congenital ichthyosiform erythroderma (BCIE). *J Invest Dermatol* 1994; **102**: 24–30.
12 Ishida-Yamamoto A, McGrath JA et al. Epidermolysis bullosa simplex (Dowling–Meara type) is a genetic disease characterized by an abnormal keratin filament network involving keratins K5 and K14. *J Invest Dermatol* 1991; **97**: 959–68.

13 Irwin McLean WH, Morley SM, Lane EB et al. Ichthyosis bullosa of Siemens (IBS) – a disease involving keratin 2e. *J Invest Dermatol* 1994; **103**: 277–81.
14 Mali JWH, Bergers AMG, Van den Hurk JJMA, Mier PD, Van den Staak WJBM. A lysosomal storage disorder of the epidermis characterized by a deficiency of alpha mannosidase and an accumulation of mannose-rich materials. *Br J Dermatol* 1976; **95**: 627–30.
15 Camissa C, Hessel A, Rossana C, Parks A. Autosomal dominant keratoderma, ichthyosiform dermatoses and elevated serum beta-glucuronidase. *Dermatologica* 1988; **177**: 341–7.
16 Holbrook KA, Dale BA, Sybert VP, Sagebiel RW. Epidermolytic hyperkeratosis: ultrastructure and biochemistry of skin and amniotic fluid cells from two affected fetuses and a newborn infant. *J Invest Dermatol* 1983; **80**: 222–7.
17 Eady RAJ, Gunner DB, Carbonne LDL et al. Prenatal diagnosis of bullous ichthyosiform erythroderma: detection of tonofilament clumps in fetal epidermis and amniotic fluid cells. *J Med Genet* 1986; **23**: 46–51.

Ichthyosis hystrix

Definition

The subgroup of ichthyosis hystrix encompasses a heterogeneous group of rare conditions, characterized by spiny hyperkeratotic scale similar to that of BIE. However, they differ from BIE in that blistering is not a feature, erythroderma is less marked and limited forms are more common. They are autosomal dominant disorders.

Clinical features

The first documented cases of apparent ichthyosis hystrix were the Lambert family of Suffolk who between 1731 and 1851 had 11 affected members through four generations[1]. The first, Edward Lambert, was presented to the Royal Society of Medicine in 1731 and some of his affected descendants, known as the 'porcupine men', made their living appearing in circuses, billed as 'a new species of man'. Contrary to reports, female family members were also affected and the ichthyosis was autosomal dominant[2]. The skin was normal at birth and dark, warty scale accumulated after 7 weeks of age. The face, palms and soles were spared. The severity of the ichthyosis varied among family members and at different stages of their lives, and seemed to lessen in later generations.

Similar cases of ichthyosis were reported during the nineteenth century, and in 1954 Ollendorff Curth and Macklin described two brothers, who had from birth 'verrucous black' scale on the scalp, neck and limbs[3,4]. They also had truncal erythema, severe palmoplantar keratoderma and keratoses. Other family members spanning five generations had focal keratoses, palmar keratoderma and 'ichthyosis

simplex' to varying degrees, and it appeared to be an autosomal dominant condition with variable expression.

Other variants of ichthyosis hystrix include the case reported by Bafverstedt of a mentally retarded man with dramatic hyperkeratotic spiny scale but mildly affected palms[5]. Ichthyosis hystrix gravior of Rheydt (a town near Düsseldorf) was described by Schnyder in 2 patients who had an ichthyosiform erythroderma with hystrix-like scale which resembled the ichthyosis of keratosis–ichthyosis–deafness (KID) syndrome[6]. These and other similar patients had mild palmoplantar hyperkeratosis and deafness, which led Traupe to suggest the name HID to describe the hystrix-like ichthyosis and deafness[7]. Zeligman reported 4 cases of ichthyosis hystrix and 1 of naevus unius lateris in 1965 and believed on the basis of their histology that in several instances they were subtypes of bullous ichthyosiform erythroderma[8].

In the authors' department this heterogeneity is borne out in 3 ichthyosis hystrix patients with diverse manifestations. A young girl had a naevoid distribution of prominent spiny scale on the trunk and limbs and severe palmar involvement. A teenage male patient had KID-like hyperkeratotic plaques with normal vision and hearing. The third, an adult man, suffered from marked hystrix scaling on the distal limbs and severe palmoplantar keratoderma which required grafting in childhood.

From the limited number of reports of ichthyosis hystrix in the literature, there appears to be both interfamilial and intrafamilial variation.

Pathology

Early reports identified the histological features of epidermolytic hyperkeratosis but with minimal acantholysis. However, in the authors' experience the light microscopic signs are non-specific, and in each of our three patients the skin biopsies showed orthokeratosis, acanthosis and scattered vacuolation in the upper epidermis. Electron microscopic studies of Curth–Macklin type ichthyosis hystrix highlighted a characteristic continuous perinuclear tonofilament shell (in contrast to the clumped filaments in EHK), conspicuous vacuoles in 30% and double nuclei in 10% of spinous and granular keratinocytes[9]. Deformed lamellar bodies were a feature in some and the major features were unchanged after retinoid therapy[10]. An unusual histological finding in a family of 8 members with ichthyosis hystrix was the presence of cornoid lamellae[11].

Genetics

Where a positive family history is available all reported types of ichthyosis hystrix have been inherited as an autosomal dominant trait and the same genetic principles apply as with BIE. Because of the considerable interfamilial variation and the frequent absence of BIE type histology, genetic counselling is difficult.

References

1 Machin J. An uncommon case of distempered skin. *Phil Trans* 1733; **37**: 299–300.
2 Penrose LS, Stern C. Reconsideration of the Lambert pedigree (Ichthyosis hystrix gravior). *Ann Hum Genet* 1957; **22**: 258–83.
3 Ollendorff Curth H, Macklin MT. The genetic basis of various types of ichthyosis in a family group. *Am J Hum Genet* 1954; **6**: 371–82.
4 Ollendorff Curth H, Allen FH, Schnyder UW, Anton-Lamprecht I. Follow up of a family suffering from ichthyosis hystrix, type Curth Macklin. *Hum Genet* 1972; **17**: 37–48.
5 Bafverstedt B. Fall von genereller, naevusartiger Hyper-keratose, Imbecillitat, Epilepsie. *Acta Derm Venereol* 1941; **22**: 207–12.
6 Schnyder UW. Ichthyosis hystrix typus Rheydt (Ichthyo-sis hystrix gravior mit praktischer Taubheit). *Z Hautkr* 1977; **52**: 763–6.
7 Traupe H. *The Ichthyoses: A Guide to Clinical Diagnosis, Genetic Counselling and Therapy.* Springer, Heidelberg, 1989.
8 Zeligman I, Pomeranz J. Variations of congenital ichthyo-siform erythroderma. *Arch Dermatol* 1965; **91**: 120–5.
9 Anton-Lamprecht I, Curth HO, Schnyder UW. Zur Ultrastruktur hereditarer Verhornungsstorungen. *Arch Derm Forsch* 1973; **246**: 77–91.
10 Kanerva L, Karvonem J, Oikarinem A et al. Ichthyosis hystrix (Curth–Macklin). *Arch Dermatol* 1984; **120**: 1218–23.
11 Braun-Falco O, Schurig V, Meurer M, Klepzig K, Ichthyo-sis hystrix mit Parakeratose nach Art der kornoiden Lamelle. *Hautarzt* 1985; **36**: 132–41.

Harlequin ichthyosis

Definition

The most extreme and distinctive form of ichthyosis was one of the first subgroups to be described in 1750, and because of its skin patterning and lethality became known as 'harlequin fetus'[1]. Since survival is now possible the term 'harlequin ichthyosis' (HI) is more appropriate. It is, fortunately, a very rare occurrence, approximately 5 cases in the UK annually.

Clinical features

The affected infant, usually premature, is encased in a grossly hyperkeratotic 'coat of armour' composed of large (2–5 cm across), thick, yellow-brown, firmly adherent plaques covering the whole body surface and severely restricting movement. Soon after birth the taut, inflexible cast splits, producing deep red

fissures extending into the dermis and a skin pattern resembling a harlequin's costume. The facial features are distorted owing to severe ectropion and conjuncti-val oedema which obscures the eye, and eclabium (eversion of the lips). The scalp feels boggy and the nose and external ears are tethered and appear rudimentary. The oedematous hands and feet may either be encased in hard, mitten-like casts or covered with a thin membrane, but the digits are well formed underneath. The skull may appear microcephalic. Additional congenital defects have been found in some.

Respiratory insufficiency results from restriction of chest movement. In infants who survive the first days, absence of effective sucking causes feeding difficulties leading to hypoglycaemia, dehydration and renal failure. Temperature instability and infection commonly supervene and may lead to rapid demise. Remarkably, several survivors have now been reported [2–6]. In these cases intensive nursing and medical care, and in all but one retinoid therapy from the outset, prolonged survival until the plate-like scale was shed over a period of weeks. In most, a severe ichthyosis resembling non-bullous ichthyosiform ery-throderma was the eventual outcome. The oldest of the survivors at 10 years of age was of normal intelligence, and continued on retinoid therapy[2]. In the case reported by Lawlor the patient was the sole survivor of 5 affected babies in a kindred with 9 other healthy children[3]. Etretinate therapy was commenced in the first week of life and was continued for 18 months. At the age of 6 years the girl was growth-retarded and had severe ichthyosiform erythroderma with limb contractures, but was mobile and of normal intelligence.

Pathology

Skin biopsy shows massive orthohyperkeratosis extending down into hair follicles and pilosebaceous units, but often no other specific changes are noted on light microscopy and the impression is of a retention ichthyosis. However, in some cases vacuoles are seen in the stratum corneum, the granular layer is reduced in thickness and rarely papillomatosis and a dermal inflammatory infiltrate are present. Pilosebaceous and sweat glands are preserved. Non-keratinizing mucous membranes are normal.

Electron microscopy of 9 cases in one study revealed lipid droplets and cellular remnants in corneocytes in all cases[7]. The lamellar bodies in spinous and granular cells were either absent or abnormal in all and failed to discharge their contents, resulting in disrupted intercellular lipid lamellae.

Biochemical findings

A variety of defects in both keratin and lipid composi-tion of stratum corneum have been reported, but no consistent abnormality has been found. The first recorded keratin defect was identified by X-ray diffraction studies which showed substitution of the usual alpha-helical pattern of epidermal keratins by a crossed beta structure[8]. Abnormal epidermal lipid deposition was found in another case[6].

A study of 9 cases of harlequin ichthyosis revealed abnormal (though variable) keratin and filaggrin expression in all which permitted a subdivision into three types of HI[7]. Type 1 cases had a normal keratin profile and positive profilaggrin staining but absent filaggrin expression, while type 2 displayed a hyper-proliferative keratin pattern in suprabasal cells (prominent keratins 6 and 16 and reduced keratins 1 and 10) again without filaggrin. The least common was type 3 with suprabasal keratins 6 and 16 expression and absence of profilaggrin staining except in intra-epidermal sweat ducts. The changes in types 2 and 3 suggested a hyperproliferative ichthyosis, but kinetic studies have yet to be done. Cultured keratinocytes showed the same morphologic features[7]. It was suggested that the failure to convert profilaggrin to filaggrin was due to an inactive protein phosphatase preventing phosphorylation. Clearly, although harlequin ichthyosis has a clinically uniform phenotype, it represents a genetically heterogeneous group of disorders with both lipid and protein metabolic defects contributing to the severe epidermal disruption.

Genetics

It appears that HI is always an autosomal recessive disorder. Each family may possess a different genetic defect but within families disease expression is consistent. Detailed genetic counselling is required for these families and prenatal diagnostic testing with identification of premature and abnormal keratinization by weeks 20–22 of gestation should be available for those who wish it[9]. On electron microscopy, atypical intraepidermal vesicles have been detected in an affected fetus at 18 weeks[10]. Consanguineous families often seem to have a disproportionately high incidence of affected offspring and in these kindred the extended family should be warned of the genetic risk of intermarriage. Harlequin ichthyosis has been reported in one of non-identical twins and in both of a male twin pair[11].

Treatment

The potential for survival of harlequin ichthyosis babies presents carers with the conflict of providing aggressive neonatal treatment for babies who survive the first few hours, while accepting the likely outcome of severe, lifelong ichthyosis. Parents and family should be informed of the implications of the condition, encouraged to consider all options and supported in the role they wish to play. Staff unfamiliar with the startling and distressing deformity also need

to be enlightened about the prognosis and practical problems that result. They often express surprise that these infants could be normal except for their skin. If survival seems possible and intensive treatment is agreed, a care plan should be drawn up within the first day of life and support provided for staff in their difficult role. There appears to be a benefit in using early retinoid therapy. For survivors, later staged plastic surgery may improve the cosmetic result, and retinoids may further reduce the degree of disability.

References

1 Waring JJ. Early mention of a harlequin fetus in America. *Am J Dis Child* 1932; **43**: 442.
2 Roberts LJ. Long term survival of a harlequin fetus. *J Am Acad Dermatol* 1989; **212**: 335–9.
3 Lawlor F. Progress of a harlequin fetus to non-bullous ichthyosiform erythroderma. *Paediatrics* 1989; **82**: 870–3.
4 Rogers M, Scarf C. Harlequin baby treated with etretinate. *Pediatr Dermatol* 1989; **6**: 216–21.
5 Ward PS, Jones RD. Successful treatment of a harlequin fetus. *Arch Dis Child* 1989; **64**: 1309–11.
6 Buxman MM, Goodkin PE, Fahrenback WH, Dimond RL. Harlequin ichthyosis with an epidermal lipid abnormality. *Arch Dermatol* 1979; **115**: 189–93.
7 Dale BA, Holbrook KA, Fleckman P et al. Heterogeneity in harlequin ichthyosis, an inborn error of epidermal keratinization: variable morphology and structural protein expression and a defect in lamellar granules. *J Invest Dermatol* 1990; **94**: 6–18.
8 Craig JM, Goldsmith LA, Baden HP. An abnormality of keratin in the harlequin fetus. *Pediatrics* 1970; **46**: 437–40.
9 Blanchet-Bardon C, Dumez Y. Prenatal diagnosis of a harlequin fetus. *Sem Dermatol* 1984; **3**: 225–8.
10 Eady RAJ, Blanchet-Bardon C, Gunner DB, Schofield OMV, Rodeck CH. Atypical intraepidermal vesicles serve as a marker for the prenatal diagnosis of harlequin ichthyosis. *J Invest Dermatol* 1990; **95**: 468 (abstract).
11 Anstey A, Judge M, Salisbury J, Meadows N. Harlequin twins. *Br J Dermatol* 1991; **125** (suppl.): 22

Netherton's syndrome

Definition

Netherton's syndrome (NS) is a multisystem disorder comprising an ichthyosiform dermatosis, hair shaft defects and atopic features. Netherton's original patient, reported in 1958, was a young girl with a generalized, scaly, erythematous 'dermatitis' similar to NBIE, paroxysmal pruritus and abnormal hair[1]. The hair was fragile and lustreless, and light microscopy revealed irregularly spaced nodose swellings along the shaft which were due to dilatation of the proximal shaft with invagination of the adjacent distal portion of hair. Netherton termed this hair shaft defect 'bamboo hair' and subsequently it was called trichorrhexis invaginata (TI). Later reports noted the association of trichorrhexis invaginata with migratory, circinate, double-edged scaly lesions called ichthyosis linearis circumflexa (ILC)[2]. The latter condition was described by Comel in 1949 but there was no comment on that patient's hair[3].

Clinical features

Skin manifestations

Generalized erythroderma of variable intensity is evident at or shortly after birth (Figures 5.6 and 5.7). Collodion baby presentation is not a feature of NS but the complications in infancy are similar and include temperature instability and hypernatraemic dehydration. Some infants, in addition, suffer from severe failure to thrive, diarrhoea and recurrent infections, and in the not-too-distant past they would have been diagnosed as having Leiner's syndrome. Congenital erythroderma of whatever cause may be associated with a transient enteropathy. A non-gluten-sensitive jejunal villous atrophy, which resolved spontaneously at 10 months of age, was found in one NS infant under the authors' care. There was and may still be a considerable mortality rate due to failure to thrive and infection in the first year of life, but in survivors of the first year erythroderma tends to improve in parallel with improving growth and development.

During childhood about half of NS patients develop typical lesions of ILC on the trunk and limbs; they may still be at risk of acute erythroderma. A typical ILC lesion is an erythematous, slightly scaly, annular or polycyclic migrating patch with an incomplete double edge of peeling scale. These lesions are episodic, transient – lasting some days – and easily missed, but similar lesions without the double-edged margin are more commonly seen.

Severely affected patients retain a fluctuating erythroderma, while others have exacerbations triggered by intercurrent illness, and rarely pustular lesions are superimposed. Between acute attacks the skin may look surprisingly normal. In a review of 43 reported cases of Netherton's syndrome, ILC was recorded in 30 of 43 cases, while congenital ichthyosiform erythroderma was the predominant skin lesion in 13[4]. Many patients are distressed by prominent facial erythrema and peeling, particularly in perioral and nasal areas. Pruritus may be troublesome, and another feature reminiscent of atopic eczema is flexural lichenification. The severity of the skin disease lessens with age in most patients.

A late complication in severe cases is painful flexural oedema and papillomatosis affecting the axillae, groin and perineum[4]. This may prove disabling, and was a premalignant lesion in 2 cases of squamous cell carcinoma of the vulva in middle-aged women with NS[5]. An adult male patient under the authors' care had similar painful epidermal hyperplasia topped with malodorous hystrix-like scale on the lower legs. A vascularizing keratitis occurred in an elderly patient with severe facial involvement and ectropion. A proportion of patients have a nail dystrophy, ranging from thickening to pterygia formation.

Hair abnormalities

The major diagnostic clue in NS is the hair shaft defect known as trichorrhexis invaginata, but it is often overlooked in infancy because scalp hair growth is poor and attributed to erythroderma. In childhood, scalp, eyebrow and even body hair remains sparse, slow-growing, lustreless and brittle, and patchy

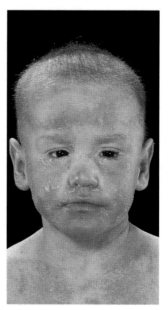

Figure 5.7 *Netherton's syndrome: same boy as in Figure 5.6, aged 5 years, exhibiting the characteristic facial appearance and short hair*

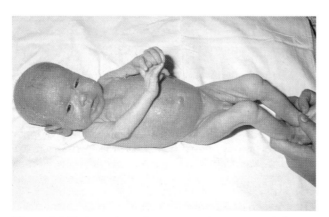

Figure 5.6 *Netherton's syndrome presenting as congenital erythroderma*

traumatic alopecia results from normal wear and tear. Terminal hair growth improves with age, but in many the hair is unruly or short and spiky and some patients may opt to wear a wig. A few older patients have clinically normal, though microscopically defective, hair. Trichorrhexis invaginata is thought to result from intermittent interrupted keratinization of the internal root sheath in the hair follicle. The focal softening with loss of splinting action allows the distal hair shaft to invaginate into the dilated proximal cup. Other common hair shaft defects are pili torti and trichorrhexis nodosa.

The proportion of scalp hair affected varies from less than 5% to approximately 50% and the only clue to the presence of hair defects may be ragged, cupped hair ends where the shaft has broken off. Clipped hairs may be more informative and examination of clipped eyebrows is recommended by some authorities. Body hair is often sparse, and broken hair shafts at follicular orifices produce a peppered appearance.

Atopic features

The majority of patients with NS have a personal or family history of atopy, especially hay fever or asthma. The question as to whether NS patients actually have atopic eczema with an ichthyosis is controversial. The pruritus, flexural accentuation, occasional eczematous-like lesions and periods of remission along with raised IgE levels suggest that they do. However, typical skin lesions are not eczematous and do not respond to appropriate eczema therapy.

Many NS patients suffer from recurrent angioedema or urticaria on ingestion of certain foodstuffs. In Greene's review the incidence was low[4], whereas in the authors' group of 8 NS patients, 6 had one or more attacks of facial angioedema, usually starting in early childhood[6]. The most common triggers were nuts and fish; hay fever occurred in 3 of these patients.

Other associated features

Transient aminoaciduria occurred in Greene's own patient and in 25% of the reviewed patients[4], but in only 1 of the authors' 8 patients during infancy (glycine and alanine aciduria). All 8 in the latter group were mildly growth-retarded. One patient was considered educationally subnormal, though an incidence of 10% with mental retardation was noted in Greene's review[4]. This is unlikely to be a primary feature and possibly results from perinatal complications.

Pathology

The histological features vary with the type and phase of the lesion sampled. Hyperkeratosis, parakeratosis and a reduced or absent granular layer occur at the spreading border and eosiniphilic material may collect within the corneal and granular layers in ILC lesions.

Psoriasiform epidermal hyperplasia, papillomatosis and a mixed perivascular inflammatory infiltrate occur in older ILC lesions and in the more diffuse scaly erythroderma. Acute erythroderma is accompanied by pronounced inflammatory changes with spongiosis and upper epidermal eosinophilic necrolysis which may lead to a subcorneal split.

Ultrastructural studies in NS have identified inclusion bodies in suprabasal keratinocytes and reduced numbers of desmosomes and lamellar bodies[7].

Microscopy of the scalp and eyebrow hair in NS patients shows, in a variable proportion of intact hairs, the 'bamboo' nodal dilatation consisting of a bulbous distal hair sitting in a socket composed of a concave proximal hair. Often only the ragged, dilated proximal end remains, and in some cases pili torti and nodal swellings are the only shaft defects seen. Scalp biopsies have shown early nodal deformity occurring at the zone of keratinization within the hair follicle and an increase in sulphydroyl groups in stained cortical cells[8].

Immunologic abnormalities

Most if not all NS patients have laboratory markers of atopy with raised IgE levels, positive skin prick responses and high specific serum IgE tests to the common aero and food allergens[6]. The skin prick test shows more variable results than the specific serum IgE assessment, but neither reliably predicts clinically important triggers of skin disease or angioedema. In 2 patients under the authors' care IgE levels have fallen from very high to almost normal during childhood. Other immune function tests show only minor and inconsistent abnormalities, although transient neutrophil chemotactic defects have occurred in at least 2 patients[4,6].

Levels of C1 esterase inhibitor were normal in 8 patients studied[6].

Genetics

Netherton's syndrome is an autosomal recessive disorder with many reports of affected siblings and a high proportion of patients coming from consanguineous families. The clinical manifestations may vary between siblings, making genetic counselling difficult. Prenatal diagnosis is not possible at present.

Differential diagnosis

Netherton's syndrome is a rare disorder with a gradual evolution of clinical manifestations. The two characteristic features, namely trichorrhexis invaginata and ILC, are delayed in onset and often subtle, so it is not surprising that diagnosis is difficult. In infancy the presumed diagnoses have included erythrodermic eczema, NBIE, hyper-IgE syndrome and acrodermatitis enteropathica. In older children and adults, NBIE is the usual misdiagnosis, but atopic eczema, peeling skin syndrome and erythrokeratoderma may be considered.

Treatment

The day-to-day treatment of patients with NS is similar to that of other patients with ichthyosiform erythroderma but the former do present some specific problems. In the neonatal period erythroderma tends to be more severe than in NBIE and hypernatraemic dehydration is a particular risk[9]. Failure to thrive is often severe in infants and necessitates intensive nutritional support.

Topical steroids have been used in infants with NS mistakenly diagnosed as having atopic eczema, but their effect is surprisingly poor, and because of the intense erythroderma and high surface area steroid toxicity is a common complication of such therapy.

An important marker of NS in older patients is the marked deterioration induced by standard retinoid therapy which is usually beneficial in other erythrodermic keratinizing disorders. Increased erythroderma, peeling and skin fragility occur, but some patients may benefit from intermittent low-dose etretinate therapy[10].

Psoralens with ultraviolet A (PUVA) therapy has been used in at least 1 patient[11], but other experimental treatments such as methotrexate have not helped.

Excision of hyperkeratotic papillomatosis lesions on the lower leg with split skin grafting from the thigh has been performed on an adult patient, but the outcome is uncertain.

References

1 Netherton EW. A unique case of trichorrhexis nodosa, 'Bamboo hairs'. *Arch Derm* 1958; **78**: 483–7.
2 Mevorah B, Frenck E, Brooke EM. Ichthyosis linearis circumflexa of Comel. A clinicostatistical approach to its relationship with Netherton's syndrome. *Dermatologica* 1974; **149**: 201–9.
3 Comel M. Ichthyosis linearis circumflexa. *Dermatologica* 1949; **98**: 133–6.
4 Greene SL, Muller SA. Netherton's syndrome; a report of a case and review of the literature. *J Am Acad Dermatol* 1985; **13**: 329–37.
5 Hintner H, Jaschke E, Fritsch P. Netherton syndrome: Abswehrschwache, generalisierte Verrukose and Karzinogenese. *Hautarzt* 1980; **31**: 428–32.
6 Judge M, Morgan G, Harper JI. A clinical and immunological study of Netherton's syndrome. *Br J Dermatol* 1994; **131**: 615–21.
7 Frenk E, Mevorah B. Ichthyosis linearis circumflexa of Comel with trichorrhexis invaginata (Netherton's syndrome). An ultrastructural study of the skin changes. *Arch Dermatol Forsch* 1972; **245**: 42–9.
8 Ito M, Ho K, Hashimoto K. Pathogenesis of trichorrhexis invaginata (Bamboo hair). *J Invest Dermatol* 1984; **83**: 1–6.
9 Jones SK, Thomson LM, Surbrugg SK, Weston WL. Neonatal hypernatraemia in two siblings with Netherton's syndrome. *Br J Dermatol* 1986; **114**: 741–3.
10 Hartschuh W, Hauber I, Petzoldt D. Successful retinoid therapy of Netherton's syndrome. *Hautarzt* 1989; **40**: 430–3.
11 Nagata T. Netherton's syndrome which responded to photochemotherapy. *Dermatologica* 1980; **161**: 51–6.

Sjögren–Larsson syndrome

Definition

Sjögren-Larsson syndrome (SLS) is an autosomal recessive condition comprising ichthyosis, spastic diplegia and mild to moderate mental retardation. In addition, a characteristic retinopathy has been noted. Although this syndrome may have been described some years before, credit goes to Sjögren and Larsson, Swedish psychiatrists, for their classic description in 1957. They reported a detailed clinical and epidemiologic study of 28 institutionalized patients from 13 families, many of them consanguineous, in an area of northwestern Sweden where inbreeding was common[1]. Similar cases were reported in the UK the same year[2] and since then over 200 cases worldwide have been documented. The incidence in Sweden has been estimated at 1 in 100 000 rising to 1 in 10 000 in the northwestern region of Vasterbotten[3]; in the UK the incidence may be 1 in 300 000, but this is probably an underestimate.

Clinical features

Skin manifestations

Although collodion baby presentation has been reported[4], it was not a feature in the authors' group of 9 patients. Usually the skin is dry and mildly erythrodermic at birth, and scaling develops within the first 3 months of life. Thereafter a mild erythema persists and a variable degree of scaling develops which is often a mixture of light peeling on the trunk and more lamellar-type ichthyosis on the lower limbs. Scaling tends to follow a cyclical pattern of accumulation and shedding and predominantly affects the limbs and face.

A velvety orange or brown lichenification, sometimes topped with verrucous hyperkeratosis, develops in the flexures, neck and periumbilical folds (Figure 5.8). This characteristic feature may even be noted during the first year of life and is helpful in diagnosis. Skin infections are rare, but diffuse lichenification becomes prominent and is embarrassing to older children in whom it may also restrict the mobility of already hypertonic limbs.

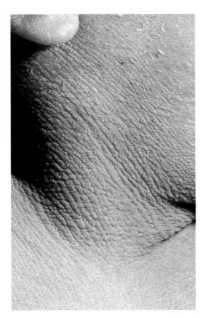

Figure 5.8 *Sjögren–Larsson syndrome: typical thickened, lichenified skin on the neck*

Neuro-ocular features

Neurological dysfunction is obvious in early infancy with delayed motor milestones and evolution of upper motor neuron signs (weakness, hypertonicity and hyper-reflexia) in the legs and rarely the arms also. The motor features are of a typical, non-progressive spastic paraparesis. Most patients learn to walk unaided or with crutches in early childhood. Areas of attenuation of the cortical white matter have been reported on computed tomographic scanning in SLS[5]. Altered posture and movement may lead to skeletal defects such as scoliosis, dislocated hips due to adductor deformity and short stature. Development of speech is also delayed.

Mild to moderate mental handicap is the rule; although many SLS patients were consigned to institutions in the past, with special training most will achieve limited independence in later life. They are notable for their cheerful, friendly disposition.

Ocular signs were reported by Jagell in 1980 and consist of glistening dots on the macula which develop during childhood and which do not seem to interfere with vision[6]. They were detected in 5 of 9 patients seen in the authors' department and disappeared in early adult life in the 2 adult patients. The lesions may result from lipid degeneration in the retinal epithelium but their content is unknown.

Pathology

Skin sections show hyperkeratosis, acanthosis and papillomatosis; no significant ultrastructural features have been recorded. Kinetic studies in 1 patient indicated a hyperproliferative epidermis[7].

Lipid metabolism

Defects in fatty acid metabolism in plasma phospholipids of patients with SLS have been reported by two groups. In 1982, Hernell found that the fatty acid metabolites of linoleic acid were markedly reduced, pointing to a deficiency or defective function of the delta 6-desaturase enzyme[8]. These observations were confirmed by Harper in 1987 but their significance was unknown[9]. More recently, Rizzo demonstrated elevated levels of plasma hexadecanol, a C16 long-chain fatty alcohol, in 5 SLS patients. This was attributed to a deficiency of fatty alcohol oxido-reductase (FAO) demonstrated in leucocytes and cultured fibroblasts from SLS skin biopsies[10]; FAO is an alcohol dehydrogenase which mediates conversion of fatty alcohols to fatty acids. Rizzo's findings have been confirmed by the authors' group[11].

The histochemical demonstration of absent alcohol dehydrogenase in the epidermis and jejunal mucosa in SLS but not in other ichthyoses provides further evidence of the importance of abnormal fatty alcohol metabolism in this syndrome[11]. It seems likely that the neurological defects may also result from abnormal lipid development in myelin.

Genetics

Though rare outside northern Sweden, SLS is a severe autosomal recessive disorder, and in view of the 1 in 4 risk of subsequent affected pregnancies, most families seek prenatal diagnosis. Fetal skin biopsy at 20–22 weeks has been successfully used to detect premature keratinization[12]. With the identification of fatty alcohol defects and FAO enzyme deficiency in fibroblasts in SLS, it is possible to apply this biochemical technique to fetal cells during the first trimester. The SLS gene has been mapped to chromosome 17p[13].

Treatment

The abnormal fatty acid profile in plasma phospholipids in 3 SLS patients prompted treatment with a 6-month course of essential fatty acid supplements, but there was minimal improvement in the skin and neurological features[9]. Reports of a beneficial effect of a diet rich in medium-chain triglycerides on the skin manifestations in SLS warrant further attention[14].

Retinoid (etretinate) therapy was very effective in relieving the scaling and disabling lichenification in 3 older children and 2 adults in the authors' group, but tolerance developed after 3 months or so and intermittent therapy seems the best option.

Intensive physiotherapy and education in early childhood clearly improve motor and social development in SLS, and orthopaedic treatment of skeletal deformities is beneficial in many cases.

References

1 Sjögren T, Larsson T. Oligophrenia in association with congenital ichthyosis and spastic disorders. *Acta Psychiatr Scand* 1957; **32** (suppl. 113): 1–112.

2 Richards BW, Rundle A, Wilding A. Congenital ichthyosis, spastic diplegia and mental deficiency. *J Ment Def Res* 1957; **1**: 118–29.

3 Jagell S, Gustavson JH, Holmgren G. Sjögren–Larsson syndrome in Sweden. A clinical, genetic and epidemiological study. *Clin Genet* 1981; **19**: 233–56.

4 Larregue M, Ottavy N, Bressieux JM, Lorette J. Bébé collodion; trente-deux nouvelles observations. *Ann Derm Venereol* 1986; **113**: 773–85.

5 Gomori JM, Leibovici V, Zlotogorski A. Computed tomography in Sjögren–Larsson syndrome. *Neuroradiology* 1987; **29**: 557–9.

6 Jagell S, Polland W, Sansgren O. Specific changes in the fundus typical for the Sjögren–Larsson syndrome. An ophthalmological study. *Acta Ophthalmol* 1980; **58**: 321–30.

7 Jagell S, Liden S. Ichthyosis in the Sjögren–Larsson syndrome. *Clin Genet* 1982; **21**: 243–52.

8 Hernell O, Holmgren G, Jagell SF. Suspected faulty fatty acid metabolism in Sjögren–Larsson Syndrome. *Paediatr Res* 1982; **16**: 45–9.

9 Harper JI. Analysis of essential fatty acid metabolism in Sjögren–Larsson syndrome. *Pediatr Dermatol News* 1987; **6**: 7–9.

10 Rizzo WB, Dammann AL, Craft DA. Sjögren–Larsson syndrome: impaired fatty alcohol oxidation in cultured fibroblasts due to deficient fatty alcohol:NAD oxidoreductase activity. *J Clin Invest* 1988; **81**: 738–44.

11 Judge MR, Lake BD, Smith VV, Besley GTN, Harper JI. Depletion of alcohol dehydrogenase activity in the epidermis and jejunal mucosa in Sjögren–Larsson syndrome. *J Invest Dermatol* 1990; **95**: 632–4.

12 Kouseff BG, Matsuoka LY, Stenn KS et al. Prenatal diagnosis of Sjögren–Larsson syndrome. *J Pediatr* 1982; **101**: 998–1001.

13 Pigg M, Jagell S, Sillen A et al. The Sjögren-Larsson syndrome gene is close to D17S805 as determined by linkage analysis and allelic association. *Nature Genet* 1994; **8**: 361–4.

14 Hooft C, Kreikemans J, van Acker K et al. Sjögren–Larsson syndrome with exudative enteropathy. Influence of medium chain triglycerides on the symptomatology. *Helv Paediatr Acta* 1967; **5**: 447–58.

Refsum's disease

Definition

Refsum's disease (RD) is a rare autosomal recessive neurocutaneous disorder, caused by defective fatty acid metabolism. Refsum, a Norwegian neurologist, reported its features in 1946 and called it 'heredopathia atactia polyneuritiformis'[1].

Clinical features

Neurological signs develop in adolescence or early adult life, and progress slowly over a period of some months. Failing vision and night blindness result from progressive retinitis pigmentosa and cataracts may also contribute. Sensorineural deafness, tinnitus and, in some, anosmia occur in the early stages. Progressive weakness, foot drop and loss of balance are due to cerebellar ataxia, a mixed sensorimotor polyneuropathy with hypertrophied peripheral nerves, and elevated cerebrospinal fluid protein levels are characteristic findings. In the early stages of evolution the neurological symptoms and signs of RD may fluctuate and patients may be labelled as neurotic. Consequent delayed diagnosis may result in severe neurological impairment, wasting and depression. Some patients develop a cardiomyopathy with serious conduction defects[2], and skeletal defects occur in others.

The ichthyosis, which either coincides with or postdates the onset of neurological signs, resembles a mild acquired ichthyosis vulgaris with a fine, white scaling most noticeable over the lower trunk but also affecting the limbs. In untreated cases lamellar-type scale develops.

An infantile form of Refsum's disease is described with neurodegenerative disease in early infancy, but ichthyosis is an unusual feature.

Pathology

Skin biopsy changes are similar to those of ichthyosis vulgaris but without the typical ultrastructural findings. An important feature is the presence of lipid droplets in the basal and suprabasal layers of the epidermis, a marker shared only with neutral lipid storage disease (Chanarin–Dorfman syndrome). Their significance may only be appreciated after special lipid stains are used. Kinetic studies in 1 patient with advanced disease showed a hyperproliferative pattern[3]. Electron microscopy reveals enlarged, distorted mitochondria[4].

Biochemical basis

In the early 1960s, an abnormal accumulation of a storage product identified as a branched-chain 20 carbon fatty acid was reported[5]. Herndon, in 1969, demonstrated impaired oxidation of phytanic acid, a long-chain branched fatty acid, in cultured fibroblasts from skin biopsies of 11 patients with RD[6]. This was due to a marked deficiency of phytanic acid oxidase, and the asymptomatic heterozygote carriers possessed half the enzyme activity.

Phytanic acid is obtained from plant chlorophyll and to a lesser extent animal sources in the diet and cannot be synthesized by human tissues. It is usually not detected in serum (normal values are below 1 mg/100 ml), but in RD it accounts for 5–30% of serum lipids and levels rise to more than 60 mg/100 ml. In tissues it replaces other fatty acids and binds to sterols resulting in lipid vacuoles in the basal epidermis. A study of phospholipid fatty acids in 1 patient revealed raised linoleic acid levels in plasma and reduced levels in red blood cells, with low levels of long straight-chain fatty acids in both[7].

Genetics

Detection of new cases of RD should prompt intensive family screening for other presymptomatic cases[8]. Prenatal testing by amniocentesis and culture of amniocytes to assay phytanic acid oxidase is theoretically possible, but the availability of effective dietary therapy reduces demand for this approach[9].

Treatment

Exclusion of sources of chlorophyll in the diet is mandatory in the treatment of RD. The major dietary exclusions are green vegetables (phytanic acid) and animal fat (phytol) and the aim of dietary treatment is to reduce daily intake of these two compounds to below 5 mg. Rapid weight loss should be avoided since it mobilizes tissue phytanic acid, and in 1 patient coincided with the onset of severe clinical manifestations[7]. A high carbohydrate intake ensures adequate energy, and when this regimen is instituted in the early stages of the disease blood levels of phytanic acid fall rapidly followed by clearance of the ichthyosis and to a variable extent reversal of recent neurological signs. Lifelong, strict adherence to the diet is necessary, and recurrence of scaling is an obvious marker of rising phytanic acid levels.

Plasmapheresis has been used to reduce phytanic acid levels rapidly in acutely ill patients at diagnosis[7,10].

References

1 Refsum S. Heredopathia atactica polyneuritiformis. *Acta Psychiatr Scand* 1946; **38** (suppl.): 1–303.
2 Leys D, Petit H, Bonte-Adnet C et al. Refsum's disease revealed by cardiac disorders. *Lancet* 1989; **i**: 621.
3 Dykes PJ, Marks R, Davies MG, Reynolds DJ. Epidermal metabolism in heredopathia atactica polyneuritiformis (Refsum's disease). *J Invest Dermatol* 1978; **70**: 126–9.
4 Blanchet-Bardon CL, Anton-Lamprecht I, Puissant A, Schnyder UW. Ultrastructural features in ichthyotic skin in Refsum's disease. In: Marks R, Dykes PJ, eds. *The Ichthyoses*. MTP Press, Lancaster, 1978; 65–9.
5 Kahlke W, Riterich R. Refsum's disease: an inborn error of lipid metabolism with storage of 3,5,11,15-tetramethyl hexadecanoic acid. Isolation and identification of the storage product. *Am J Med* 1965; **39**: 237–41.
6 Herndon JH, Steinberg D, Uhlendorf BW. Refsum's disease: defective oxidation of phytanic acid in tissue cultures derived from homozygotes and heterozygotes. *New Engl J Med* 1969; **281**: 1034–8.
7 Ramsey BC, Meeran K, Woodrow D et al. Cutaneous aspects of Refsum's disease. *J Roy Soc Med* 1991; **84** (9): 559–60.
8 Britton TC, Gibberd FB. A family with heredopathia atactica polyneuritiformis (Refsum's disease). *J Roy Soc Med* 1988; **81**: 602–3.
9 Poll-The BT, Poulos A, Sharp P et al. Ante-natal diagnosis of infantile Refsum's disease. *Clin Genet* 1985; **27**: 524–6.
10 Gibberd FB, Page NGR, Billimoria JD, Retsas J. Heredopathia atactica polyneuritiformis (Refsum's disease) treated by diet and plasma exchange. *Lancet* 1979; **i**: 575–8.

Keratitis–ichthyosis–deafness syndrome

Definition

The combination of keratitis, ichthyosis and deafness was first reported in 1915 as a generalized congenital keratoderma[1], and the acronym KID was coined in 1981 by Skinner[2]. However, the skin disease combines features of a hystrix-like ichthyosis and an erythrokeratoderma, and keratitis is not present in all cases. The pattern of inheritance is uncertain as most cases have been sporadic.

Clinical features

Many affected neonates have generalized erythema and some also have diffuse scaling. The typical skin changes gradually develop during infancy with linear and spiny hyperkeratosis in the flexures, elbows and knees and hystrix-like scaling on the limbs[3]. Scattered follicular hyperkeratoses appear on the trunk. Fixed, well-demarcated hyperkeratotic plaques arise on the scalp and face and some patients have a leonine facies[4]. Later, keratotic nodules may develop on the scalp, face and trunk, and in-situ and invasive squamous cell carcinomas arising in chronic keratotic lesions have been reported in several KID patients in early adult life[5,6]. Squamous carcinoma of the tongue has occurred in 2 children[7].

Most patients have extensive scarring alopecia and loss of eyebrows due to follicular hyperkeratosis. A reticulated palmoplantar keratoderma is a characteristic feature and progressive nail dystrophy may lead to nail loss. Acneiform eruptions over the upper trunk are common, and chronic deep abscesses with discharging sinuses (similar to hidradenitis suppurativa) are a distressing complication in some older patients. Many KID patients have had chronic resistant granulomatous fungal infections and candidal overgrowth which contribute to the nail dystrophy and body odour. Premature dental decay, short stature and cryptorchidism are occasional complications.

Rapidly progressive sensorineural deafness develops in infancy. In the most severe cases, progressive corneal vascularization occurs in childhood, often after a febrile illness, leading to pannus formation and blindness by adolescence. A progressive peripheral neuropathy, with an onset in early adulthood, has occurred in some reported cases of KID[4] and it results in severe disability. The 'tight heel cords' noted in some older patients may be an early sign of neuropathy. Intelligence is normal and it is no surprise that the combined handicaps of deafness, blindness and disfigurement impose severe limitations and hardship on the patient and family.

Pathology

There are no typical skin biopsy changes but orthohyperkeratosis and spiky acanthosis are seen, and epidermal dysplasia, often with vacuoles, in the upper epidermal layers is evident. Long-standing proliferating or invasive keratoses should be examined for signs of malignancy.

Genetics

Of the reported cases of probable KID syndrome, the majority have been sporadic, but an affected father-daughter pair[5] suggested autosomal dominant inheritance and one instance of affected siblings implied an autosomal recessive transmission[8]. Because of the rarity of this syndrome and its variable neonatal signs, prenatal diagnosis by fetal skin biopsy would probably be unreliable.

References

1 Burns FS. A case of generalized congenital keratoderma with unusual involvement of eyes, ears and nasal and buccal mucous membranes. *J Cut Dis* 1915; **33**: 255–60.
2 Skinner BA, Greist MC, Norins AL. The keratitis, ichthyosis and deafness (KID) syndrome. *Arch Dermatol* 1981; **117**: 285–9.
3 Langer K, Konrad K, Wolff K. Keratitis, ichthyosis and deafness (KID) syndrome: report of three cases and a review of the literature. *Br J Dermatol* 1990; **122**: 689–97.
4 Rycroft RJG, Moynahan EJ, Wells RS. Atypical ichthyosiform erythroderma, deafness and keratitis: a report of two cases. *Br J Dermatol* 1976; **94**: 211–17.
5 Grob JJ, Breton A, Bonafe JL, Sauvan-Ferdani M, Bonerandi JJ. Keratitis, ichthyosis and deafness (KID) syndrome. Vertical transmission and death from multiple squamous cell carcinomas. *Arch Dermatol* 1987; **123**: 777–82.
6 Hazen PG, Carney P, Lynch WS. Keratitis, ichthyosis and deafness syndrome with development of multiple cutaneous neoplasms. *Cutis* 1989; **28**: 190–1.
7 Lancaster L, Fournet BLF. Carcinoma of the tongue in a child. *J Oral Surg* 1969; **27**: 269–70.
8 Legrand I, Litoux P, Quere M, Stalder JF, Ertus M. Un syndrome rare oculo-auriculo-cutane (syndrome du Burns). *J Fr Ophthalmol* 1982; **5**: 441–5.

The trichothiodystrophies: IBIDS, PIBIDS and Tay's syndrome

Definition

The trichothiodystrophies are a rare and heterogeneous group of disorders which are known by several different names. Pollitt reported in 1968 a sibling pair with a combination of brittle hair due to trichorrhexis nodosa and altered amino acid composition, intellectual impairment and short stature[1]. Further reports highlighted the alternating birefringence and low sulphur content of the hair[2] which led to the term 'trichothiodystrophy'. In 1971 Tay reported 3 siblings who, in addition to these problems, had a generalized ichthyosiform erythroderma[3]. Decreased fertility in affected members of a large Amish kindred was attributed to the disorder[4]. The acronym IBIDS evolved to represent Ichthyosis, Brittle hair, Impaired intelligence, Decreased fertility and Short stature[5]. Photosensitivity was a feature in some patients, hence PIBIDS. These autosomal recessive disorders are presumed to be due to defects of protein metabolism and DNA repair.

Clinical features

The IBIDS syndrome may present with a collodion membrane or congenital erythroderma and evolve during infancy into an ichthyosis. Skin manifestations vary widely, from generalized fine scaling on a background erythroderma similar to NBIE, to a lamellar ichthyosis. Additional features in some patients are palmoplantar hyperkeratosis which may cause pulp atrophy and flexion contractures, hypoplastic aural cartilage, cataracts and severe nail dystrophy[5]. An elfin-like facies, chin recession and an aged appearance are typical.

Scalp and eyebrow hair is sparse, short and unruly. Mild to moderate intellectual impairment is the rule and hypogonadism leads to delayed puberty and infertility. All appear to have severe growth failure (height below the third centile), and congenital cataracts, skeletal defects, dental anomalies and neurological signs (cerebellar dysfunction, seizures, nerve deafness) have been described. An increased incidence of asthma has been noted and frequent respiratory infections and bronchiectasis developed in 1 patient though no immune defect was found[5]. A friendly disposition is characteristic.

Marked photosensitivity was reported in 15 patients with features of IBIDS but their ichthyosis resembled ichthyosis vulgaris[6]. This variant was called PIBIDS and felt to be an entity distinct from IBIDS, though this has not been the authors' experience.

Pathology

In most cases skin biopsy has shown changes similar to those of NBIE with hyperkeratosis, acanthosis and a normal or reduced granular layer. Hair microscopy shows pili torti, trichorrhexis nodosa and trichoschisis (transverse fractures). Polarizing light reveals alternating light and dark bands which give rise to the term 'tiger tail' hair.

Levels of the sulphur-containing amino acids of hair, cystine and proline are reduced to approximately half normal, but circulating levels are normal.

DNA repair studies

The result of DNA repair studies on skin fibroblasts and lymphocytes from patients with the PIBIDS variant showed markedly reduced levels of unscheduled DNA synthesis on UV light exposure[6]. The response pattern was similar to that seen in xeroderma pigmentosum (XP), complementation group D. Similar results have been obtained in IBIDS patients. In 1 patient with PIBIDS the repair defect complemented all known XP groups and was ascribed to a novel nucleotide excision repair gene defect[7]. In spite of these DNA repair defects, patients with PIBIDS or IBIDS have not developed skin malignancies which are typical of xeroderma pigmentosum.

Genetics

The trichothiodystrophies are heterogeneous autosomal recessive disorders due to differing gene defects. Some appear to involve XP genes but others clearly do not[7]. Prenatal diagnosis by fetal hair analysis has been carried out in a severely affected family[8] and molecular techniques should soon be available.

References

1 Pollitt RJ, Jenner FA, Davies M. Sibs with mental and physical retardation and trichorrhexis nodosa with abnormal amino acid composition of the hair. *Arch Dis Child* 1968; **43**: 211–16.
2 Brown AC, Belser RB, Crounse RG, Wehr BF. A congenital hair defect; trichoschisis with alternating birefringence and low sulfur content. *J Invest Dermatol* 1970; **54**: 496–509.
3 Tay CH. Ichthyosiform erythroderma, hair shaft abnormalities, mental and growth retardation, a new recessive disorder. *Arch Dermatol* 1971; **104**: 4–13.
4 Jackson CE, Weiss L, Watson JHL. Brittle hair with short stature, intellectual impairment and decreased fertility. An autosomal recessive syndrome in an Amish kindred. *Pediatrics* 1974; **54**: 201–7.
5 Jorizzo JL, Atherton DJ, Crounse RG, Wells RS. Ichthyosis, brittle hair, impaired intelligence, decreased fertility and short stature (IBIDS). *Br J Dermatol* 1982; **106**: 705–10.
6 Rebora A, Crovato F. PIBI(D)S syndrome; trichothiodystrophy with xeroderma pigmentosum (group D) mutation. *J Am Acad Dermatol* 1987; **16**: 940–7.
7 Stefanini M, Vermeulen W, Weeda G et al. A new nucleotide excision repair gene associated with the disorder trichothiodystrophy. *Am J Hum Genet* 1993; **53**: 817–21.
8 Blanchet-Bardon C. Prenatal diagnosis in Tay's syndrome. *17th World Congress in Dermatology*, Berlin, 1987.

Conradi–Hünermann syndrome, X-linked dominant ichthyosis

Definition

The condition termed X-linked dominant ichthyosis is a distinctive skin disorder which is usually associated with skeletal (chondrodysplasia punctata) and ocular defects. There are three subgroups of the chondrodysplasia punctata (CP) syndrome defined on the pattern of defects and the mode of inheritance. The rhizomelic type of CP is autosomal recessive and generally lethal in infancy, while the Conradi–Hünermann variant is either autosomal dominant or X-linked dominant[1]. Ichthyosiform erythroderma followed by a mosaic pattern ichthyosis occurs in the X-linked dominant form and this is often referred to as the Conradi–Hünermann syndrome (CHS)[2]. Females only are affected as male fetuses do not survive.

Clinical features

Affected babies are usually premature with either a collodion membrane or generalized erythroderma. Within the first year, linear and swirling patterns of erythroderma and scaling, following the lines of Blaschko, are apparent. Intervening areas of skin are unaffected. Recurrent infections (especially in the flexures) can be troublesome, and scalp and eyebrow hair growth are sparse. The X-linked dominant ichthyosis improves with age and residual signs are often subtle in adult life: they include swirls of fine scale, linear pigmentary change, follicular atrophoderma and cicatricial alopecia.

Other variable features include rounded or asymmetric facies with frontal bossing, a broad, flat nasal bridge, congenital asymmetric cataracts (mosaic lens involvement), short stature, asymmetric shortening of a limb and other skeletal defects. Chondrodysplasia punctata is a stippled calcification of long bone epiphyses and a characteristic radiological finding in infancy which usually resolves by later childhood.

Pathology

Biopsy of ichthyotic skin shows changes similar to those of ichthyosis vulgaris but without the typical ultrastructural features. Older lesions show prominent perifollicular atrophy. Epidermal calcification, needle-like inclusions in the granular layer and reduced numbers of Langerhans' cells have also been reported [3,4].

Biochemical basis

A partial deficiency of a peroxisomal enzyme, dihydroxyacetone phosphate acyltransferase (DHAPAT), has been identified in cultured fibroblasts from patients with both rhizomelic chondrodysplasia punctata and X-linked dominant ichthyosis [5]. This peroxisomal enzyme is responsible for synthesis of a group of phospholipids called plasmalogens, and deficiency of these compounds may lead to the skin changes and other manifestations of this disease. In addition, an increased level of plasma phytanic acid or urinary pipecolic acid has been found in some patients, but apart from confirming a peroxisomal defect, the significance of these results is unknown. Clofibrate has been shown to increase the number of peroxisomes in hepatocytes, but a therapeutic trial did not affect the skin disease in a patient under the authors' care.

The occurrence of epiphyseal and sometimes epidermal calcification in X-linked ichthyosis suggests that calcium metabolism may be abnormal, but baseline calcium studies are normal.

Genetics

The mosaic pattern of the ichthyosis in CHS reflects the two populations of skin cells that result from the X chromosome alleles, one normal and the other containing the genetic defect. X-linked dominant ichthyosis shows variable penetrance and is lethal in male embryos. However, a male infant with typical features of X-linked dominant CP syndrome and erythroderma in association with severe hydrocephalus and skeletal defects survived for 2 days [4].

Before undertaking genetic counselling it is important to examine all members of the extended family for subtle dysmorphism, residual skin signs, subclinical cataracts and a history of radiological abnormalities. It is also important to rule out fetal warfarin or hydantoin toxicity which can mimic autosomal dominant CP.

Studies using DNA linkage to locate the gene defect on the X chromosome are in progress. Prenatal testing, assaying DHAPAT, may be possible. The variability of disease expression and change with age make decisions on prenatal diagnosis difficult.

References

1 Spranger JW, Opitz JM, Bidder U. Heterogeneity of chondrodysplasia punctata. *Hum Genet* 1971; **11**: 190–212.
2 Happle R. X-linked dominant chondrodysplasia punctata. Review of the literature and report of a case. *Hum Genet* 1979; **53**: 65–73.
3 Kolde G, Happle R. Histologic and ultrastructural features of the ichthyotic skin in X-linked linked dominant chondrodysplasia punctata. *Acta Derm Venereol* 1984; **64**: 389–94.
4 De Raeve L, Song M, De Dobbeleer G, Spehl M, Van Regemorter N. Lethal course of X-linked dominant chondrodysplasia punctata in a male newborn. *Dermatologica* 1989, **178**: 167–70.
5 Clayton PT, Kalter DC, Atherton DA, Besley GT, Broadhead DM. Peroxisomal enzyme deficiency in X-linked dominant Conradi–Hünermann syndrome. *J Inher Metab Dis* 1989, **12**: 358–60.

Neutral lipid storage disease, Chanarin–Dorfman syndrome

Definition

The association of an autosomal recessive ichthyosis and leucocyte lipid vacuolation affecting 2 sisters was first described in 1966 by Rozenszajn [1]. Dorfman, reporting on 4 cases including a follow-up of the 2 sisters, recognized that this was a specific multisystem lipoidosis [2], and Chanarin in 1975, describing a similar case, referred to it as neutral lipid (triglyceride) storage disease (NLSD) [3]. The triglyceride deposition in white blood cells and several organs results in a combination of skin, hepatic, muscle and ocular abnormalities. Neutral lipid storage disease occurs mainly in people of Arabic descent, especially where consanguinity is common. It is rare (fewer than 20 reported cases), but some cases may be misdiagnosed.

Clinical features

Affected newborns are either erythrodermic or collodion babies. The pattern of skin disease thereafter resembles mild to moderate non-bullous ichthyosiform erythroderma, with fine, white scaling on a pink background which improves in summertime. Pruritus is often troublesome. Mild ectropion and focal lichenification over joints are common, and palmoplantar hyperkeratosis with nail dystrophy has been reported.

Muscle involvement ranges from an asymptomatic or subclinical myopathy with elevated muscle enzymes in a majority of patients to marked proximal myopathy in a few older cases. Hepatomegaly and abnormal liver enzymes due to fatty infiltration are common in childhood. Splenomegaly and malabsorption, due to intestinal mucosal lipid deposition, are occasional features. Cataracts of the nuclear type may be detected from infancy but rarely affect vision. Nerve deafness, ataxia, microcephaly and mental retardation have been reported, but most patients are intellectually normal.

Pathology

A notable feature in NLSD (seen to a lesser extent in heterozygote carriers) is the presence of lipid droplets, visible on light microscopy, in circulating polymorphs (neutrophils, eosinophils and basophils) and monocytes, but not in lymphocytes, red cells or platelets. The vacuoles stain with oil red O and Sudan black, confirming their lipid nature, and this feature has been termed 'Jordan's anomaly'. Electron microscopy shows non-membrane-bound cytoplasmic lipid droplets. Careful inspection of a fresh blood film is a simple diagnostic test for NLSD and may help to detect carriers. It should be done routinely in all patients with congenital ichthyosis.

Biopsies of muscle, liver and skin also contain numerous lipid droplets. Skin biopsy shows acanthosis and hyperkeratosis and discloses closely packed lipid droplets of varying size in basal, granular and adnexal keratinocytes and in dermal fibroblasts, smooth muscle cells and endothelium. Lipid vacuoles are also seen in the epidermis, but not in other tissues, in Refsum's disease. Ultrastructurally, epidermal lamellar bodies and intercellular lipid lamellae are disrupted by electron lucent inclusions and this lipid metabolic defect is presumed to be responsible for the ichthyosis[4]. Lipid vacuoles are present in muscle fibres and hepatocytes and mild hepatic fibrosis is common.

Biochemistry

Blood lipid analysis is normal in NLSD and scale lipids show a raised triglyceride content. Histochemical studies on cultured fibroblasts and keratinocytes confirm that the stored lipid is composed of neutral lipid or triglyceride. Studies have shown a six-fold increase in fibroblast triglyceride synthesis and a complete failure of endogenous triglyceride breakdown[5]. Exogenous triglyceride metabolism was normal and a defect in mitochondrial fatty acid oxidation was suspected. Dietary manipulation is unhelpful.

Differential diagnosis

Muscle carnitine deficiency and Wolman's disease should be excluded, as they share some of the features of NLSD.

Genetics

Most NLSD patients come from Mediterranean regions, often remote inbred communities, and are of Arab descent. The disease is clearly autosomal recessive, and heterozygotic carriers may be identified by detection of lipid vacuoles in leucocytes on a fresh blood film. This screening test should be offered to members of the extended family. Prenatal diagnosis using fetal skin biopsy is theoretically possible, and identification of the lipid metabolic defect in cultured cells may allow for early prenatal diagnosis in the near future.

References

1 Rozenszajn L, Klazman A, Yaffe D, Efrati P. Jordan's anomaly in white blood cells. *Blood* 1966; **28**: 258–65.
2 Dorfman ML, Hershko C, Eisenberg S, Sagher F. Ichthyosiform dermatosis with systemic lipidosis. *Arch Dermatol* 1974; **110**: 261–6.
3 Chanarin I, Patel A, Slavin G et al. Neutral lipid storage disease, a new disorder of lipid metabolism. *Br Med J* 1975; **1**: 553–5.
4 Elias PM, Williams ML. Neutral lipid storage disease: defective lamellar body contents and intracellular dispersion. *Arch Dermatol* 1985; **121**: 1000–8.
5 Radom J, Salvayre R, Maret A, Negre A, Douste-Blazy L. Metabolism of neutral lipids in cultured fibroblasts from multisystemic (type 3) lipid storage myopathy. *Eur J Biochem* 1987; **164**: 703–8.

Other ichthyotic disorders

CHILD syndrome

The CHILD syndrome is a very rare multisystem developmental disorder which is thought to be an X-linked dominant trait as the female to male ratio is 28:1. Isolated cases of a striking congenital unilateral dermatosis and hypoplasia had been reported since the 1960s[1], and in 1980 the acronym CHILD for Congenital Hemidysplasia, Ichthyosiform erythroderma and unilateral Limb Defects (mainly hypoplasia) was suggested[2].

The skin lesions are noted in the first days of life as hyperkeratotic crusting plaques covering most of one side of the body with sharp demarcation at the midline. Linear bands of normal skin on the affected side and of ichthyotic skin on the 'normal' side may occur and suggest a mosaic somatic mutation. The skin lesions may improve with time. Various other defects include congenital heart disease, spina bifida, renal defects, unilateral alopecia, nail dystrophy and skeletal defects[3].

Ultrastructural features noted in skin have included stratum corneum lipid vacuolation and disrupted lamellar bodies[3]. The cause is unknown but altered epidermal and fibroblast proliferation and increased synthesis of prostaglandin E_2 associated with a peroxisomal defect have been reported[4].

The occurrence of the syndrome in siblings has raised the possibility of autosomal recessive inheritance, but Happle favoured X-linked dominant expression and postulated that the unilateral and mosaic distribution was due to the Lyon effect of random X chromosome inactivation[2]. Alternatively, a teratogenic insult early in the first trimester may account for the range of defects.

References

1 Rossman RE, Shapiro EM, Freeman RG. Unilateral ichthyosisform erythroderma. *Arch Dermatol* 1963; **88**: 567–71.
2 Happle R, Koch H, Renz W. The CHILD syndrome: congenital hemidysplasia, ichthyosiform erythroderma and limb defects. *Eur J Pediatr* 1980; **134**: 27–33.
3 Hebert AA, Esterly NB, Holbrook KA, Hall JC. The CHILD syndrome. Histologic and ultrastructural studies. *Arch Dermatol* 1987; **123**: 503–9.
4 Emami S, Rizzo WB, Hanley KP et al. Peroxisomal abnormality in fibroblasts from involved skin of CHILD syndrome. *Arch Dermatol* 1992; **128**: 1213–22.

Multiple sulphatase deficiency

Multiple sulphatase deficiency[1,2] is an exceedingly rare autosomal recessive disorder caused by deficiency of two or more sulphatase enzymes, usually aryl sulphatases A, B and C and steroid sulphatase. This, in effect, leads to a combination of overlap features typical of mucopolysaccharidosis, metachromatic leucodystrophy and recessive X-linked ichthyosis[1]. Progressive neurological degeneration occurs from infancy and is often fatal in childhood. Sulphatase deficiency is confirmed by assay on fibroblasts or fresh leucocytes.

References

1 Burch M, Fensom AH, Jackson M, Pitts-Tucker T, Congdon PJ. Multiple sulphatase deficiency presenting at birth. *Clin Genet* 1986; **30**: 409–15.
2 Burk RD, Valle D, Thomas GH et al. Early manifestations of multiple sulphatase deficiency. *J Pediatr* 1984; **104**: 574–8.

Ichthyosis follicularis with alopecia and photophobia

Ichthyosis follicularis with alopecia and photophobia (IFAP) is a syndrome consisting of extensive, non-inflammatory follicular hyperkeratosis with congenital, generalized, non-cicatricial alopecia affecting the whole body, and severe photophobia[1]. It is sometimes called MacLeod's syndrome[2]. There are widespread keratotic papules on the head, trunk and limbs, especially the knees and elbows, with prominent follicular spiny projections over extensor surfaces. Generalized xerosis and pruritus are common. The keratoses may improve with age. Teeth, nails and sweating are normal and the palms and soles are spared. Histology of the skin in 2 cases revealed follicular plugging and hyperkeratosis with absence of sebaceous glands and hair follicles, but normal sweat glands[1].

Photophobia is due to keratitis and corneal erosions. Additional features described in some patients included atopy, recurrent chest infections, growth retardation and seizures.

The IFAP syndrome can be distinguished from keratosis follicularis spinulosa decalvans and keratosis pilaris rubra atrophicans facei (ulerythema ophryogenes) in which a non-congenital, inflammatory, scarring alopecia occurs. Keratosis follicularis spinulosa decalvans and the KID syndrome both feature ocular disease, but palmoplantar hyperkeratosis is characteristic of each. The IFAP syndrome has been noted in siblings and all patients have been males, so an X-linked recessive inheritance is likely.

References

1 Eramo LR, Esterly NB, Zieserl EJ, Lee Stock E, Herrmann J. Ichthyosis follicularis with alopecia and photophobia. *Arch Dermatol* 1985; **121**: 1167–74.
2 MacLeod JMH. Three cases of ichthyosis follicularis associated with baldness. *Br J Dermatol* 1909; **21**: 165–89.

Familial peeling skin syndrome

Familial peeling skin syndrome is not a true ichthyosis as it causes periodic or continual shedding of large sheets of stratum corneum rather than scaling. Variously known as keratolysis exfoliativa congenita or deciduous skin, the label 'familial continual skin peeling' was suggested in 1969 in a case report of 4 affected siblings[1].

Continuous and generalized non-inflammatory, superficial peeling starts either at birth or in childhood, and persists with only slight seasonal variation. Thin flakes of varying size and shape result and peeling can be produced by rubbing. The palms and soles are spared and hair, nails and teeth are normal.

Histologically, a lesion showed hyperkeratosis and splitting at the corneal–granular interface. Reduced desmosomal plates and irregular intercellular lamellae at the junction of the stratum corneum and stratum granulosum have been reported[2]. An intracellular cytoplasmic split in the lower stratum corneum was identified on electron microscopy[3].

Some confusion concerning the existence of an inflammatory type of familial continual skin peeling has arisen. Continuous peeling was reported in siblings in association with congenital ichthyosiform erythroderma[4], but Traupe suggested that this condition resembled the exfoliative lesions seen in Netherton's syndrome[5].

References

1 Kurban AK, Azar HA. Familial continual skin peeling. *Br J Dermatol* 1969; **81**: 191–5.

2 Abdel-Hafez K, Safer AM, Selim MM, Rehak A. Familial continual skin peeling. *Dermatologica* 1983; **166**: 23–31.

3 Silverman AK, Ellis CN, Beais TF, Woo TY. Continual skin peeling syndrome. An electron microscopic study. *Arch Dermatol* 1986; **122**: 71–5.

4 Mevorah B, Frenk E, Saurat JH, Siegenthaler G. Peeling skin syndrome: a clinical, ultrastructural and biochemical study. *Br J Dermatol* 1987; **116**: 117–25.

5 Traupe H. *The Ichthyoses: A Guide to Clinical Diagnosis, Genetic Counselling and Therapy.* Springer, Heidelberg, 1989.

Isolated genetic disorders with ichthyosis

There are several case reports of congenital ichthyoses occurring in association with extracutaneous defects which do not fit within the recognized classification of inherited ichthyoses.

Ichthyosis and renal disease

Ichthyosis associated with renal disease was reported by Passwell in 3 siblings of a consanguineous family[1]. Their skin was red with fine scaling, and atrophic changes with small blisters occurred over the dorsal hands and feet. Skin biopsy revealed vacuolation in basal keratinocytes, reminiscent of neutral lipid storage disease, and collagen disruption. They had a generalized aminoaciduria, dwarfism and mental retardation.

A congenital ichthyosis with renal parenchymal disease, growth retardation and hypogonadism was reported in 3 siblings of a family by Rayner[2], while another family had renal disease, prolinuria, nerve deafness and a poorly defined ichthyosis which appeared to be autosomal dominant[3].

Ichthyosis and deafness

Congenital ichthyosis with neural deafness has been frequently recorded. In Baden's report of a young man, generalized fine scaling and keratosis pilaris developed in early infancy and were associated with red, scaly plaques on the arms, moderate sensorineural deafness from childhood, pes cavus and ocular albinism[4]. The patient later developed perioral rugae and multifocal alopecia, and many of his features resembled those of KID syndrome. Senter's case with so-called atypical ichthyosiform erythroderma and neurosensory deafness was more akin to the KID syndrome[5]. A 65-year-old woman who had lifelong follicular and acral warty keratoses with deforming palmoplantar keratoderma, severe alopecia and squamous cell carcinomas may also have had a variant of the KID syndrome[6]. Mallory's patient, an infant with ichthyosis and deafness, may have had KID syndrome, but he died of malnutrition due to Hirschsprung's disease[7]. A further patient with ichthyosis, deafness and mental retardation had in addition dental and skeletal defects and developed thyroid cancer[8].

Ichthyosis and other neurological disorders

Ichthyosis associated with other neurological disorders was reported in 2 brothers with mild ichthyosis, adult-onset cerebellar degeneration and hepatosplenomegaly. There was no evidence of X-linked ichthyosis and no apparent lipid storage disorder[9].

Jagell reported a cluster of patients in Sweden with autosomal recessive congenital ichthyosis, alopecia, eclabium, ectropion and mental retardation which differed from Sjögren–Larsson syndrome[10]. A young female with features of Sjögren–Larsson syndrome but with normal fatty alcohol metabolism was noted to have defective lamellar bodies thought to be due to a novel metabolic disorder[11].

Ichthyosis and skeletal defects

Ichthyosis and skeletal defects are not uncommonly associated. The ichthyosis–cheek–eyebrow (ICE) syndrome reported in 5 subjects in four generations of one family consisted of ichthyosis vulgaris, fullness of the cheeks and thinning of the eyebrows[12]. Other dysmorphic features occurred and skeletal abnormalities included kyphoscoliosis. Cortical thickening, arthrogryposis and osteopetrosis have also been recorded in single case reports [13–15].

Ichthyosis and immune defects

Ichthyoses with immune defects includes Nezelof's syndrome[16] and a case report of a child with ichthyosiform erythroderma, congenital alopecia and deafness with recurrent infections who had a neutrophil chemotaxis defect[17]. Abnormal T lymphocytes were reported in another case[18].

Miscellaneous

Congenital ichthyosis has been reported in association with biliary atresia and in several patients with ectodermal defects[19]. An autosomal dominant syndrome in 3 members of a family included ichthyosis, abnormal platelet function, asplenism, migraine and dyslexia[20].

References

1 Passwell J, Zipperkowski L, Katznelson D et al. A syndrome characterized by congenital ichthyosis with atrophy, mental retardation, dwarfism and generalized aminoaciduria. *J Pediatr* 1973; **82**: 466–70.

2 Rayner A, Lampert RP, Rennet OM. Familial ichthyosis, dwarfism, mental retardation and renal disease. *J Pediatr* 1978; **92**: 766–8.

3 Goyer RA, Reynolds J, Burke J, Burholder P. Hereditary renal disease with neurosensory hearing loss, prolinuria and ichthyosis. *Am J Med Sci* 1968; **256**: 166–79.

4 Baden HP, Bronstein BR. Ichthyosiform dermatosis and deafness. *Arch Dermatol* 1988; **124**: 102–6.

5 Senter TP, Jones KL, Sakati N. Atypical ichthyosiform erythroderma and neurosensory deafness: a distinct syndrome. *J Pediatr* 1978; **92**: 68–72.

6 Welton DG. A peculiar combination of ectodermal defects with squamous cell carcinomas. *Cutis* 1975; **16**: 829–37.

7 Mallory SB, Haynie LS, Williams ML, Hall W. Ichthyosis, deafness and Hirschsprung's disease. *Pediatr Dermatol* 1989; **6**: 24–7.

8 Ruzika T, Goerz G, Anton-Lamprecht I. Syndrome of ichthyosis congenita, neurosensory deafness, oligophrenia, dental hypoplasia, brachydactyly, clinodactyly, accessory cervical ribs and thyroid cancer. *Dermatologica* 1981; **162**: 124–36.

9 Dykes PJ, Marks R, Harper PS. A syndrome of ichthyosis, hepatosplenomegaly and cerebellar degeneration. *Br J Dermatol* 1979; **100**: 585–90.

10 Jagell SF, Holmgren G, Hofer PA. Congenital ichthyosis, alopecia, eclabion, ectropion and mental retardation. *Clin Genet* 1987; **31**: 102–8.

11 Koone MD, Rizzo WB, Elias PM et al. Ichthyosis, mental retardation and asymptomatic spasticity. *Arch Dermatol* 1990; **126**: 1485–90.

12 Sidransky E, Feinstein A, Goodman RM. Ichthyosis-cheek-eyebrow (ICE) syndrome, a new autosomal dominant disorder. *Clin Genet* 1987; **31**: 137–42.

13 Koller E, Maureseth K, Haneberg B, Aarskog D. Familial syndrome of diaphyseal cortical thickening of the long bones, bowed legs, tendency to fracture and ichthyosis. *Pediatr Radiol* 1979; **8**: 179–82.

14 Baraitser M, Burn J, Fixsen J. A recessively inherited windmill-vane camptodactyly/ichthyosis syndrome. *J Med Genet* 1983; **20**: 125–7.

15 Dowd PM, Munro DD. Ichthyosis and osteopetrosis. *J Roy Soc Med* 1983; **76**: 423–6.

16 Nezelof C, Jammet ML, Lortholary P, Labrunes B, Lamy M. L'Hypoplasie hereditaire du thymus. *Arch Franc Pediat* 1964; **21**: 897–920.

17 Pincus SH, Thomas IT, Clark RA, Ochs HD. Defective neutrophil chemotaxis with variant ichthyosis, hyper IgE and recurrent infections. *J Pediatr* 1975; **87**: 908–11.

18 Hendrickx GF, Zegers BJ, Van Elden L, Stoop JW. Congenital ichthyosis, immunodeficiency and abnormal T cells. *Int J Dermatol* 1979; **18**: 731–42.

19 Baden HP, Imber M. Ichthyosis with an unusual constellation of ectodermal dysplasias. *Clin Genet* 1989; **35**: 455–61.

20 Stormorken H, Sjaastad O, Langslet A et al. A new syndrome: thrombocytopathia, muscle fatigue, asplenia, miosis, migraine, dyslexia and ichthyosis. *Clin Genet* 1985; **28**: 367–74.

Chapter 6

Erythrokeratodermas, follicular keratoses, palmoplantar keratodermas and porokeratoses

D. G. Paige and J. I. Harper

Introduction

The erythrokeratodermas, follicular keratoses, palmoplantar keratodermas, Darier's disease and porokeratoses are disorders of keratinization and are listed in Table 6.1.

Erythrokeratodermas

The erythrokeratodermas are a group of rare genodermatoses characterized by well-demarcated, erythematous, hyperkeratotic plaques. Three entities are recognized (Table 6.2); although other variants have been described [1–3], the relationship and significance of these is uncertain.

Erythrokeratoderma variabilis

Synonyms: *Keratosis rubra figurata, Mendes da Costa syndrome*

Clinical features

Skin lesions are normally present in the first year of life but may rarely occur later in childhood. Transient, irregularly shaped patches of erythema occur at any site and appear to migrate slowly over the body. They normally last from hours to days and may be accompanied by some fine scaling. Changes in ambient temperature, emotional upsets or external pressure may induce new lesions. Patients also develop more fixed geographic, hyperkeratotic plaques, most commonly on the extensor surfaces, buttocks and face.

These are well demarcated and range from red to yellowish-brown in colour. They are somewhat more persistent, but they may vary both in size and thickness. Palmoplantar keratoderma is rarely associated [4]. The condition normally continues into adult life. The clinical features are variable both within a single family and an individual patient [4–8].

Pathology

Light microscopy reveals non-specific compact hyperkeratosis with a varying degree of 'basket-weave' hyperkeratosis and parakeratosis. There is underlying acanthosis and papillomatosis. A sparse, mononuclear perivascular infiltrate is seen in the upper dermis. Electron microscopy has shown a decrease in keratinosomes (membrane coating granules) in the granular layer [9,10] in some patients, but this has not been found in other reports [11,12]. A dense perinuclear tonofilament and keratohyalin granule complex has been described [12], but this finding is not consistent. Immunohistochemical studies have revealed abnormal basal cytokeratin staining [13] and an increase in suprabasal involucrin [14] although the epidermal proliferation rate is normal.

Genetics

The inheritance is autosomal dominant. Van der Schroeff et al [15] described a large Dutch family in whom the disorder showed close linkage with the Rh blood group system, which is located at 1p36.2–34. A maximum log of the odds (LOD) score of 5.5 was found at a recombination fraction of 0.03. Only 1 recombinant was found among 27 informative

Table 6.1 *Disorders of keratinization (excluding the ichthyoses, Chapter 5)*

Erythrokeratodermas
    Erythrokeratoderma variabilis
    Erythrokeratoderma *en cocardes*
    Erythrokeratoderma progressiva symmetrica

Follicular keratoses
    Keratosis pilaris
    Keratosis pilaris atrophicans
    Erythromelanosis follicularis faciei et colli

Darier's disease
    Acrokeratosis verruciformis of Hopf

Palmoplantar keratodermas
    Diffuse palmoplantar keratodermas
        Tylosis; Thost–Unna syndrome
        Epidermolytic (Vörner) type
        Progressive type; Greither's syndrome
        Gamborg–Nielsen type
        Mal de Meleda
        Papillon–Lefèvre syndrome
        Pachonychia congenita
    Mutilating keratodermas
        Vohwinkel's syndrome
        Olmsted's syndrome
    Localized palmoplantar keratodermas
        Punctate palmoplantar keratoderma
        Keratosis punctata of the palmar creases
        Focal acral hyperkeratosis/acrokeratoelastoidosis
        Striate palmoplantar keratoderma
        Oculocutaneous tyrosinaemia
    Miscellaneous palmoplantar keratodermas

Porokeratoses
    Porokeratosis of Mibelli
    Linear porokeratosis
    Disseminated superficial actinic porokeratosis
    Palmoplantar porokeratosis

patients. Subsequent study of a second Dutch kindred brought the maximum LOD score to 9.93, for linkage between erythrokeratoderma variabilis and Rh at a recombination fraction of 0.03[15].

Treatment

Oral retinoids are effective [13,16]. Ultraviolet B therapy may also be beneficial.

Table 6.2 *The erythrokeratodermas*

Erythrokeratoderma variabilis
Erythrokeratoderma *en cocardes*
Erythrokeratoderma progressiva symmetrica

References

1 Beare JM, Nevin NC, Frogatt P et al. Atypical erythrokeratoderma with deafness, physical retardation and peripheral neuropathy. *Br J Dermatol* 1972; **87**: 308–14.
2 Giroux JM, Barbeau A. Erythrokeratoderma with ataxia. *Arch Dermatol* 1972; **106**: 183–8.
3 Schnyder VW, Wissler H, Wendt G. Eine weitere Form von atypischer Erythrokeratodermie mit Schwerborigkeit und cerebraler Schadigung. *Helv Paediatr Acta* 1968; **23**: 220–30.
4 Brown J, Kierland RR. Erythrokeratodermia variabilis. *Arch Dermatol* 1966; **93**: 194–201.
5 Cram DL. Erythrokeratoderma variabilis and variable circinate erythrokeratodermas. *Arch Dermatol* 1970; **101**: 68–73.
6 Gewirtzman GB, Winkler NW, Dobson RL. Erythrokeratoderma variabilis. A family study. *Arch Dermatol* 1978; **114**: 259–61.
7 Hacham-Zadeh S, Even-Paz Z. Erythrokeratoderma variabilis in a Jewish Kurdish family. *Clin Genet* 1978; **13**: 404–8.
8 Luy JT, Jacobs AH, Nickoloff BJ. A child with erythematous and hyperkeratotic patches. *Arch Dermatol* 1988; **124**: 1271–7.
9 Rappaport IP, Goldes GA, Goltz RW. Erythrokeratoderma variabilis treated with isotretinoin – a clinical histological and ultrastructural study. *Arch Dermatol* 1986; **122**: 441–5.
10 Vandersteen PR, Muller SA, Erythrokeratoderma variabilis. *Arch Dermatol* 1971; **103**: 362–70.
11 Jurecka W. Erythrokeratodermia variabilis. *Arch Dermatol* 1986; **122**: 1356.
12 Macfarlane AW, Chapman SJ, Verbov JL. Is erythrokeratoderma one disorder? A clinical and ultrastructural study of two siblings. *Br J Dermatol* 1991; **124**: 487–91.
13 McFadden N, Oppedal BR, Ree K et al. Erythrokeratoderma variabilis: immunohistochemical and ultrastructural studies of the epidermis. *Acta Derm Venereol* 1987; **67**: 284–8.
14 Kanitakis J, Zambruno G, Viac J et al. Involucrin expression in keratinization disorders of the skin – a preliminary study. *Br J Dermatol* 1987; **117**: 479–86.
15 Van der Schroeff JG, Van Leeuwen-Cornelisse I, Van Haeringen A et al. Further evidence for localization of the gene of erythrokeratoderma variabilis. *Hum Genet* 1988; **80**: 97–8.
16 Marks R, Finlay AY, Holt PJA. Severe disorders of keratinization: effects of treatment with Tigason (etretinate). *Br J Dermatol* 1981; **104**: 667–73.

Erythrokeratoderma *en cocardes*

Synonym: *Degos syndrome*

Clinical features

Erythrokeratoderma *en cocardes* is similar to erythrokeratoderma variabilis (EKV) in that fixed, erythematous, hyperkeratotic plaques appear in infancy, commonly on extensor surfaces. However, this condition is also characterized by intermittent annular lesions which show central scaling with surrounding erythema, giving a target-like appearance. The eruption may clear at times but tends to progress during childhood. Intercurrent infection may exacerbate the condition, whereas sunlight tends to improve it. There is no associated palmoplantar keratoderma, although intermittent peeling of the palmar skin may be seen[1,2].

Pathology

Light microscopy findings are similar for both types of lesion, and consist of hyperkeratosis with underlying acanthosis and a mild perivascular monocytic infiltrate in the upper dermis[3].

Genetics

Kelly et al described a family of 31 members spanning five generations where 12 members were affected. This family showed an autosomal dominant inheritance. Degos's original family also showed dominant inheritance over two generations. The relationship to EKV is uncertain as linkage studies have not yet been reported.

Differential diagnosis

Erythema perstans and tinea corporis must be excluded.

Treatment

Treatment is as for EKV.

References

1 Cram DL. Erythrokeratoderma variabalis and variable circinate erythrokeratodermas. *Arch Dermatol* 1970; **101**: 68–73.
2 Degos R, Delzant O, Morival H. Erythème desquamatif en plaques congénital et familial (génodermatose nouvelle?). *Bull Soc Fr Dermat Syph* 1947; **54**: 4–42.
3 Kelly LJ, Koscard E. Congenital ichthyosis with erythema annulare centrifugum. A new form of ichthyosis affecting 12 members of a family of 31 in 5 generations. *Dermatologica* 1970; **140**: 75–83.

Erythrokeratoderma progressiva symmetrica

Synonym: *Gottron's syndrome*

Clinical features

Erythrokeratoderma progressiva symmetrica (EPS) usually appears in early childhood and is characterized by fixed, large, well-defined, hyperkeratotic plaques. These plaques are normally symmetrical with a somewhat orange colour. Lesions are commonly on the limbs, buttocks, shoulders and fingers and occasionally involve the face. An erythematous, palmoplantar keratoderma is seen in about 50% of cases. The plaques tend to extend during the first decade of life and then remain stable. There is some tendency to improvement after puberty, but lesions persist into adult life[1].

Pathology

Light microscopy is non-specific and shows hyperkeratosis and patchy parakeratosis overlying an acanthotic epidermis. Vacuolation around the nuclei has been reported in the granular layer. A sparse, lymphohistiocytic, perivascular infiltrate is seen in the upper dermis. Electron microscopy shows markedly swollen mitochondria in the granular cells and vacuolation in the cells of the lower stratum corneum. Desmosomes, keratohyalin granules and tonofilament bundles appear normal[2]. Epidermal proliferation is increased owing to shortening of the interphase[3].

Genetics

In 1982 Ruiz-Maldonado reported 10 cases of EPS[1]. Four of these were sporadic cases, 2 of them from consanguineous parents. However, the other 6 cases were from three families (in which 16 relatives were affected) and the condition followed an autosomal dominant inheritance pattern. The clinical severity showed marked variation within individual families. Rodriguez-Pichardo reported 1 sporadic case and a kindred with 7 affected members spanning five generations that followed an autosomal dominant pattern[4]. Reviewing all the reported cases, it appears that the inheritance is autosomal dominant, although 30–40% of these were sporadic cases and presumably new mutations. MacFarlane et al described 2 sisters born to non-consanguineous, unaffected parents. The younger sister developed EKV at the age of 17 months, whereas the elder sister developed the clinical signs of EPS at the age of 6 years. The skin ultrastructural findings were identical although the epidermal proliferation rate was not measured. These workers conjectured that EKV and EPS might be different phenotypic expressions of a single genetic disorder[5].

Treatment

Oral retinoids produce a good response[1].

References

1 Ruiz-Maldonado R, Tamayo L, Del Castillo V et al. Erythrokeratodermia progressive symmetrica. Report of 10 cases. *Dermatologica* 1982; **164**: 133–41.

2 Nazzaro V, Blanchet-Bardon C. Progressive symmetric erythrokeratoderma. Histological and ultrastructural study of patient before and after treatment with etretinate. *Arch Dermatol* 1986; **122**: 434–40.

3 Hopsu-Havu VK, Tuohimaa P. Erythrokeratodermia congenitalis progressiva symmetrica (Gottron). An analysis of kinetics of epidermal cell proliferation. *Dermatologica* 1971; **142**: 137–44.

4 Rodriguez-Pichardo A, Garcia-Bravo B, Sanchez-Pdreno P et al. Progressive symmetric erythrokeratodermia. *J Am Acad Dermatol* 1988; **19**: 129–30.

5 MacFarlane AW, Chapman SJ, Verbov JL. Is erythrokeratoderma one disorder? A clinical and ultrastructural study of two siblings. *Br J Dermatol* 1991; **124**: 487–91.

Follicular keratoses

The follicular keratoses are a large group of skin disorders characterized by keratinous plugging in follicular orifices, which may be associated with perifollicular erythema and scarring alopecia. This group is normally discussed separately from conditions of follicular hyperkeratosis (e.g. Darier's disease, follicular ichthyosis and pityriasis rubra pilaris) and inflammatory skin conditions with a follicular distribution (e.g. follicular psoriasis). This separation is somewhat artificial, as it is based in part on the extent and severity of the lesions and the associated features. The aetiology of the follicular keratoses is poorly understood and considerable overlap exists in the present clinical classification (Table 6.3).

Keratosis pilaris

Clinical features

Keratosis pilaris is a common condition characterized by the appearance of greyish-white plugs of keratin in follicular orifices, which may contain damaged hair[1]. The cause is unknown. The condition usually starts in childhood and increases in incidence until the end of the second decade, and then tends to decrease in later life. Its distribution is commonly on the upper, outer surfaces of the arms and thighs, and less frequently affects the face. Rarely it can be generalized. The affected areas often show complete sparing of some follicles. Some cases have a degree of perifollicular erythema. It is often this latter feature, particularly when severe and involving the face, that

Table 6.3 *Follicular keratoses*

Keratosis pilaris
Keratosis pilaris atrophicans
Erythromelanosis follicularis faciei et colli

causes concern. An 'atypical keratosis pilaris', which has an erythematous base and extensively involves the trunk, has been reported in a number of institutionalized patients with various forms of mental retardation[2]. Similar findings were reported in 51 patients with Down's syndrome[3]. Most of those affected were male, aged between 20 and 40 years.

Pathology

Light microscopy reveals a plug of keratin within the follicular opening. Mild, non-specific inflammatory changes may be seen in the upper dermis.

Genetics

Keratosis pilaris is a common disorder affecting up to 40% of the population. It shows an increased incidence in patients with autosomal dominant ichthyosis vulgaris (74%)[4] and possibly in patients with atopic dermatitis[5], although the association in this latter group has been disputed by Mevorah et al[4]. It is generally believed that keratosis pilaris shows an autosomal dominant inheritance pattern with variable penetrance[6]. Some authors have argued that keratosis pilaris is indeed part of the phenotype of ichthyosis vulgaris[7]. However, the genetic relationship between keratosis pilaris, ichthyosis vulgaris and atopic dermatitis has yet to be elucidated.

Treatment

Keratosis pilaris often causes anxiety to parents of affected children. Reassurance is essential, and the fact that the condition tends to improve with age should be emphasized. Treatment is unsatisfactory. The regular application of an emollient ointment is recommended. Keratolytic preparations and other abrasive agents are usually disappointing and tend to cause unacceptable irritation and soreness of the skin.

References

1 Forman L. Keratosis pilaris. *Br J Dermatol* 1954; **66**: 279–82.

2 Coombs FP, Butterworth T. Atypical keratosis pilaris. *Arch Derm Syphilol* 1950; **62**: 305–13.

3 Finn OA, Grant PW, McCallum DI et al. A singular dermatosis of mongols. *Arch Dermatol* 1978; **114**: 1493–4.

4 Mevorah B, Marazzi A, Frenk E. The prevalence of accentuated palmoplantar markings and keratosis pilaris in atopic dermatitis, autosomal dominant ichthyosis and control dermatological patients. *Br J Dermatol* 1985; **112**: 679–85.

5 Hanifin JM, Rajka G. Diagnostic features of atopic dermatitis. *Acta Derm Venereol* 1980; **92** (suppl.): 44–7.

6 Griffiths WAD, Leigh IM, Marks R. Keratosis pilaris. In: Champion RH, Burton JL, Ebling FJG, eds. *Textbook of Dermatology*, vol. 3. 5th ed. Blackwell, Oxford, 1992; 1352.

7 Kuokkanen K. Ichthyosis vulgaris. *Acta Derm Venereol* 1969; **49** (suppl. 62): 5–35.

Keratosis pilaris atrophicans

Three subtypes of this condition are said to occur based on the variation in clinical features. They all have in common the triad of follicular keratoses, inflammation and atrophy. At present it is not clear whether they reflect a *spectrum* of a single disorder or whether they exist as separate disease entities (Table 6.4). Certainly some patients appear to overlap this clinical classification.

Clinical features

Ulerythema ophryogenes

In ulerythema ophryogenes[1,2], from early childhood keratosis pilaris with varying degrees of perifollicular erythema occurs on the lateral portion of the eyebrows and progresses to the cheeks. The erythematous component is variable but normally pronounced. Keratosis pilaris may also be seen on the upper arms, thighs and buttocks. The atrophic nature of the process leads to loss of the lateral eyebrows and may progress to involve the medial portion as well. Associations with Noonan's syndrome[3] and dysmorphic facies, motor delay and mental retardation[2] have been reported.

Keratosis pilaris decalvans

Keratosis pilaris decalvans [4–6] starts in infancy with keratosis pilaris on the face. This becomes more extensive during childhood, affecting the limbs, scalp and neck. By late childhood a significant degree of atrophy occurs, leading to scarring alopecia of the scalp and eyebrows. The condition is more severe in males. Various associations have been reported with this disorder but their significance is unclear. Photophobia and palmoplantar keratoderma appear most common. Corneal abnormalities, deafness, mental retardation and nail abnormalities are less frequently associated. There is some clinical overlap with the X-linked recessive IFAP syndrome (ichthyosis follicularis, atrichia and photophobia)[7]. The presence of pustulation, with a polymorphonuclear neutrophil infiltrate and a lack of follicular plugging histologically, are more in favour of the diagnosis of folliculitis decalvans.

Table 6.4 *Subtypes of keratosis pilaris atrophicans*

Ulerythema ophryogenes (keratosis pilaris atrophicans faciei)
Keratosis pilaris decalvans (keratosis follicularis spinulosa decalvans)
Atrophoderma vermiculata

Atrophoderma vermiculata

Atrophoderma vermiculata[8] manifests itself somewhat later, towards the end of the first decade of life, with small, erythematous follicular plugs affecting the cheeks. It extends back towards the ears and can rarely involve the forehead. This stage is short-lived and atrophy rapidly ensues, leaving numerous small, irregularly shaped pits or scars on the cheeks. Keratosis pilaris may be found on the limbs, but atrophy at these sites is most uncommon.

Pathology

The pathological findings are similar in all three of these conditions and vary depending on the biopsy site and the time-course of the disease. Early changes are similar to keratosis pilaris. Later on in the disease, light microscopy shows follicular plugging with keratin, epithelial cysts and an atrophic epidermis. In the dermis there is a perifollicular and perivascular lymphocytic infiltrate which progresses to sclerosis of the dermal collagen and skin appendages with time.

Genetics

Most cases appear to occur sporadically. However, Frosch described 4 members of a German family over three generations with atrophoderma vermiculata showing autosomal dominant inheritance[8]. A similar but smaller pedigree was described by Voge[9]. The original paper describing ulerythema ophryogenes reported three families spanning only two generations, suggesting autosomal dominant transmission[10]. Mertens reported 15 patients with ulerythema from five families suggesting a dominant inheritance and also commented on an increase incidence of atopy[11].

Keratosis pilaris decalvans is probably inherited as an X-linked dominant trait, with more severe manifestations appearing in males, especially when the condition is associated with photophobia and/or palmoplantar keratoderma[12,13]. Kuokkanen described a Finnish pedigree with 3 affected males and 3 less severely affected females over three generations and suggested X-linked inheritance, but the numbers are too small to exclude an autosomal dominant pattern[5]. The relationship to the IFAP syndrome is unclear.

Treatment

No effective treatment exists for these follicular disorders. Topical treatments, as used for keratosis pilaris, are frequently ineffective[2]. There is the occasional anecdotal report of some improvement with systemic retinoids (etretinate), but generally the response to this drug is very disappointing. Dermabrasion or collagen implants may help the cosmetic appearance of facial pitting. These disorders follow a chronic course, but they may improve spontaneously to some degree in the third and fourth decades.

References

1 Davenport DD. Ulerythema ophryogenes. Review and report of a case. Discussion of relationship to certain other skin disorders and association with internal abnormalities. *Arch Dermatol* 1964; **89**: 74–80.
2 Burnett JW, Schwartz MF, Berberian BJ. Ulerythema ophryogenes with multiple congenital anomalies. *J Am Acad Dermatol* 1988; **18**: 437–40.
3 Snell JA, Mallory SB. Ulerythema ophryogenes in Noonan syndrome. *Pediatr Dermatol* 1990; **7** (1): 77–8.
4 Rand R, Baden HP. Keratosis follicularis spinulosa decalvans. *Arch Dermatol* 1983; **119**: 22–6.
5 Kuokkanen K. Keratosis follicularis spinulosa decalvans in a family from northern Finland. *Acta Derm Venereol* 1971; **51**: 146–50.
6 Stevanovic DV. Keratosis follicularis spinulosa decalvans with birefringent hairs. An association with variable keratoderma. *Dermatol Monatsschr* 1988; **174**: 736–40.
7 Traupe H. The ichthyosis follicularis, atrichia and photophobia (IFAP) syndrome. In: *The Ichthyoses. A Guide to Clinical Diagnosis, Genetic Counselling and Therapy.* Springer, Heidelberg, 1989; 203–6.
8 Frosch PJ, Brumage MR, Schuster-Pavlovic C et al. Atrophoderma vermiculatum. *J Am Acad Dermatol* 1988; **18**: 538–42.
9 Vogel L. Atrophoderma vermiculata. *Dermatol Wochensche* 1950; **122**: 669–74.
10 Taenzer P. Über das Ulerythema ophryogenes, eine noch nicht beschriebene Hautkrankheit. *Monatsschr Prakt Dermatol* 1889; **8**: 197–208.
11 Mertens RLJ. Ulerythema ophryogenes and atopy. *Arch Dermatol* 1969; **97**: 662–3.
12 Siemens HW. Keratosis follicularis spinulosa decalvans. *Arch Dermatol Syphilol* (Berlin) 1926; **151**: 384–6.
13 Voss M. Keratosis follicularis – new genetic aspects. *Hautarzt* 1991; **42**: 319–21.

Erythromelanosis follicularis faciei et colli

Erythromelanosis follicularis faciei et colli is a rare disorder of unknown aetiology characterized by follicular keratosis, hyperpigmentation and erythema.

Clinical features

The condition was first described in 6 Japanese men in 1960 by Kitamura[1]. It has since been described in a number of Caucasians [2–4]. The onset is normally in the second decade of life, but it may appear in early childhood. It is considerably more common in males, although a number of cases have now been reported in females [3, 5, 6]. Lesions arise symmetrically on the cheeks or neck and may then spread to involve the chin or temples, and in one case the auricles and eyebrows[7]. A unilateral presentation is also possible. Lesions show a red-brown pigmentation, fine telangiectasia and scaling, and follicular papules. Keratosis pilaris at other sites is common. The erythematous component blanches, leaving a brownish discolouration.

Pathology

Light microscopy shows non-specific changes of dilated follicles with keratin plugs, mild hyperkeratosis and acanthosis. There is a mild dilation of the capillaries and moderate perivascular, lymphocytic infiltrate around the follicles of the upper dermis with some dermal oedema. There is pronounced melanin pigmentation in the basal layer.

Genetics

No familial cases have been described to date, and although many authors regard erythromelanosis follicularis as a variant of keratosis pilaris, the sexual predilection and presence of pigmentation may distinguish this as a separate entity.

Treatment

Treatment is difficult. Topical retinoic acid has been tried, with little improvement[3].

References

1 Kitamura K, Kato H, Mishima Y et al. Erythromelanosis follicularis faciei. *Hautartz* 1960; **9**: 391–3.
2 Mishima Y, Rudner E. Erythromelanosis follicularis faciei et colli. *Dermatologica* 1966; **132**: 269–87.
3 Andersen BL. Erythromelanosis follicularis faciei et colli. *Br J Dermatol* 1980; **102**: 323–5.
4 Watt TL, Kaiser JS. Erythromelanosis follicularis faciei et colli. *J Am Acad Dermatol* 1981; **5**: 533–4.
5 McGillis ST, Tuthill RJ, Ratz JL et al. Unilateral erythromelanosis follicularis faciei et colli in a young girl. *J Am Acad Dermatol* 1991; **25** (2): 430–2.
6 Alcalay J, Ingber A, Halevi S et al. Erythromelanosis follicularis faciei in women. *Br J Dermatol* 1986; **114**: 267.
7 Seki T, Takahashi S, Morohashi M. A case of erythromelanosis follicularis faciei with a unique distribution. *J Dermatol* 1991; **18** (3): 167–70.

Darier's disease

Synonyms: *Darier–White disease, keratosis follicularis*

Darier's disease is characterized by abnormal follicular keratinization in a seborrhoeic distribution. It was first described by Darier[1] and White[2] in 1889.

Clinical features

Patients usually present in childhood or as teenagers with hyperkeratotic, follicular papules in the seborrhoeic areas[3,4]. Males and females are equally affected. Papules are not entirely follicular but also occur around sweat ducts and salivary ducts. The lesions have a somewhat greasy, crusted appearance with a yellowish-brown hue. Common sites are the axillae, groin, natal cleft, neck, seborrhoeic areas of the trunk, and the face, especially the scalp margin (Figure 6.1). The papules may coalesce to form confluent, boggy, papillomatous masses which can become malodorous. The lesions are frequently itchy but rarely painful. Most patients note that heat or increased sweating can exacerbate the condition. Sunlight may also exacerbate the disease, although a small percentage of patients notice improvement after sun exposure. Scalp involvement is common but only rarely leads to alopecia.

Small keratotic papules and pitting are commonly seen on the palms and soles and can be an isolated finding in 'unaffected' relatives. Haemorrhagic macules are also occasionally seen on the palms and soles and may follow trauma[5]. Nails are frequently involved and may show red or white longitudinal lines, longitudinal ridging, V-shaped notching at the free nail margin, subungual hyperkeratoses and increased fragility with painful splitting. Oral mucosal lesions are seen in 15–50% of patients and manifest as fine white papules. Salivary gland involvement may also occur[6]. An increased susceptibility to cutaneous viral infections occurs, especially to herpes simplex virus[7,8]. However, a consistent underlying immune defect has not been demonstrated.

Neuropsychiatric features have been documented in 25% of affected patients in a large Danish study, with mental retardation in 10% and various psychiatric illnesses in another 15%[9]. Epilepsy and spinocer-ebellar tract degeneration have also been recorded. There are several reports of multiple bone cysts occurring in patients with Darier's disease[10] and one report of kyphoscoliosis[11].

The clinical severity of Darier's disease varies considerably, from isolated nail splitting to severe, widespread disease. The disease follows a chronic relapsing course throughout life. The pattern of the disease can show clinical variability. Although most patients show a seborrhoeic distribution, flexural, hypertrophic and bullous forms of the disease exist. The bullous and flexural forms can cause diagnostic confusion with Hailey–Hailey disease, but the early age of onset, the hand changes and a more seborrhoeic distribution favour the diagnosis of Darier's disease. There is also a naevoid, unilateral form, but such patients do not have a positive family history and they are not known to produce children with the more generalized form. They are probably better classified separately as having dyskeratotic, acantholytic epidermal naevi.

Pathology

Light microscopy shows focal acantholytic dyskeratosis, which is not specifically diagnostic of Darier's disease[12]. Suprabasal clefts are formed by acantholysis. Hyperkeratosis, acanthosis and papillomatosis occur. *Corps ronds* (groups of large cells with darkly staining nuclei surrounded by a clear halo) are found in the upper prickle layer and granular layer, and reflect premature partial keratinization. They give rise to the *grains* (small, shrunken cells) in the cornified layer. A mild, non-specific inflammatory infiltrate may be seen in the upper dermis.

Electron microscopy shows stretching of the tonofilaments and their separation from desmosomes[13]. The number of desmosomes is reduced. The reason for the focal loss of cell adhesion is not as yet understood. Studies of desmosomal proteins, cell adhesion and epidermal keratins have not revealed any primary abnormalities responsible for causing Darier's disease, although it seems likely that a structural abnormality within the cytoskeleton exists [14–17].

Genetics

Several large kinships have been reported [18–20] and show an autosomal dominant pattern of inheritance, but considerable phenotypic variation exists, sometimes even within one family. Darier's disease has also been reported in monozygotic twins, arising as a new mutation[21]. The disease does not appear to skip generations. Many cases are sporadic. Burge reported a large series in which 46 out of 163 patients with Darier's disease had no family history[3]. These individuals followed the same clinical course as the familial cases.

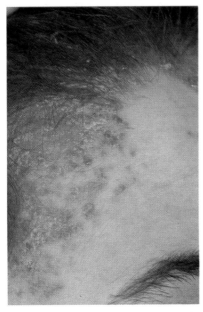

Figure 6.1 *Darier's disease: encrusted papular rash on the scalp and hairline resembling seborrhoeic dermatitis*

Darier's disease has been mapped to chromosome 12q 23–24.1[22].

Differential diagnosis

The differential diagnosis includes Hailey–Hailey disease and acrokeratosis verruciformis.

Treatment

General advice should be given on avoiding exacerbating factors such as heat and sunlight. Topical steroids may help with the pruritus but have no effect on the disease. Antibiotics and antiseptics help decrease odour. Systemic retinoids are the most effective treatment, but may not be justified in patients with mild disease[13,23]. Hypertrophic disease is particularly resistant to treatment. A variety of surgical treatments have been tried in difficult cases, such as dermabrasion and treatment with carbon dioxide laser.

References

1 Darier J. Psorospermose folliculaire végétante. *Ann Dermatol Syphilol* 1889; **10**: 597–612.

2 White JC. A case of keratosis (ichthyosis) follicularis. *J Cutan Genitourin Dis* 1889; **7**: 201–9.

3 Burge SM, Wilkinson D. Darier-White disease: a review of the clinical features in 163 patients. *J Am Acad Dermatol* 1992; **27** (1): 40–50.

4 Wilkinson JD, Marsden RA, Dawber RPR. Review of Darier's disease in the Oxford region. *Br J Dermatol* 1977; **97** (suppl. 15): 15–16 (abstract).

5 Coulson IH, Misch KJ. Haemorrhagic Darier's disease. *J Roy Soc Med* 1989; **82**: 365–6.

6 Macleod RI, Munro CS. The incidence and distribution of oral lesions in patients with Darier's disease. *Br Dent J* 1991; **171** (5): 133–6.

7 Carney JF, Caroline NL, Nankervis GA et al. Eczema vaccinatum and eczema herpeticum in Darier's disease. *Arch Dermatol* 1973; **107**: 613–14.

8 Claudy AL, Gaudin OG, Granouillet R. Pox virus infection in Darier's disease. *Clin Exp Dermatol* 1982; **7**: 261–6.

9 Svendsen IB, Albrectsen B. The prevalence of dyskeratosis follicularis in Denmark. An investigation of the heredity in 22 families. *Acta Derm Venereol* 1959; **39**: 256–69.

10 Menne T, Nielsen AO. Bone cysts and spontaneous fractures in two siblings with dyskeratosis follicularis Darier. *Acta Derm Venereol* 1978; **58**: 366–7.

11 Judge MR, Harper JI. Familial Darier's disease with skeletal and neurological complications. *Br J Dermatol* 1991; **125** (38): 51–2.

12 Ackerman AB. Focal acantholytic dyskeratosis. *Arch Dermatol* 1972; **106**: 702–6.

13 Lauharanta J, Kanerva L, Turjanmaa K et al. Clinical and ultrastructural effects of acitretin in Darier's disease. *Acta Derm Venereol* 1988; **68**: 492–8.

14 Burge SM, Garrod DR. An immunohistochemical study of desmosomes in Darier's disease and Hailey–Hailey disease. *Br J Dermatol* 1991; **124**: 242–51.

15 Setoyama M, Choi KC, Hashimoto K et al. Desmoplakin I and II in acantholytic dermatoses. Preservation in pemphigus vulgaris and pemphigus erythematosus and dissolution in Hailey–Hailey disease and Darier's disease. *J Dermatol Sci* 1991; **2** (1): 9–17.

16 Burge SM, Fenton DA, Dawber RPR et al. Darier's disease: an immunohistochemical study using monoclonal antibodies to human cytokeratins. *Br J Dermatol* 1988; **118**: 629–40.

17 Burge SM, Cederholm-Williams SA, Garrod DR et al. Cell adhesion in Hailey–Hailey disease and Darier's disease: immunocytological and explant-tissue-culture studies. *Br J Dermatol* 1991; **125**: 426–35.

18 Beck AL, Finocchio AF, White JP. Darier's disease: a kindred with a large number of cases. *Br J Dermatol* 1977; **97**: 335–9.

19 Hitch JM. Callaway JL, Moseley V. Familial Darier's disease (keratosis follicularis) *South Med J* 1941; **34**: 578–86.

20 Getzler NA, Flint A. Keratosis follicularis. *Arch Dermatol* 1966; **93**: 545–9.

21 Mohd KN. Darier's disease in twins. *Int J Dermatol* 1984; **23**: 339–40.

22 Parfitt E, Burge S, Craddock N et al. The gene for Darier's disease maps between D12578 and D12579. *Hum Molec Genet* 1994; **3** (1): 35–8.

23 Burge SM. Darier's disease and other dyskeratoses: response to retinoids. *Pharmacol Ther* 1989; **40**: 75–90.

Acrokeratosis verruciformis

Synonym: *Hopf's disease*

Clinical features

Acrokeratosis verruciformis [1–3] affects both sexes equally and is characterized by flesh-coloured, warty, hyperkeratotic papules on the backs of the hands and feet, and on the elbows, knees and forearms. The lesions may blister and small keratoses may be noted on the palms. The nails may be thickened and white. The onset is in early infancy but is occasionally delayed until middle age. Malignant change has been reported by two authors[1,4].

Pathology

Histological examination reveals hyperkeratosis, acanthosis and a prominent granular layer. Less frequently papillomatosis and pointed epidermal upgrowths are seen[5]. The presence of suprabasal clefting suggests an overlap with a limited form of Darier's disease.

Genetics

Acrokeratosis verruciformis is inherited as an autosomal dominant condition in most pedigrees[2,4], although sporadic cases may occur. In view of the clinical similarities with Darier's disease, it has been proposed that the two conditions may form part of a single genetic disorder[6,7]. Herndon described a family of which 7 members had typical acrokeratosis verruciformis, 2 had possible Darier's disease and 3 had white nails, subungual hyperkeratoses and punctate keratoses of the palms[6].

References

1 Dogliotti M, Schmaman A. Acrokeratosis verruciformis: malignant transformation. *Dermatologica* 1971; **143**: 95–9.
2 Rook A, Stevanovic D. Acrokeratosis verruciformis. *Br J Dermatol* 1957; **69**: 450–1.
3 Niedelmann ML, McKusick VA. Acrokeratosis verruciformis (Hopf). A follow-up study. *Arch Dermatol* 1962; **86**: 779–82.
4 Panja RK. Acrokeratosis verruciformis (Hopf) – a clinical entity? *Br J Dermatol* 1977; **96**: 643–52.
5 Schueller WA. Acrokeratosis verruciformis of Hopf. *Arch Dermatol* 1972; **106**: 81–3.
6 Herndon JH, Wilson JD. Acrokeratosis verruciformis (Hopf) and Darier's disease. Genetic evidence for a unitary origin. *Arch Dermatol* 1966; **93**: 305–10.
7 Krause W, Ehlers G. Über die beziehung zwischen acrokeratosis verruciformis Hopf und dyskeratosis follicularis vegetans Darier. *Hautarzt* 1969; **20**: 397–403.

Palmoplantar keratoderma

Synonyms: *Keratoderma, palmoplantar hyperkeratosis, tylosis*

The term 'palmoplantar keratoderma' (PPK) covers a number of different skin disorders characterized by diffuse or focal abnormalities in keratinization of the palms and soles. Only the hereditary types are considered here. They are separated on the basis of clinical appearance, inheritance, aetiology (where known) and associated features. Palmoplantar keratoderma may be part of a more widespread disorder of keratinization, such as the dominantly inherited bullous ichthyosis and Dowling–Meara epidermolysis bullosa. Isolated cases or pedigrees of PPK occur in association with abnormalities in other systems (e.g. bone, hair, teeth, neurological system, eyes, internal malignancy). Their relationship to the genetic basis of these dermatoses is uncertain (see page 114). The different types of PPK are listed in Table 6.5.

Thost–Unna syndrome

Clinical features

Thost–Unna syndrome or tylosis [1, 2] is the most common variety of PPK and presents in infancy with a diffuse yellowish palmoplantar hyperkeratosis with an erythematous margin. It is confined to the palms and soles with no progression to the extensor surfaces. Complications include fissuring (Figure 6.2) hyperhidrosis, secondary dermatophyte infection and thick-

Table 6.5 *Hereditary palmoplantar keratodermas*

Diffuse palmoplantar keratodermas
    Thost–Unna syndrome (tylosis)
    Epidermolytic (Vörner) type
    Progressive type (Greither's syndrome)
    Gamborg–Nielsen type
    Mal de Meleda
    Papillon–Lefèvre syndrome
    Pachonychia congenita
Mutilating keratodermas
    Vohwinkel's syndrome
    Olmsted's syndrome
Localized palmoplantar keratodermas
    Punctate palmoplantar keratoderma
    Keratosis punctata of the palmar creases
    Focal acral hyperkeratosis (acrokeratoelastoidosis)
    Striate palmoplantar keratoderma
    Oculocutaneous tyrosinaemia
Miscellaneous palmoplantar keratodermas

ening of the nails. There is little tendency to improvement.

Pathology

Histological examination of the skin shows marked hyperkeratosis, acanthosis and hypergranulosis.

Genetics

Family studies confirm autosomal dominant inheritance with a high degree of penetrance [1, 2]. There is no evidence of a more severe homozygous form in those families with two affected parents. Linkage has been demonstrated to the keratin gene clusters on 12q and 17q[3]. A mutation in the V1 region of keratin 1, an area critical for keratin desmosome interactions, has been described in one pedigree[4].

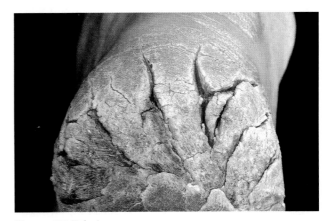

Figure 6.2 *Tylosis*

Treatment

Topical agents such as salicylic acid preparations used under occlusion may help. Antiseptics or Whitfield's ointment (benzoic acid compound ointment) may help the secondary infection. Systemic retinoids are most effective in severe disease.

References

1 Nielsen PG. Two different clinical and genetic forms of hereditary palmoplantar keratoderma in the northernmost county of Sweden. *Clin Genet* 1985; **28**: 361–6.
2 Nielsen PG. Hereditary palmoplantar keratoderma and dermatophytosis. *Int J Dermatol* 1988; **27**: 223–31.
3 Kelsell DP, Stevens HP, Ratnavel R et al. Genetic linkage studies in non-epidermolytic palmoplantar keratoderma; evidence for heterogeneity. *Hum Mol Genet* 1995; **4** (6): 1021–5.
4 Kimonis V, DiGovanna JJ, Yang J-M et al. A mutation in the V1 end domain of keratin 1 causes non-epidermolytic palmar-plantar keratoderma. *J Invest Dermatol* 1994; **103**: 764–9.

Epidermolytic (Vörner) palmoplantar keratoderma

Epidermolytic palmoplantar keratoderma (EPPK) [1–3] is a clinically similar disorder to the diffuse Thost–Unna type except that these patients do not always have hyperhidrosis and they may develop blisters. Knuckle pad-like lesions over the dorsal aspect of the finger joints have also been reported[4]. The disorder is characterized by pathological changes which are similar to those of bullous ichthyosis; epidermolytic hyperkeratosis is seen on light microscopy, with evidence of tonofilament clumping and irregular keratohyalin granules on ultrastructural analysis. In one patient a tonotubular cytoskeleton has been reported[5].

Genetics

The pedigrees of the epidermolytic variant show the same autosomal dominant inheritance and penetrance[2,3]. Point mutations in the palm and sole specific keratin K9 have been shown to be responsible for EPPK, with linkage demonstrated to chromosome 17q12–21[6]. There may also be an autosomal recessive variant of EPPK. Alsaleh described two children, born to consanguineous unaffected Arab parents, suffering from EPPK[7].

Treatment

The treatment is the same as for Thost–Unna syndrome. However, systemic retinoid therapy may cause problems of excessive peeling. Excision and skin grafting have been tried in very severe cases[8].

References

1 Moriwaki S, Tanaka T, Horiguchi Y et al. Epidermolytic hereditary palmoplantar keratoderma. *Arch Dermatol* 1988; **124**: 555–9.
2 Berth-Jones J, Hutchinson PE. A family with palmoplantar epidermolytic hyperkeratosis. *Clin Exp Dermatol* 1989; **14**: 313–16.
3 Kanitakis J, Tsoitis G, Kanitakis C. Hereditary epidermolytic palmoplantar keratoderma (Vörner type) *J Am Acad Dermatol* 1987; **17**: 414–22.
4 Nogita T, Nakagawa H, Ishibashi Y. Hereditary epidermolytic palmoplantar keratoderma with knuckle pad-like lesions over the finger joints. *Br J Dermatol* 1991; **125**: 496.
5 Wevers A, Kuhn A, Mahrle G. Palmoplantar keratoderma with tonotubular keratin. *J Am Acad Dermatol* 1991; **24**: 638–42.
6 Reis A, Hennies H-C, Langbein L et al. Keratin 9 gene mutations in epidermolytic palmoplantar keratoderma (EPPK). *Nature Genet* 1994; **6**: 174–9.
7 Alsaleh QA, Teebi AS. Autosomal recessive epidermolytic palmoplantar keratoderma. *J Med Genet* 1990; **27**: 519–22.
8 Tropet Y, Zultak M, Blanc D et al. Surgical treatment of epidermolytic hereditary palmoplantar keratoderma. *J Hand Surg* (Am) 1989; **14**: 143–9.

Progressive diffuse PPK

Synonym: *Greither's syndrome*

The progressive type of diffuse PPK [1–3] was first described in 1952. It presents in infancy and is characterized by a diffuse keratoderma with hyperhidrosis, similar to the Thost–Unna type. Hyperkeratotic lesions progress and spread onto the dorsal surface of the hands and appear on the extensor surfaces of the knees and elbows. Both males and females are affected and there is some tendency to improve in later life.

Genetics

Greither's PPK, as originally described, is extremely rare; although a number of patients exist with PPK spreading onto the dorsa of the hands and feet, they do not have lesions on the elbows and knees. Kansky described a large Yugoslavian pedigree of 48 members spanning five generations[2]. Seventeen individuals were affected; 1 had just hyperkeratosis of the knees (HOK), 12 had a diffuse PPK and 4 members suffered with both. Interestingly, one family with both PPK and HOK showed the ability to pass on either lesion or both of them to their children. Another family showed one offspring with PPK and HOK, when the affected parent had only PPK. Also the cases seen in the later generations were much fewer in number and developed less severe disease, which may suggest the gene was becoming less penetrant. However, this could also be explained by a decrease in manual work in this population (which may contribute to disease severity) or may reflect a change in marriage patterns causing less chance of homozygous expression. Too few cases exist in the literature with both PPK and HOK, to be certain that the inheritance is autosomal dominant. Greither's syndrome has been linked to 1p36.2–34, the same locus as erythrokeratoderma variabilis[4].

Treatment

Treatment is as for Thost–Unna syndrome.

References

1 Greither A. Keratosis extremitatum progrediens mit dominatem Erbang. *Hautarzt* 1952; **3**: 198–203.
2 Kansky A, Arzensek J. Is palmoplantar keratoderma of Greither's type a separate nosologic entity? *Dermatologica* 1979; **158**: 244–8.
3 Salomon T. Uber einige Falle von Keratosis extremitatum hereditaria progrediens mit dominatum Erbang (Greither). *Z Haut-Geschl Krankh* 1960; **29**: 289–98.
4 Gedde-Dahl TJ, Rogde S, Helsing P et al. Greither's disease and erythrokeratoderma variabilis (EKH) caused by the same mutation on chromosome 1. *Human Genome Mapping Workshop 93 P* 1993; **1** (abstract).

Diffuse recessive PPK

Synonym: *Gamborg–Nielsen PPK*

Nielsen's study of 72 families in north Sweden reported two pedigrees in which 6 children were affected with a very severe form of diffuse PPK (which in one case was mutilating)[1]. One family showed 3 affected children born to unaffected first-cousin parents. A second family showed 3 affected children from unaffected, unrelated parents. Five of the affected cases had a total of 9 children, all of whom were unaffected. Autosomal recessive inheritance is likely in these cases. Nielsen also reported a number of dominant pedigrees in the same study with a milder PPK. Five children, who had both parents affected with the condition, showed no evidence of a more severe PPK and thus it seems likely that the recessive form is a separate genodermatosis.

Five of Nielsen's original patients subsequently had skin biopsies. After histological review it was felt this condition was more likely to be a variant of the recessive mal de Meleda than the dominant Thost–Unna PPK, but the evidence was not conclusive[2].

References

1 Nielsen PG. Two different clinical and genetic forms of hereditary palmoplantar keratoderma in the northernmost county of Sweden. *Clin Genet* 1985; **28**: 361–6.
2 Kastl I, Anton-Lamprecht I, Nielsen PG. Hereditary palmoplantar keratosis of the Gamborg Nielsen type. *Arch Dermatol Res* 1990; **282**: 363–70.

Mal de Meleda

Synonyms: *Meleda disease, keratoderma palmoplantaris transgrediens*

Mal de Meleda is a rare PPK first described by Hovorka in 1897 in a small population from the Yugoslavian island of Meleda[1]. A number of cases have also been reported originating from the Greek island of Naxos.

Clinical features

Erythema of the palms and soles appears in early infancy. This soon progresses to a predominantly diffuse PPK. The lesions may spread to the dorsal surfaces of the hands and feet and show a marked erythematous background. Plaques may also appear on knees and elbows and thus mimic the dominant conditions, symmetrical progressive erythrokeratoderma or Greither's syndrome. The fingers are often short and stumpy. Hyperhidrosis, perioral erythema and nail dystrophy may also be seen. Cardiovascular abnormalities are also common in this condition [1–5].

Pathology

The skin is histologically different from the dominant diffuse PPK[6]. There is marked acanthosis, hyperkeratosis with some parakeratosis, and a prominent perivascular, lymphocytic and histiocytic infiltrate.

Genetics

The inheritance is autosomal recessive.

Treatment

A good response to etretinate has been reported[7].

References

1 Hovorka O, Ehlers E. Mal de Meleda. *Arch Derm Syph (Berlin)* 1897; **40**: 251.
2 Brunner MJ, Fuhrman DL. Mal de Meleda. Report of a case and results of treatment with vitamin A. *Arch Dermatol Syphilol* 1950; **61**: 820–3.
3 Niles HD, Klumpp MM. Mal de Meleda. Review of the literature and report of four cases. *Arch Dermatol Syphilol* 1939; **39**: 409–21.
4 Salamon T, Berberovic L, Topic B et al. Mal de Meleda. Data and remarks on a series. *G Ital Dermatol Venereol* 1988; **123**: 649–55.
5 Protonotarios N, Tsatsopoulou A, Patsourakos P et al. Cardiac abnormalities in familial palmoplantar keratosis. *Br Heart J* 1986; **56**: 321–6.
6 Salamon T, Lazovic O. Contribution au problème de la maladie de Mijet (Mal de Meleda). *J Genet Hum* 1961; **10**: 172–201.
7 Brambilla L, Pigatto PD, Boneschi V et al. Unusual cases of Meleda keratoderma treated with aromatic retinoid etretinate. *Dermatologica* 1984; **168**: 283–6.

Papillon–Lefèvre syndrome

Synonym: *Palmoplantar keratoderma with periodontosis*

Papillon–Lefèvre syndrome (PLS) was first described in 1924 and is characterized by the association of a diffuse PPK and periodontosis with an increased frequency of cutaneous infection.

Clinical features

Erythema followed by a diffuse PPK appears in early childhood. Involvement of the sides of the hands and feet, the elbows and the knees may follow, thus mimicking mal de Meleda[1]. Hyperhidrosis is common and recurrent bacterial infections of the skin and gums are seen. 'Systemic' infections are also more common, and liver and lung abscesses have been reported[2]. Mild mental retardation may be a feature. Some patients show a spontaneous improvement with age, but this is not universal. Unless treatment is initiated early, severe gingivitis leads to premature loss of both deciduous and permanent teeth, usually in the first decade. Dural calcification has been noted in a number of cases[3].

A clinical variant has been described in a community from southern India. Haim and Puliyel reported a number of cases in which PLS features were seen in association with pes planus, onychogryphosis, arachnodactyly and acro-osteolysis[4,5]. Trattner reported a case of PLS with acro-osteolysis and clubbed nails[6]. These PLS-like cases were from consanguineous marriages and presumably were autosomal recessive. They may represent allelic forms of PLS.

A family showing possible autosomal recessive inheritance has been described, in which PPK was associated with hypodontia, hypotrichosis and cystic lesions of the eyelids[7].

Pathology

Light microscopy shows hyperkeratosis, a degree of parakeratosis and marked acanthosis with a moderate perivascular lymphocytic infiltrate (similar to mal de Meleda). Electron microscopy shows a decrease in tonofilaments, irregular keratohyalin granules and vacuolation in the stratum corneum[8]. Abnormalities in the immune system have been described, particularly in neutrophil phagocytosis and chemotaxis, but T-cell and B-cell dysfunction has also been documented [9–11]. Interestingly, Stalder reported a family in which affected members showed a spontaneous recovery in neutrophil phagocytosis despite receiving no treatment[12]. Other patients appear to have normal immune function tests. It remains unclear how common immune abnormalities are in patients with PLS and what role they play in pathogenesis.

Genetics

Papillon–Lefèvre syndrome is an autosomal recessive condition[1]. Gorlin estimated that 2–4 people per 1000 are heterozygous carriers for this condition[3].

Treatment

Synthetic retinoids offer the best therapy. Etretinate [2, 13, 14] isotretinoin[15] and acitretin[8] have all proved successful in terms both of improving the skin and of decreasing gingivitis, thus preserving the teeth. Improvement may be maintained for a number of years after cessation of therapy. Failure to treat early may lead to the necessity for dental clearance and recurrent courses of antibiotics.

References

1 Haneke E. The Papillon–Lefèvre syndrome: keratosis palmoplantaris with periodontopathy. *Hum Genet* 1979; **51**: 1–35.
2 Bergman R, Friedman-Birnbaum R. Papillon–Lefèvre syndrome: a study of the long-term clinical course of recurrent pyogenic infections and the effects of etretinate treatment. *Br J Dermatol* 1988; **119**: 731–6.
3 Gorlin RJ, Sedano H, Anderson VE. The syndrome of palmoplantar hyperkeratosis and premature periodontal destruction of the teeth: a clinical and genetic analysis of the Papillon–Lefèvre syndrome. *J Pediatr* 1964; **65**: 895–908.
4 Haim S, Munk J. Keratosis palmoplantaris congenita, with periodontosis, arachnodactyly and peculiar deformity of the terminal phalanges. *Br J Dermatol* 1965; **77**: 42–54.
5 Puliyel JM, Iyer KSS. A syndrome of keratosis palmoplantaris congenita, pes planus, onychogryphosis, periodontosis, arachnodactyly and a peculiar acroosteolysis. *Br J Dermatol* 1986; **115**: 243–8.
6 Trattner A, David M, Sandbank M. Papillon–Lefèvre syndrome with acroosteolysis. *J Am Acad Dermatol* 1991; **24**: 835–58.
7 Schopf E, Schulz HJ, Passarge E. Syndrome of cystic eyelids, palmoplantar keratosis, hypodontia and hypotrichosis as a possible autosomal recessive trait. *Birth Def* 1971; **7**: 219–21.
8 Nazzaro V, Blanchet-Bardon C, Mimoz C. Papillon–Lefèvre syndrome. Ultrastructure study and successful treatment with acitretin. *Arch Dermatol* 1988; **124**: 533–9.
9 Haneke E, Hornstein OP, Lex C. Increased susceptibility to infections in the Papillon–Lefèvre syndrome. *Dermatologica* 1975; **150**: 283–6.
10 Djawari D. Deficient phagocytic function in Papillon–Lefèvre syndrome. *Clin Exp Immunol* 1980; **40**: 407–10.
11 Vandyke T, Taubman M, Ebersole J. The Papillon–Lefèvre syndrome: neutrophil dysfunction with severe periodontal disease. *Clin Immunol Immunopathol* 1984; **31**: 419–29.
12 Stalder JF, Huu TP, Dreno B et al. Defective leucocyte adhesion in Papillon–Lefèvre syndrome (letter). *Br J Dermatol* 1989; **121**: 668–9.

13 Gelmetti C, Nazzaro V, Cerri D et al. Long-term preservation of permanent teeth in a patient with Papillon–Lefèvre syndrome treated with etretinate. *Pediatr Dermatol* 1989; **6**: 222–5.
14 Driban NE, Jung JR. Treatment of Papillon–Lefèvre syndrome with etretinate. *J Am Acad Dermatol* 1988; **18**: 583–4.
15 Nguyen TQ, Greer KE, Fisher GB et al. Papillon–Lefèvre syndrome – report of two patients treated successfully with isotretinoin. *J Am Acad Dermatol* 1986; **15**: 46–9.

Pachyonychia congenita

Clinical features

Pachyonychia congenita [1–4] is a rare ectodermal disorder characterized by the triad of diffuse PPK, dystrophic nails and leucoplakia of the tongue. Hyperhidrosis and blistering of the palms and soles are frequently present, and follicular keratoses may be seen on the knees and elbows. Nail changes are variable but classically show a wedge-shaped elevation of yellowish nail plates due to onychogryphosis. Onset is normally in the first few years of life, although the disorder may appear in the second or third decade[5,6].

The above spectrum of signs has been referred to as type 1 pachyonychia congenita (Jadassohn-Lewandowsky syndrome)[1]. Further subtypes have been proposed for families with additional clinical features [2–4]. In type 2 pachyonychia congenita (Jackson–Lawler syndrome) there is, in addition, multiple epidermoid cysts and natal teeth but no oral leucoplakia. Type 3 (Schäfer–Brünauer syndrome) is the same as type 1 but with leucokeratosis of the cornea. Feinstein has described a type 4 variant with the features of type 1 plus laryngeal lesions with hoarseness, mental retardation and alopecia.

Pathology

Light microscopy shows hyperkeratosis, acanthosis and occasional keratotic plugging of the sweat ducts. Electron microscopy shows an increase in tonofibrils in the basal, spinous and granular layers with oedema and large keratohyalin granules in the granular layer[6].

Genetics

The vast majority of patients show autosomal dominant inheritance with a high degree of penetrance[2,4]. There have been two reports of possible autosomal recessive inheritance[7,8].

The two major subtypes of pachyonychia congenita are caused by mutations in keratin 16 (the Jadassohn-Lewandosky form) and keratin 17 (the Jackson-Lawler form)[9]. Keratin 6A has also been implicated highlighting the genetic heterogeneity of this group of disorders[10].

Treatment

Systemic retinoid therapy (isotretinoin) has been reported [6]. Some improvement was noted in the keratotic papules on the knees and the oral leucoplakia. However, the most disabling feature, severe PPK, showed no change.

References

1 Jadassohn J, Lewandowsky F. Pachyonychia congenita. In: Neisser A, Jacobs E, eds. *Ikonographia Dermatologica*, vol. 1. Urban & Schwarzenberg, Baltimore, 1906; 29.
2 Jackson ADM, Lawler SD. Pachyonychia congenita: a report of six cases in one family, with a note on linkage data. *Ann Eugen* 1951; **16**: 142–6.
3 Schönfield PHIR. The pachyonychia congenita syndrome. *Acta Derm Venereol* 1980; **60**: 45–9.
4 Feinstein A, Friedman J, Schewach-Millet M. Pachyonychia congenita. *J Am Acad Dermatol* 1988; **19**: 705–11.
5 Paller AS, Moore JA, Scher R. Pachonychia congenita tarda. A late onset form of pachonychia congenita. *Arch Dermatol* 1991; **127**: 701–3.
6 Thomas DR, Jorizzo JL, Brysk MM et al. Pachonychia congenita. Electron microscopic and epidermal glycoprotein assessment before and during isotretinoin treatment. *Arch Dermatol* 1984; **120**: 1475–9.
7 Chong-Hai T, Rajagopalan DDM. Pachyonychia congenita with recessive inheritance. *Arch Dermatol* 1977; **113**: 685–6.
8 Haber RM, Rose TH. Autosomal recessive pachyonychia congenita. *Arch Dermatol* 1986; **122**: 919–23.
9 McLean WH, Rugg EL, Lunny DP et al. Keratin 16 and keratin 17 mutations cause pachonychia congenita. *Nature Genet* 1995 **9**: 273–6.
10 Bowden PE, Haley JL, Kansky A et al. Mutation of a type II keratin gene (K6A) in pachyonychia congenita. *Nature Genet* 1995; **10**(3): 363–5.

Vohwinkel's syndrome

Synonym: *Keratoderma hereditaria mutilans*

Vohwinkel's syndrome[1,2] is a mutilating keratoderma which was first described in 1929. It presents in infancy or early childhood with a diffuse palmoplantar keratoderma, affecting both males and females.

Clinical features

Fine surface depressions are found, giving a honeycomb appearance. Distinctive linear or starfish-shaped keratoses may involve the elbows, knees and the dorsa of the hands and feet, but are not universally present. The nails are usually normal. During later childhood ainhum-like constriction bands appear and may lead to strangulation and autoamputation of the toes and fingers. Associations with alopecia, deafness, inguinal and perianal keratoses, spastic paraplegia and myopathy have been recorded in isolated case reports, but their significance is unclear.

Pathology

Histological examination shows extreme hyperkeratosis and a sparse, perivascular lymphocytic infiltrate in the dermis.

Genetics

The pattern of disease in both Cole's family (3 affected members over two generations) and Rivers' family (4 affected members over three generations) strongly suggests a highly penetrant autosomal dominant disorder. Sporadic cases may also occur, presumably as new mutations[3].

Treatment

Oral systemic retinoids[1,4] are effective, and surgery may be beneficial[4].

References

1 Rivers JK, Duke EE, Justus DW. Etretinate: management of keratoma hereditaria mutilans in four family members. *J Am Acad Dermatol* 1985; **13**: 43–9.
2 Cole RD, McCauley MG, Way BH. Vohwinkel's keratoma hereditaria mutilans. *Int J Dermatol* 1984; **23**: 131–4.
3 Schamroth JM. Mutilating keratoderma. *Int J Dermatol* 1986; **25**: 249–51.
4 Camisa C, Rossana C. Variant of keratoderma hereditaria mutilans (Vohwinkel's syndrome). Treatment with orally administered isotretinoin. *Arch Dermatol* 1984; **120**: 1323–8.

Olmsted's syndrome

A few, mostly sporadic, cases of mutilating keratoderma have been described in association with periorificial keratotic plaques and nail dystrophy under the name of Olmsted's syndrome [1–3]. Many of the clinical features in the hands and feet are identical to Vohwinkel's keratoderma. Atherton reported 2 cases of Olmsted's syndrome, in a 4-year-old boy and his mother. However, although the parent had a mutilating palmoplantar keratoderma, she had no facial lesions. The relationship between Olmsted's syndrome and Vohwinkel's keratoderma remains unclear.

A possible variant has been described in which an infant presented with a palmoplantar keratoderma (non-mutilating), periorificial lesions, nail dystrophy, alopecia and severe corneal epithelial dysplasia[4].

References

1 Olmsted HC. Keratodermia palmaris et plantaris congenitalis. *Am J Dis Child* 1927; **33**: 757–64.
2 Atherton DJ, Sutton C, Jones BM. Mutilating palmoplantar keratoderma with periorificial keratotic plaques. *Br J Dermatol* 1990; **122**: 245–52.
3 Poulin Y, Perry HO, Muller SA. Olmsted syndrome – congenital palmoplantar and periorificial keratoderma. *J Am Acad Dermatol* 1984; **10**: 600–10.
4 Judge MR, Misch K, Wright P, Harper JI. Palmoplantar and periorificial keratoderma with corneal epithelial dysplasia: a new syndrome. *Br J Dermatol* 1991; **125**: 186–8.

Localized palmoplantar keratodermas

Localized palmoplantar keratodermas are a group of disorders separated on clinical grounds. The terminology is confusing, reflecting the difficulty in precise classification. Oculocutaneous tyrosinaemia should be considered in all focal keratodermas as its treatment is entirely different, and if instigated early, can prevent long-term ocular damage.

Punctate palmoplantar keratoderma

Synonyms: *Buschke–Fischer syndrome, Brauer's syndrome, keratosis palmaris et plantaris papulosa*

Punctate palmoplantar keratoderma[1,2] is a rare type of keratoderma which usually presents between the ages of 15 and 30 years.

Clinical features

Numerous small, circular or oval, hyperkeratotic papules appear on the palms and the soles. They range from flesh-coloured to yellowish-brown in appearance, and vary in size from pinhead up to 1–2 cm in diameter. The lesions also vary in character from translucent to small papules to hard warty masses, but the type of lesion tends to breed true in familial cases. The lesions are usually asymptomatic but they can be mildly tender. The central part of the lesion may fall out, leaving a shallow depression with a keratotic margin.

Pathology

Histological analysis reveals an acanthotic epidermis with marked hyperkeratosis and some areas of parakeratosis. The stratum corneum may invaginate the epidermis. Ultrastructural studies have reported a decrease in tonofilaments and perinuclear vacuolization in the granular layer[2].

Genetics

Most of the reported cases are sporadic. Since Brauer's original case[3] a number of pedigrees have been recorded with autosomal dominant inheritance [1, 2, 4, 5]; however, Nielsen's review showed that only 6 cases out of 25 affected patients had a positive family history. A number of features have been reported in association with punctate PPK, especially in the sporadic form, although internal malignancy has also been reported in familial cases[1,6]. As few cases have been described, it remains unclear whether the different clinical patterns reflect genotypic or phenotypic variation.

Treatment

Topical keratolytics are of minimal value. Oral retinoids may produce a marked improvement in some cases[7].

References

1 Nielsen PG. Punctate palmoplantarkeratoderma associated with Morbus Bechterew and HLA B27. *Acta Derm Venereol* 1988; **68**: 346–50.
2 Salamon T, Stolic V, Lazovic-Tepavac O et al. Peculiar findings in a family with keratodermia palmo-plantaris papulosa Buschke–Fischer–Brauer. *Hum Genet* 1982; **60**: 314–19.
3 Brauer A. Ueber eine besondere Form des heriditaren Keratomas. (Keratoma disseminatum hereditarium palmare et plantare.) *Arch Derm Syph* (Berlin) 1913; **114**: 211–36.
4 Michael JC. Keratoderma disseminatum palmaris et plantaris. Its mode of inheritance. *Arch Dermatol Syph* (Chicago) 1933; **27**: 78–88.
5 Brown FC. Punctate keratoderma (letter). *Arch Dermatol* 1971; **104**: 682–3.
6 Bennion SD, Patterson JW. Keratosis punctata palmaris et plantaris and adenocarcinoma of the colon. *J Am Acad Dermatol* 1984; **10**: 587–91.
7 Christiansen JV. Keratodermia punctate hereditaria treated with etretinate. *Acta Derm Venereol* 1983; **63**: 181–2.

Keratosis punctata of the palmar creases

Keratosis punctata of the palmar creases[1] is a rare condition characterized by hard, hyperkeratotic plugs confined to the palmar creases. The lesions are normally asymptomatic and rarely may involve the soles. The onset is normally in childhood or young adults and affects both males and females. The condition is largely confined to people of Afro-Caribbean origin.

Histologically, a parakeratotic or hyperkeratotic plug is seen overlying a depressed area of epidermis with loss of the granular layer. A sparse mononuclear infiltrate may be seen in the upper dermis.

Most cases are sporadic, although autosomal dominant inheritance may occur[2]. The relationship with other punctate PPK is uncertain.

References

1 Weiss RM, Rasmussen JE. Keratosis punctata of the palmar creases. *Arch Dermatol* 1980; **116**: 669–71.
2 Griffiths WAD, Leigh IM, Marks R. Keratosis punctata of the palmar creases. In: Champion RH, Burton, JL, Ebling FJG, eds. *Textbook of Dermatology*, vol. 3. 5th ed. Blackwell, Oxford, 1992; 1381.

Acrokeratoelastoidosis

Synonym: *Focal acral hyperkeratosis*

Clinical features

Costa first described in 1953 a condition called acrokeratoelastoidosis [1–4], predominantly affecting Afro-Caribbeans. Polygonal, firm, hyperpigmented papules appear on the lateral borders of the hands and feet, usually before the age of 20 years. The papules may also involve the wrist creases, the dorsal surface of the interphalangeal joints and the skin between the digits. A mild, diffuse PPK may also be present[5]. The lesions are predominantly a cosmetic problem.

Pathology

Histological examination shows focal hyperkeratosis over a depression in an acanthotic epidermis. Dermal capillaries may be dilated but no inflammatory infiltrate is seen. Costa's original cases and those described by other authors showed fragmentation of the elastic fibres in the dermis[2,6]. However, both Matthews and Dowd described a number of clinically identical cases who did not show this latter histological finding, and the term 'focal acral hyperkeratosis' has been proposed for this group[4,7]. Degenerative collagenous plaques[8] of the hands (due to sun damage) have a similar clinical appearance, but they are not found on the feet, there is no family history, they do not appear in childhood, and the skin usually shows other evidence of solar damage.

Genetics

Jung reported a large kindred (86) in 1973 with 21 affected members over four generations showing autosomal dominant inheritance with nearly complete penetrance but variable expression[9]. Other dominant kinships have been described as well as a number of sporadic cases. Jung's kindred were studied by Greiner in 1983[10]. A loose linkage was found to *ACP1* (acid phosphatase 1), *Jk* (blood group Kidd) and *IGKC* (immunoglobulin chain constant region). The lod scores did not reach significance, but as all three of these markers are on the short arm of chromosome 2, it is suggested that the acrokeratoelastoidosis gene may also be in this region. Dowd's series of 15 patients showed 8 sporadic cases and 7 familial cases with probable autosomal dominant inheritance. A female preponderance (12 out of 15 patients) was also noted.

Treatment

A good response to etretinate has been reported[11].

References

1 Costa OG. Acrokeratoelastoidosis: a hitherto undescribed skin disease. *Dermatologica* 1953; **107**: 164–8.
2 Costa OG. Acrokeratoelastoidosis. *Arch Dermatol Syphilol* 1954; **70**: 228–31.
3 Harper JI, Smith N. Acrokeratoelastoidosis: mother and two daughters. *Br J Dermatol* 1981; **105** suppl. (19): 101–2.
4 Dowd PM, Harman RRM, Black MM. Focal acral hyperkeratosis. *Br J Dermatol* 1983; **109**: 97–103.
5 Highet AS, Rook A, Anderson JR. Acrokeratoelastoidosis. *Br J Dermatol* 1982; **106**: 337–44.
6 Jung EG, Beil FU, Anton-Lamprecht I et al. Akrokeratoelastoidosis. *Hautarzt* 1974; **25**: 127–33.
7 Matthews CNA, Harman RRM. Acrokerato-elastoidosis (without elastorrhexis). *Proc Roy Soc Med* 1974; **67**: 57–8.
8 Koscard E. Keratoelastoidosis marginalis of the hands. *Dermatologica* 1964; **131**: 169–75.
9 Jung EG. Acrokeratoelastoidosis. *Humangenetik* 1973; **17**: 357–8.
10 Greiner J, Krüger J, Palden L et al. A linkage study of acrokeratoelastoidosis. Possible mapping to chromosome 2. *Hum Genet* 1983; **63**: 222–7.
11 Handfield-Jones S, Kennedy CTC. Acrokeratoelastoidosis treated with etretinate. *J Am Acad Dermatol* 1987; **17**: 881–2.

Striate palmoplantar keratoderma

Synonyms: *Keratosis palmoplantaris areata/striata, Siemens' syndrome, Brunauer–Fuhs type*

Clinical features

Striate palmoplantar keratoderma[1,2] usually presents in patients 10–30 years old with linear (striata) and/or circular islands (areata) of hyperkeratosis on the palms and soles. It may occur on a background of mild, diffuse thickening. Lesions are frequently painful or tender and tend to occur at pressure areas. The severity often relates to the degree of mechanical trauma or friction.

Considerable clinical variability exists between different pedigrees and even within an individual family[3]. Siemens' original family showed some members with striate lesions, some with circular islands and others with a diffuse PPK[4]. Families who show only circular lesions at pressure points (often in early childhood) are referred to by some as having circumscribed PPK[5] or nummular PPK[6], but it remains uncertain whether this is a distinct entity. Wachters proposed the term 'keratosis palmoplantaris varians' to encompass these variations.

Pathology

Light microscopy is non-specific and shows a marked hyperkeratosis, acanthosis, hypergranulosis and a degree of papillomatosis [1, 2, 6]. Tezuka's case had similar findings, but for a complete absence of keratohyalin granules except in the acrosyringium[5].

Genetics

A number of families with striate PPK have been described showing an autosomal dominant inheritance [1, 2, 4, 6]. Cascado reported a large pedigree with 36 affected members over five generations.

Egelund reported a family with striate PPK in association with hair, teeth and hearing abnormalities[7]. Its relationship to isolated striate PPK remains uncertain. Nesbitt described 3 siblings with striate PPK in association with hyperkeratosis on the palms and soles, and on the knees and elbows[8]. Linkage has been reported to a cluster of genes for desmosomal caherins, desmogleins and desmocollins on chromosome 18q12[9].

Treatment

Topical and oral retinoids help [1, 2].

References

1 Ortega M, Quintana J, Camacho F. Keratosis palmoplantar striata (Brunauer–Fuhs type) *Acta Derm Venereol* 1983; **63**: 273–5.
2 Cascado M, Jiminez-Acosta F, Borbujo J et al. Keratoderma palmoplantaris striata. *Clin Exp Dermatol* 1989; **14**: 240–2.
3 Sutton-Williams GD. Keratosis palmo-plantaris varians mit helicotrichie. *Arch Klin Exp Derm* 1969; **236**: 97–106.
4 Siemens HW. Keratosis palmo-plantaris striata. *Arch Derm Syphilol* (Berlin) 1929; **157**: 392–408.
5 Tezuka T. Circumscribed, palmoplantar keratoderma. Unusual histological findings. *Dermatologica* 1982; **165**: 30–8.
6 Wachters DHJ, Frensdorf EL, Hausman R et al. Keratosis palmoplantaris nummularis ('hereditary painful callosities'). *J Am Acad Dermatol* 1983; **9**: 204–9.
7 Egelund E, Frentz G. A case of hyperkeratosis palmoplantaris striata combined with pili torti, hypohidrosis, hypodontia and hypacusis. *Acta Otolaryngol* 1982; **94**: 571–3.
8 Nesbitt LT, Rothschild H, Ichinose H et al. Acral keratoderma. *Arch Dermatol* 1975; **111**: 763–8.
9 Hennies H-C, Küster W, Mischke D et al. Localisation of a locus for the striated form of palmoplantar keratoderma to chromosome 18q near the desmosomal cadherin gene cluster. *Hum Mol Genet* 1995; **4** (6): 1015–20.

Oculocutaneous tyrosinaemia

Synonyms: *Tyrosinaemia type II, Richner–Hanhart syndrome*

The clinical syndrome of oculocutaneous tyrosinaemia was first described by Richner in 1938 and Hanhart in 1947 but its relation to tyrosine metabolism was not determined until 1973 [1–3]. It is now known to be an inborn error of tyrosine metabolism due to a deficiency of hepatic tyrosine aminotransferase (TAT).

Clinical features

Oculocutaneous tyrosinaemia is characterized by a triad of skin, eye and neurological changes [1–4]. Skin lesions usually appear in the first year of life. A circumscribed, painful PPK appears over the pressure areas with a distinctive erythematous background (Figure 6.3). The lesions sometimes blister and the hyperkeratosis may disintegrate, leaving shallow erosions. They range in size from a few millimetres to 2–3 cm. Ocular lesions tend to appear in the first few months of life, initially as photophobia and hyperlacrimation. Dendritic corneal opacities may also be present, which if untreated can progress to neovascularization, corneal scarring and glaucoma. Neurological changes are very variable; if present, mild mental impairment is most common, but poor motor coordination, gross mental retardation and self-mutilation have also been recorded in a few patients.

A number of recorded cases have only one or two of the above clinical features[5,6]. It has been estimated that 80% of cases have skin involvement, 75% eye disease and 60% mental retardation.

Pathology

A marked hyperkeratosis is seen on light microscopy. Ultrastructural study shows a thickened granular layer with an increase in tonofibrils and keratohyalin. Tubular structures are seen within the dense tonofibril masses. It has been suggested that the high levels of intracellular tyrosine may modulate the tonofibril cross-linking[7], but Saijo has since reported that there is no specific increase in tyrosine levels in lesional skin, just a mild increase in all amino acids[8].

The pathogenesis of the tissue damage in this disorder remains unclear. Plasma tyrosine, tyrosine metabolites (phenolic acids) and high cerebrospinal fluid tyrosine levels have all been implicated, but the evidence is not conclusive[4]. The clinical variability is also difficult to explain. The biochemical pathways not involving the deficient hepatic TAT may be of more importance. Mitochondrial transaminases can metabolize tyrosine to a degree and induction of these enzymes may be a crucial factor. High tyrosine levels can drive the catecholamine synthesis pathway which is normally subject to negative feedback control.

Genetics

The condition is autosomal recessive. In 1986 the *TAT* gene was mapped to the long arm of chromosome 16 (16q22–24)[9]. In 1987, Natt reported a patient with multiple congenital anomalies and oculocutaneous tyrosinaemia. A large 27-kilobase deletion involving the *TAT* allele was inherited from his mother. The loss of the second *TAT* allele was from a small de novo interstitial deletion in his paternally inherited chromosome 16. Three additional loci assigned to 16q22 were studied and the haptoglobin locus was found to be codeleted. The *TAT* gene site was narrowed to 16q22.1–q22.3[10]. In 1988, Westphal described two restriction fragment length polymorphisms (*Msp* I and *Hae* III) associated with the *TAT* locus. With these they were able to demonstrate delineation of the mutant alleles in each parent and thus provide the possibility of prenatal diagnosis in this particular family[11].

Treatment

A diet low in tyrosine and phenylalanine leads to rapid resolution of ocular and dermatological symptoms, even when the plasma tyrosine level is still considerably above the normal range (i.e. above 120 μmol/l) [12–14]. Supplementation with carbohydrate, lipid, vitamins and minerals is needed to prevent the formation of a catabolic state. If tyrosine levels do not fall satisfactorily, very low-protein diets with amino acid supplementation may be needed. Treatment prevents long-term ocular damage, but it remains unclear how this may influence mental development, especially as some patients do not develop any neurological problems. Barr reported 2 infants followed up for 10 years whose treatment regimen led to plasma tyrosine levels ranging between 300 μmol/l and 800 μmol/l, still well above the normal range[14]. Although their psychomotor development remained normal, the optimal strictness of dietary management and the possible damaging effects of mildly raised tyrosine levels remain unclear.

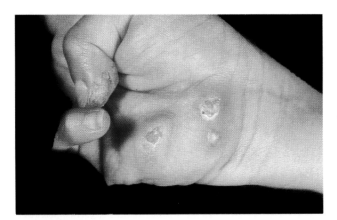

Figure 6.3 *Tyrosinaemia type II: circumscribed painful lesions on an erythematous background*

References

1 Goldsmith LA, Kang E, Bienfang DC et al. Tyrosinemia with plantar and palmar keratosis and keratitis. *J Pediatr* 1973; **5**: 798–805.

2 Zaleski WA, Hill A, Kushniruk W. Skin lesions in tyrosinosis: response to dietary treatment. *Br J Dermatol* 1973; **88**: 335–40.

3 Buist NRM, Kenneway NG, Fellman JH. Disorders of tyrosinemia. *Lancet* 1973; **i**: 620–1.

4 Goldsmith LA, Laberge C. Tyrosinemia and related disorders. In: Scriver CR et al, eds. *The Metabolic Basis of Inherited Disease*, vol. 1. 6th ed. McGraw-Hill, New York, 1989; 547–54.

5 Rehak A, Selim MM, Yadav G. Richner-Hanhart syndrome (tyrosinaemia II): report of four cases without ocular involvement. *Br J Dermatol* 1981; **104**: 469–75.

6 Waardenburg PJ, Franceschetti A, Klein D. In: *Genetics and Ophthalmology*, vol. 1. CC Thomas, Springfield, 1961; 515–17.

7 Bonhert A, Anton-Lamprecht I. Richner-Hanhart's syndrome: ultrastructural abnormalities of epidermal keratinization indicating a causal relationship to high intracellular tyrosine levels. *J Invest Dermatol* 1982; **79**: 68–74.

8 Saijo S, Kudoh K, Kuramoto Y et al. Tyrosinemia II: report of an incomplete case and studies on the hyperkeratotic stratum corneum. *Dermatologica* 1991; **182**: 168–71.

9 Barton DE, Yang-Feng TL, Francke U. The human tyrosine aminotransferase gene mapped to the long arm of chromsome 16 (region 16q22–24) by somatic cell hybrid analysis and in situ hybridization. *Hum Genet* 1986; **72**: 221–6.

10 Natt E, Westphal E, Toth-Fejel SE et al. Inherited and *de novo* deletion of the tyrosine aminotransferase gene locus at 16q22.1–22.3 in a patient with tyrosinemia type II. *Hum Genet* 1987; **77**: 352–8.

11 Westphal E, Natt E, Grimm T et al. The human tyrosine aminotransferase gene: characterization of restriction fragment length polymorphisms and haplotype analysis in a family with tyrosinemia type II. *Hum Genet* 1988; **79**: 260–4.

12 Machino H, Miki Y, Kawatsu T et al. Successful dietary control of tyrosinemia II. *J Am Acad Dermatol* 1983; **9**: 533–9.

13 Ney D, Bay C, Schneider JA et al. Dietary management of oculocutaneous tyrosinemia in an 11 year old child. *Am J Dis Child* 1983; **137**: 995–1000.

14 Barr DGD, Kirk JM, Laing SC. Outcome in tyrosinaemia type II. *Arch Dis Child* 1991; **66**: 1249–50.

Miscellaneous palmoplantar keratodermas

A number of pedigrees and isolated cases of PPK have been reported in association with other 'systemic' features (Table 6.6). Their relationship to the above dermatoses is uncertain.

Porokeratoses

The porokeratoses are a group of clinically variable dermatoses which share a similar histological picture of cornoid lamella.

Porokeratosis of Mibelli

Clinical features

Porokeratosis of Mibelli[1,2] usually presents in childhood with single or multiple papules which slowly enlarge outwards to form annular, keratotic plaques. A disseminated form has been described in infancy associated with craniosynostosis[3] (Figure 6.4). Lesions have a raised, firm keratotic edge which may be associated with longitudinal furrowing. The centre of the lesions is usually atrophic but rarely can be hypertrophic. The extremities, neck and face are the most commonly affected sites but the genitalia and mucous membranes may also be involved. Males are more commonly and more severely affected than females (ratio 3:1). The lesions may undergo malignant change to squamous cell or basal cell carcinomas[4].

Pathology

Skin biopsy should be through the edge of a lesion and serial sections cut, or the distinctive histological change of cornoid lamella may be missed[5,6]. This is found at the level of the raised border and consists of an invagination of epidermis containing a column of parakeratosis. The granular layer is absent and the underlying keratinocytes are degenerate with pyknotic nuclei. A mild to moderate lymphocytic infiltrate is seen in the upper dermis. Sections through the centre of a lesion show an atrophic or acanthotic epidermis. The aetiology of this condition is unknown, although it has been proposed that the condition reflects a mutant or neoplastic clonal expansion of epidermal cells[5,7]. Chromosomal instability is frequently seen in lesional skin, and cultured fibroblasts show evidence of hypersensitivity to X-ray irradiation[8]. Lesions may appear or become widespread in immunosuppressed patients, although the exact mechanism is unclear[9,10].

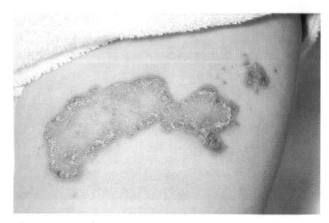

Figure 6.4 *Porokeratosis in an infant with craniosynostosis*

Table 6.6 *Miscellaneous abnormalities reported to occur in association with palmoplantar keratoderma*

Associated feature	Inheritance	Reference
Deafness	Autosomal dominant	1–3
Neuropathy	Autosomal dominant	4–6
	Possible X-linked	7
Clinodactyly	Autosomal dominant	8–9
Malignancy	Autosomal dominant	10–14
	Non-familial	15–16
Dental abnormalities	Autosomal dominant	17
	Autosomal recessive	see Papillon–Lefèvre syndrome
Scleroatrophy	Autosomal dominant	18–20
Gingival hyperkeratosis	Autosomal dominant	21–22

References

1 Bitici OO. Familial hereditary, progressive sensori-neural hearing loss with keratosis palmaris et plantaris. *J Laryng Otol* 1975; **89**: 1143–6.

2 Hatomachi A, Nakagawa S, Ueki S et al. Diffuse palmoplantar keratoderma with deafness. *Arch Dermatol* 1982; **118**: 605–7.

3 Gloor M, Gross M, Happle R et al. Familial circumscribed plantar keratosis with sensorineural hearing loss and sporadic CHILD syndrome. *Hautarzt* 1989; **40**: 304–7.

4 Rabbiosi G, Borroni G, Pinelli P et al. Palmoplantar keratoderma and Charcot–Marie–Tooth disease. *Arch Dermatol* 1980; **116**: 789–90.

5 Tolmie JL, Wilcox DE, McWilliam R et al. Palmoplantar keratoderma, nail dystrophy, and hereditary motor and sensory neuropathy: an autosomal dominant trait. *J Med Genet* 1988; **25**: 754–7.

6 Powell FC, Venencie PY, Gordon H et al. Keratoderma and spastic paralysis. *Br J Dermatol* 1983; **109**: 589–96.

7 Fitzsimmons JS, Fitzsimmons EM, McLachlan JI et al. Four brothers with mental retardation, spastic paraplegia and palmoplantar hyperkeratosis. A new syndrome? *Clin Genet* 1983; **23**: 329–35.

8 Aguirre-Negrette MG, Hernández A, Ramírez-Soltero et al. Keratosis palmaris et plantaris with clinodactyly. A direct autosomal dominant genodermatosis. *Dermatologica* 1981; **162**: 300–3.

9 Anderson IF, Klintworth GK. Hypovitaminosis-A in a family with tylosis and clinodactyly. *Br Med J* 1961; **1**: 1293–7.

10 Howel-Evans W, McConnell RB, Clarke CA et al. Carcinoma of the oesophagus with keratosis palmaris et plantaris (tylosis): a study of two families. *Quart J Med* 1958; **27**: 413–29.

11 Tyldesley WR. Oral leukoplakia associated with tylosis and oesophageal carcinoma. *J Oral Path* 1974; **3**: 62–70.

12 Shine I, Allison PR. Carcinoma of the oesophagus with tylosis (keratosis palmaris et plantaris). *Lancet* 1966; **i**: 951–3.

13 Yesudian P, Premalatha S, Thambiah AS. Genetic tylosis with malignancy: a study of a south Indian pedigree. *Br J Dermatol* 1980; **102**: 597–600.

14 Bennion SD, Patterson JW. Keratosis punctata palmaris et plantaris and adenocarcinoma of the colon. *J Am Acad Dermatol* 1984; **10**: 587–91.

15 Murata Y, Kumano K, Tani M. Acquired diffuse keratoderma of the palms and soles with bronchial carcinoma: report of a case and review of the literature. *Arch Dermatol* 1988; **124**: 497–8.

16 Breathnach SM, Wells GC. A distinctive pattern of palmar keratoderma frequently associated with malignancy. *Clin Exp Dermatol* 1980; **5**: 181–9.

17 Koch H, Hübner U, Schaarschmidt E et al. Keratosis palmoplantaris mit Trommelschlegelfingern, Hypotrichose, Hypohidrose und Zahndysplasie. *Hautarzt* 1991; **42**: 399–401.

18 Huriez C, Deminatti M, Agache P et al. Une génodysplasie non encore individualisée: la génodermatose sclérotrophiante et kératodermique des extrémités fréquemment dégénérative. *Sem Hôp Paris* 1968; **44**: 481–8.

19 Fischer S. La génodermatose scléroatrophiante et kératodermique des extrémités (au sujet de trois nouveaux cas familiaux). *Ann Dermatol Vénéréol* 1978; **105**: 1079–82.

20 Mennecier M. Individualisation d'une nouvelle entité: la génodermatose sclérotrophiante et kératodermique des extrémités fréquemment dégénérative: étude clinique et génétique (possibilité de linkage avec le système MNSs) *MD Thesis*, Lille University, 1967.

21 Young WG, Newcomb GM, Daley TJ. Focal palmoplantar and gingival hyperkeratosis syndrome: report of a family with cytologic, ultrastructural, and histochemical findings. *Oral Surg* 1982; **53**: 473–82.

22 Laskaris G, Vareltzidis A, Avgerinou G. Focal palmoplantar and oral mucosa hyperkeratosis syndrome: a report concerning five members of a family. *Oral Surg* 1980; **50**: 250–3

Genetics

Familial cases show an autosomal dominant inheritance with a decreased penetrance in females[2]. Sporadic cases also exist[11]. A variety of chromosomal abnormalities have been reported in this condition with a possible linkage to chromosome 3 [12–14]. Scappaticci reported 4 cases with particular involvement of the chromosome region 3p14–12 (a common fragile site in humans) and proposed that this instability predisposed to malignant transformation[13].

Treatment

Topical fluorouracil[15] has proved to be of some use in limited disease. Retinoid therapy may be of benefit in the more widespread cases[16], although it can also exacerbate the condition[17].

References

1 Virgili A, Strumia R. Annular hyperkeratosis. Porokeratosis of Mibelli. *Arch Dermatol* 1986; **122**: 586–7.
2 Bloom D, Abramowitz EW. Porokeratosis Mibelli: report of three cases in one family: histologic studies. *Arch Derm Syph* 1943; **47**: 1–15.
3 Judge MR, Michaels M, Sams VR et al. Disseminated porokeratosis in an infant with craniosynostosis. *Br J Dermatol* 1990; **123**: 249–54.
4 Goerttler EA, Jung EG. Porokeratosis of Mibelli and skin cancer: a critical review. *Humangenetik* 1975; **26**: 291–6.
5 Reed RJ, Leone P. Porokeratosis – a mutant clonal keratosis of the epidermis. Histogenesis. *Arch Derm* 1970; **101**: 340–7.
6 Mann PR, Cort DF, Airburn EA et al. Ultrastructural studies on two cases of porokeratosis of Mibelli. *Br J Dermatol* 1974; **90**: 607–17.
7 Otsuka F, Shima A, Ishibashi Y. Porokeratosis has neoplastic clones in the epidermis: microfluorometric analysis of DNA content of epidermal cell nuclei. *J Invest Dermatol* 1989; **92** (suppl. 5): 231–3S.
8 Watanabe R, Ishibashi Y, Otsuka F. Chromosomal instability and cellular hypersensitivity to X-radiation of cultured fibroblasts derived from porokeratosis patient's skin. *Mutat Res* 1990; **230** (2): 273–8.
9 MacMillan AL, Roberts SO. Porokeratosis of Mibelli after renal transplantation. *Br J Dermatol* 1974; **90**: 45–51.
10 Rothman IL, Wirth PB, Klaus MV. Porokeratosis of Mibelli following heart transplant. *Int J Dermatol* 1992; **31** (1): 52–4.
11 Bhutani LK, Kanwar AJ, Singh OP. Porokeratosis of Mibelli with unusual features. *Dermatologica* 1977; **155**: 296–300.
12 Taylor AMR, Harnden DG, Fairburn EA. Chromosomal instability and malignant disease in patients with porokeratosis of Mibelli. *Br J Cancer* 1973; **28**: 88.
13 Scappaticci S, Lambiase S, Orecchia G et al. Clonal chromosomal abnormalities with preferential involvement of chromosome 3 in patients with porokeratosis of Mibelli. *Cancer Genet Cytogenet* 1989; **43**: 89–94.
14 Otsuka F, Watanabe R, Kawashima M et al. Porokeratosis with large skin lesions. Histologic, cytologic and cytogenetic study of three cases. *Acta Derm Venereol* 1991; **71** (5): 437–40.
15 McDonald SG, Peterka ES. Porokeratosis (Mibelli): treatment with topical 5-fluorouracil. *J Am Acad Dermatol* 1983; **8**: 107–10.
16 Danno K, Yamamoto M, Yokoo T. Etretinate treatment in disseminated porokeratosis. *J Dermatol* 1988; **15**: 440–4.
17 Knobler RM, Neumann RA. Exacerbation of porokeratosis during etretinate therapy. *Acta Derm Venereol* 1990; **70**: 319–22.

Linear porokeratosis

Clinically, linear porokeratosis presents in childhood with papular linear lesions or a linear arrangement of annular lesions and thus may mimic a linear verrucous epidermal naevus[1,2]. Histological study shows typical cornoid lamellae. Most cases are sporadic. It has been described in monozygotic twins with a distribution following Blaschko's lines[3]. Malignant change may occur[4].

Treatment

Cryotherapy, diamond fraise dermabrasion[5] and carbon dioxide laser[6] have been tried with some success.

References

1 Karadaglic DL, Berger S, Jankovic D et al. Zosteriform porokeratosis of Mibelli. *Int J Dermatol* 1988; **27**: 589–90.
2 Rahbari H, Cordero AA, Mehregan AH. Linear porokeratosis. A distinctive clinical variant of porokeratosis of Mibelli. *Arch Dermatol* 1974; **109**: 526–8.
3 Guillot P, Taieb A, Fontan I et al. Linear porokeratosis of Mibelli in monozygotic twin girls. *Ann Dermatol Venereol* 1991; **118**: 519–24.
4 Lozinski AZ, Fisher BK, Walter JB et al. Metastatic squamous cell carcinoma in linear porokeratosis of Mibelli. *J Am Acad Dermatol* 1987; **16**: 448–51.
5 Cohen PR, Held JL, Katz BE. Linear porokeratosis: successful treatment with diamond fraise dermabrasion. *J Am Acad Dermatol* 1990; **23**: 975–7.
6 Barnett JH. Linear porokeratosis: treatment with the carbon dioxide laser. *J Am Acad Dermatol* 1986; **14**: 902–4.

Disseminated superficial actinic porokeratosis

Disseminated superficial actinic porokeratosis (DSAP) is more common than porokeratosis of Mibelli and is characterized by the development of numerous small, superficial porokeratotic plaques, confined to sun-exposed areas, which histologically show typical cornoid lamellae [1–3]. They begin to develop after childhood and are usually apparent by middle age, showing exacerbations in the summer. The lesions can be induced experimentally with ultraviolet light exposure[4]. Autosomal dominant inheritance is seen in some families but many cases are sporadic[5]. The link with malignancy is less certain than with porokeratosis of Mibelli[1].

Rarely patients have been reported with DSAP and linear lesions of porokeratosis[6] and Happle has proposed that this may reflect a somatic recombination[7].

References

1 Shumack SP, Commens CA. Disseminated superficial actinic porokeratosis: a clinical study. *J Am Acad Dermatol* 1989; **20**: 1015–22.
2 Chernosky ME, Freeman RG. Disseminated superficial actinic porokeratosis (DSAP). *Arch Dermatol* 1967; **96**: 611–24.
3 Shumack S, Commens C, Kossard S. Disseminated superficial actinic porokeratosis. A histological review of 61 cases with particular reference to lymphocytic inflammation. *Am J Dermatopathol* 1991; **13**: 26–31.
4 Chernosky ME, Anderson DE. Disseminated superficial actinic porokeratosis: clinical studies and experimental production of lesions. *Arch Dermatol* 1969; **99**: 401–7.
5 Anderson DE, Chernosky ME. Disseminated superficial actinic porokeratosis. Genetic aspects. *Arch Dermatol* 1969; **99**: 408–12.
6 Feldman SR, Crosby DL, Tomsick RS. Scaly atrophic lesions both scattered and in linear arrays. Disseminated superficial actinic porokeratosis in a patient with linear porokeratosis. *Arch Dermatol* 1991; **127**: 1219–22.
7 Happle R. Somatic recombination may explain linear porokeratosis associated with disseminated superficial actinic porokeratosis. *Am J Med Genet* 1991; **39**: 237.

Palmoplantar porokeratosis

Palmoplantar porokeratosis is a rare autosomal dominant variant of porokeratosis that presents at or shortly after puberty with minute, spiny hyperkeratotic lesions on the palms and soles [1–3]. Histological examination shows a columnar parakeratosis similar to the cornoid lamella of porokeratosis. The condition appears to be more common in males.

A variant of palmoplantar porokeratosis called porokeratosis plantaris, palmaris et disseminata (PPPD) has been described in 8 patients spanning four generations[4]. A palmoplantar porokeratosis developed in late teenage years followed by further lesions developing on both sun-exposed and unexposed parts of the body. This disorder appeared consistent with either X-linked or autosomal dominant inheritance. Further cases of PPPD have been reported which showed DNA aneuploidy in lesional epidermis, and the development of squamous cell carcinomas[5,6].

References

1 Lestringant GG, Berge T. Porokeratosis punctata palmaris et plantaris. A new entity? *Arch Dermatol* 1989; **125**: 816–19.
2 Chernosky ME. Porokeratosis. *Arch Dermatol* 1986; **122**: 869–70.
3 Brown F. Punctate keratoderma. *Arch Dermatol* 1971; **104**: 682–3.
4 Guss SB, Osbourn RA, Lutzner MA. Porokeratosis plantaris, palmaris et disseminata: a third type of porokeratosis. *Arch Dermatol* 1971; **104**: 366–73.
5 Beers B, Jaszcz W, Sheetz K et al. Porokeratosis palmaris et plantaris disseminata. Report of a case with abnormal DNA ploidy in lesional epidermis. *Arch Dermatol* 1992; **128** (2): 236–9.
6 Ruocco V, Satriano RA, Florio M et al. Porokeratosis palmaris et plantaris disseminata with squamous cell carcinoma. *G Ital Dermatol Venereol* 1990; **125**: 53–8.

Chapter 7

Metabolic disorders

L. G. Rabinowitz

There are numerous inherited metabolic disorders, many of which have clearly described dermatologic manifestations (Table 7.1). Although the dermatologic features may be prominent, they often do not receive much attention, probably because they are usually absent at initial presentation and because they tend to be less serious problems than the other features of these diseases. This chapter focuses on selected diseases that have significant skin, hair and/or nail changes.

Phenylketonuria

Definition

Phenylketonuria (PKU) [1–6] was the first inborn error of amino acid metabolism to be clearly defined. It has been the model for newborn biochemical screening. There are eight types of hyperphenylalaninaemia; this discussion is limited to classic PKU, which was first described by Folling in 1934. This error is due to the deficiency of phenylalanine hydroxylase. Without this enzyme there is no conversion of phenylalanine to tyrosine. The result is an accumulation of phenylalanine and its metabolites in blood, tissues and urine.

Clinical features

Some of these metabolites are responsible for the characteristic musty odour in PKU patients. It is primarily phenylacetic acid that causes this odour. The mousy or musty odour may be noted in the urine and sweat.

Patients with PKU are normal at birth. Within a short time they may develop one or more of the typical features of this disease. Severe mental retardation is seen in every untreated patient. It is usually apparent by 4–24 months of life. Severe mental retardation led to institutionalization of most PKU patients prior to the discovery that dietary restriction of phenylalanine could prevent this problem. In the past, 1% of institutionalized mentally retarded patients were patients with PKU.

Hypopigmentation is seen in 90% of patients. Most caucasians with PKU are blond, blue-eyed and fair-skinned. Studies reveal a normal number of melanocytes but decreased mature melanosomes in these patients. Almost all patients with PKU have pigment dilution of hair, skin and eyes, since tyrosine is needed for melanin production and is diminished in PKU. This leads to increased photosensitivity and increased problems with sunburn. The classic explanation for this has been that phenylalanine inhibits tyrosinase. One study done by a group at the Wistar Institute in Philadelphia on a hamster melanoma cell line revealed that the pigment abnormality was due to the very low tyrosine levels and the restriction of tyrosine uptake by phenylalanine. The pigment dilution is usually reversible with diet therapy, that is, phenylalanine restriction or tyrosine supplementation.

Dermatitis or eczema is seen in 10–50% of untreated patients, primarily during the first year of life. Some of these patients have true atopic dermatitis while others have ill-defined, irregular patterns. There is usually no family history of atopy. The eczema clears with dietary phenylalanine restriction and will flare within a day if phenylalanine blood levels increase. Although most patients do not have eczema past 4–5 years of age, it

Table 7.1 *Inherited metabolic diseases with dermatologic features*

Disease	Clinical features
Disorders of amino acid metabolism	
Phenylketonuria	Hypopigmentation, eczema, pseudoscleroderma
Tyrosinaemia type II (see Chapter 6)	Hyperkeratotic palms and soles
Alkaptonuria	Blue-black (ochronotic) discolouration of cartilage, cerumen, eyes and skin
Albinism (see Chapter 13)	Hypopigmentation
Prolidase deficiency [1]	Leg ulcers, telangiectases, maculopapular lesions, purpura, poliosis
Biotinidase deficiency [2]	Dermatitis, candidiasis, alopecia
Homocystinuria [3]	Hypopigmentation, malar flush, telangiectases, livedo reticularis
Hartnup disease [4] (see Chapter 12)	Pellagra-like rash, photosensitivity
Urea cycle disorders	
Argininosuccinic aciduria	Trichorrhexis nodosa
Disorders of carbohydrate metabolism	
Glycogen storage diseases	Lesions secondary to hyperlipidaemia and hyperuricaemia (xanthomas and gouty tophi)
Disorders of lipid metabolism	
Refsum's disease (see Chapter 5)	Ichthyosis
Hyperlipoproteinaemias	Xanthomas
Disorders of lysosomal enzymes	
Hunter's syndrome [5]	Pebbly nodules over scapulae and upper arms, thickened skin, hirsutism
GM_1 gangliosidosis [6]	Extensive and unusual mongolian spots
Fabry's disease	Angiokeratomas, hypohidrosis
Fucosidosis [7]	Angiokeratomas
Multiple sulphatase deficiency (see Chapter 5)	Ichthyosis

References

1 Der Kaloustian VM, Freij BJ, Kurban AK. Prolidase deficiency: an inborn error of metabolism with major dermatological manifestations. *Dermatologica* 1982; **164**: 293–304.
2 Williams ML, Packman S, Cowan MJ. Alopecia and periorificial dermatitis in biotin-responsive multiple carboxylase deficiency. *J Am Acad Dermatol* 1983; **9**: 97–103.
3 Brenton DP, Cusworth DC, Dent CE et al. Homocystinuria. Clinical and dietary studies. *Quart J Med* 1966; **35**: 325–45.
4 Wilcken B, Yu JS, Brown DA. Natural history of Hartnup disease. *Arch Dis Child* 1977; **52**: 38–40.
5 Prystowsky S, Maumanee IH, Freeman RG et al. A cutaneous marker in the Hunter syndrome. A report of four cases. *Arch Dermatol* 1977; **113**: 602–5.
6 Weissbluth M, Esterly NB, Caro W. Report of an infant with GM_1 gangliosidosis type I and extensive and unusual mongolian spots. *Br J Dermatol* 1981; **104**: 195–200.
7 Dvoretzky I, Fisher BK. Fucosidosis. *Int J Derm* 1979; **18**: 213–16.

may persist into adulthood in some. Several studies on small groups of patients have attempted to elucidate this dermatologic feature of PKU. The results of Fisch's group in Minnesota are as follows: phenylalanine and tyrosine levels in cultured skin fibroblasts have been measured and are the same in eczema patients with or without PKU; histopathologic and electron microscopic findings are identical in eczema patients with or without PKU and reveal a nonspecific dermatitis; patch tests with 50% phenylalanine in petrolatum under occlusion for 48 hours failed to produce a reaction in PKU patients and controls. Thus, it has been difficult to prove that the eczematous condition in PKU is due to elevated phenylalanine levels or hypersensitivity to phenylalanine.

Pseudoscleroderma is another dermatologic feature of PKU. It is much rarer than eczema and hypopigmentation, but has been reported in a number of cases. This feature occurs during early childhood and develops slowly, affecting the thighs and buttocks first, then the trunk and proximal extremities. The process begins deep in the muscle and subcutis, and eventually involves the dermis. There may be myositis and muscle cramps also. The aetiology of Pseudoscleroderma is unknown; perhaps it is due to a toxic metabolite. It may resolve with diet therapy. Pseudoscleroderma differs from true scleroderma in that it occurs early in life; it spares hands and feet, having a truncal distribution; and there is no visceral involvement. Leg contractures are occasionally seen. The histopathology differs from true scleroderma in that there is a proliferation of histiocytes and fibroblasts, there are fragmented elastic fibres, and there is muscle fibre atrophy. Both pseudoscleroderma and scleroderma have appendageal atrophy and a variable inflammatory infiltrate.

Approximately 80% of patients have an abnormal electroencephalogram and seizures. Skeletal changes include microcephaly, partial syndactyly, kyphosis and pes planus. Dental findings include widely spaced incisors. These patients also develop various behavioural disturbances such as hyperactivity, depression, anxiety, decreased concentration ability and learning disabilities.

Genetics

Phenylketonuria is a classic autosomal recessive disease. Linkage analysis using DNA polymorphisms can lead to prenatal diagnosis and carrier detection. The cloned gene for phenylalanine hydroxylase is on chromosome 12q.

Treatment

The infant with PKU is immediately placed on a low phenylalanine diet which prevents most of the associated abnormalities. The diet is usually continued throughout childhood, thus preventing mental retardation and the other complications.

Although maternal PKU is not dermatologically related, it is the major PKU problem today. Treated PKU women are more likely to have children. If the mother's diet is not well controlled prior to, or during, early pregnancy there is great risk to the fetus. The increased PHE levels in the blood can cause microcephaly, mental retardation, congenital heart disease and low birthweight in these infants. The exact mechanism is unknown. New concerns about PKU mean new strategies are needed: patient education, diet intervention and pregnancy planning. Maternal PKU is currently being studied in several centres throughout the world.

References

1 Fleisher TL, Zeligman I. Cutaneous findings in phenylketonuria. *Arch Derm* 1960; **81**: 64–9.
2 Ghavami M, Levy H, Erbe R. Prevention of fetal damage through dietary control of maternal hyperphenylalaninemia. *Clin Obst Gynecol* 1986; **29**: 580–5.
3 Lidsky AS, Guttler F., Woo SLC. Prenatal diagnosis of classic phenylketonuria by DNA analysis. *Lancet* 1985; **i**: 549–51.
4 Jablonska S, Stachow A, Suffczynska M. Skin and muscle indurations in phenylketonuria. *Arch Derm* 1967; **95**: 443–50.
5 Fisch R, Tsai M, Gentry W. Studies of phenylketonurics with dermatitis. *J Am Acad Dermatol* 1981; **4**: 284–90.
6 Farishian R, Shittaker J. Phenylalanine lowers melanin synthesis in mammalian melanocytes by reducing tyrosine uptake: implications for pigment reduction in phenylketonuria. *J Invest Dermatol* 1980; **74**: 85–9.

Alkaptonuria

Definition

Alkaptonuria [1–5] is a rare disease due to deficiency of homogentisic acid oxidase. This results in elevated levels of homogentisic acid in the urine, skin and connective tissue. Homogentisic acid is a metabolic product of phenylalanine and tyrosine and is excreted in the urine. The relationship between the enzyme defect and the clinical features is unknown.

Clinical features

There is a classic triad that characterizes this disease. Homogentisic aciduria is present, which results in urine that darkens on standing or when alkaline. Another feature is ochronosis, which is pigment deposition in various tissues, especially eyes, ears, skin, cartilage, heart, kidneys and prostate. It develops after homogentisic acid is oxidized and polymerized. The polymer has not been well characterized. Thirdly, there is a crippling arthritis which develops in adulthood and is due to cartilaginous involvement of joints.

There are different presentations at different ages. In infancy, dark urine may be the presenting sign. Diapers (napkins) may discolour, especially after laundering with alkaline soap. If urine is acidic, this change will not be seen. The next change seen is black cerumen, which is usually noted by 5 years of age. Between the ages of 8 and 10 years, pigmentation of the axillae occurs with staining of the undergarments. This disease is harmless in childhood. Patients over 20 years old, however, develop the auricular pigmentation and thickening, eye pigmentation of the sclerae, corneas, lids and conjunctivae, and the crippling arthropathy.

Involvement of the tympanic membranes and ossicles can lead to deafness. Facial pigmentation on the nose and cheeks in a 'butterfly' distribution is common. Nail discolouration may be seen as well.

The arthritis may be crippling. It is worse in males and affects the back, knees, shoulders and hips. Intervertebral discs are pigmented and become calcified, resulting in vertebral collapse. One possible mechanism for the arthritis is that homogentisic acid inhibits lysyl hydroxylase. This decreases hydroxylysine levels, altering the collagen structure. The type II collagen in articular cartilage is normally rich in hydroxylysine; its inadequate production results in abnormal type II collagen and cartilage.

Pathology

The skin discolouration is due to ochronotic pigment granules which are deposited in the dermis, cartilage and tendons. The histopathology of ochronosis reveals pigmentation and pigment granules in endothelial cells, basement membrane and secretory cells of eccrine sweat glands, macrophages and elastic fibres. Collagen bundles are also pigmented and become swollen and degenerated.

Genetics

Alkaptonuria is a typical autosomal recessive disease. Rarely it can be associated with other genetic disorders such as Gilbert's syndrome and sucrase-isomaltase deficiency.

Treatment

Dietary restriction of phenylalanine and tyrosine may be helpful.

References

1 O'Brien WM, La Du BN, Bunim JJ et al. Biochemical, pathologic and clinical aspects of alcaptonuria, ochronosis and ochronotic arthropathy. *Am J Med* 1963; **34**: 813.
2 Srsen S. Alkaptonuria. *Johns Hopkins Med J* 1979; **145**: 217–26.
3 O'Brien WM, Banfield WG, Sokoloff L et al. Studies on the pathogenesis of ochronotic arthropathy. *Arthritis Rheum* 1961; **4**: 137.
4 Murray JC, Lindberg KA, Pinnell SR. In vitro inhibition of chick embryo lysyl hydroxylase by homogentisic acid. A proposed connective tissue defect in alkaptonuria. *J Clin Invest* 1977; **59**: 1071.
5 Brown NK, Smuckler EA. Alkaptonuria and Gilbert's syndrome. *Am J Med* 1970; **48**: 759.

Argininosuccinic aciduria

Definition

A rare metabolic disease, argininosuccinic aciduria (ASA) is due to a deficiency of a urea cycle enzyme, argininosuccinase, resulting in elevated levels of argininosuccinic acid, ammonia and citrulline[1]. There are three forms of ASA. There is a neonatal form which is fatal, a subacute form seen in infancy, and a delayed onset form. The third type is the only one with hair abnormalities[2].

Clinical features

Clinical features include mental retardation, hepatomegaly, seizures, ataxia and lethargy. The sole dermatologic finding is trichorrhexis nodosa, manifested by friable, brittle hair. It is not seen in other urea cycle disorders. Trichorrhexis nodosa is seen in half the patients with ASA; the other half have normal hair. This finding is not related to disease severity. It usually involves only scalp hair but other areas may be involved. Mechanical trauma contributes to breakage.

Pathology

Microscopically, one sees nodular protrusions along hairs and frayed ends, much like a straw broom. This involves the proximal part of the hair shaft. The cortex swells and splits with fracturing through the centre of the node. The pathogenesis is unknown. Amino acid analysis of hair has not helped to elucidate the aetiology of trichorrhexis nodosa in this disease. There is a report of a patient who had low cystine levels in the hair. The condition seems to improve with age.

Genetics

Disease inheritance is autosomal recessive. The argininosuccinate lyase gene has been cloned and is located on the 7q chromosome.

Treatment

There is no effective treatment. Improvement of abnormal hair may be seen with advancing age.

References

1 Walser M. Urea cycle disorders and other hereditary hyperammonemic syndromes. In: Stanbury JB, Wyngaarden JB, Fredrickson DS, Goldstein JL, Brown MS, eds. *The Metabolic Basis of Inherited Disease*. McGraw-Hill, New York, 1983; 402–38.
2 Potter JL, Timmons GD, Silvidi AA. Argininosuccinic aciduria: the hair abnormality revisited. *Am J Dis Child* 1980; **134**: 1095–6.

Hyperlipoproteinaemias

The hyperlipoproteinaemias, also known as hyperlipidaemias, consist of a group of disorders characterized by elevated serum cholesterol levels, elevated triglyceride levels, or both [1–4]. These are inherited disorders and can be classified into five groups, hyperlipoproteinaemias I–V. Each entity has its own specific features. All types of hyperlipoproteinaemia may have the cutaneous lesions known as xanthomas (see below).

Xanthomas

Xanthomas are the most characteristic skin manifestation of the hyperlipoproteinaemias. Xanthomas are papules, nodules or tumours that contain lipid. They may be found anywhere on the cutaneous surface; the location can be helpful in discerning which type of hyperlipoproteinaemia is present. Regression or disappearance of xanthomas may be seen when lipid levels are reduced.

Plane xanthomas are fairly flat to slightly elevated yellowish plaques which are most commonly seen in the palmar and digital creases.

Xanthelasmata are located on the eyelids and are superficial lesions. They may be associated with normal lipid levels or type II hyperlipoproteinaemia.

Eruptive xanthomas are usually reddish-yellow papules that appear in crops, particularly on the buttocks and extensor surfaces of the extremities. They are associated with hypertriglyceridaemia and are commonly seen in patients with diabetes and in hyperlipoproteinaemia types I, III, IV and V. Oestrogen, retinoids and corticosteroids can cause these lesions as well.

Tendinous xanthomas tend to be nodular and have a predilection for extensor tendons of the knees, elbows, hands and feet. They are skin-coloured or yellowish, mobile subcutaneous nodules. These usually indicate the existence of hypercholesterolaemia, and appear in types II and III.

Tuberous xanthomas are large tumours, often flesh-coloured or yellow, present on extensor surfaces of the elbows, knees, hands or buttocks. They are usually associated with hypertriglyceridaemia and are seen in types II, III and IV hyperlipoproteinaemia. They may be confluent.

References

1 Hobbs H, Leitersdorf E, Goldstein J, Brown M, Russell D. Multiple crm- mutations in familial hypercholesterolemia: evidence for 13 alleles, including four deletions. *J Clin Invest* 1988; **81**: 909–17.
2 Parker F. Xanthomas and hyperlipidemias. *J Am Acad Dermatol* 1985; **13**: 1–30.
3 Haber C, Kwiterovich P. Dyslipoproteinemia and xanthomatosis. *Pediatr Dermatol* 1984; **1**: 261–80.
4 Cruz P, East C, Bergstresser P. Dermal, subcutaneous, and tendon xanthomas: diagnostic markers for specific lipoprotein disorders. *J Am Acad Dermatol* 1988; **19**: 95–111.

Type I hyperlipoproteinaemia

Synonym: *Burger–Grutz syndrome*

Clinical features

Type I hyperlipoproteinaemia is characterized by excess chylomicrons. It is manifested by hypertriglyceridaemia. The predominant skin lesions are eruptive xanthomas. Lipaemia retinalis can be seen in the eyes of patients with this form of hyperlipidaemia. Hepatosplenomegaly, pancreatitis and abdominal pain can also be seen in these patients. The age groups affected include infants and teenagers. Although the disorder appears early in life, with advancing age these patients have elevated levels of very low-density lipoproteins (VLDL) as well (type V pattern).

This type of hyperlipoproteinaemia is due to impaired lipoprotein lipase activity. This leads to impaired removal of chylomicrons, chylomicron remnants and endogenous VLDL.

Genetics

Type I hyperlipoproteinaemia is an autosomal recessive disorder.

Treatment

The choice of therapy for all of these disorders depends upon the underlying lipid abnormality. Treatment can help reduce atherosclerosis, hepatosplenomegaly and abdominal pain. Diet and antihyperlipidaemic medications are the mainstays of treatment.

For type I disease, a low-fat diet and medium-chain triglycerides can be beneficial.

Type II hyperlipoproteinaemia

Clinical features

Type II hyperlipoproteinaemia is characterized by elevation of serum cholesterol levels. In addition to premature coronary artery disease, liver disease accompanied by jaundice and pruritus may be pres-

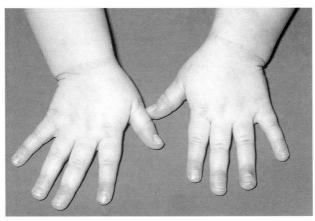

Figure 7.1 *'Bracelet' xanthelasma in a child with familial hypercholesterolaemia (type II hyperlipoproteinaemia) (Courtesy of Dr J Harper)*

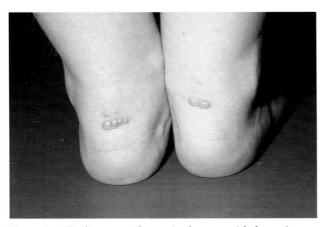

Figure 7.2 *Tendinous xanthomas in the same girl shown in Figure 7.1*

ent. Cutaneous findings include tendinous, tuberous and plane xanthomas (Figures 7.1 and 7.2). Palmar xanthomas are seen too.

An increase in low-density lipoproteins (LDL) (beta-lipoproteins) are seen in the type IIa form of hyperlipoproteinaemia, whereas type IIb has increased LDL and VLDL.

Genetics

Transmitted as an autosomal dominant trait, this type occurs in about 1 in 500 people. There is a genetic mutation which affects the formation of LDL receptors. At least eight mutant alleles have been identified. Several phenotypic genetic conditions are categorized as familial hypercholesterolaemia.

Treatment

Dietary therapy consists of a low-energy, low-carbohydrate, low-alcohol, low-cholesterol diet. Intake of unsaturated fats rather than saturated fats would be helpful. Drugs such as clofibrate, cholestyramine, colestipol, gemfibrozil and nicotinic acid may help reduce high lipid levels.

Type III hyperlipoproteinaemia

Clinical features

Also known as 'broad beta' disease, type III hyperlipoproteinaemia is seen primarily in adults. It is rare in children. Elevated levels of cholesterol and triglycerides are present. There is increased incidence of coronary artery disease. Diabetes mellitus is frequently seen in these patients. Plane xanthomas as well as tendinous and tuberous xanthomas may be noted.

There are elevated concentrations of remnant lipoproteins (intermediate density lipoprotein, IDL) and reductions in LDL and HDL. The alterations seen in VLDL and IDL are due to a genetically controlled abnormality of apoprotein E.

Genetics

Inheritance of this disorder is autosomal recessive.

Treatment

The same dietary manipulations as for type II disease are beneficial here. Clofibrate is also useful.

Type IV hyperlipoproteinaemia

Clinical features

Type IV disease is characterized by an increase in VLDL levels and, thus, hypertriglyceridaemia. There may be mild elevation in cholesterol levels as well. The disorder is seen predominantly in adults and can be manifested by obesity, hepatosplenomegaly, lipaemia retinalis, abdominal pain, premature coronary artery disease and xanthomas. The eruptive and tuberous xanthomas are the most common skin lesions seen in this disorder.

Genetics

Inheritance of type IV disease is autosomal dominant.

Treatment

A diet low in energy, carbohydrates, fat and alcohol can help lower lipid levels. Clofibrate and gemfibrozil are useful adjuncts.

Type V hyperlipoproteinaemia

Clinical features

Type V hyperlipoproteinaemia is characterized by increased levels of chylomicrons as well as VLDLs. Triglycerides are elevated. The disorder is seen mostly in adults, and obesity, hepatosplenomegaly, lipaemia retinalis and various xanthomas are present. It is very rare to see this form in children. Eruptive and tuberous xanthomas as well as xanthelasma are common. Lipoprotein lipase deficiency is the basic abnormality in this form of hyperlipidaemia.

Genetics

Inheritance is autosomal recessive.

Treatment

Treatment is the same as for type IV disease.

Fabry's disease

Synonym: *Angiokeratoma corporis diffusum*

Definition

Fabry's disease [1–4] is a rare inborn error of metabolism of glycosphingolipids, resulting from deficiency of alpha-galactosidase A, a lysosomal acid hydrolase.

Clinical features

The major features of Fabry's disease are angiokeratomas (Figure 7.3), hypertension and uraemia. This genetic disorder has an incidence of 1 in 40 000 persons. The clinical features are due to the accumulation of a neutral glycosphingolipid (GSL), ceramide trihexoside. The accumulation of GSL in body fluids

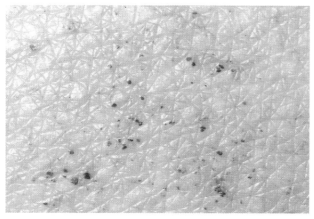

Figure 7.3 *Fabry's disease: angiokeratomas (Courtesy of Dr J Harper)*

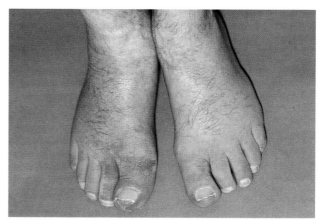

Figure 7.4 *Fabry's disease (same patient as in Figure 7.3): dry, dusky red, painful feet*

and lysosomes leads to the development of multiple angiokeratomas, and to ocular, cardiac, renal and central nervous system dysfunction. Glycolipid deposition increases with increasing age of the patient.

Clinically there may be debilitating pain and paraesthesia of the extremities (Figure 7.4), in addition to abdominal pain, nausea, vomiting and diarrhoea. Corneal and lens opacities are characteristic. Whorled corneal opacities ('corneal verticillata') are seen in over 90% of patients. Joint deformities of the hands are also commonly seen.

The angiokeratomas appear during childhood and increase in size and number over time. They are dark-red papules ranging in size from punctate to a few millimetres in diameter. The distribution of these lesions includes the lower abdomen, perineum, upper thighs and periumbilical skin. The head and neck are spared, as are the palms and soles. The lesions are usually symmetrical. Mucosal involvement is common. Hypohidrosis is extremely common in these patients.

Cardiac involvement leads to cardiomegaly, myocardial ischaemia, conductive abnormalities and heart failure. Renal involvement can lead to renal failure, with initial presentations of proteinuria and hypertension. Death usually results from renal failure.

Pathology

Fabry's disease is due to an alpha-galactosidase A deficiency. This enzyme deficiency leads to the abnormal deposition of neutral glycosphingolipids in most visceral tissues throughout the body. The deposits of trihexosyl ceramide are found mainly in the lysosomes of vascular endothelial cells. Lipid-laden foamy macrophages in the bone marrow suggest the diagnosis.

Lipid deposits in the skin are seen mainly in endothelial cells and pericytes of the capillaries. They are also seen in fibroblasts and the arrector muscles of the hair.

Genetics

The disorder is X-linked recessive, localized to chromosome Xq22. Hemizygous males have the severest form of the disease with complete penetrance. There is variable expression in heterozygous females; they may be asymptomatic, have an attenuated form of the disease, or – rarely – may be severely affected. Corneal opacities are the most common presentation in the mildly affected females.

Treatment

Prognosis is usually grave in males, with death in the third or fourth decade from vascular accident or renal failure. Therapy is not specific. The renal disease may require haemodialysis or perhaps renal transplantation; however, reaccumulation of ceramide has been reported in the transplanted kidney. Pain can be treated with phenytoin (diphenylhydantoin) or carbamazepine. Reduction of ceramide levels may be achieved by plasmapheresis, but this has a transient effect. A promising therapeutic modality is that of enzyme replacement. Prenatal diagnosis is possible.

References

1 Paller A. Metabolic disorders characterized by angiokeratomas and neurologic dysfunction. *Neurol Clin* 1987; **5**: 441–5.
2 Crovato F, Rebora A. Angiokeratoma corporis diffusum and normal enzyme activities. *J Am Acad Dermatol* 1985; **12**: 885–6.
3 Desnick RJ, Grabowki GA. Advances in the treatment of inherited metabolic diseases. *Adv Hum Genet* 1981; **11**: 281–369.
4 Maizel SE, Simmons RL, Kjellstrand CK et al. Ten year experience in renal transplantation for Fabry's disease. *Transplant Proc* **13**: 57–59.

Chapter 8

Ectodermal dysplasias

M. Pinheiro and N. Freire-Maia

Introduction

Ectodermal dysplasias (EDs) form a large and complex nosologic group whose delineation and classification were proposed by Freire-Maia[1,2]. It encompasses two groups. To group A belong all the conditions with defects in at least *two* of the 'classic' structures – hair, teeth, nails and sweat glands – with or without malformations and other dysplasia defects; to group B belong the conditions with defects in only *one* of the four above-mentioned structures plus at least one other ectodermal defect.

A condition characterized by only ectodermal signs is called a pure ectodermal dysplasia; if it combines ectodermal signs and malformations, it is termed an ectodermal dysplasia–malformation syndrome, or ectodermal dysplasia syndrome for short. Pure ectodermal dysplasias and ectodermal dysplasia syndromes compose the large group of ectodermal dysplasias *sensu lato*.

The above-mentioned structures – hair, teeth, nails and sweat glands – are numbered 1, 2, 3 and 4, and the several subgroups of group A are called 1–2, 1–3, 1–4, 2–3, 2–4, 3–4, 1–2–3, 1–2–4, 1–3–4, 2–3–4 and 1–2–3–4, or, if one prefers, tricho-odontic subgroup, tricho-onychial subgroup, trichodyshidrotic subgroup, etc. This arbitrary clinical classification and the definition of ectodermal dysplasia given above will eventually be replaced by others based on pathogenesis, as yet poorly known in this nosologic group.

The conditions belonging to group B are termed by the number corresponding to the affected structure (1, 2, 3 or 4) and by number 5, indicative of the other ectodermal defect. Therefore, conditions belonging to this group are termed 1–5, 2–5, 3–5 or 4–5, or, if one prefers, trichic subgroup, odontic subgroup, etc.

This review of ectodermal dysplasias belonging to group A is summarized in Tables 8.3 and 8.4 at the end of this chapter. Bibliographical reference is given only for the conditions not mentioned either in the authors' previous reviews [3–5] or in McKusick's *Mendelian Inheritance in Man* (MIM)[6]. The presence of a condition in McKusick is denoted by its MIM number. The criteria used for accepting a genetic cause – autosomal dominant (AD), autosomal recessive (AR) or X-linked (XL) – as 'proved' or merely 'possible' (AD? AR? XL?) for a given condition are those presented on pages 187–8 of the authors' book on the ectodermal dysplasias[3]. The data presented permit the following comments.

The total number of conditions is 146, including 'aetiological heterogeneity'. In previous reviews, conditions that seemed clinically very similar but had different causes were presented under the same heading. Here they are presented separately: see, for instance, dyskeratosis congenita (Table 8.3: subgroup 1–2–3–4; conditions 6, 7 and 8). Some conditions have changed subgroup and some have changed name. One condition suffered both changes: hypotrichosis–hypodontia, formerly part of the 1–2 subgroup, now belongs to subgroup 1–2–3 with the name Winter–MacDermot–Hill syndrome. For a full comparison see Freire-Maia and Pinheiro [3–5].

The 146 conditions are distributed within the 11 subgroups previewed in Freire-Maia's 1971 classification[1], but there is a wide diversity of numbers in the different subgroups. Those presenting the largest numbers (10 or more) are 1–2–3 with 38, 1–2 with 30, 1–2–3–4 with 28, 1–3 with 14, and 1–3–4 with 11. The numbers in the other subgroups are: 1–2–4 and 2–3 with 7 each, 1–4 with 6, 2–4 and 3–4 with 2 each, and 2–3–4 with 1. This extreme diversity is certainly not due to chance and does not appear to reflect ascertainment bias.

Autosomal dominant and autosomal recessive conditions are present in very similar numbers (respectively 43 and 42).

Among conditions with unknown cause, there are some (23) with no suggestion at all of a genetic cause, and others with suggestion of AD, AR and XL causes (7, 22 and 11, respectively). Note that 9 of these conditions appear to have two possible causes: 8 as AD? and XL?, and 1 as AR? and XL? The relative excess of AR? and XL? seems to reflect the greater difficulty in determining AR and XL inheritance than AD inheritance. The total number of conditions with unknown causes – including both possible (AD? AR? XL?) and totally unknown (?) – is 54 (37% of the total).

Summing up proved and possible causes, the numbers of AD conditions range from 43 to 50, those of AR from 42 to 64, those of XL from 7 to 18, and the unknown ones from 23 to 54.

The above data show that 23/146 (16%) and 54/146 (37%) of all EDs have causes either totally unknown or poorly suggested.

Each of the four signs used for the classification (trichodysplasia, dental defects, onychodysplasia and dyshidrosis) is present in 7 out of the 11 subgroups. They are respectively present in 134, 113, 101 and 57 conditions. This distribution does not seem to be a random one.

Comparison of the number of currently known EDs with those presented in previous reviews reveals a remarkable increase (from 32 to 146; Table 8.1).

Of the 146 currently known EDs, 8 well-known conditions are described here to give an idea of the extensive clinical variation found among them (Table 8.2).

References

1 Freire-Maia N. Ectodermal dysplasias. *Hum Hered* 1971; **21**: 309–12.
2 Freire-Maia N. Ectodermal dysplasias revisited. *Acta Genet Med Gemell* 1977; **26**: 121–31.
3 Freire-Maia N, Pinheiro M. *Ectodermal Dysplasias: A Clinical and Genetic Study*. Alan R. Liss, New York; 1984.
4 Freire-Maia N, Pinheiro M. Ectodermal dysplasias – a review of the conditions described after 1984 with an overall analysis of all the conditions belonging to this nosologic group. *Rev Brasil Gen* 1987; **10**: 403–14.
5 Freire-Maia N, Pinheiro M. Ectodermal dysplasias – some recollections and a classification. *Birth Def Orig Art Ser* 1988; **24**: 3–14.
6 McKusick VA. *Mendelian Inheritance in Man. Catalogs of Autosomal Dominant, Autosomal Recessive and X-Linked Phenotypes*. 11th ed. Johns Hopkins University Press, Baltimore; 1994.

Table 8.1 *Number of known EDs from 1971 to 1995*

Reference	No. of conditions	No. of subgroups
Freire-Maia (1971) [1]	32	8
Freire-Maia (1977) [2]	57	10
Freire-Maia and Pinheiro (1984) [3]	117	11
Freire-Maia and Pinheiro (1988)* [4]	131	11
Freire-Maia and Pinheiro (1987) [5]	145	11
This chapter**	146	11

* Review performed in 1985.
** Three 'conditions' referred to in previous reviews [4, 5] have been deleted for different reasons: triphalangeal thumbs–onychodystrophy–deafness (subgroup 2–3) is now accepted as a single condition (DOOR syndrome); the condition formerly labelled dentoungular dysplasia with hypothyroidism (subgroup 2–3) has been identified as ANOTHER syndrome (subgroup 1–3–4); and Marshall's syndrome I (subgroup 2–4) is generally not accepted as being a typical ED.

References

1 Freire-Maia N. Ectodermal dysplasias. *Hum Hered* 1971; **21**: 309–12.
2 Freire-Maia N. Ectodermal dysplasias revisited. *Acta Genet Med Gemell* 1977; **26**: 121–31.
3 Freire-Maia N, Pinheiro M. *Ectodermal Dysplasias: A Clinical and Genetic Study*. Alan R. Liss, New York, 1984.
4 Freire-Maia N, Pinheiro M. Ectodermal dysplasias – some recollections and a classification. *Birth Def Orig Art Ser* 1988; **24**: 3–14.
5 Freire-Maia N, Pinheiro M. Ectodermal dysplasias – a review of the conditions described after 1984 with an overall analysis of all the conditions belonging to this nosologic group. *Rev Brasil Genēt* 1987; **10**: 403–14.

Table 8.2 *The eight selected ectodermal dysplasias discussed in this chapter*

Condition	MIM no.
Christ–Siemens–Touraine syndrome	305100
Fischer–Jacobsen–Clouston syndrome	129500
Ellis–van Creveld syndrome	225500
Ectrodactyly–ectodermal dysplasia–cleft lip/palate syndrome	129900
Hypertrichosis and dental defects	See text
Coffin–Siris syndrome	135900
Growth retardation–alopecia–pseudoanodontia–optic atrophy (GAPO)	230740
Johanson–Blizzard syndrome	243800

Christ–Siemens–Touraine syndrome

Synonyms: *Hypohidrotic X-linked ectodermal dysplasia; sex-linked ectodermal dysplasia; ectodermal dysplasia, anhidrotic (EDA); ectodermal polydysplasia; anhidrosis–hypotrichosis–anodontia syndrome; anhidrosis hypotrichotica sexoligata; etc.*

Clinical features

The clinical features of Christ–Siemens–Touraine syndrome are illustrated in Figure 8.1.

Hair: fine and dry; hypochromic; hypotrichosis of scalp and body; absent or scanty eyebrows and lashes; moustache and beard generally normal. Structural changes.

Teeth: hypodontia; peg-shaped incisors and/or canines; persistence of deciduous teeth; delayed eruption; occasional anodontia.

Nails: generally normal; sometimes dystrophic or absent at birth, or fragile and brittle with incomplete development and celonychia.

Sweat: hypohidrosis with or without hyperthermia; reduced response to pilocarpine by iontophoresis; absence or decreased number of epidermal ridge sweat pores. The main danger in infancy is brain damage (and even death) due to hyperthermia.

Skin: thin, smooth and dry due to hypoplasia or absence of sebaceous glands; occasional pigmentation and dermatoglyphic changes; absent or supernumerary areolae and nipples.

Hearing: occasional conductive loss. Otitis media.

Eyes: photophobia; decreased function of the lacrimal glands; aplasia or hypoplasia of lacrimal ducts.

Face: highly characteristic, mainly in males: thick and prominent lips; depressed nasal bridge ('saddle' nose); frontal bossing; hypoplasia of the maxilla; wrinkles beneath or around the eyes, nose and mouth; and minor alterations of the auricles. The periorbital region is often more darkly pigmented than the rest of the body.

Psychomotor and growth development: normal. Brain damage due to hyperthermia may occur.

Limbs: normal.

Other findings: aplasia or hypoplasia of sebaceous and mucous glands of respiratory tract (leading to atrophic rhinitis, chronic pharyngitis and laryngitis, causing dysphonia and/or hoarseness) and gastrointestinal tract (reduced salivary production and feeding problems); aplasia or hypoplasia of breasts; abnormal immunoglobulin production.

On the basis of data obtained in the Oxford Regional Hospital Board area, Stevenson and Kerr[1] obtained the following estimates: approximate relative reproductive fitness 0.6; crude frequency among living males 9×10^{-6}; birth frequency among living males 10×10^{-6}; mutation rate $1–5 \times 10^{-6}$.

Genetics

The mode of inheritance is X-linked recessive; roughly 70% of heterozygous women have partial or mild manifestations (minor form) of the syndrome (hypotrichosis, hypodontia, microdontia, hypohidrosis, patchy mosaic distribution of body hair and of sweat pores, slight darkening around eyes, oligohydramnios, dry palms, etc.) [2–9].

Comments

Thurnam in 1848 seems to have been the first author to describe Christ–Siemens–Touraine syndrome (CST)[10]. Bernard et al[11] reported a kindred with 6 severely affected women in three generations with a CST-like syndrome, severe retardation of psychomotor development, and early death. They suggested that CST might be due to different alleles with different degrees of expression and penetrance. Their pedigree is compatible both with X-linked and autosomal dominant inheritance.

There is interfamily clinical heterogeneity both among men and women, all situations being compatible with X-linked inheritance. Different alleles at the same locus or two or more X-linked loci may be involved in what may really be a small group of similar conditions.

Severe illnesses were described among affected boys; roughly 30% of them died in early childhood in a sample studied by Clarke et al[12].

Chautard-Freire-Maia et al[13] presented evidence against linkage with Xg. The CST locus is now known

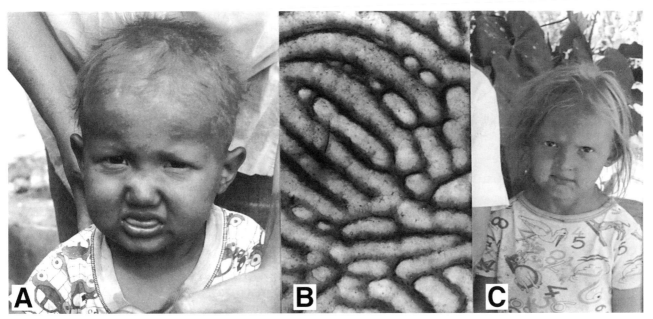

Figure 8.1 *Christ–Siemens–Touraine syndrome. (A) Hypotrichosis, hypochromic hair, abnormal auricles, depressed nose ('saddle' nose), protruding lips and hypoplastic mandible. (B) Absence of sweat pores in an affected man. (C) Carrier girl showing some signs of the syndrome*

to be on the proximal part of the X chromosome long arm and its probable assignment is Xq 12.2–13.1[14].

The syndrome is also discussed in references 15–27.

References

1 Stevenson AC, Kerr CB. On the distributions of frequencies of mutation to genes determining harmful traits in man. *Mutation Res* 1967; **4**: 339–52.

2 Pinheiro M, Freire-Maia N. Christ–Siemens–Touraine syndrome – a clinical and genetic analysis of a large Brazilian kindred. III. Carrier detection. *Am J Med Genet* 1979; **4**: 129–34.

3 Nakata M, Koshiba H, Eto K, Nance WE. A genetic study of anodontia in X-linked hypohidrotic ectodermal dysplasia. *Am J Hum Genet* 1980; **32**: 908–19.

4 Pinheiro M, Ideriha MT, Chautard-Freire-Maia EA, Freire-Maia N, Primo-Parmo SL. Christ–Siemens–Touraine syndrome. Investigations on two large Brazilian kindreds with a new estimate of the manifestation rate among carriers. *Hum Genet* 1981; **57**: 428–31.

5 Sofaer JA. A dental approach to carrier screening in X-linked hypohidrotic ectodermal dysplasia. *J Med Genet* 1981; **18**: 459–60.

6 Sofaer JA. Hypodontia and sweat pore counts in detecting carriers of X-linked hypohidrotic ectodermal dysplasia. *Br Dental J*, 1981; **151**: 327–30.

7 Airenne P. X-linked hypohidrotic ectodermal dysplasia in Finland. A clinical, radiographic and genetic study. *Academic Dissertation*, University of Helsinki, 1981.

8 Freire-Maia N, Pinheiro M. Carrier detection in Christ–Siemens–Touraine syndrome (X-linked hypohidrotic ectodermal dysplasia). *Am J Hum Genet* 1982; **34**: 672–4.

9 Freire-Maia N, Pinheiro M. Ectodermal dysplasias in females. *J Med Genet* 1982; **19**: 316.

10 Thurnam J. Two cases in which the skin, hair and teeth were very imperfectly developed. *Proc Roy Med Chir Soc* 1848; **31**: 71–82.

11 Bernard R, Giraud F, Touby M, Hartung M. A propos de sept observations de dysplasie ectodermique chez des sujets de sexe feminin dont six dans la même famille. Discussion génétique. *Arch Franc Péd* 1963; **20**: 1051–61.

12 Clarke A, Phillips DIM, Brown R, Harper PS. Clinical aspects of X-linked hypohidrotic ectodermal dysplasia. *Arch Dis Child* 1987; **62**: 989–96.

13 Chautard-Freire-Maia EA, Primo-Parmo SL, Pinheiro M, Freire-Maia N. Further evidence against linkage between Christ–Siemens–Touraine syndrome (*CST*) and *XG* loci. *Hum Genet* 1981; **57**: 205–6.

14 Human Gene Mapping 9.5. New Haven Conference. Update to the Ninth International Workshop on Human Gene Mapping. *Cytogenet Cell Genet* 1988; **49** (1–3): 1–258.

15 Simpson JL, Allen FH Jr, New M, German J. Absence of close linkage between the locus for Xg and the locus for anhidrotic ectodermal dysplasia. *Vox Sang* 1969; **17**: 465–7.

16 Mochizuki Y, Teramura F, Kawai K. A family of congenital anhidrotic ectodermal dysplasia. *Ann Paed Japon* 1971; **17**: 31–9.

17 Pinheiro M, Freire-Maia N. Christ–Siemens–Touraine syndrome – a clinical and genetic analysis of a large Brazilian kindred. I. Affected females. *Am J Med Genet* 1979; **4**: 113–22.

18 Pinheiro M, Freire-Maia N. Christ–Siemens–Touraine syndrome – a clinical and genetic analysis of a large Brazilian kindred. II. Affected males. *Am J Med Genet* 1979; **4**: 123–8.

19 Fuenmayor HM, Roldan-París L, Bermúdez H. Ectodermal dysplasia in females and inversion of chromosome 9. *J Med Genet* 1981; **18**: 214–17.

20 Söderholm A-L, Kaitila I. Expression of X-linked hypo-hidrotic ectodermal dysplasia in six males and in their mothers. *Clin Genet* 1985; **28**: 136–44.

21 Happle R, Frosch PJ. Manifestation of the lines of Blaschko in women heterozygous for X-linked hypohidrotic ectodermal dysplasia. *Clin Genet* 1985; **27**: 468–71.

22 Buckle VJ, Edwards JH, Evans EP et al. Comparative maps of human and mouse X chromosomes (abstract). *Cytogenet Cell Genet* 1985; **40**: 594–5.

23 Clarke A, Sarfarazi M, Thomas NST, Roberts K, Harper PS. X-linked hypohidrotic ectodermal dysplasia: DNA probe linkage analysis and gene localization. *Hum Genet* 1987; **75**: 378–80.

24 Bixler D, Saksena S, Ward RE. Characterization of the face in hypohidrotic ectodermal dysplasia by cephalometric and anthropometric analysis. In: Salinas CF, Opitz JM, Paul NW, eds. *Recent Advances in Ectodermal Dysplasias. Birth Defects: Original Article Series*, 1988; **24**: 197–203.

25 Coston GN, Salinas CF. Speech characteristics in patients with hypohidrotic ectodermal dysplasias. In: Salinas CF, Opitz JM, Paul NW, eds. *Recent Advances in Ectodermal Dysplasias. Birth Defects: Original Article Series* 1988; **24** (2): 229–34.

26 Tanner BA. Psychological aspects of hypohidrotic ectodermal dysplasia. In: Salinas CF, Opitz JM, Paul NW, eds. *Recent Advances in Ectodermal Dysplasias. Birth Defects: Original Article Series* 1988; **24** (2): 263–75.

27 Zonana J, Clarke A, Sarfarazi M et al. X-linked hypohidrotic ectodermal dysplasia: localization within the region Xq11–21.1 by linkage analysis and implications for carrier detection and prenatal diagnosis. *Am J Hum Genet* 1988; **43**: 75–85.

Fischer–Jacobsen–Clouston syndrome

Synonyms: *Hidrotic ectodermal dysplasia; Clouston syndrome; Waldeyer–Fischer syndrome; Jacobsen syndrome; Jacobsen–Clouston–Weech syndrome; hereditary dystrophy of the hair and nails*

Clinical features

Hair: dry, fine, usually blond, slow-growing; slight to severe hypotrichosis; absent or scanty eyebrows and lashes. Escobar et al[1] demonstrated a biochemical defect in the keratin of the integumentary system.

Teeth: generally normal; occasionally hypodontia, anodontia, widely spaced teeth, natal teeth, carious teeth (see Comments).

Nails: the defects vary considerably and several degrees of dystrophy are frequently found in the same hand. Nails are thickened and slightly discoloured; striated longitudinally; there may be paronychia, a tendency toward horny hypertrophy, convex ends, and anonychia.

Sweat: normal.

Skin: dry and rough; tendency toward scaliness; hyperpigmentation of some areas, especially over the joints; thick, dyskeratotic palms and soles.

Hearing: normal.

Eyes: generally normal. Occasionally strabismus, cataract and myopia.

Face: normal.

Psychomotor and growth development: generally normal; occasionally mental deficiency and short stature.

Limbs: generally normal; occasionally tufting of terminal phalanges and clubbing of fingers.

Other findings: occasionally thickening of the skull bones.

Genetics

The mode of inheritance is autosomal dominant.

Comments

Contrary to the opinion of Witkop et al[2], dental abnormalities also occur in this condition [3–5]. However, hair and nail defects are the most common and important findings.

Rajagopalan and Tay[6] described a Chinese family from Malaysia with 15 affected members over five generations.

Both the words 'hidrotic' and 'hydrotic' have been used in describing this condition. The first relates to *sweat* and the second to *water*[7]; the first term is, therefore, the correct one[8].

Of the two cases described by Weech[9], case 2 probably presented this condition, and *not* hypodontia and nail dysgenesis (tooth and nail syndrome)[10]. Case 1 was probably Christ–Siemens–Touraine syndrome.

Rousset[11] described 6 men and 1 woman over four generations with a dysplasia similar to Fischer–Jacobsen–Clouston syndrome, and which may be summarized as follows: hair – trichorrhexis nodosa, hypotrichosis, atrichia; teeth – widely spaced, pointed canines; nails – thick, brittle and upturned at the free margins. This condition seems to be due to an autosomal dominant gene with incomplete penetrance and variable expression.

The syndrome is also discussed in references 12–20.

References

1 Escobar V, Goldblatt LI, Bixler D, Weaver D. Clouston syndrome: an ultrastructural study. *Clin Genet* 1983; **24**: 140–6.

2 Witkop CJ Jr, Brearley LJ, Gentry WC. Hypoplastic enamel, onycholysis, and hypohidrosis inherited as autosomal dominant trait. A review of ectodermal dysplasia syndromes. *Oral Surg Oral Med Oral Pathol* 1975; **39**: 71–86.

3 Jacobsen AW. Hereditary dystrophy of the hair and nails. *J Am Med Assoc* 1928; **90**: 686–9.

4 Clouston HR. A hereditary ectodermal dystrophy. *Canad Med Assoc J* 1929; **21**: 18–31.

5 Aceves-Ortega R, Madrigal LR. Displasia ectodermica hidrotica. *Dermatologica* 1977; **21**: 12–21.

6 Rajagopalan K, Tay CH. Hidrotic ectodermal dysplasia. Study of a large Chinese pedigree. *Arch Dermatol* 1977; **113**: 481–5.

7 Taylor NB. *Stedman's Medical Dictionary.* Baltimore, Williams & Wilkins, 1957.

8 Freire-Maia N, Pinheiro M. Ectodermal dysplasias in females. *J Med Genet*, 1982; **19**: 316.

9 Weech AA. Hereditary ectodermal dysplasia (congenital ectodermal defect). A report of two cases. *Am J Dis Child* 1929; **37**: 766–90.

10 Witkop CJ Jr. Genetic disease of the oral cavity. In: Tiecke RW, ed. *Oral Pathology.* McGraw-Hill, New York; 1965.

11 Rousset MJ. Génodermatose difficilement classable (Trichorrhexis nodosa) prédominant chez les mâles dans quatre générations. *Bull Soc Fr Dermat Syphil* 1952; **59**: 298–300.

12 Fischer E. Ein Fall von erblicher Haararmut und die Art ihrer Vererbung. Ein Beitrag zur Familienanthropologie. *Archiv Rass Gesellschaftsbiol* 1910; **7**: 50–6.

13 Clouston HR. The major forms of hereditary ectodermal dysplasia. *Canad Med Assoc J* 1939; **40**: 1–7.

14 Joachim H. Hereditary dystrophy of the hair and nails in six generations. *Ann Intern Med* 1936; **10**: 400–2.

15 Wilkey WD, Stevenson GH. A family with inherited ectodermal dystrophy. *Canad Med Assoc J* 1945; **53**: 226–30.

16 Klein D. Cas observé. Une famille alsacienne de dysplasie ectodermique. *J Génét Hum* 1954; **3**: 210–13.

17 Williams M, Fraser FC. Hydrotic ectodermal dysplasia – Clouston's family revisited. *Canad Med Assoc J* 1967; **96**: 36–8.

18 McNaughton PZ, Pierson DL, Rodman OG. Hidrotic ectodermal dysplasia in a black mother and daughter. *Arch Dermatol* 1976; **112**: 1448–50.

19 Giraud F, Mattei JF, Rolland M, Ghiglione C, Santi PP de, Sudan N. La dysplasie ectodermique de type Clouston. *Arch Franc Pédiatr* 1977; **34**: 982–93.

20 Hazen PG, Zamora I, Bruner WE, Muir VA. Premature cataracts in a family with hidrotic ectodermal dysplasia. *Arch Dermatol* 1980; **116**: 1385–7.

Ellis–van Creveld syndrome

Synonyms: *Chondroectodermal dysplasia; mesoectodermal dysplasia*

Clinical features

The clinical features of Ellis–van Creveld syndrome are illustrated in Figure 8.2.

Hair: thin, brittle, sparse, and hypochromic; absent or scanty eyebrows and lashes.

Teeth: natal teeth; precocious exfoliation; hypodontia (deciduous and permanent teeth); occasionally hypoplastic enamel.

Nails: dysplastic (brittle, furrowed and underdeveloped).

Sweat: normal. See Comments.

Skin: occasional different alterations (hypotrophy, eczema, petechiae, etc.) are described in different patients. See Comments.

Hearing: normal.

Eyes: occasional strabismus, cataract, coloboma of the iris, microphthalmia, exophthalmia, etc. See Comments.

Face: broad nose; occasional change in the upper lip ('partial hare-lip', 'lip-tie', etc.), frontal bossing and hypertelorism.

Psychomotor and growth development: short-limb dwarfism; occasional mild mental retardation. See Comments.

Limbs: bilateral postaxial polydactyly (generally of the hands); brachymetacarpy; fusion of the hamate and capitate bones of the wrist; clubfoot; genua valga; syndactyly.

Other findings: congenital heart defect; respiratory difficulties (due to thoracic and tracheobronchial abnormalities); gingivolabial fusion; occasional cleft palate; genitourinary tract anomalies; lordosis.

Genetics

The mode of inheritance is autosomal recessive.

Comments

Four cardinal signs are important for the diagnosis:

1. Bilateral postaxial polydactyly.
2. Chondrodysplasia of the long bones resulting in acromelic dwarfism.
3. Ectodermal defects (generally in the hair, teeth and nails.
4. Congenital heart defect.

According to Pilotto[1], only 12 of the 204 patients described in the literature up to 1978 (including his own) were analysed for sweating. Ten of them were euhidrotic. The 2 patients reported to be hypohidrotic by Lodin and Sjögren[2] probably did not have the Ellis–van Creveld syndrome since they did not have polydactyly, fusion of the hamate and capitate and other typical skeletal abnormalities.

It is doubtful whether skin alterations and mental retardation really represent signs of the syndrome or merely coincidental findings. Skin alterations of different types have been found in only 5 of 204 patients; mental retardation, always mild, was mentioned in only 10 patients. Although 16 of 204 patients had eye abnormalities, no single anomaly was typical of the syndrome[1].

According to Pilotto[1], the following abnormalities were found (with their respective frequencies): trichodysplasia (51%), hypodontia of deciduous teeth (88%), hypodontia of permanent teeth (12%), natal teeth (23%), onychodystrophy (93%), congenital heart defect (69%), polydactyly of the hands (96%), polydactyly of the feet (33%), synostosis of hamate and

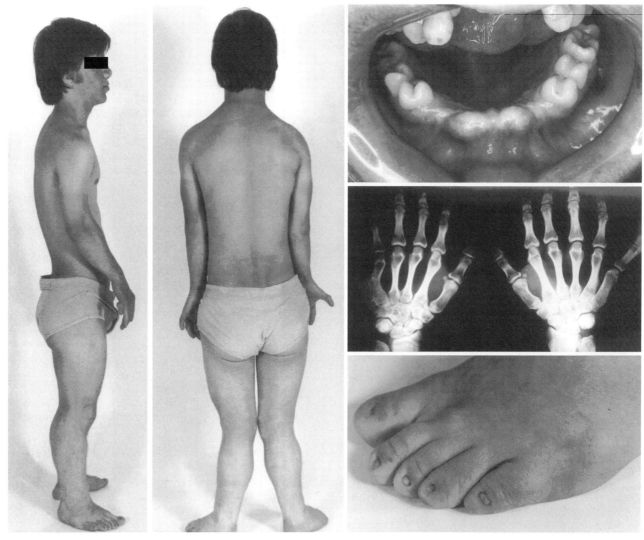

Figure 8.2 *Ellis–van Creveld syndrome. Acromelic dwarfism, lordosis, polydactyly, fusion of hamate and capitate bones of the wrist, genua valga, onychodystrophy, dental abnormalities and gingivolabial fusions (courtesy of Dr R. F. Pilotto)*

capitate (29%), pseudo cleft lip (13%) and gingivolabial alterations (55%).

Ellis–van Creveld syndrome is also classified among the chondrodystrophies or osteochondrodysplasias [3–8].

The largest kindred so far described is that investigated by McKusick et al[9] in an inbred religious isolate (the old-order Amish).

The syndrome is also discussed in references 10–16.

References

1 Pilotto RF. Estudo genético-clínico da síndrome de Ellis–van Creveld. *MSc Thesis*, Federal University of Paraná, Curitiba, Brazil, 1978.
2 Lodin H, Sjögren I. Chondro-ectodermal dysplasia (Ellis–van Creveld's syndrome). Two certain and two probable cases in the same family. *Acta Paediatr* 1964; **53**: 583–90.
3 Smith DW. Recognizable patterns of malformations in childhood. *Birth Def Orig Art Ser* 1969; **5** (2): 255–72.
4 Smith DW. *Recognizable Patterns of Human Malformation. Genetic, Embryologic and Clinical Aspects*. WB Saunders, Philadelphia, 1970.
5 Smith DW. *Recognizable Patterns of Human Malformation. Genetic, Embryologic and Clinical Aspects*. 3rd ed. WB Saunders, Philadelphia, 1982.
6 Lamy ME. Hereditary disorders of bones – an overview. *Birth Def Orig Art Ser* 1969; **5** (4): 8–16.
7 Maroteaux P. Spondyloepiphyseal dysplasias and metatrophic dwarfism. *Birth Def Orig Art Ser* 1969; **5** (4): 35–47.
8 Rimoin DL, Hall J, Maroteaux P. International nomenclature of constitutional diseases of bone with bibliography. *Birth Def Orig Art Ser* 1979; **15** (10).
9 McKusick VA, Egeland JA, Eldridge R, Krusen DE. Dwarfism in the Amish. I. The Ellis–van Creveld syndrome. *Bull Johns Hopkins Hosp* 1964; **115**: 306–36.
10 Ellis RWB, van Creveld S. A syndrome characterized by

ectodermal dysplasia, polydactyly, chondro-dysplasia and congenital morbus cordis. Report of three cases. *Arch Dis Child* 1940; **15**: 65–84.

11 Weiss H, Crosset AD Jr. Chondroectodermal dysplasia. Report of a case and review of the literature. *J Pediatr* 1955; **46**: 268–75.

12 Agostinelli O. La condrodisplasia ectodermica di Ellis-van Creveld. *Gazz Int Medico-Chirurg Inter Prof* 1970; **75**: 131–53.

13 Pinsky L. The polythetic (phenotypic community) system of classifying human malformation syndromes. *Birth Def Orig Art Ser* 1977; **13** (3A): 13–30.

14 Waldrigues A, Grohmann LC, Takahashi T, Reis HMP. Ellis-van Creveld syndrome. An inbred kindred with five cases. *Rev Brasil Pesq Méd Biol*, 1977; **10**: 193–8.

15 Da-Silva EO, Janovitz D, Albuquerque SC. Ellis-van Creveld syndrome: report of 15 cases in an inbred kindred. *J Med Genet* 1980; **17**: 349–56.

16 Rosemberg S, Carneiro PC, Zerbini MCN, Gonzalez CH. Chondroectodermal dysplasia (Ellis–van Creveld) with anomalies of CNS and urinary tract. *Am J Med Genet*, 1983; **15**: 291–5.

Ectrodactyly–ectodermal dysplasia–cleft lip/palate syndrome, Rüdiger–Haase–Passarge type

Synonyms: *Ectrodactyly–ectodermal dysplasia–clefting syndrome*

Clinical features

Figure 8.3 shows a baby with ectrodactyly–ectodermal dysplasia–cleft lip/palate (EEC) syndrome, Rüdiger–Haase–Passarge type.

Hair: hypotrichosis of scalp and body; fair and dry; scanty or absent eyebrows and lashes.

Teeth: anodontia; hypodontia; microdontia; enamel hypoplasia; poorly formed; increased caries; peg-shaped incisors.

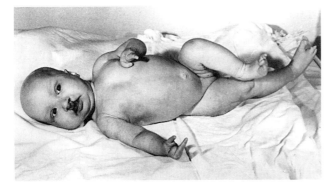

Figure 8.3 *Ectrodactyly–ectodermal dysplasia–cleft lip/palate (EEC) syndrome, Rüdiger–Haase–Passarge type. Note hypotrichosis, cleft lip, and split hands and feet (courtesy of Dr E. Passarge)*

Nails: dysplastic, thin, brittle and striated; pitted and terminated irregularly.

Sweat: occasionally hypohidrosis without hyperthermia.

Skin: dry, translucent, dystrophic; palmoplantar hyperkeratosis; eczematous patches; pigmented naevi; hypoplastic nipples and areolae.

Hearing: occasionally conductive loss.

Eyes: tear-duct anomalies; speckled iris; photophobia; strabismus; blepharitis; clouding of the cornea; congenital adhesions between the eyelids.

Face: cleft lip; broad nose; abnormal auricles; pointed chin; malar hypoplasia.

Psychomotor and growth development: occasionally mental retardation.

Limbs: ectrodactyly (split hands/feet); syndactyly; clinodactyly.

Other findings: cleft palate; genitourinary anomalies; rhinitis; respiratory infections.

Genetics

The mode of inheritance is autosomal dominant. See Comments.

Comments

Similar to ectrodactyly–ectodermal dysplasia–cleft lip/palate syndrome (the so-called 'complete form') are other conditions, sometimes called 'incomplete forms', which must be used in the differential diagnosis[1]. The main syndromes clinically close to EEC are ectrodactyly–cleft palate syndrome (ECP), AD (MIM 129830); ectrodactyly–cleft lip/palate–hand/foot deformity–mental retardation syndrome (Rosselli–Gulienetti syndrome), AR (MIM 225000); hypohidrotic ectodermal dysplasia–cleft lip/palate syndrome (Rapp–Hodgkin syndrome), AD (MIM 129400); lacrimo-auriculo-dento-digital syndrome (LADD), AD (MIM 149730); ectrodactyly–tear duct anomaly syndrome, AD; odontotrichomelic syndrome, AR? (MIM 273400); and ectrodactyly–ectodermal dysplasia with normal lip and palate, AR. The following conditions mentioned above and accepted as ectodermal dysplasias according to our definition are listed in Table 8.3: Rosselli–Gulienetti syndrome (subgroup 1–2–3–4, no. 5), Rapp–Hodgkin syndrome (subgroup 1–2–3–4, no. 11), odontotrichomelic syndrome (subgroup 1–2–3, no. 4), and ectrodactyly–ectodermal dysplasia with normal lip and palate (subgroup 1–2, no. 19). Note also that there is an EEC syndrome due to an AR cause (subgroup 1–2–3–4, no. 13).

The EEC syndrome has been identified with the odontotrichomelic syndrome by some investigators [2–4]. However, others [1, 5–14] did not agree with this identification. In spite of some similarities (as between other ectodermal dysplasias), the differences suggest that it is more reasonable to treat them as separate entities[15]. The main differences between the two syndromes are related to limb anomalies.

The syndrome is also discussed in references 16–21.

References

1 Richieri-Costa A, Vilhena-Moraes SA de, Ferrareto I, Masiero D. Ectodermal dysplasia/ectrodactyly in mono-zygotic female twins. Report of a case – review and comments of the ectodermal dysplasia/ectrodactyly (cleft lip/palate) syndromes. *Rev Brasil Genét* 1986; **9**: 349–74.

2 Brill CB, Hsu LYF, Hirschhorn K. The syndrome of ectrodactyly, ectodermal dysplasia and cleft lip and palate: report of a family demonstrating a dominant pattern. *Clin Genet* 1972; **3**: 295–302.

3 Rosenmann A, Shapira T, Cohen MM Jr. Ectrodactyly, ectodermal dysplasia and cleft palate (EEC syndrome). *Clin Genet* 1976; **9**: 347–53.

4 Schnitzler A, Schubert B, Larget-Piet L, Berthelot J, Cleirens S, Taviaux D. Le syndrome de Rüdiger (syndrome EEC). A propos d'un cas associé à un eczéma atopique. *Ann Dermatol Venereol* 1978; **105**: 201–6.

5 Freire-Maia N. Ectodermal dysplasias. *Hum Hered* 1971; **21**: 309–12.

6 Freire-Maia N. Ectodermal dysplasias revisited. *Acta Genet Med Gemell* 1977; **26**: 121–31.

7 Preus M, Fraser FC. The lobster claw defect with ectodermal defects, cleft lip–palate, tear duct anomaly and renal anomalies. *Clin Genet* 1973; **4**: 369–75.

8 Witkop CJ Jr, Brearley LJ, Gentry WC. Hypoplastic enamel, onycholysis, and hypohidrosis inherited as autosomal dominant trait. A review of ectodermal dysplasia syndromes. *Oral Surg Oral Med Oral Pathol* 1975; **39**: 71–86.

9 Pinsky L. The community of human malformation syndromes that shares ectodermal dysplasia and deformities of the hands and feet. *Teratology* 1975; **11**: 227–42.

10 Pinsky L. The polythetic (phenotypic community) system of classifying human malformation syndromes. *Birth Def Orig Art Ser* 1977; **13** (3A): 13–30.

11 Rapone-Gaidzinski R. Displasias ectodérmicas – revisão clínico-genética com especial referência ao problema da sudorese. *MSc Thesis*, Federal University of Paraná, Curitiba, Brazil, 1978.

12 Cohen MM Jr. Syndromes with cleft lip and cleft palate. *Cleft Pal J* 1978; **15**: 306–28.

13 Cohen MM Jr. Ectrodactyly–ectodermal dysplasia–clefting syndrome. In: Bergsma D, ed. *Birth Defects Compendium*, 2nd ed. Alan R. Liss, New York; 1979.

14 Da-Silva EO, Alves JG, Almeida E. Is the EEC syndrome genetically heterogeneous? *Rev Brasil Genét* 1984; **7**: 735–42.

15 Pinheiro M, Freire-Maia N. EEC and odontotrichomelic syndromes. *Clin Genet* 1980; **17**: 363–4.

16 Rüdiger RA, Haase W, Passarge E. Association of ectrodactyly, ectodermal dysplasia, and cleft lip–palate. *Am J Dis Child* 1970; **120**: 160–3.

17 Bixler D, Spivack J, Bennett J, Christian JC. The ectrodactyly-ectodermal dysplasia-clefting (EEC) syndrome. *Clin Genet* 1972; **3**: 43–51.

18 Fried K. Ectrodactyly–ectodermal dysplasia–clefting (EEC) syndrome. *Clin Genet* 1972; **3**: 396–400.

19 Swallow JN, Gray OP, Harper PS. Ectrodactyly, ectodermal dysplasia and cleft lip and palate (EEC syndrome). *Br J Dermatol* 1973; **89**: 54–6.

20 Robinson GC, Wildervanck LS, Chiang TP. Ectrodactyly, ectodermal dysplasia, and cleft lip–palate syndrome. Its association with conductive hearing loss. *J Pediatr* 1973; **82**: 107–9.

21 Rollnick BR, Hoo JJ. Genitourinary anomalies are a component manifestation in the ectodermal dysplasia, ectrodactyly, cleft lip/palate (EEC) syndrome. *Am J Med Genet* 1988; **29**: 131–6.

Hypertrichosis and dental defects

Synonyms: *see Comments*

Clinical features

Hair: generalized hypertrichosis (except on palms, soles and mucous membranes).

Teeth: occasionally persistence of deciduous teeth, delayed eruption, hypodontia, anodontia, and supernumerary teeth.

Nails: normal.

Sweat: normal.

Skin: normal.

Hearing: normal.

Eyes: normal. See Comments.

Face: normal.

Psychomotor and growth development: normal. See Comments.

Limbs: normal.

Other findings: see Comments.

Genetics

The mode of inheritance is autosomal dominant. See Comments.

Comments

Danforth[1] and Felgenhauer[2] described a number of cases (mother and daughter; grandfather, daughter and son; father and son; and sporadic cases). Freire-Maia et al[3] described a Brazilian mother and son (Figure 8.4). The mother had hypertrichosis on scalp, face, axillae and pubic areas. The boy also had dental abnormalities (supernumerary teeth, persistence of deciduous teeth, and delayed eruption of permanent teeth), growth retardation, low intelligence quotient (IQ), photophobia, hypotension and delayed sexual maturation. His low IQ was probably cultural. The reason for the photophobia could not be elucidated. The boy's hypotension, shortness of stature and delayed sexual maturation could have been due to adrenal hypoplasia not related to the hypertrichosis gene.

The above description refers only to a condition characterized by hypertrichosis and dental defects. It

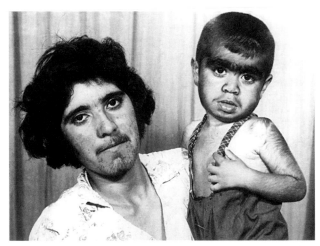

Figure 8.4 *Hypertrichosis and dental defects. Mother and son*

should not obscure the fact that hypertrichosis *sensu lato* is actually a group of conditions rather than a single entity. Hypertrichosis may be congenital or not, localized or generalized, isolated or associated with other traits (metabolic errors, dysplasias and/or malformations). Sometimes it is part of ectodermal dysplasias (as we define them) such as gingival fibromatosis and hypertrichosis; Coffin–Siris syndrome; hairy elbows dysplasia; hypomelanosis of Ito; syndrome of accelerated skeletal maturation, failure to thrive and peculiar face; and congenital lymphoedema, hypoparathyroidism, nephropathy, prolapsing mitral valve and brachytelephalangy (see Table 8.3). Therefore, the whole group of hypertrichotic conditions (ectodermal dysplasias and others) seems to be larger than that composed by the seven conditions mentioned above.

It would be difficult to attempt to disentangle the whole group into more than seven entities because most of the reported cases are poorly described, phenotypic overlap between apparently different conditions is plausible, the existence of clinical variants of the same condition is possible, and many situations are not covered by the authors' definition of ectodermal dysplasia. However, this 'splitting' task will probably prove to be as important here as it has been in other conditions.

The condition here called 'hypertrichosis and dental defects' has been described several times, but it is doubtful whether all the synonyms applied to hypertrichosis *sensu lato* would really apply to it. Some of these synonyms are congenital hypertrichosis lanuginosa syndrome, hypertrichosis universalis (MIM 145700), hypertrichosis universalis congenita and edentate hypertrichosis.

Hypertrichosis is also discussed in references 4–6.

References

1 Danforth CH. Studies on hair with special reference to hypertrichosis. *Arch Dermatol* 1925; **12**: 380–401.

2 Felgenhauer W-R. Hypertrichosis lanuginosa universalis. *J Génét Hum* 1969; **17**: 1–43.

3 Freire-Maia N, Felizali J, Figueiredo AC de, Opitz JM, Parreira M, Maia NA. Hypertrichosis lanuginosa in a mother and son. *Clin Genet* 1976; **10**: 303–6.

4 Berres HH, Nitschke R. Vergleichende klinische und morphologische Untersuchungen zwischen einem Neugeborenen mit Hypertrichosis universalis und gleichaltrigen hautgesunden Kindern. *Z Kinderheilk* 1968; **102**: 327–40.

5 Cat I, Marinoni LP, Moreira CA, Giraldi DJ, Costa O, Braga H. Hipertricose lanuginosa universal. *J Pediatr* 1971; **36**: 26–8.

6 Suskind R, Esterly NB. Congenital hypertrichosis universalis. *Birth Def Orig Art Ser* 1971; **7** (8): 103–6.

Coffin–Siris syndrome

Synonyms: *Mental retardation with absent fifth fingernails and terminal phalanx; syndrome of absent fifth fingernails and toenails, short distal phalanges and lax joints; fifth digit syndrome*

Clinical features

Hair: sparse scalp hair; bushy eyebrows and lashes; hirsutism of limbs, forehead and back.

Teeth: delayed eruption; microdontia; enamel hypoplasia.

Nails: absent or hypoplastic fifth fingernails and toenails; other nails occasionally hypoplastic or absent.

Sweat: normal.

Skin: dermatoglyphic changes; transverse crease.

Hearing: normal.

Eyes: blepharoptosis, hypophoria, hypermetropia and astigmatism have been found in one patient.

Face: coarse appearance with thick lips, wide mouth and nose, anteverted nostrils and low nasal bridge.

Psychomotor and growth development: postnatal growth deficiency; developmental delay; mental retardation; hypotonia.

Limbs: lax joints; clinodactyly of the fifth fingers; absence of terminal phalanges of fifth fingers and toes; aplasia or variable hypoplasia of middle and proximal phalanges of other fingers and toes; slender metacarpals and metatarsals; bilateral or unilateral dislocation of radial heads; small or absent patella; coxa valga.

Other findings: recurrent respiratory tract infections and feeding problems in infancy; umbilical and inguinal hernias; cleft palate; anomalies of number of vertebrae; short sternum; microcephaly; malrotation of the intestines; perforated gastrointestinal ulcers; congenital heart defect.

Genetics

The mode of inheritance is unknown. See Comments.

Comments

The first three cases (three unrelated girls from non-consanguineous parents) were described by Coffin and Siris[1]. Carey and Hall[2] reported a brother-and-sister pair from normal, non-consanguineous parents. Richieri-Costa et al[3] described the first case from consanguineous (first cousin) parents. All the other cases are sporadic. The fathers of two of the three girls (cases 1 and 2) described by Coffin and Siris[1] and of the girl (case 2) described by Weiswasser et al[4] were mildly and differently affected (bushy eyebrows, also present in two brothers; ptosis of one eyelid; iris coloboma of one eye; slightly small fingernails and toenails). A number of relatives on the paternal side of the boy described by Tunnessen et al[5] were said to present 'small nails'.

Weiswasser et al[4] noted some differences between the cases described by Senior[6] and those of Coffin and Siris[1]; they stated that 'it is unclear whether some of the patients described by Senior represent variations in the clinical spectrum of the Coffin–Siris syndrome'. However, Holmes et al[7] accepted all of these patients as having the same syndrome.

Mattei et al[8] identified the Coffin–Siris syndrome with the Coffin–Lowry syndrome (MIM 303600); this confusion was due to the fact that Dr Siris was a co-author of Dr Coffin in the description of both syndromes[1,9]. Gorlin[10] noticed this confusion and clarified some points regarding nosology in this area:

1. These two syndromes are different.
2. Coffin–Lowry syndrome is due to an X-linked gene.
3. The cause of Coffin–Siris syndrome is unknown; it may be heterogeneous, with some cases representing examples of the fetal hydantoin syndrome, or due to an autosomal recessive gene.
4. Some of the patients described in the literature, such as those of Senior[6], possibly present a mild form of the Coffin–Siris syndrome.

The syndrome is also discussed in references 11–14.

References

1 Coffin GS, Siris, E. Mental retardation with absent fifth fingernail and terminal phalanx. *Am J Dis Child* 1970; **119**: 433–9.
2 Carey JC, Hall BD. The Coffin–Siris syndrome. Five new cases including two siblings. *Am J Dis Child* 1978; **132**: 667–71.
3 Richieri-Costa A, Monteleone-Neto R, Gonzalez ML. Coffin–Siris syndrome in a Brazilian child with consanguineous parents. *Rev Brasil Genét* 1986; **9**: 169–77.
4 Weiswasser WH, Hall BD, Delavan GW, Smith DW. The Coffin–Siris syndrome: two new cases. *Am J Dis Child* 1973; **125**: 838–40.
5 Tunnessen WW, McMillan JA, Levin MB. The Coffin–Siris syndrome. *Am J Dis Child* 1978; **132**: 393–5.
6 Senior B. Impaired growth and onychodysplasia – short children with tiny toenails. *Am J Dis Child* 1971; **122**: 7–9.
7 Holmes LB, Moser HW, Halldorsson S, Mack C, Pant SS, Matzilevich B. Syndrome of absent fifth fingernails and toenails, short distal phalanges, and lax joints. In: *Mental Retardation – An Atlas of Disease with Associated Physical Abnormalities*. Macmillan, New York; 1972.
8 Mattei JF, Laframboise R, Rouault F, Giraud F. Coffin–Lowry syndrome in sibs. *Am J Med Genet* 1981; **8**: 315–19.
9 Coffin GS, Siris E, Wegienka LC. Mental retardation with osteocartilaginous anomalies. *Am J Dis Child* 1966; **112**: 205–13.
10 Gorlin RJ. Lapsus – Caveat Emptor: Coffin–Lowry syndrome vs Coffin–Siris syndrome – an example of confusion compounded. *Am J Med Gent* 1981; **10**: 103–4.
11 Bartsocas CS, Tsiantos AK. Mental retardation with absent fifth fingernail and terminal phalanx. *Am J Dis Child* 1970; **120**: 493–4.
12 Feingold M. The Coffin–Siris syndrome. *Am J Dis Child* 1978; **132**: 660–1.
13 Kessel A, Bodurtha J, Berman W, Hartenberg M. Coffin–Siris syndrome – GI tract anomaly responsible for feeding difficulties. *Am J Hum Genet* 1985; **37** (4): A62.
14 De Bassio WA, Kemper TL, Knoefel JE. Coffin–Siris syndrome. Neuropathologic findings. *Arch Neurol* 1985; **42**: 350–3.

Growth retardation–alopecia–pseudoanodontia–optic atrophy (GAPO)

Synonyms: *Pseudoanodontia, growth retardation and alopecia; pseudoanodontia, cranial deformity, blindness, alopecia and dwarfism; dwarfism, alopecia, anodontia and cutis laxa*

Clinical features

Some of the clinical features of growth retardation–alopecia–pseudoanodontia–optic atrophy (GAPO) can be seen in Figure 8.5.

Hair: severe alopecia of body and scalp hair (some hair, present at birth, is lost during infancy); sparse or absent eyebrows and lashes.

Teeth: pseudoanodontia (all buds are present) of both primary and permanent dentition with absence of alveolar ridges.

Nails: occasionally hyperconvexity on fingers and toes.

Sweat: normal.

Skin: dry; redundant; fragile with inadequate wound healing (small, depressed scars); depigmented areas; unusual wrinkles; leather-like and thick on nape and upper back; abnormal dermatoglyphics have been described.

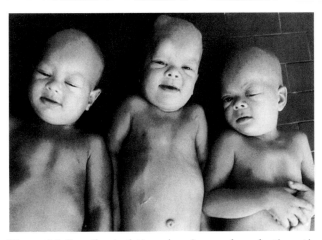

Figure 8.5 *Growth retardation–alopecia–pseudoanodontia–optic atrophy (GAPO). Three brothers: note pectus excavatum in the three, umbilical hernia in the second (present but not seen in the other two) and sequelae of neurosurgery performed to alleviate intracranial hypertension in the second (courtesy of Dr E. O. da-Silva)*

Hearing: sensorineural hypoacusia.

Eyes: progressive optic atrophy; glaucoma; keratoconus; nystagmus; photophobia.

Face: small and characteristic with disproportionate craniofacial relationship, micrognathia, frontal bossing, high forehead, hypertelorism, prominent globes (shallow orbits), protruding and thickened lips, depressed nasal bridge, minor malformations in the auricles, and wide anterior fontanelle.

Psychomotor and growth development: severe growth retardation (proportionate dwarfism); occasionally mental retardation; retarded bone age in infancy; delayed bone maturation through childhood and adolescence.

Limbs: symmetrical proximal shortening of humeri; hyperextensible fingers; second and third toes smaller than the fourth; brachychiry; wide gap between hallux and second toe.

Other findings: dilated scalp veins; increased aminoaciduria; hepatosplenomegaly; bilateral choanal atresia; hyperplasia of sublingual connective tissue; hypoplasia of mammary glands; pectus excavatum; umbilical hernia; high arched palate. The patients seem to have a shortened life expectancy.

Genetics

The mode of inheritance is autosomal recessive.

Comments

Andersen and Pindborg[1] described an isolated case in a non-inbred girl; Epps et al[2] described a boy and a girl in an inbred sibship of nine; Fuks et al[3] reported a girl in an inbred sibship of four; Wajntal et al[4] redescribed the patients of Epps et al[2]; Shapira et al[5] redescribed the patient of Fuks et al[3], but the coefficient of inbreeding of the sibship given by Fuks et al[3] seems to be the correct one (3/16 instead of 1/8). Gorlin[6] described a girl in a non-inbred sibship of three; Da-Silva[7] described a girl in an apparently non-inbred sibship of six (an affected sister died before ascertainment of the family); Gagliardi et al[8] described three boys, the only children of a normal consanguineous couple; Tipton and Gorlin[9] redescribed the patient of Gorlin[6] and reviewed the literature; Manouvrier-Hanu et al[10] described a girl born from first-cousin parents and belonging to a sibship of three.

This progeria-like condition was diagnosed as Rothmund–Thomson syndrome in the report by Epps et al[2], but this was duly corrected by Wajntal et al[4].

References

1 Andersen TH, Pindborg JJ. A case of total 'pseudo-anodontia' in combination with cranial deformity, dwarfism, and ectodermal dysplasia (in Danish). *Odont Tidskr* 1947; **55**: 484–93.

2 Epps DE, Mendonça BB, Olazabal LC, Billerbeck AEC, Wajntal A. Poiquiloderma congênito familiar (S. de Rothmund–Thomson). *Ciência Cult* 1977; **29** (suppl.): 740.

3 Fuks A, Rosenmann A, Chosack A. Pseudoanodontia, cranial deformity, blindness, alopecia, and dwarfism: a new syndrome. *J Dent Child* 1978; **45**: 155–8.

4 Wajntal A, Epps DR, Mendonça BB, Billerbeck AEC. Nova síndrome de displasia ectodérmica: nanismo, alopecia, anodontia e cutis laxa. *Ciência Cult* 1982; **34** (suppl.): 705.

5 Shapira Y, Yatziv S, Deckelbaum R. Growth retardation, alopecia, pseudoanodontia and optic atrophy. *Syndrome Ident* 1982; **8** (1): 14–16.

6 Gorlin RJ. Thoughts on some new and old bone dysplasias. In: Papadatos CJ, Bartsocas CS, eds. *Skeletal Dysplasias*. Alan R. Liss, New York, 1982.

7 Da-Silva EO. Dwarfism, alopecia, pseudoanodontia and other anomalies: report of a case. *Rev Brasil Genét* 1984; **7**: 743–7.

8 Gagliardi ART, Gonzalez CH, Pratesi R. GAPO syndrome: report of three affected brothers. *Am J Med Genet* 1984; **19**: 217–23.

9 Tipton RE, Gorlin RJ. Growth retardation, alopecia, pseudo-anodontia and optic atrophy–the GAPO syndrome. Report of a patient and review of the literature. *Am J Med Genet* 1984; **19**: 209–16.

10 Manouvrier-Hanu S, Largilliere C, Benaliona M, Farriaux J-P, Fontaine G. The GAPO syndrome. *Am J Med Genet* 1987; **26**: 683–8.

Johanson–Blizzard syndrome

Synonyms: *Nasal alar hypoplasia, hypothyroidism, pancreatic achylia, congenital deafness; syndrome of congenital aplasia of the alae nasi, deafness, hypothyroidism, dwarfism, absent permanent teeth and malabsorption*

Clinical features

Hair: sparse, dry and fine or coarse; marked frontal upsweep.

Teeth: hypodontia of both dentitions; peg-shaped teeth; small; widely spaced teeth.

Nails: normal.

Sweat: normal.

Skin: pale and smooth; *café au lait* spots on the lower limbs and abdomen; patches of vitiligo on the lower back and abdomen; midline scalp defects (aplasia cutis congenita); tiny nipples with almost no areolae; transverse palmar creases.

Hearing: congenital sensorineural deafness.

Eyes: aplasia of the inferior puncta; strabismus.

Face: aplastic alae nasi give the nose a beak-like appearance.

Psychomotor and growth development: generally severely retarded (normal intelligence has also been observed); delayed bone age; hypotonia; abnormal electroencephalogram; occasionally akinetic seizures; hyperextensibility.

Limbs: normal.

Other findings: microcephaly; hypothyroidism; exocrine pancreatic insufficiency; malabsorption; imperforate anus; genitourinary defects (rectovaginal fistula; double or septate vagina; single urogenital orifice; clitoromegaly; immature ovaries; micropenis); failure to thrive/oedema; epiphyseal dysgenesis; nasolacrimocutaneous fistulae; highly arched palate.

Genetics

The mode of inheritance is autosomal recessive.

Comments

Johanson and Blizzard described this condition in three unrelated women from normal, non-consanguineous parents[1]. Day and Israel[2] reviewed the literature and added two new cases. Consanguinity was found in about half the cases.

The syndrome is also discussed in references 3–6.

References

1 Johanson A, Blizzard R. A syndrome of congenital aplasia of the alae nasi, deafness, hypothyroidism, dwarfism, absent permanent teeth, and malabsorption. *J Pediatr* 1971; **79**: 982–7.

2 Day DW, Israel JN. Johanson-Blizzard syndrome. *Birth Def Orig Art Ser* 1978; **14** (6B): 275–87.

3 Mardini MK, Ghandour M, Sakati NA, Nyhan WL. Johanson–Blizzard syndrome in a large inbred kindred with three involved members. *Clin Genet* 1978; **14**: 247–50.

4 Daentl DL, Frias JL, Gilbert EF, Opitz JM. The Johanson–Blizzard syndrome: case report and autopsy findings. *Am J Med Genet* 1979; **3**: 129–35.

5 Baraitser M, Hodgson SV. The Johanson–Blizzard syndrome. *J Med Genet* 1982; **19**: 302–10.

6 Moeschler JB, Lubinsky MS. Johanson–Blizzard syndrome with normal intelligence. *Am J Med Genet* 1985; **22**: 69–73.

Ectodermal dysplasia centres

In the early 1990s two centres for the study of ectodermal dysplasia were created. One is in the USA, and provides assistance and information to families with affected members: it is The National Foundation for Ectodermal Dysplasias, 219 East Main, PO Box 114, Mascoutah, Illinois 62258, telephone (618) 566–2020. The other centre is in Brazil: The Center for the Study of Ectodermal Dysplasias, Federal University of Paraná, Caixa Postal 19071, 81531 Curitiba, Paraná, telephone (041) 366–3144, ext. 255 The aims of the Brazilian centre are research, genetic counselling, assistance to researchers and the diffusion of knowledge through books, reviews, letters, etc. Workers at the centre have already described 18 new conditions, published two books and seven other reviews on this nosologic group, and responded to consultations from about 30 countries. It is, therefore, an international reference centre.

The ectodermal dysplasias are summarized in Tables 8.3 and 8.4.

Acknowledgements

The authors, who are research fellows of the National Council for Scientific and Technologic Development (Brasília, Brazil), wish to thank that institution for financial help for their research, and Miss Irene Sedoski for secretarial assistance.

Table 8.3 *List of conditions with indication of cause. The number of the condition in the McKusick catalogues, if listed, is given in parentheses*

| Conditions | AD | AR | XL | Unknown | | | |
				?	AD?	AR?	XL?
Subgroup 1–2–3–4							
1. Christ–Siemens–Touraine (CST) syndrome (305100)			XR				
2. AR hypohidrotic ectodermal dysplasia (224900)		×					
3. Focal dermal hypoplasia (FDH) (305600)			XD^l				
4. Xeroderma–talipes–enamel defect					×		
5. Rosselli–Gulienetti syndrome (225000)		×					
6. Dyskeratosis congenita, Scoggins type (127550)	×						
7. Dyskeratosis congenita, AR type (224230)		×					
8. Dyskeratosis congenita, Zinsser–Cole–Engman type (305000)			×				
9. Pachyonychia congenita, Jadassohn–Lewandowsky type (167200)	×						
10. Pachyonychia congenita, Jackson–Lawler type (167210)	×						
11. Rapp–Hodgkin syndrome (129400)					×		
12. Ectrodactyly–ED–cleft lip/palate (EEC) syndrome, Rüdiger–Haase–Passarge type (129900)	×						
13. Ectrodactyly–ED–cleft lip/palate (EEC) syndrome, AR type [1–3]		×					
14. Ankyloblepharon–ectodermal defects–cleft lip and palate (AEC) syndrome (106260)	×						
15. Zanier–Roubicek syndrome	×						
16. Tricho-onychodental (TOD) dysplasia	×						
17. Jorgenson syndrome					×		XD
18. Carey syndrome				×			
19. Camarena syndrome					×		XD
20. Keratitis–ichthyosis–deafness (KID) (242150)		×					
21. Anonychia with flexural pigmentation (106750)	×						
22. Hypohidrotic ED with papillomas and acanthosis nigricans						×	
23. Odonto-onychohypohidrotic dysplasia with midline scalp defect (129550)	×						
24. Odonto-onychodermal dysplasia (257980)		×					
25. Tricho-odonto-onycho-hypohidrotic dysplasia with cataract						×	
26. Papillon–Lefèvre syndrome (245000)		×					
27. Hypomelanosis of Ito (146150)	×						
28. Ulnar–mammary syndrome of Pallister (181450)	×						
Total	11	7	3	1	3	3	2
Subgroup 1–2–3							
1. Rothmund–Thomson syndrome (268400)		×					
2. Fischer–Jacobsen–Clouston syndrome (129500)	×						
3. Coffin–Siris syndrome (135900)					×	×	XD
4. Odontotrichomelic syndrome (273400)						×	
5. Trichodento-osseous (TDO) syndrome, Lichtenstein type (190320)	×						
6. Trichodento-osseous (TDO) syndrome, Leisti–Sjöblom type (190320)	×						

Table 8.3 *Continued*

Conditions	AD	AR	XL	Unknown			
				?	AD?	AR?	XL?
Subgroup 1–2–3 (continued)							
7. Trichodento-osseous (TDO) syndrome, Shapiro type (190320)	×						
8. Incontinentia pigmenti (308300)			XD[1]				
9. Cranioectodermal syndrome (218330)						×	
10. Fried's tooth and nail syndrome		×					
11. Hypodontia and nail dysgenesis (189500)	×						
12. Dento-oculocutaneous syndrome (200970)						×	
13. Trichorhinophalangeal (TRP) syndrome, Giedion type (275500)						×	
14. Trichorhinophalangeal (TRP) syndrome, Murdoch–Gorlin type (190350)	×						
15. Ellis–van Creveld syndrome (225500)		×					
16. Cystic eyelids–palmoplantar keratosis–hypodontia–hypotrichosis		×					
17. Šalamon syndrome		×					
18. Tricho-oculodermovertebral syndrome		×					
19. Oculodentodigital (ODD) syndrome, O'Rourk–Bravos type (164200)				×			
20. Arthrogryposis and ectodermal dysplasia				×			
21. Tricho-odonto-onychodermal syndrome				×			
22. Tricho-odonto-onychial dysplasia (275450)						×	
23. Odonto-onychodysplasia with alopecia		×					
24. Schinzel–Giedion syndrome (269150)		×					
25. Growth retardation–alopecia–pseudoanodontia–optic atrophy (GAPO) (230740)		×					
26. Ectodermal dysplasia with pillous anomaly and syndactyly		×					
27. Côté–Katsantoni syndrome		×					
28. Dermo-odontodysplasia (125640)	×						
29. Tricho-odonto-onychodysplasia with pili torti					×		XD
30. Mesomelic dwarfism–skeletal abnormalities–ectodermal dysplasia				×			
31. Ectodermal dysplasia syndrome with tetramelic deficiencies (Schinzel–Klingenberg syndrome)				×			
32. Pilodentoungular dysplasia with microcephaly		×					
33. Trichodermodysplasia with dental alterations					×		XD
34. Oculotrichodysplasia (OTD) (257960)		×					
35. Brittle hair–intellectual impairment–decreased fertility–short stature (BIDS syndrome) (234050)		×					
36. Dolichocephaly–dental defects–trichodysplasia	×						
37. Cortes–Lacassie syndrome				×			
38. Winter–MacDermot–Hill syndrome [4]						×	XD
Total	8	14	1	6	4	6	4
Subgroup 1–2–4							
1. Regional ectodermal dysplasia with total bilateral cleft				×			
2. Leucomelanoderma–infantilism–mental retardation–hypodontia–hypotrichosis (246500)		×					

Table 8.3 *Continued*

Conditions	AD	AR	XL	Unknown			
				?	AD?	AR?	XL?
Subgroup 1–2–4 (continued)							
3. Premolar aplasia–hyperhidrosis–canities prematura (PHC) syndrome (112300)	×						
4. Congenital insensitivity to pain with anhidrosis of Swanson (256800)		×					
5. Lenz–Passarge dysplasia			XD				
6. Ectodermal dysplasia with palatal paralysis				×			
7. Alopecia–anosmia–deafness–hypogonadism (147770)	×						
Total	2	2	1	2	0	0	0
Subgroup 1–3–4							
1. Fischer syndrome	×						
2. Trichodysplasia–onychogryposis–hypohidrosis–cataract				×			
3. Alopecia–onychodysplasia–hypohidrosis–deafness				×			
4. Hayden's syndrome				×			
5. Alopecia–onychodysplasia–hypohidrosis				×			
6. Alopecia, nail dystrophy, ophthalmic complications, thyroid dysfunction, hypohidrosis, ephelides and enteropathy, and respiratory tract infections (ANOTHER) (225050)						×	
7. Ectodermal dysplasia with severe mental retardation				×			
8. Alopecia universalis–onychodystrophy–total vitiligo						×	
9. Dermotrichic syndrome			XR				
10. Linear skin atrophy–scarring alopecia–anonychia–tongue lesion				×			
11. Viljoen–Winship syndrome [5]				×			
Total	1	0	1	7	0	2	0
Subgroup 2–3–4							
1. Amelo-onychohypohidrotic dysplasia (104570)	×						
Total	1	0	0	0	0	0	0
Subgroup 1–2							
1. Orofaciodigital (OFD) syndrome, Papillon-Léage–Psaume type (311200)			XD[1]				
2. Oculodentodigital (ODD) syndrome, AD type (164200)	×						
3. Oculodentodigital (ODD) syndrome, AR type		×					
4. Hallermann–Streiff syndrome, AR type (234100)		×					
5. Hallerman–Streiff syndrome, Koliopoulos–Palimeris type (234100)					×		
6. Gorlin–Chaudhry–Moss syndrome (233500)						×	
7. Mikaelian's syndrome (224800)		×					
8. Gingival fibromatosis–sparse hair–malposition of teeth		×					

Table 8.3 *Continued*

Conditions	AD	AR	XL	Unknown			
				?	AD?	AR?	XL?
Subgroup 1–2 (continued)							
9. Hypertrichosis–dental defects	×						
10. Gingival fibromatosis–hypertrichosis (135400)	×						
11. Gingival fibromatosis–hypertrichosis, recessive type?						×	
12. Pili torti–enamel hypoplasia (261900)		×					
13. Walbaum–Dehaene–Schlemmer syndrome		×					
14. Brachymetapody–anodontia–hypotrichosis–albinoidism (211370)						×	
15. Agammaglobulinaemia–thymic dysplasia–ectodermal dysplasia				×			
16. Johanson–Blizzard syndrome (243800)		×					
17. Trichodental dysplasia	×						
18. Acrorenal field defect–ectodermal dysplasia–lipoatrophic diabetes (AREDYLD) (207780)		×					
19. Ectrodactyly–ectodermal dysplasia with normal lip and palate (129810)	×						
20. Ectodermal dysplasia–ectrodactyly–macular dystrophy (EEM) (225280)		×					
21. Hypotrichosis and dental defects				×			
22. Cleft lip/palate–oligodontia–syndactyly–hair alterations					×		XD
23. Migratory ichthyosiform rash–retinal coloboma–mental retardation–seizures (280000)				×			
24. Pilodental dysplasia with refractive errors (262020)						×	
25. Uncombable hair–retinal pigmentary dystrophy–juvenile cataract–brachymetacarpia	×						
26. Familial clefting syndrome with ectropion and dental anomaly (119580)	×						
27. Ichthyosiform erythroderma with hair abnormality, mental retardation and growth retardation (IBIDS syndrome) (242170)						×	
28. Dubowitz's syndrome (223370)		×					
29. Spinocerebellar ataxia–monilethrix–typical facial features–dental anomalies				×			
30. Growth retardation, ocular abnormalities, microcephaly, brachydactyly, oligophrenia (GOMBO) syndrome [6]						×	
Total	7	10	1	4	2	6	1
Subgroup 1–3							
1. Hairy elbows dysplasia (139600)	×						
2. Palmoplantar hyperkeratosis and alopecia (104100)	×						
3. Curly hair–ankyloblepharon–nail dysplasia syndrome CHANDS (214350)		×					
4. Onychotrichodysplasia with neutropenia (258360)		×					
5. Pili torti and onychodysplasia	×						
6. Agammaglobulinaemia–dwarfism–ectodermal dysplasia						×	

Table 8.3 *Continued*

| Conditions | AD | AR | XL | Unknown | | | |
				?	AD?	AR?	XL?
Subgroup 1–3 (continued)							
7. Tricho-onychodysplasia with xeroderma		×					
8. Skeletal anomalies–ectodermal dysplasia–growth and mental retardation				×			
9. Sabinas' brittle hair and mental deficiency syndrome (211390)		×					
10. Syndrome of accelerated skeletal maturation, failure to thrive and peculiar face						×	
11. Congenital lymphoedema–hypoparathyroidism–nephropathy–prolapsing mitral valve–brachytelephalangy (247410)						×	XR
12. Bartsocas–Papas syndrome (263650)		×					
13. Digitorenocerebral syndrome (222760)		×					
14. Onychodystrophy and aplasia/hypoplasia of distal phalanges	×						
Total	4	6	0	1	0	3	1
Subgroup 1–4							
1. Focal facial dermal dysplasia (136500)	×						
2. Facial ectodermal dysplasia (Setleis syndrome) (227260)						×	
3. Trichofaciohypohidrotic syndrome							XR
4. Dry skin and extranumerary areolae	×						
5. Short stature–kidney insufficiency–ophthalmologic anomaly–growth retardation–ectodermal dysplasia (SKORED)							XR
6. Mental retardation–atrichia–digital anomalies–dwarfism–septal defects (RADS)				×			
Total	2	0	0	1	0	1	2
Subgroup 2–3							
1. Deafness–onycho-osteodystrophy–mental retardation (DOOR) (220500)		×					
2. Deafness and onychodystrophy (124480)	×						
3. Ectodermal defect with skeletal abnormalities				×			
4. Weyers' acrofacial dysostosis (193530)	×						
5. Odonto-onychodysplasia	×						
6. Kirghizian's dermato-osteolysis (221810)						×	
7. Corneodermato-osseous syndrome (122440)	×						
Total	4	1	0	1	0	1	0
Subgroup 2–4							
1. Naegeli–Franceschetti–Jadassohn dysplasia (161000)	×						
2. Amelocerebrohypohidrotic syndrome (226750)						×	XR
Total	1	0	0	0	0	1	1

Table 8.3 *Continued*

Conditions	AD	AR	XL	Unknown			
				?	AD?	AR?	XL?
Subgroup 3–4							
1. Absence of dermal ridge patterns, onychodystrophy and palmoplantar anhidrosis	×						
2. Pachyonychia congenita, AR type [7, 8]		×					
Total	1	1	0	0	0	0	0

AD, autosomal dominant; AR, autosomal recessive; ED, ectodermal dysplasia; XD, X-linked dominant; XD^l, XD with lethality in males; XL, X-linked; XR, X-linked recessive.

References

1 Romagnoli G, Zunin C. L'associazione displasia ectodermica, ectrodattilia e labio-palatoschisi. La sindrome EEC. *Pathologica* 1974; **66**: 95–103.
2 Gemme G, Bonioli E, Ruffa G, Grosso P. La sindrome EEC. Descrizione di due casi in una stessa famiglia. *Min Pediatr* 1976; **28**: 36–43.
3 Schmidt M, Salzano FM. Síndrome EEC com possível herança autossômica recessiva em gêmeos. *Ciência Cult* 1988; **40** (suppl.): 853.
4 Winter RM, MacDermot KD, Hill FJ. Sparse hair, short stature, hypoplastic thumbs, single upper central incisor and abnormal skin pigmentation: a possible (new) form of ectodermal dysplasia. *Am J Med Genet* 1988; **29**: 209–16.
5 Viljoen DL, Winship WS. A new form of hypohidrotic ectodermal dysplasia. *Am J Med Genet* 1988; **31**: 25–32.
6 Verloes A, Delfortrie J, Lambotte C. GOMBO syndrome of growth retardation, ocular abnormalities, microcephaly, brachydactyly, and oligophrenia: a possible (new) recessively inherited MCA/MR syndrome. *Am J Med Genet* 1989; **32**: 15–18.
7 Chong-Hai T, Rajagopalan K. Pachyonychia congenita with recessive inheritance. *Arch Dermatol* 1977; **113**: 685–6.
8 Haber RM, Rose TH. Autosomal recessive pachyonychia congenita. *Arch Dermatol* 1986; **122**: 919–23.

Table 8.4 *Number of ectodermal dysplasias in the different subgroups of group A and their cause*

Subgroups	No. of conditions	AD	AR	XL	Unknown			
					?	AD?	AR?	XL?
1–2–3–4	28	11	7	3	1	3	3	2
1–2–3	38	8	14	1	6	4	6	4
1–2–4	7	2	2	1	2	0	0	0
1–3–4	11	1	0	1	7	0	2	0
2–3–4	1	1	0	0	0	0	0	0
1–2	30	7	10	1	4	2	6	1
1–3	14	4	6	0	1	0	3	1
1–4	6	2	0	0	1	0	1	2
2–3	7	4	1	0	1	0	1	0
2–4	2	1	0	0	0	0	1	1
3–4	2	1	1	0	0	0	0	0
Total	146	42	41	7	23	9	23	11

Note: In the section labelled 'unknown' the suggested genetic inheritance is sometimes repeated in more than one column, hence the apparent discrepancy in totalling the figures.

Chapter 9

Neurocutaneous syndromes

R. Ruiz-Maldonado and L. Tamayo

Introduction

The common ectodermal origin of the epidermis and the nervous system explains the frequent association of abnormalities in the two organ systems. The classification of the neurocutaneous syndromes is complex. The authors prefer a clinical classification as detailed in Table 9.1. Each category is then further subdivided into those associated with (a) central nervous system alterations and (b) peripheral nervous system alterations.

In this chapter the three main neurocutaneous syndromes – neurofibromatosis, tuberous sclerosis and incontinentia pigmenti – are described in detail. Other neurocutaneous syndromes are documented in Tables 9.4–9.12 at the end of this chapter.

Table 9.1 *Classification of neurocutaneous syndromes*

I	With pigmentary changes
II	With vascular malformations
III	With altered keratinization
IV	With metabolic disorders
V	With hair abnormalities
VI	With connective changes
VII	With hamartomas
VIII	Neurocutaneous dysmorphic syndromes
IX	Peripheral neuropathies with skin alterations

Neurofibromatosis

Definition

Neurofibromatosis is a genetically determined, complex, multisystem disorder, with predominant nervous and cutaneous tissue alterations. Two distinct forms are recognized: neurofibromatosis type I or von Recklinghausen's disease, with a prevalence in the USA of 1 in 2500–3300 individuals, and neurofibromatosis type II (bilateral acoustic neurofibromatosis), which is considerably less frequent. Other possible variants of neurofibromatosis exist[1].

Clinical features

Neurofibromatosis type I may be diagnosed when two or more of the following features are present: six or more *café au lait* spots with a diameter greater than 5 mm (Figure 9.1); freckling in the axillae (Figure 9.2); two or more neurofibromas of any type (Figure 9.3) or one plexiform neurofibroma (Figures 9.4 and 9.5); optic glioma; two or more iris hamartomas (Lisch nodules); a distinctive osseous lesion (sphenoid dysplasia, thinning of long-bone cortex) or a first-degree relative with neurofibromatosis according to the previous criteria. The main features of neurofibromatosis I appear in Table 9.2.

Neurofibromatosis type II may be diagnosed when one of the following features is present: the presence of bilateral eighth cranial nerve tumours visualized by computerized tomography or magnetic resonance

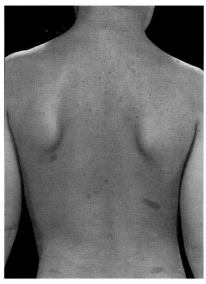

Figure 9.1 *Multiple* café au lait *spots: a characteristic feature of neurofibromatosis (courtesy of Dr J. Harper)*

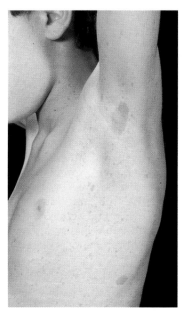

Figure 9.2 *Freckling of the axillary area in a child with neurofibromatosis type I (courtesy of Dr J. Harper)*

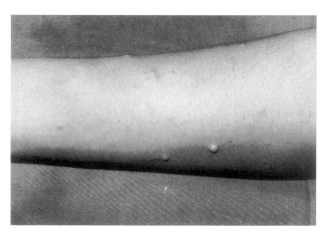

Figure 9.3 *Multiple cutaneous neurofibromas on the arm*

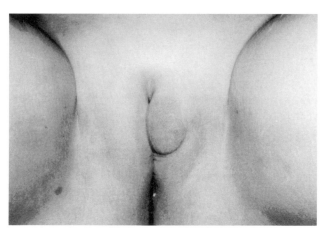

Figure 9.4 *Plexiform neurofibroma in the genital area*

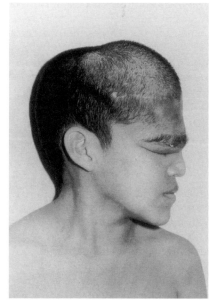

Figure 9.5 *Large plexiform neurofibroma on the scalp causing considerable disfigurement*

imaging; a first-degree relative with neurofibromatosis and either a unilateral eighth nerve tumour or any of the following: neurofibroma, meningioma, glioma, schwannoma or juvenile posterior subcapsular lenticular opacity[2].

Pathology

Cutaneous *café au lait* spots may have giant pigment particles known as macromelanosomes. These are inconstant and non-specific. In neurofibromatosis, cutaneous nodular or plexiform neurofibromas are

Table 9.2 *Clinical features of neurofibromatosis I*

Cutaneous	Central nervous system	Skeletal	Other features
Café au lait spots	Intellectual impairment	Short stature	Phaeochromocytoma
Giant melanotic macule	Epilepsy	Marcrocephaly	Endocrine dysfunction
Palmar melanotic macule	CNS tumours (optic	Kyphoscoliosis	Digestive,
Neurofibromas – pendulous	glioma, astrocytoma,	Pseudoarthritis	nasopharyngeal,
or plexiform	meningioma,	Segmental hypertrophy	respiratory and
Juvenile xanthogranuloma	neurofibroma,	Cystic and erosive lesions	urinary tract
Pruritus	acoustic neuroma,	Bowing of the tibia	alterations
	neurolemmoma,	Twisted ribs	Renal artery stenosis
	schwannoma)		Cardiac abnormalities
	Lisch nodules		

often observed; malignant transformation may occur. In both neurofibromatosis I and II, central nervous system tumours are schwannomas, gliomas and meningiomas.

Genetics

Neurofibromatosis I (NF-I) accounts for 85% of all neurofibromatosis. Its genetic locus has been identified in the proximal long arm of chromosome 17[3,4]. It is inherited as an autosomal dominant trait with variable penetrance and expression, and a spontaneous mutation rate of around 50%. The fact that some cases of NF-I may have minimal clinical expression makes mandatory a meticulous cutaneous, ophthalmological, audiological and skeletal examination, as well as computerized tomography (CT) or magnetic resonance imaging (MRI) of the brain. Examination and investigation of the parents and siblings are essential before making the diagnosis of a new mutation. Long-term follow-up should always be maintained since a number of alterations, in particular of a tumoral nature, may manifest later in life. The risk of having a second affected child for the healthy parents of a new mutation is nearly that for the general population (1 in 10 000)[5]. The risk of an affected individual passing the disease on to the offspring of either sex is 50%. Penetrance of an NF-I mutation is nearly 100%, therefore an offspring of NF-I mutation will probably either manifest the NF-I mutation or not bear the mutation. On the other hand, parents at risk of NF-I may manifest the typical disease, a partial expression of the mutant gene, or no expression of the mutant gene. In the latter situation there may be non-penetrance, which is unlikely, or absence of the mutant gene[5]. No known factors contribute to generate or aggravate the signs and symptoms of NF, although hormonal or growth factors may contribute to tumour formation. Prenatal diagnosis is possible but not an option for the 50% of cases who represent new mutations.

Neurofibromatosis II (NF-II) has the same mode of inheritance, high spontaneous mutation rate, high penetrance and variable expression as NF-I. The gene for NF-II is located near the centre of the long arm of chromosome 22[6]. Unlike NF-I, NF-II is often undetected until adolescence or later. In a recent report of a large family, nearly half the patients remained asymptomatic during their first 30 years of life[6]. The above facts stress the importance of a reserved prognosis and genetic counselling in persons at risk of NF-II.

Differential diagnosis

Confusion in the diagnosis of NF-I may occur in cases with minimal or atypical lesions. Albright's syndrome or polyostotic fibrous dysplasia presents with large *café au lait* spots with ragged contour, and precocious puberty. Noonan's syndrome may share with neurofibromatosis skeletal abnormalities, short stature, mild mental retardation and seizures. Patients with this syndrome have a characteristic facies. The association of Noonan's syndrome and neurofibromatosis has been reported[7]. In children the most frequent diagnostic problem is the evaluation of *café au lait* spots in an otherwise normal child with no family history of NF. More than six *café au lait* spots or a single large macule are not necessarily diagnostic of neurofibromatosis, particularly in non-caucasian individuals. Cutaneous neurofibromas in the absence of other features are similarly not necessarily diagnostic of neurofibromatosis.

Treatment

Periodic clinical examination is mandatory in patients with proved or suspected NF. Large neurofibromas may be excised for medical or cosmetic reasons. Other tumours, benign and malignant, will be treated according to location, symptoms and biological behaviour. Denervation was reported to result in fewer and smaller neurofibromas[8]. Osseous lesions may require rehabilitation and/or surgery. Symptomatic treatment is recommended for seizures, pruritus, pain, hypertension and headache. Ketotifen in the authors' experience has no effect in neurofibromatosis. In NF-II early diagnosis of acoustic neuroma provides the best therapeutic results. Treatment decisions should be based on the patient's age, neurological condition, level of hearing, tumour size and growth, and social, psychological, and occupational factors[2]. The course of the disease varies considerably in individual patients. The prognosis depends upon the extent of involvement[9]. Computed tomographic scans and magnetic resonance imaging with gadolinium enhancement are useful tools in the evaluation of patients with NF[10]. Support groups for NF patients and their families exist in several countries.

References

1 Crowe FW, Schull WJ, Neel JV. *A Clinical, Pathological and Genetic Study of Multiple Neurofibromatosis.* C Thomas, Springfield, 1956.
2 Martuza RL, Eldridge R. Neurofibromatosis 2 (bilateral acoustic neurofibromatosis). *New Engl J Med* 1988; **318**: 684–8.
3 Barker D, Wright T, Neuyen K et al. Gene for von Recklinghausen neurofibromatosis in the pericentromeric region of chromosome 17. *Science* 1987; **236**: 1100–2.
4 Seizinger BR, Rouleau GA, Ozelius LJ et al. Genetic linkage of von Recklinghausen neurofibromatosis to the nerve growth factor receptor gene. *Cell* 1987; **49**: 589–94.
5 Riccardi VM, Lewis RA. Penetrance of von Recklinghausen neurofibromatosis: a distinction between predecessors and descendants. *Am J Hum Genet* 1988; **42**: 284–9.
6 Werteleck W, Rouleau GA, Superneau DW et al. Neurofibromatosis 2: clinical and DNA linkage studies of a large kindred. *New Engl J Med* 1988; **319**: 278–83.
7 Mendez HMM. The neurofibromatosis–Noonan syndrome. *Am J Med Genet* 1985; **21**: 471–6.
8 Riccardi VM, Powell PP. Denervation in von Recklinghausen's neurofibromatosis (NF-1) leads to fewer and smaller neurofibromas. *Neurology* 1988; **38**: 1810.
9 Soerensen SA, Mulvihill JJ, Nielsen A. Long-term follow up of von Recklinghausen neurofibromatosis. Survival and malignant neoplasms. *New Engl J Med* 1986; **314**: 1010–15.
10 Truhan AP, Filipek PA. Magnetic resonance imaging. Its role in the neurodiagnostic evaluation of neurofibromatosis, tuberous sclerosis, and Sturge–Weber syndrome. *Arch Dermatol* 1993; **129**: 219–26.

Tuberous sclerosis

Synonym: *Bourneville–Pringle disease, epiloa*

Definition

Tuberous sclerosis (TS) is a genetically determined disease characterized by connective tissue hamartomatous proliferations, white cutaneous macules, embryogenic tumours, seizures and mental retardation. All proliferative lesions may originate from immature Schwann cells[1].

The point prevalence of TS in the USA has been estimated to be 1 in 9407 with an incidence of 0.56 cases for 100 000 person years in Rochester, Minnesota, between 1950 and 1980[2].

Clinical features

The classical clinical triad in TS is angiofibroma (misnamed adenoma sebaceum) (30–80%), mental retardation (50–60%) and seizures (80–85%). Gomez proposed criteria for the diagnosis of TS[3]. In the authors' opinion none of the criteria listed by Gomez, if present as an isolated feature, is sufficient to make

Table 9.3 *Tuberous sclerosis. The definitive diagnosis of TS requires the presence of at least one major and one minor diagnostic feature; the probable diagnosis of TS requires one major diagnostic feature*

Major diagnostic features	Minor diagnostic features
Hypomelanotic macules	Infantile spasm
Facial angiofibromas	Mental retardation
Periungual fibromas	Seizures
Fibrous (shagreen) patches	Gingival fibromas
Retinal hamartoma	Dental enamel pits
Cortical tuber	Multicystic kidneys
Renal cysts or angiomyolipomas	Cardiac rhabdomyoma
Subependymal glial nodule	Intracranial calcification
First-degree relative with tuberous sclerosis	Radiological lung changes
	Patch of depigmented hair

the definitive diagnosis of TS, with the possible exception of facial angiofibromas. The combination of a major and a minor feature for a definitive diagnosis of TS and the presence of one major feature for the suspected diagnosis of TS is suggested (Table 9.3).

The most characteristic and evident lesions of TS are cutaneous. The earliest and most constant cutaneous manifestations are the 'ash-leaf' achromic macules (Figure 9.6), which are found in up to 90% of patients and may be isolated or multiple. Achromic macules are not always ash-leaf shaped, and sometimes number hundreds, with a 'raindrop' appearance. Rarely achromic macules may appear months or years after birth[4]. In patients with fair skin a Wood's light examination may help to identify hypochromic macules. A patch of depigmented hair (poliosis) is present in around 20% of cases of TS and is usually present at birth.

Facial angiofibromas, present in up to 80% of patients, first appear in infancy or childhood as tiny skin-coloured or erythematous pinhead nodules with a butterfly distribution. With time they increase in number, size and colour, becoming an aesthetic nuisance (Figure 9.7).

Periungual fibromas are also characteristic of TS. They first appear in adolescence or adulthood in 15–20% of patients as fleshy, hard nodules, more frequently on the proximal aspect of the toenails (see Chapter 16, Figure 16.5).

The fibrous or shagreen patch is present in 20–25% of patients as a firm, slightly raised skin plaque measuring 1 cm or more. Most often it is present on the back.

Skin tags are found on the neck and in the axillae, from adolescence onwards.

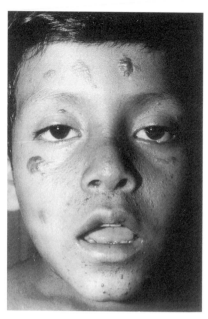

Figure 9.7 *Numerous angiofibromas with centrofacial distribution and small shagreen patches on forehead and cheeks*

Gingival hyperplasia, often aggravated by phenytoin, is another characteristic feature of TS.

Retinal hamartomas or phacomas are present in around 50% of patients.

Neurological alterations are frequent and severe. Mental retardation is found in up to 60% of patients, and seizures in up to 85%[3].

Intracranial calcification (subependymal), cranial vault sclerosis, cortical tubers, dilatation of the lateral ventricles and diffuse demyelination of the brain are frequent alterations, identified by CT or preferably MRI.

Hamartomatous tumours are frequent in TS. These include cardiac rhabdomyomas, detected by echocardiography, which occur in over 50% of infants. These tumours may result in early death; however, recent evidence suggests that in the majority these tumours regress in early infancy. Renal involvement includes angiomyolipomas or cysts. Rarely, haemangiomas of the liver and spleen and thyroid adenomas may occur.

Cystic lung disease or pulmonary lymphangiomyomatosis affects around 1% of patients.

Pathology

Hypochromic macules have a normal number of melanocytes of reduced size and content of melanin. Angiofibromas of the face were previously considered to be sebaceous adenomas owing to the large size of sebaceous glands normally present on the face. Shagreen patches correspond to connective tissue naevi. Central nervous system tumours are hamartomas composed of neuronal and glial tissue.

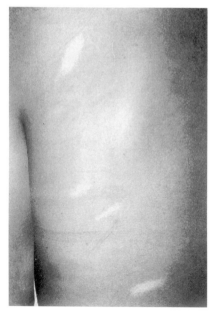

Figure 9.6 *Multiple 'ash-leaf' hypomelanotic macules*

Genetics

Tuberous sclerosis is a genetically determined disease transmitted as an autosomal dominant trait with high penetrance and variable expression. A high mutation rate (50%) is observed. A gene responsible for TS in some patients, 'tuberin', was identified on chromosome 16. Tuberin encodes a 198 kDa protein of unknown function[5]. Several families have been reported with more than one affected child but with no signs of TS in either parent on full examination[3,6]. The risk of an affected parent with TS having a child with the disease is 50%. Before excluding the possibility of TS in either parent, a complete cutaneous, neurological and ophthalmological examination should be performed, complemented by a cranial CT scan and/or gadolinium enhanced MRI. First-degree relatives should also be carefully examined.

Asymptomatic offspring of parents with TS should undergo periodic clinical and CT scanning, since a number of markers for TS from hypochromic macules to hamartomas may develop years after birth.

Prenatal diagnosis of TS has been possible when a fetus at risk has been examined with an ultrasound scan of the brain or a two-dimensional echocardiogram of the heart[7]. A DNA marker link to TS may in the future allow the identification of non-expressing individuals with TS[3]; however, there is some question of genetic heterogeneity in TS with chromosome 9 also being implicated.

Differential diagnosis

Hypochromic macules in otherwise normal infants and children are a frequent finding and correspond to hypochromic naevi. A periungual fibroma alone is not necessarily a marker for TS. The same is true for shagreen patches or connective tissue naevi.

As indicated in Table 9.3, a definitive diagnosis must be based on the presence of at least one major and one minor diagnostic feature.

Treatment

Treatment of TS involves medical, surgical and psychosocial care. Symptoms, in particular seizures, are often difficult to control and require appropriate anticonvulsant therapy. Intracranial tumours may be removed if symptomatic and operable. Renal function should be evaluated twice a year since renal involvement is one of the most frequent causes of death. Cutaneous facial angiofibromas are often of cosmetic concern to the patient and the family. They may be palliatively treated with dermabrasion or laser therapy. Periungual fibromas are easily excised.

Psychosocial management of the patient and family is one of the most relevant aspects of a disease that is not curable and tends to worsen with time. Support groups exist in several countries.

The prognosis of TS depends on the severity of the disease. Involvement of brain, kidneys, heart and lungs is usually indicative of a poor prognosis.

References

1 Mori M, Ikeda T, Onoe T. Blastic Shwann cells in renal tumor of tuberous sclerosis complex. *Acta Pathol Japonica* 1971; **21**: 121–9.
2 Wiederholdt WC, Gomez MR, Kurland LT. Incidence and prevalence of tuberous sclerosis in Rochester, Minnesota, 1950 through 1982. *Neurology* 1985; **35**: 600–3.
3 Gomez MR. Tuberous sclerosis. In: Gomez MR, Adams RD, eds. *Neurocutaneous Diseases. A Practical Approach.* Butterworth, Boston, 1987; 30–52.
4 Oppenheimer EY, Rosman NP, Dooling EC. The late appearance of hypopigmented maculae in tuberous sclerosis. *Am J Dis Child* 1985; **139**: 408–9.
5 European Chromosome 16 Tuberous Sclerosis Consortium. Identification and characterization of the tuberous sclerosis gene on chromosome 16. *Cell* 1993; **75**: 1305–15.
6 Hunt A. Tuberous sclerosis: a survey of 97 cases. III Family aspects. *Dev Med Child Neurol* 1983; **25**: 346–9.
7 Muller G, De Jong C, Falk V et al. Antenatal ultrasonographic findings in tuberous sclerosis. *S Afr Med J* 1986; **69**: 633–8.

Incontinentia pigmenti

Synonym: *Bloch–Sulzberger syndrome*

Definition

Incontinentia pigmenti (IP) is an inherited disorder involving ectodermal and mesodermal tissues. The most striking manifestations are cutaneous and the vast majority of patients are female.

Clinical features

In the newborn infant the cutaneous lesions are initially vesicles and then verrucous lesions which follow linear or whorled lines (lines of Blaschko). At this stage blood eosinophilia is a frequent feature. On the vertex of the scalp there is sometimes a cicatricial area devoid of hair (aplasia cutis). The vesicular and verrucous lesions spontaneously disappear during the first year of life and are replaced by lines of hyperpigmentation in capricious figures like a china vase (Figure 9.8). As the child grows older the cutaneous hyperpigmentation fades, and may disappear by adolescence. A variety of ocular alterations are present in around 30% of patients; severe alterations are found in about 15%. The most typical anomaly is detachment of a dysplastic retina with a retrolental mass (retrolental fibroplasia) which may be confused with a retinoblastoma. Other possible alterations are microphthalmos, uveitis, cataract, optic atrophy, pigmentary retinopathy, abnormal iris pigmentation, chorio-

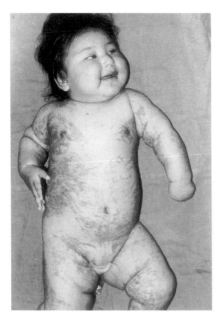

Figure 9.8 *Hyperpigmented verrucous lesions following the lines of Blaschko*

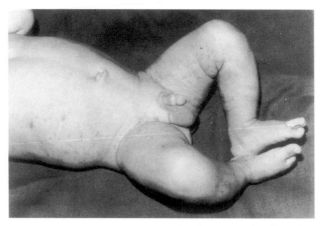

Figure 9.9 *Incontinentia pigmenti in a boy 3 months old with minor cutaneous involvement*

retinitis, vascular changes, papillitis, corneal clouding and other minor anomalies[1].

Neurological complications may be present in 30–50% of patients, the most frequent being psychomotor retardation, seizures, spastic paralysis and microcephaly[1].

Bony abnormalities are present in around 20% of cases. Dental alterations in over 50% of patients are a helpful clue once the cutaneous lesions have faded. There may be conical crown deformity, partial or complete anodontia and delayed dentition. Nails may occasionally be dystrophic[1].

Pathology

The vesicular lesions are intraepidermal and filled with eosinophils. The verrucous lesions show acanthosis, hyperkeratosis with parakeratosis, and dyskeratotic cells. Pigmented lesions show diminished melanocytes and melanin-loaded macrophages in the papillary dermis. Dyskeratotic cells may also be seen.

Genetics

Incontinentia pigmenti is an X-linked dominant condition usually lethal for hemizygous males. The gene for the familial form of IP maps to the telomeric portion of the Xq28 region[1]. In the largest series of cases 90% of patients were female[2]. One surviving male has been reported to have had an affected daughter[3], and two cases of transmission from mother to son have been described[4]. The disease tends to increase in severity from mother to offspring. An explanation for IP in a surviving male (Figure 9.9) would be mosaicism[5]. Partial cutaneous involvement in a strip pattern is explained through the random X chromosome inactivation or Lyon hypothesis.

On the basis of an X-linked dominant type of inheritance, an affected woman with two female and two male children could expect one boy to be hemizygous and die in utero, the other to be healthy; one girl would have IP and the other girl would be unaffected. In other words, a woman with IP has a 1 in 4 risk of the pregnancy terminating in a spontaneous miscarriage, and half of her female offspring will have IP. When a boy is born with IP, chromosomal analysis should be done to exclude XXY or other abnormal karyotype.

Spontaneous mutations do occur in IP in less than a third of cases. If a child with IP is born from apparently healthy parents it is of the utmost importance to perform a detailed physical examination of the mother, other daughters, the maternal grandmother and maternal aunts in order to detect minor markers of IP such as a small area of aplasia cutis, or dental or ocular anomalies. A history of miscarriages in the apparently healthy mother of a child with IP is suggestive of IP in the mother.

Chromosomal instability has been reported in several families with IP. Chromosomal aberrations are similar to those observed in Fanconi's anaemia and ataxia-telangiectasia. Chromosomal instability in IP may increase the risk of cancer; 6 patients with IP and malignant tumours have been reported[6].

Differential diagnosis

A typical case of IP can hardly be confused with other conditions. In the newborn infant the presence of grouped vesicles on an inflammatory background may suggest herpes simplex infection. Verrucous naevi of the epidermolytic hyperkeratosis type may present with vesicles and have a linear distribution.

Pigmented lesions in IP may be confused with melanocytic naevi.

The Naegeli–Franceschetti–Jadassohn syndrome has been confused with IP. Pigmentation in this syndrome first appears during the second or third year of life, is finely reticular and associated with palmoplantar keratoderma and hypohidrosis. Teeth may be abnormal.

Treatment

No treatment is necessary for the cutaneous lesions. Dental rehabilitation may improve the function and aspect of teeth.

References

1 Smahi A, Hyden-Granskog C, Peterlin B et al. The gene for the familial form of incontinentia pigmenti (IP2) maps to the distal part of Xq28. *Hum Molec Genet* 1994; **3**: 273–8.

2 Carney RG. Incontinentia pigmenti: a world statistical analysis. *Arch Dermatol* 1976; **112**: 535–42.

3 Sommer A, Liu PH. Incontinentia pigmenti in father and his daughter. *Am J Hum Genet* 1984; **17**: 655–9.

4 Hecht F, Hecht BK, Austin WJ. Incontinentia pigmenti in Arizona Indians including transmission from mother to son inconsistent with the half chromatid mutation model. *Clin Genet* 1982; **21**: 293–6.

5 Lenz W. Half chromatid mutations may explain incontinentia pigmenti in males. *Am J Hum Genet* 1975; **27**: 690–1.

6 Roberts WM, Jenkins JJ, Moorehead EL et al. Incontinentia pigmenti, a chromosomal instability syndrome, is associated with childhood malignancy. *Cancer* 1988; **62**: 2370–2.

Other neurocutaneous syndromes

Other neurocutaneous syndromes are summarized in Tables 9.4–9.12.

Table 9.4 *Genetically determined neurocutaneous syndromes with pigmentary changes*

Syndrome	Main clinical features	Mode of inheritance
1. Central neurocutaneous syndromes with cutaneous hyperpigmentation		
Neurofibromatosis types I and II(von Recklinghausen's disease, bilateral acoustic neurofibromatosis)	See text	Autosomal dominant
Incontinentia pigmenti (Bloch–Sulzberger syndrome)	See text	X-linked dominant
Xeroderma pigmentosum (De Sanctis–Cacchione syndrome)	Facial freckles, keratosis, telangiectasia, cutaneous tumours, microcephaly, mental retardation seizures, spinocerebellar degeneration, short stature, gonadal hypoplasia	Autosomal recessive [1]
Cardiomyopathic lentiginosis	Multiple lentigines, obstructive cardiomyopathy, small stature, deafness, mental retardation	Autosomal dominant [2]
Seckel's syndrome	Brown pigmentation, grey hair, skin atrophy, bird-headed dwarfism, skeletal and dental defects, mental retardation	Autosomal recessive [3]
Hyperpigmentation, leucodystrophy, adrenal atrophy (Siemmerling–Creutzfeld syndrome)	Addisonian cutaneous hyperpigmentation	X-linked recessive [4]
Centrofacial lentiginosis (Touraine's syndrome)	Centrofacial pigmented freckles, mental retardation, epilepsy, endocrine dysfunction	Autosomal dominant [5]
Dyskeratosis congenita (Zinsser–Cole–Engman) Syndrome)	Poikiloderma, oral leucoplakia, dystrophy of nails, occasional mental retardation	Partial X-linked recessive [6]

Table 9.4 *Continued*

Syndrome	Main clinical features	Mode of inheritance
1. Central neurocutaneous syndromes with cutaneous hyperpigmentation – (continued)		
Ruvalcaba–Myhre syndrome	Pigmented macules over the glans penis, macrocephaly, delayed motor development, mental retardation, colonic polyps, ocular alterations	Probably autosomal dominant [7]
Phacomatosis pigmentovascularis	See Chapter 11	
2. Central neurocutaneous syndromes with hypopigmentation		
Hypomelanosis of Ito	Cutaneous pigmentation in whorls, streaks or patches, mental–motor retardation (58%), seizures (28%), abnormal EEG (28%), microcephaly (19%), hypotonia (14%), skeletal alterations (22%), ocular alterations (17%)	Most cases sporadic Exceptionally autosomal dominant [8]
Oculocerebral hypopigmentation (Cross's syndrome, Kramer's syndrome)	Generalized hypopigmentation, microphthalmia, microcornea, nystagmus, gingival fibromatosis, mental retardation	Autosomal recessive [9]
Neuroectodermal melanolysosomal disease (Elejalde's syndrome)	Cutaneous hypopigmentation, silver-coloured hair, epilepsy, mental retardation, cerebellar ataxia	Autosomal recessive [10]
3. Peripheral neurocutaneous syndromes with hypopigmentation		
Oculocutaneous albinism	Complete or partial depigmentation of hair, vellus, skin and iris. Nystagmus, strabismus, photophobia, deafness	X-linked recessive [11]
Waardenburg's syndromes I and II	White forelock and eyelashes, leucoderma, heterochromia iridis, dystopia canthorum (type I), deafness, vestibular symptoms	Autosomal dominant [12]
Chédiak–Higashi syndrome	Silvery-grey hair and skin, photophobia, nystagmus, recurrent infections	Autosomal recessive [13]
4. Central neurocutaneous syndromes with hyper-and hypopigmentation		
Neurodyschromic syndrome type I	Congenital hypopigmented and hyperpigmented macules, mental and growth retardation	Autosomal dominant [14]
Neurodyschromic syndrome type II	Hypo- and hyperpigmentation, progressive spastic paraparesis, peripheral neuropathy	Autosomal recessive [15]
Mukamel's syndrome	Cutaneous hypo- and hyperpigmentation, grey hair, mental retardation, spastic paraparesis, microcephaly, skeletal alterations	Autosomal recessive [16]
Rothmund–Thompson syndrome (poikiloderma congenitale)	Cutaneous reticular hypo- and hyperpigmentation, telangiectasia and atrophy, cataracts, skeletal alterations, hypogonadism. Rarely microcephaly, cortical atrophy and mental deficiency	Autosomal recessive [17]

References to Table 9.4

1 Kraemer KH, Lee M, Scotto J. Xeroderma pigmentosum: cutaneous, ocular and neurologic abnormalities in 830 published cases. *Arch Dermatol* 1987; **123**: 241–50.

2 Sevanez H, Mane-Garzon F, Kolski R. Cardio-cutaneous syndrome (the 'LEOPARD' syndrome). Review of the literature and a new family. *Clin Genet* 1976; **9**: 266–76.

3 Fitch N, Pinsky L, Lachance RC. A form of bird-headed dwarfism with features of premature senility. *Am J Dis Child* 1970; **120**: 260–4.

4 Aubourg PR, Sack GH, Meyers DA et al. Linkage of adrenoleukodystrophy to a polymorphic DNA probe. *Ann Neurol* 1987; **21**: 349–52.

5 Docin I, Galaction-Niteler O, Sirjita N et al. Centrofacial lentiginosis. A survey of 40 cases. *Br J Dermatol* 1976; **94**: 39–43.

6 Schneider A, Mayer U, Gebhart E et al. Clastogen-induced fragility may differentiate pancytopenia of congenital dyskeratosis from Fanconi's anemia. *Eur J Pediatr* 1988; **148**: 37–9.

7 Di Liberti JH, D'Agostino AN, Ruvalcaba RHA et al. A new lipid storage myopathy observed in individuals with the Ruvalcaba–Myhre–Smith syndrome. *Am J Med Genet* 1984; **18**: 163–7.

8 Ruiz-Maldonado R, Toussaint S, Tamayo L, Laterza AM, del Castillo V. Hypomelanosis of Ito: diagnostic criteria and report of 41 cases. *Pediatr Dermatol* 1992; **9**: 1–9.

9 Patton MA, Baraitser M, Heagerty AHM et al. An oculocerebral hypopigmentation syndrome: a case report with clinical, histochemical and ultrastructural findings. *J Med Genet* 1987; **24**: 118–22.

10 Elejalde BR, Holguin J, Valencia A et al. Mutations affecting pigmentation in man I. Neuroectodermal melanolysosomal disease. *Am J Hum Genet* 1979; **3**: 65–80.

11 Winship I, Gericke G, Beighton P. X-linked inheritance of ocular albinism with late onset sensorineural deafness. *Am J Med Genet* 1984; **19**: 797–83.

12 Ortonne JP. Piebaldism, Wardenburg's syndrome, and related disorders: 'Neural crest depigmentation syndromes'. *Dermatol Clin* 1988; **6**: 205–16.

13 Blumme RS, Wolf SM. The Chediak–Higashi syndrome: studies in four patients and review of the literature. *Medicine* 1972; **51**: 247–80.

14 Westerhoff W, Beemer FA, Cormane RH et al. Hereditary congenital hypopigmented and hyperpigmented macules. *Arch Dermatol* 1978; **114**: 931–6.

15 Abdallat A, Davies SM, Farrage J et al. Disordered pigmentation, spastic paraparesis, and peripheral neuropathy in three siblings. A new neurocutaneous syndrome. *J Neurol Neurosurg Psychiat* 1980; **43**: 962–6.

16 Mukamel M, Weitz R, Metzker A et al. Spastic paraparesis, mental retardation and cutaneous pigmentation disorder. A new syndrome. *Am J Dis Child* 1985; **139**: 1090–2.

17 Starr DG, McClure JP, Connor JM. Non dermatological complications and genetic aspects of the Rothmund–Thomson syndrome. *Clin Genet* 1985; **27**: 102–4.

Table 9.5 *Neurocutaneous syndromes with vascular changes*

Syndrome	Main clinical features	Mode of inheritance
1. Central neurocutaneous vascular syndromes		
Encephalotrigeminal angiomatosis (Sturge–Weber syndrome)	See Chapter 11	
Retinocerebellar–medullar angiomatosis (von Hippel–Lindau disease)	See Chapter 11	
Ataxia-telangiectasia (Louis-Bar syndrome)	See Chapter 18	
Riley–Smith syndrome	Subcutaneous haemangiomas, macrocephaly, pseudopapilloedema	Autosomal dominant [1]
Bannayan–Zonana syndrome	Cutaneous haemangiomas, lymphangiomas and lipomas, macrocephaly	Autosomal dominant [2]
Van Bogaert–Diury syndrome	Mottled vascular skin naevi, seizures, mental retardation, pyramidal symptoms	X-linked recessive, autosomal recessive [3]
Hereditary neurocutaneous haemangioma	Port-wine stain at various skin sites, arteriovenous malformations in the brain, spinal cord and meninges	Autosomal dominant [4]
Familial cavernous haemangioma of brain, retina and skin	Cavernous haemangiomas in central nervous system, retina and skin, seizures, intracranial haemorrhage and calcifications	Autosomal dominant [5]
Lymphocerebral syndrome	Lymphoedema of the feet, cerebrovascular malformations	Autosomal dominant [6]
Lymphoedema–microcephaly	Lymphoedema, microcephaly, coarse skin and hair follicles	Autosomal dominant [7]
Malignant atrophic papulosis (Degos's disease)	Atrophic, porcelain-coloured papules on skin and mucosae CNS infarcts, headache, seizures, hydrocephalus, lethargy	Autosomal dominant or sporadic [8]
2. Peripheral neurocutaneous vascular syndromes		
Hereditary haemorrhagic telangiectasia (Rendu–Osler–Weber syndrome)	Telangiectasia of skin and mucosae Angiomas of brain and spinal cord	Autosomal dominant [9]
Angiokeratoma corporis diffusum (Fabry's disease)	Angiokeratoma, pain, renal lesions, peripheral neuritis, cerebrovascular accidents	X-linked recessive [10]
Angioneurotic oedema	Oedema of skin and mucous membranes, intracranial hypertension, mental confusion, coma	Autosomal dominant [11]

References

1 Riley HD, Smith WR. Macrocephaly, pseudopapilledema and multiple hemangiomata: a previously undescribed heredofamilial syndrome. *Pediatrics* 1960; **26**: 293–300.
2 Miles JH, Zonana I, Mcfarlane J et al. Macrocephaly with hamartomas: Bannayan–Zonana syndrome. *Am J Med Genet* 1984; **19**: 225–34.

3 Van Bogaert L. Pathologie des angiomatoses. *Acta Neurol Psychiat Belg* 1950; **50**: 525–610.

4 Zaremba J, Stepien M, Jelowicka M et al. Hereditary neurocutaneous angioma: a new genetic entity? *J Med Genet* 1979; **16**: 443–7.

5 Dobyns WB, Michels VV, Groover RV et al. Familial cavernous malformations of the central nervous system and retina. *Ann Neurol* 1987; **21**: 578–83.

6 Avasthey P, Roy SB. Primary pulmonary hypertension, cerebrovascular malformation, and lymphedema of the feet in a family. *Br Heart J* 1968; **30**: 769–75.

7 Leung AKC. Dominantly inherited syndrome of microcephaly and congenital lymphedema with normal intelligence. *Am J Med Genet* 1987; **26**: 231.

8 Rosemberg S, Lopez MBS, Sotto MN et al. Childhood Degos disease with prominent neurological symptoms: report of a clinicopathological case. *J Child Neurol* 1988; **3**: 42–6.

9 McCaffrey TV, Kern EB, Lake CF. Management of epistaxis in hereditary hemorrhagic telangiectasia: review of 80 cases. *Arch Otolaryngol* 1977; **103**: 627–30.

10 Tagliavini F, Pietrini V, Gemignani F et al. Anderson–Fabri disease: neuropathological and neurochemical investigations. *Acta Neuropath* 1982; **56**: 93–8.

11 Hartmann L. L'oedeme agioneurotique héréditaire. A propos de 185 malades et 40 familles. *Bull Acad Nat Med* 1983; **167**: 343–51.

Table 9.6 *Neurocutaneous syndromes with altered keratinization*

Syndrome	Main clinical features	Mode of inheritance
1. *Central neurocutaneous syndromes with altered keratinization*		
Sjögren–Larsson syndrome Refsum's disease Rud's syndrome Brittle hair–ichthyosis–dwarfism (BID) syndrome Ichthyosis and neutral lipid storage disease Tay's syndrome Keratitis–ichthyosis–deafness (KID) syndrome	See Chapter 5	
Neuropathy and palmoplantar keratoderma Darier's disease	See Chapter 6	
2. *Peripheral neurocutaneous syndromes with altered keratinization*		
Bart–Pumphrey syndrome	Knuckle pads, leuconychia, deafness	Autosomal dominant [1]
Bitici's syndrome	Tylosis, sensorineural deafness	Autosomal dominant [2]

References

1 Bart RS, Pumphrey RE. Knuckle pads, leukonychia and deafness – a dominantly inherited syndrome. *New Engl J Med* 1967; **276**: 202–7.

2 Bitici OO. Familial hereditary, progressive sensori-neural hearing loss with keratosis palmaris et plantaris. *J Laryng Otol* 1975; **89**: 1143–6.

Table 9.7 *Neurocutaneous syndromes with metabolic changes*

Syndrome	Main clinical features	Mode of inheritance
1. Central neurocutaneous metabolic syndromes		
Phenylketonuria (phenylpyruvic oligophrenia)	Atopic-like dermatitis, fair skin and hair, mental retardation, seizures, hyperreflexia	Autosomal recessive [1]
Homocystinuria (cystathionine beta-synthase deficiency)	Malar flush, fine sparse hair, mental deterioration, lens dislocation, epilepsy	Autosomal recessive [2]
Sphingomyelinosis (Niemann–Pick disease types A, B, C)	Yellowish-brown waxy skin, mental retardation, muscle weakness, seizures, spasticity, hepatosplenomegaly	Autosomal recessive [3]
Glucocerebrosidosis (Gaucher's disease types I, II, III)	Hyperpigmentation of hands and face, muscular hypertonia, laryngeal spasm, hypoaesthesia, catatonia and death	Autosomal recessive [4]
Alpha-aminoaciduria (Hartnup disease)	Pellagroid lesions, cerebellar ataxia, psychic disturbances, mental retardation, seizures	Autosomal recessive [5]
Lipogranulomatosis (Farber's disease, ceramidase deficiency)	Swollen joints, subcutaneous nodules, hoarse cry, hyporeflexia, progressive paralysis, mental deterioration and death	Autosomal recessive [6]
Cerebral cholesterinosis (cerebrotendinous xanthomatosis)	Tendon xanthomas, xanthelasma, ataxia, seizures, mental retardation, cataracts	Autosomal recessive [7]
Lipoid proteinosis (Urbach–Wiethe disease)	Clear-yellowish tumours in eyelids, lips and skin, hoarseness, symmetric calcification of hippocampal gyrus, epilepsy, mental retardation	Autosomal recessive [8]
Tyrosinaemia II (Richner–Handhart syndrome)	Focal palmoplantar keratoderma, corneal opacities, keratitis and ulcers, mental retardation and neurological damage	Autosomal recessive [9]
Fucosidosis (alpha-L-fucosidase deficiency)	Cutaneous angiokeratomas, severe motor and mental retardation	Autosomal recessive [10]
Mucopolysaccharidosis II (Hurler–Scheie syndrome, alpha-L-iduronidase deficiency)	Coarse, thick skin with 'orange peel' aspect, hirsutism, progressive mental deterioration, coarse facies, stiff joints, hepatosplenomegaly	Autosomal recessive [11]
Mucopolysaccharidosis IIA (Hunter's syndrome, gargoylism)	Thick, ridged skin over the fingers, pebbly papules over the scapula, hirsutism, mental, ocular and acoustic deterioration, coarse facies, hepatosplenomegaly	Autosomal recessive [12]
Multiple carboxylase deficiency (neonatal) (holocarboxylase synthetase deficiency)	Scaly erythematous rash, acidosis, vomiting, hypotonia, seizures, coma and death	Autosomal recessive [13]
Multiple carboxylase deficiency (infantile) (biotinidase deficiency)	Erythematous scaly rash, hair loss, seizures, ataxia, hypotonia, deafness	Autosomal recessive [14]

continued

Table 9.7 *Continued*

Syndrome	Main clinical features	Mode of inheritance
2. *Peripheral neurocutaneous metabolic syndromes*		
Amyloid neuropathy (several forms)	Trophic ulcers, deafness, analgesia, anaesthesia	Autosomal dominant [15]
Purinosis (Lesch–Nyhan syndrome, hypoxanthine guanine phosphoribosyl transferase deficiency)	Self-inflicted ulcerations and mutilations, oligophrenia, spastic cerebral palsy, choreoathetosis	X-linked recessive [16]
Porphyric neuropathy (in porphyria variegata) (protoporphyrinogen oxidase deficiency)	Thick, hyperpigmented skin, vesicles, crusts, hypertrichosis. Peripheral neuritis, abdominal pain, mental confusion, Wernicke's encephalopathy, bulbar palsy	Autosomal dominant [17]
Heredopathia atactica polyneuritiformis (Refsum's disease, phytanic acid oxidase deficiency)	Ichthyotic skin, cerebellar ataxia, retinitis pigmentosa, areflexia, distal paresis	Autosomal recessive [18]

References

1 Guttler F, Woo SLC. Molecular genetics of PKU. *J Inher Metab Dis* 1986; **9** (suppl.): 58–68.
2 Abbott MH, Folstein SE, Abbey H et al. Psychiatric manifestations of homocystinuria due to cystathionine beta-synthase deficiency: prevalence, natural history, and relationship to neurologic impairment and vitamin B(6)-responsiveness. *Am J Med Genet* 1987; **26**: 959–69.
3 Brady RO. Sphingomyelin lipoidoses: Niemann–Pick disease. In Stanbury JB et al, eds. *The Metabolic Basis of Inherited Disease.* 5th ed. McGraw-Hill, New York, 1983; 731.
4 Beutler E, Kuhl W, Sorge J. Glucocerebrosidase 'processing' and gene expression in various forms of Gaucher disease. *Am J Hum Genet* 1985; **37**: 1062–70.
5 Wilcken B, Yu JS, Brown DA. Natural history of Hartnup disease. *Arch Dis Child* 1977; **52**: 38–40.
6 Antonarakis SE, Valle D, Moser HW et al. Phenotypic variability in siblings with Farber disease. *J Pediat* 1984; **104**: 406–9.
7 Berginer VM, Salen G, Shefer S. Long-term treatment of cerebrotendinous xanthomatosis with chenodeoxycholic acid. *New Engl J Med* 1984; **311**: 1649–52.
8 Haneke E, Hornstein OP, Meisel-Stosiek M et al. Hyalinosis cutis et mucosae in siblings. *Hum Genet* 1984; **68**: 342–5.
9 Natt E, Kao FT, Rettenmeier R et al. Assignment of the human tyrosine aminotransferase gene to chromosome 16. *Hum Genet* 1986; **72**: 225–8.
10 Fukushima H, Wet JR, O'Brien JS. Molecular cloning of a CDNA for human alpha-L-fucosidase. *Proc Nat Acad Sci* 1985; **82**: 1262–5.
11 Roubicek M, Gehler J, Spranger J. The clinical spectrum of alpha-L-iduronidase deficiency. *Am J Med Genet* 1985; **20**: 471–81.
12 Chase DS, Morris AH, Ballabio A et al. Genetics of Hunter syndrome: carrier detection, new mutations, segregation and linkage analysis. *Ann Hum Genet* 1986; **50**: 349–60.
13 Sweetman L, Nyhan WL. Inheritable biotin-treatable disorders and associated phenomena. *Ann Rev Nutr* 1986; **6**: 317–43.
14 Thy LP, Zielinska B, Zammarchi E et al. Multiple carboxylase deficiency due to deficiency of biotinidase. *J Neurogenet* 1986; **3**: 357–63.
15 Sack GH, Dumars KW, Gummerson KS et al. Three forms of dominant amyloid neuropathy. *Johns Hopkins Med J* 1981; **149**: 239–47.
16 Gibbs RA, Caskey CT. Identification and localization of mutations at the Lesch–Nyhan locus by ribonuclease A cleavage. *Science* 1987; **236**: 303–5.
17 Mustajoki P, Tenhunen R, Niemi KM et al. Homozygous variegate porphyria: a severe skin disease of infancy. *Clin Genet* 1987; **32**: 300–5.
18 Poulos A, Pollard AC, Mitchell JD et al. Patterns of Refsum disease: phytanic acid oxidase deficiency. *Arch Dis Child* 1984; **59**: 222–9.

Table 9.8 *Neurocutaneous syndromes with hair abnormalities*

Syndrome	Main clinical features	Mode of inheritance

1. Central neurocutaneous hair syndromes

With hypertrichosis:

Syndrome	Main clinical features	Mode of inheritance
De Lange's syndrome	Generalized hypertrichosis and cutis marmorata, long eyebrows and lashes, low hairline, characteristic facies, increased muscular tone, seizures, mental retardation	Autosomal recessive or sporadic [1]
Leprechaunism (Donohue's syndrome)	Redundant skin, absence of subcutaneous fat tissue, hypertrichosis, hyperinsulinaemia, mental and growth retardation, characteristic aspect	Autosomal recessive [2]

With hypotrichosis:

Syndrome	Main clinical features	Mode of inheritance
Kinky hair syndrome (Menkes' syndrome, defective copper metabolism)	Sparse, short, fragile, kinky hair (pili torti). Pale skin, mental retardation, spasticity, seizures, lethargy, hypothermia	X-linked recessive [3]
Kinky hair, photosensitivity and mental retardation	Kinky hair, broken eyebrows and lashes, mental retardation	Autosomal recessive [4]
Alopecia, epilepsy and oligophrenia (Moynahan's syndrome)	Delayed hair growth, epilepsy, oligophrenia, microcephaly	Autosomal dominant [5]
Atrichia, cysts and mental retardation (Castillo's syndrome)	Dystrophic hair forming keratinous cysts, alopecia of scalp, eyebrows and lashes, severe mental retardation	Autosomal recessive [6]
Marinesco–Sjögren syndrome	Short, sparse, fine and hypopigmented hair, ichthyosis. Progressive mental retardation, cerebellar ataxia, nystagmus, dysarthria, cataracts, decreased fertility	Autosomal recessive [7]
Keratosis follicularis decalvans and nervous system alterations*	Generalized keratosis follicularis decalvans of scalp, eyebrows and lashes, nail defects, dwarfism, cerebral atrophy seizures, psychomotor retardation, eye defects	X-linked recessive [8]
Cerebellar trigeminal dermal dysplasia	Parieto-occipital symmetric alopecia, cerebellar ataxia, atresia of the fourth ventricle, corneal opacities, mental retardation	Not conclusively established [9]
Hair–brain syndrome* (Sabinas' syndrome, Pollitt's syndrome, BIDS syndrome; amino acid metabolic alteration, trichothiodystrophy)	Brittle, sparse hair (trichorrhexis nodosa), mental retardation, short stature, decreased fertility	Autosomal recessive [10]
Universal congenital alopecia (UCA) and neurologic abnormalities (AMR syndrome)*	Universal congenital alopecia, microcephaly, seizures, psychomotor and physical retardation, skeletal alterations	Autosomal recessive or autosomal dominant [11]
Pili torti mental retardation	Sparse scalp hair (pili torti), malformed ears, syndactylism, mental retardation, cleft lip and palate	Autosomal recessive [12]

Table 9.8 *Continued*

Syndrome	Main clinical features	Mode of inheritance
Coffin–Siris syndrome	Sparse hair, hypoplastic nails, body hypertrichosis, microcephaly, mental retardation	Autosomal dominant or autosomal recessive [13]
GAPO syndrome*	Growth retardation, alopecia, pseudoanodontia, optic atrophy, cerebrovascular anomalies	Autosomal recessive [14]
Cardiofaciocutaneous syndrome	Skin lesions in 95% of patients: sparse, early, friable hair, patchy alopecia, eczema, ichthyosis Congenital heart defects, craniofacial dysmorphisms, mental retardation and brain abnormalities	Autosomal dominant [15, 16]

2. *Peripheral neurocutaneous hair syndromes*

Syndrome	Main clinical features	Mode of inheritance
Syndrome of alopecia and deafness*	Scalp and body alopecia (pili torti), neurosensory deafness, hypogonadism	Autosomal recessive [17]
Kinky hair and giant axonal neuropathy (altered microfilaments)	Kinky hair, chronic polyneuritis, impaired mental function, hypotonia, muscle weakness, dysaesthesia	Not established [18]

* Includes several conditions with minor variants.

References

1 Hawley PP, Jackson LG, Kurnit DM. Sixty-four patients with Brachmann–de Lange syndrome: a survey. *Am J Med Genet* 1985; **20**: 453–9.
2 Cantani A, Ziruolo MG, Tacconi ML. A rare polydysmorphic syndrome: leprechaunism – review of forty-nine cases reported in the literature. *Ann Genet* 1987; **30**: 221–7.
3 Moore CM, Howell RR. Ectodermal manifestations in Menkes disease. *Clin Genet* 1985; **28**: 532–40.
4 Calderon R, Gonzalez-Cantu N. Kinky hair, photosensitivity, broken eyebrows and eyelashes, and non-progressive mental retardation. *J Pediatr* 1979; **95**: 1007–8.
5 Pfeiffer RA, Volklein J. Congenital universalis alopecia, mental deficiency, and microcephaly in two sibs. *J Med Genet* 1982; **19**: 388–9.
6 Castillo VD, Ruiz-Maldonado R, Carnevale A. Atrichia with cysts and mental retardation. *Mod Probl Pediat* 1975; **17**: 21–4.
7 Walker PD, Blitzer MG, Shapira E. Marinesco–Sjögren syndrome: evidence for a lysosomal storage disorder. *Neurology* 1985; **35**: 415–19.
8 Cantu JM, Hernandez A, Larracilla J et al. A new X-linked recessive disorder with dwarfism, cerebral atrophy, and generalized keratosis follicularis. *J Pediatr* 1974; **84**: 564–70.
9 Pascual-Castroviejo I. Displasia cerebrotrigeminal. In: *Neurología infantil*. Científico Medica, Barcelona, 1983; 680.
10 McKusick VA. *Mendelian Inheritance in Man*. 8th ed. Johns Hopkins University Press, Baltimore, 1988; 976.
11 Wessel HB, Barmade MA, Hashida Y. Congenital alopecia, seizures and psychomotor retardation in three siblings. *Pediat Neurol* 1987; **3**: 101–7.
12 Zlotogora J, Zilberman Y, Tenenbaum A et al. Cleft lip and palate, pili torti, malformed ears, partial syndactily of fingers and toes, and mental retardation: a new syndrome? *J Med Genet* 1987; **24**: 291–3.
13 DeBassio WA, Kemper TL, Knoefel JE. Coffin–Siris syndrome: neuropathologic findings. *Arch Neurol* 1985; **42**: 350–3.
14 Manouvrier-Hanu S, Larguilliere C, Benalioua M et al. The GAPO syndrome. *Am J Med Genet* 1987; **26**: 683–8.
15 Young TL, Ziylan S, Schaffer DB. The ophthalmologic manifestations of the cardiofaciocutaneous syndrome. *J Pediat Ophthal Strab* 1993; **30**: 48–52.
16 Raymond G, Holmes LB. Cardio-facio-cutaneous syndrome (CFC). Neurological features in two children. *Dev Med Child Neurol* 1993; **35**: 727–41.
17 Cremers CWJ, Geerts SJ. Sensorineural hearing loss and pili torti. *Ann Otol Rhinolaryng* 1979; **88**: 100–4.
18 Fois A, Balestri P, Farnetani MA et al. Giant axonal neuropathy. Endocrinological and histological studies. *Eur J Pediatr* 1985; **144**: 274–80.

Table 9.9 *Neurocutaneous syndromes with connective tissue changes*

Syndrome	Main clinical features	Mode of inheritance
Central neurocutaneous connective tissue syndromes		
Tuberous sclerosis (Bourneville–Pringle disease)	See text	
Cutis verticis gyrata	Scalp with corrugated folds producing a cerebriform aspect, epilepsy, mental retardation	Autosomal recessive [1]
De Barsy's syndrome	Wrinkled, inelastic, translucent skin, progeroid aspect. Corneal opacities, mental and motor retardation	Autosomal recessive
Flynn–Aird syndrome	Acral skin atrophy, ulcerations, ichthyosis, alopecia, dementia, seizures, peripheral neuritis	Autosomal dominant [3]
Facial hemiatrophy (Parry–Romberg syndrome, scleroderma *en coup de sabre*	Unilateral facial and scalp atrophy, hyperpigmentation, alopecia of skin and subcutaneous tissue	? Autosomal dominant. Most cases sporadic [4]
Wrinkly skin syndrome	Wrinkled skin, hypotonia, microcephaly, chorioretinitis, mental retardation	Autosomal recessive [5]
Lupus erythematosus	Facial erythema and vasculitis, seizures, meningitis, ataxia, paraplegia, chorea, psychosis	? Autosomal dominant [6]

References

1 Akesson HO. Cutis verticis gyrata and mental deficiency in Sweden II. Genetic aspects. *Acta Med Scand* 1965; **177**: 459–64.
2 Pontz BF, Zepp F, Stoss H. Biochemical, morphological and immunological findings in a patient with cutis laxa-associated inborn disorder (De Barsy syndrome). *Eur J Pediatr* 1986; **145**: 428–34.
3 Flynn P, Aird RB. A neuroectodermal syndrome of dominant inheritance. *J Neurol Sci* 1965; **2**: 161–82.
4 Lewkonia RM, Lowry RB. Progressive hemifacial atrophy (Parry–Romberg syndrome). Report with review of genetics and nosology. *Am J Med Genet* 1983; **14**: 385–90.
5 Casamassima AC, Wesson SK, Conlon CJ et al. Wrinkly skin syndrome: phenotype and additional manifestations. *Am J Med Genet* 1987; **27**: 885–93.
6 Green JR, Montasser M, Woodrow JC. The association of HLA-linked genes with systemic lupus erythematosus. *Ann Hum Genet* 1986; **50**: 93–6.

Table 9.10 *Neurocutaneous syndromes with hamartomas*

Syndrome	Main clinical features	Mode of inheritance
Central neurocutaneous-hamartomatous syndromes		
Organoid naevus syndrome (Schimmelpenning–Feuerstein–Mims–Solomon)	Linear sebaceous naevus along the lines of Blaschko. Ocular and cerebral defects	Autosomal dominant [1, 2] ? Dominant lethal gene
Basal cell naevus syndrome	Naevi-like basal cell carcinomas, pinhead-size palmoplantar pits, odontogenic mandibular cysts, bifurcated ribs. Calcification of falx cerebri, dura and choroides, mental retardation, medulloblastoma, ocular anomalies	Autosomal dominant [3]
Multiple hamartoma syndrome (Cowden syndrome)	Fibromas, trichilemmomas, acrokeratosis, malignant tumours, meningiomas, neuromas, retinal gliomas	Autosomal dominant [4]
Neurocutaneous lipomas (Krabbe–Bartle syndrome)	Multiple cutaneous lipomas. Mental retardation, spinal, meningeal and encephalic lipomas	Autosomal dominant or sporadic [5]
Encephalocraniocutaneous lipomatosis	Large, subcutaneous lipomas on the scalp with overlying skin devoid of hair, pterygium-like lesions on the sclera, skin tags, epilepsy, intellectual impairment	Sporadic [6]
Delleman's syndrome	Orbital cysts, skin appendages, aplasia, seizures, psychomotor retardation, ocular, skeletal, genital and dental anomalies	Not established [7]

References

1 Bouwes Bavinck JN, van de Kamp JJP. Organoid naevus phakomatosis: Schimmelpenning–Feuerstein–Mims syndrome. *Br J Dermatol* 1985; **113**: 491–2.
2 Happle R. Cutaneous manifestation of lethal genes. *Hum Genet* 1986; **72**: 280.
3 Berlin NI, Van Scott EJ, Clendenning WE et al. Basal-cell nevus syndrome. *Ann Intern Med* 1966; **64**: 403–21.
4 Starink TM, van der Veen JPW, Arwert F et al. The Cowden syndrome: a clinical and genetic study in 21 patients. *Clin Genet* 1986; **29**: 222–33.
5 Haberland C, Perou M. Encephalocraniocutaneous lipomatosis. A new example of ectomesodermal dysgenesis. *Arch Neurol* 1970; **22**: 144–55.
6 Fishman MA, Chang CSC, Miller JE. Encephalocraniocutaneous lipomatosis. *Pediatrics* 1978; **61**: 580–2.
7 Delleman JW, Oorthuys EM, Bleeker EM et al. Orbital cyst in addition to congenital cerebral and focal dermal malformations: a new entity. *Clin Genet* 1984; **25**: 470–2.

Table 9.11 *Neurocutaneous dysmorphic syndromes*

Syndrome	Main clinical features	Mode of inheritance
Chromosome 21 trisomy (Down's syndrome)	Soft, hyperelastic, thick skin, characteristic palmar ridge, mental retardation, muscular hypotonia	Chromosomal [1]
Focal dermal hypoplasia	Fat herniation of epidermis, papillomas, telangiectasia, syndactyly, body asymmetry, mental retardation, microcephaly, craniostenosis	X-linked dominant [2]
Cockayne's syndrome	Facial sun-induced erythema, atrophy and telangiectasia. 'Mickey Mouse' appearance, physical and mental retardation	Autosomal recessive [3]
Aplasia cutis congenita (congenital absence of skin)	Ulcerated or cicatricial areas on scalp or body, involving the skin or deeper structures. Seizures, spastic paralysis, mental retardation, hydrocephalus, cerebral cortical atrophy	Autosomal dominant or autosomal recessive [4]
Oculoauriculovertebral dysplasia (Goldenhar's syndrome)	Preauricular appendages, preauricular fistulas, epibulbar dermoids, vertebral anomalies, epilepsy, mental retardation	Autosomal recessive [5]

References

1 Zeligman I, Scalia SP. Dermatologic manifestations of mongolism. *Arch Dermat Syphilol* 1954; **69**: 342–4.
2 Ruiz-Maldonado R, Carnevale A, Tamayo L et al. Focal dermal hypoplasia. *Clin Genet* 1974; **6**: 36–45.
3 Lehman AR, Francis AJ, Giannelli F. Prenatal diagnosis of Cockayne disease. *Lancet* 1985; **i**: 486–8.
4 Sybert VP. Aplasia cutis congenita: a report of 12 new families and review of the literature. *Pediatr Dermatol* 1985; **3**: 1–14.
5 Boles DJ, Bodurtha J, Nance WE. Goldenhar complex in discordant monozygotic twins: a case report and review of the literature. *Am J Med Genet* 1987; **28**: 103–9.

Table 9.12 *Peripheral neuropathies with skin changes*

Syndrome	Main clinical features	Mode of inheritance
1. Primary peripheral neuropathies with skin changes		
Hereditary sensory neuropathy type I (Thevenard's syndrome, ulceromutilating acropathy)	Calluses, blisters, ulcers and necrosis on the soles, osteolysis and deformity. Sensory loss, hyporeflexia; anhidrosis	Autosomal dominant [1]
Hereditary sensory neuropathy type II (Morvan's disease, syringomyelia of infancy; absence of myelinated fibres)	Recurrent paronychia, ulcers, mutilation of fingers and plantar ulcers. Sensory loss, hyporeflexia, anhidrosis	Autosomal recessive [2]
Hereditary sensory neuropathy type III (familial dysautonomia, Riley–Day syndrome; deficient dopamine beta-hydroxylase)	Generalized heat or exercise-induced erythema, autonomic disturbances, areflexia, anaesthesia	Autosomal recessive [3]
Hereditary sensory neuropathy type IV (neural crest syndrome)	Blond hair, anhidrosis, anaesthesia of acral portions with trophic ulcerations, seizures, mental retardation	Autosomal recessive [4]
Congenital insensitivity to pain (congenital pain asymbolia)	Burns, abrasions, lacerations, ulceration of cornea, nasal septum and lips	Autosomal recessive [5]
Melkersson–Rosenthal syndrome	Recurrent angioneurotic oedema of the lips, scrotal tongue, facial paralysis	Autosomal dominant or sporadic [6]
2. Secondary peripheral neuropathies with skin changes		
Diastematomyelia (middle cutaneous and spinal defects)	Dermal sinus, port-wine naevus, lipoma, tuft of hair, dimple, pigmented naevus, glioma. Meningitis, spina bifida, compression of spinal cord, motor and sensory impairment	Autosomal recessive or multifactorial [7]

References

1 Berginer V, Baruchin A, Ben-Yakar Y et al. Plantar ulcers in hereditary sensory neuropathy. *Int J Dermatol* 1984; **23**: 664–8.
2 Axelrod FB, Pearson J. Congenital sensory neuropathies. Diagnostic distinction from familial dysautonomia. *Am J Dis Child* 1984; **138**: 947–54.
3 Axelrod FB, Pearson J, Tepperberg J et al. Congenital sensory neuropathy with skeletal dysplasia. *J Pediatr* 1983; **102**: 727–30.
4 Lee EL, Oh GC, Lam KL et al. Congenital sensory neuropathy with anhidrosis: a case report. *Pediatrics* 1976; **57**: 259–62.
5 Thrush DC. Congenital insensitivity to pain. A clinical, genetic and neurophysiological study in four children from the same family. *Brain* 1973; **96**: 369–86.
6 Lygidakis C, Tsankanikas C, Llias A et al. Melkersson–Rosenthal's syndrome in four generations. *Clin Genet* 1979; **15**: 189–92.
7 Kapasalökis Z. Diastematomyelia in two sisters. *J Neurol* 1964; **21**: 66–7

Chapter 10

Disorders of collagen and elastin

P. Beighton

Introduction

Significant skin involvement is a feature of a number of genetic disorders of collagen and elastin. These disorders are listed in Table 10.1.

The biomolecular basis of the heritable disorders of collagen and elastin is currently the focus of great scientific interest and much research endeavour. This difficult subject has been reviewed in *Connective Tissue and Its Heritable Disorders*[1] and in *McKusick's Heritable Disorders of Connective Tissue*[2].

The nosology of the collagen and elastin disorders is complex; for the sake of clarity the format promulgated following the International Congress of Human Genetics, Berlin, 1986, is employed throughout this chapter[3]. A molecular nosology of the heritable disorders of connective tissue, aimed at facilitating genotype-phenotype correlations, has also been published[4]. The code numbers from *Mendelian Inheritance in Man* (MIM) have been quoted where relevant in the tables and text[5].

References

1 Royce PM, Steinmann B *Connective Tissue and Its Heritable Disorders*. Wiley-Liss, New York, 1993.
2 Beighton P. (ed) *McKusick's Heritable Disorders of Connective Tissue*. 5th ed. Mosby, St Louis, 1993.
3 Beighton P, de Paepe A, Danks D et al. International Nosology of Heritable Disorders of Connective Tissue, Berlin, 1986. *Am J Med Genet* 1988; **29**: 581–94.
4 Beighton P, De Paepe A, Hall JG et al. Molecular nosology of heritable disorders of connective tissue. *Am J Med Genet* 1992; **42** (4): 431–48.
5 McKusick VA. *Mendelian Inheritance in Man*. 11th ed. Johns Hopkins Press, Baltimore, 1994.

Table 10.1 *Genetic disorders of collagen and elastin with significant skin involvement*

Ehlers–Danlos syndrome
Cutis laxa
Pseudoxanthoma elasticum
Dermatofibrosis lenticularis disseminata with
    osteopoikilosis (Buschke–Ollendorff syndrome)
Wrinkly skin syndrome
Connective tissue naevi
    Familial cutaneous collagenoma
    Familial reactive collagenosis
    Elastoma perforans serpiginosa
Connective tissue disorders with minor skin
    involvement
    Marfan's syndrome
    Osteogenesis imperfecta
    Spondyloepiphyseal dysplasia with joint laxity

Ehlers–Danlos syndrome

Definition

The Ehlers–Danlos syndrome (EDS) is a heterogeneous disorder of connective tissue which is characterized by the triad of skin hyperextensibility, connective tissue fragility and articular hypermobility. Cutaneous scarring, especially over bony prominences, and a variable propensity to bruising are important features.

Table 10.2 *Forms of Ehlers–Danlos syndrome*

Type		Mode of inheritance	MIM no.
EDS I	Gravis type	AD	130000
EDS II	Mitis type	AD	130010
EDS III	Hypermobile type	AD	130020
EDS IV	Vascular	Heterogeneous	
	IV-A Acrogeric type	AD	130050
	IV-B Acrogeric type	AR	225350
	IV-C Ecchymotic type	AD	130050
EDS V	X-linked type	XL	305200
EDS VI	Ocular-scoliotic type	AR	225400
EDS VII	Arthrochalasis multiplex congenita	Heterogeneous	
		AD	130060
		AR	225410
EDS VIII	Periodontitis type	AD	130080
EDS IX	Vacant (formerly occipital horn syndrome, or X-linked cutis laxa, now recategorized as a disorder of copper transport)		304150
EDS X	Fibronectin abnormality	AR	225310
EDS XI	Vacant (formerly familial joint instability, now recategorized with the familial articular hypermobility syndromes)		147900

AD, autosomal dominant; AR, autosomal recessive.

The archaic synonym 'cutis hyperelastica', which was sometimes used for EDS, has now been relegated to oblivion. Cutis laxa and the familial joint hypermobility syndrome are specifically excluded from the EDS group of disorders.

More than a thousand affected persons have now been reported, and EDS has moved from obscurity to prominence. The conventional numerical and descriptive designations of the various forms of EDS, together with their mode of inheritance and MIM number, as they appear in the Berlin nosology, are listed in Table 10.2.

Historical background

Early cases were described by Ehlers in 1901 and Danlos in 1908 and the conjoined eponym was firmly established by Frederick Parkes Weber in 1936.

Ehlers–Danlos syndrome can be diagnosed retrospectively in a Spanish sailor, George Albes, who was presented at the Academy of Leyden in 1657 by a Dutch surgeon, Job van Meekren. Skin-stretching fairground exhibitionists of the last century who had EDS included Felix Wehle, the India-Rubber Man, and Etta Lake, the Elastic Lady. The first complete description of the condition was given by Tschernogobow, when he presented two patients at the Moscow Dermatological and Venereological Society in 1892. The paper was published in Russia but owing to language difficulties this contribution was overlooked in Europe, and eponymous priority was accorded to Ehlers and Danlos.

Edvard Ehlers (1863–1937)

Ehlers was an eminent Danish dermatologist (Figure 10.1). He was appointed as chief of the dermatological polyclinic at the Fredericks Hospital, Copenhagen, in

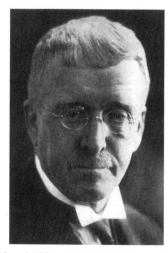

Figure 10.1 *Edvard Ehlers (1863–1937). From Beighton P, Beighton G* The Man Behind the Syndrome. *Springer Verlag, Berlin, 1986*

1906 and subsequently became president of the International Union against Venereal Disease.

Ehlers was a tall man, with fair hair, intellectual charm and a distinguished manner. He spoke several languages and had considerable organizational abilities. Ehlers was a Francophile and frequently participated in clinical meetings of the French Dermatological Society in Paris. He was honoured by the French government for his activities during World War I, which involved the evacuation of wounded French servicemen to Denmark. Ehlers died in Denmark in 1937, after a brief illness.

Henri-Alexandre Danlos (1844–1912)

Danlos was a French physician with a special interest in dermatology and therapeutics (Figure 10.2). He was appointed as consultant physician at the Hôpital Tenon, Paris, in 1881 and subsequently moved to a similar post at the Hôpital St Louis, where he spent the rest of his career.

Danlos was an innovator in the treatment of skin conditions with arsenicals, mercurials and radiation. He conducted meticulous studies in this field and published numerous papers on his findings. His scientific work received recognition in 1904 when he was elected president of the Medical Society of Paris and two years later he became secretary of the Parisian Dermatological Society.

Danlos had a painful chronic illness, and was depressed and withdrawn. Indeed, it is said that despite his professional successes, he was never seen to smile! He died in 1912 at the age of 68 years.

Clinical features

The cardinal manifestations of EDS are hyperextensibility of the skin, hypermobility of the joints and fragility of the connective tissues. Easy bruising and dystrophic scarring are the external sequelae of this latter problem (Figures 10.3–10.5). The clinical features are very variable but they are present to some degree in all affected persons. The various forms of EDS are defined clinically on a basis of the extent and severity of these changes, together with additional involvement of other systems in some instances. Further subcategorization is possible in terms of the mode of genetic transmission and underlying biomolecular defect.

The major clinical manifestations of the various forms of EDS are listed in Table 10.3.

A general review of EDS can be found in the book *Hypermobility of Joints*[1]. Skin involvement in EDS is discussed in detail below.

Skin hyperextensibility

Skin hyperextensibility varies in degree between affected individuals and may differ at different sites of the body. In the more severely affected person, a fold of skin can be stretched for several centimetres without discomfort and on release the skin springs back to resume its former position. In some individuals with EDS the skin seems to be loosely attached to the underlying tissues, and when friction is applied there is a sensation of the skin 'coming away'. The skin has been described as feeling loose, like that of a puppy. The thickness of the fold of skin that can be lifted is dependent upon the properties of the underlying tissues; in some patients the fold is

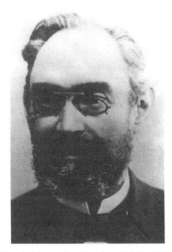

Figure 10.2 *Henri-Alexandre Danlos (1844–1912). From Beighton P, Beighton G The Man Behind the Syndrome. Springer Verlag, Berlin, 1986*

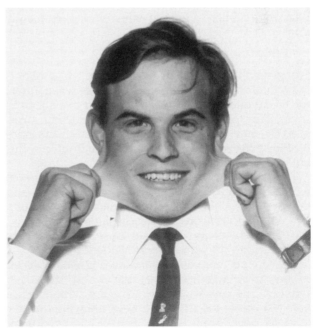

Figure 10.3 *EDS: skin hyperextensibility. From Beighton P, Price A, Lord S et al Ann Rheum Dis 1969; **28**: 228–45, by permission of Oxford University Press*

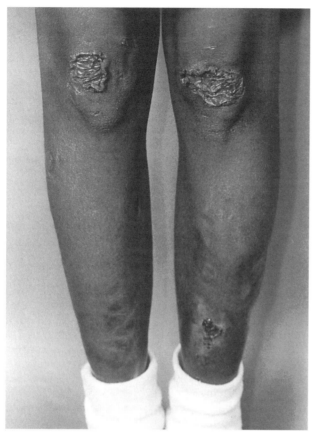

Figure 10.4 *EDS: the knees and shins of this affected girl bear the characteristic scars. From Winship I S Afr Med J 1985; 67: 509–11, by permission*

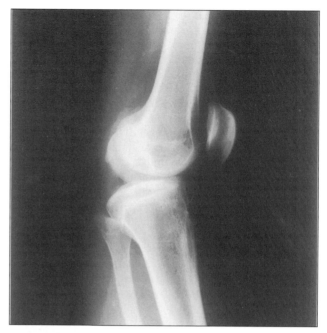

Figure 10.5 *EDS: lateral radiograph of the knee demonstrating articular hypermobility. Calcified subcutaneous spheroids are evident in the soft tissues. From Beighton P, Lea-Thomas M Clin Radiol 1969; 20: 354–61*

thick and rubbery, while in others it is surprisingly thin.

Skin fragility

The generalized connective tissue fragility in EDS is most evident in the skin, which splits when direct force is applied or tears when subjected to a shearing stress. This feature is very variable in different forms of EDS; some persons experience numerous episodes of skin splitting, while others have little trouble of this kind.

The lacerations usually occur on exposed surfaces where there are underlying bony prominences, and the forehead, elbows, knees and shins are most often affected. Subcutaneous fat has a cushioning effect and the relative paucity of fat at those sites probably contributes to the skin splitting tendency.

The wounds are painless and do not usually bleed to any great extent, but they gape, and often heal slowly. If the cuts are repaired surgically the stitches may tear out of the adjacent tissues, allowing the scar to break open. Scars tend to distract and eventually become wide and thin, with a 'cigarette paper' or papyraceous appearance. The scars are often darkly pigmented with telangiectasia within their borders.

Skin haematomas

A bleeding diathesis is a very variable facet of EDS. It is severe in EDS IV (arterial or ecchymotic type) and mild or absent in other forms of the disorder. The pathogenesis of the abnormal bleeding is uncertain, but the dermal consequences of this problem are the presence of bruises in all stages of resolution and darkening of the scars. It is noteworthy that the abnormal bruising has led to a misdiagnosis of battered child syndrome on several occasions.

Pseudotumours

Fleshy, heaped-up molluscoid pseudotumours often form at the sites exposed to trauma, notably the knees and elbows. These lesions vary in diameter from a few millimetres to 1–2 centimetres. They are present in the majority of affected persons and were a feature of the original case described by Danlos in 1906. It is possible that they are the result of an abnormal response to superficial tissue which has been implanted during skin splitting.

Large pseudotumours are sometimes found over the tendo Achillis and in association with hallux valgus. These swellings are apparently due to overgrowth of tissue around bursae which have previously been inflamed.

A third variety of pseudotumour occurs when preexisting scar tissue becomes heaped-up and hypertrophic. These lesions may be flabby and impart a sensation akin to that of an empty grape-skin.

Table 10.3 *Clinical manifestations of Ehlers–Danlos syndrome*

Type	Clinical features
EDS I	Cardinal manifestations in severe degree
EDS II	Cardinal manifestations in mild degree
EDS III	Marked articular hypermobility Moderate dermal hyperextensibility Minimal scarring
EDS IV	Variable stigmata Severe bruising, hyperpigmentation and/or scarring Thin skin with prominent venous plexus Vascular rupture Colonic perforation Characteristic facial appearance
EDS V	Cardinal manifestations in moderate degree X-linked inheritance
EDS VI	Cardinal manifestations in severe degree Eye involvement (microcornea, scleral perforation, retinal detachment) Scoliosis
EDS VII	Cardinal manifestations with marked articular hypermobility Short stature Micrognathia
EDS VIII	Cardinal manifestations in moderate degree Aggressive periodontitis, gingival recession, early tooth loss
EDS X	Cardinal manifestations but skin texture normal Petechiae Striae distensae Platelet aggregation defect corrected by fibronectin

Subcutaneous spheroids

Many affected persons have multiple small, hard, mobile spheroids beneath their skin, particularly in the forearms and shins. These subcutaneous lesions are a few millimetres in diameter, and they feel like hard grains of rice or small pieces of shot. They may be very numerous, but invariably many more of them can be demonstrated radiographically than can be located by palpation (Figure 10.5). It is probable that they represent lobules of fatty tissue which have lost their blood supply owing to trauma and then become fibrosed and calcified.

Other skin manifestations

The skin of many patients has a soft, velvety or doughy consistency. On palpation it resembles chamois leather, and has been described by an enthusiastic author as 'the skin you love to feel'. The skin is often very white but the extremities readily become cyanosed, probably due to stasis of blood in small venules. True acrocyanosis and Raynaud's phenomenon also occur, and chilblains have been reported in some patients.

In some individuals the skin is particularly thin and the venous plexus is easily visible. These features are characteristic of the EDS IV group of patients who are at high risk from the lethal complications of EDS. However, dilated capillaries are frequently found on the cheeks of patients with other forms of the condition. The veins of the legs may be prominent, not only from varicosities but also because of a lack of subcutaneous fat.

Many patients seem to have an undue liability to infection of the skin and cellulitis is not uncommon. This problem may be due to the laxity of the subcutaneous tissues which allows uninterrupted spread of the infection.

Striae gravidarum are consistently absent in EDS; this feature may be related to the mechanical properties of the connective tissues.

Pathology

From the clinical manifestations of EDS it is evident that the basic defect resides in the connective tissues, but despite many decades of research and speculation, surprisingly little is known about the nature of the primary abnormality.

At the ultrastructural level the only significant changes which have been detected in the skin have been abnormally large collagen fibrils, which are often irregular in shape. This feature is very variable and in many affected persons the ultrastructure of the skin is normal. The vast majority of reports of studies of this type have concerned persons with the common EDS types I, II and III, and even within these categories the changes are not consistent. For this reason ultrastructural investigations are of little value for diagnosis, or for the specific discrimination of the different forms of EDS. The rare type IV EDS is an exception, in that collagen fibres are frequently small and variable in size; nevertheless these changes are also inconsistent and far from being diagnostic.

Investigations of the biochemical and molecular basis of EDS have met with limited success, but progress in the near future is anticipated[2]. It is noteworthy that the pathogenesis of the common EDS types I, II and III remains unknown, while in type IV, which is comparatively rare, considerable heterogeneity is apparent at a biomolecular level. Abnormalities that have been elucidated thus far are listed in Table 10.4.

Genetics

Ehlers–Danlos syndrome is very heterogeneous; nine major types have been delineated and in some instances further subcategorization is possible in terms of the mode of inheritance or the biomolecular defect.

Heterogeneity in the EDS was first documented in the mid-1960s following investigations of large series of patients in the UK. Types I–IV were differentiated by their clinical stigmata, while type V was distinguished by an X-linked mode of inheritance[3,4] (Figure 10.6).

In the years that followed, types VI–XI were delineated and in some instances subcategorized on a basis of biomolecular abnormalities[5]. Several putative additional forms of EDS have also been reported, but these disorders have not yet been formally assimilated into the EDS nosology.

Gene mapping studies have localized *COL3A1* (EDS IV) to 2q31, *COL1A1* (EDS VII-A) to 17q21.31–22.05, *COL1A2* (EDS VII-B) to 7q21.3–22.1 and *Fibronectin-1* (? EDS X) to 2q34–36.

It must be emphasized that the vast majority of patients with EDS have the autosomal dominant (AD) forms I, II or III and that the other types are rare. It is also of practical importance that there is considerable phenotypic overlap, and that precise diagnostic categorization of a sporadic case can be very difficult indeed.

The potentially lethal complications of arterial and bowel rupture in EDS IV necessitate diagnostic precision in this entity; in this respect investigations of type III collagen may be helpful. Further difficulties in the context of genetic counselling arise from the fact that EDS IV is genetically heterogeneous as autosomal dominant and recessive forms have been documented.

In view of the complexity of both connective tissue structure and the collagen molecule, it is probable that a wide assortment of disparate defects can produce

Table 10.4 *Pathogenesis of Ehlers–Danlos syndrome*

Type		Abnormality
EDS IV		Type III collagen abnormal in all forms (COL3A1) [1]
EDS VI		
	A	Decreased lysyl hydroxylase activity
	B	Normal lysyl hydroxylase activity?
EDS VII		
	A	Structural defect of pro-alpha 1 (COL1A1) [1]
	B	Structural defect of pro-alpha 2 (COL1A2) [1]
	C	Procollagen N proteinase deficiency?
EDS X		Fibronectin-1 abnormality?

Reference

1 Superti-Furga A, Steinmann B, Ramirez F, Byers PH. Molecular defects of type III procollagen in Ehlers-Danlos syndrome type IV. *Hum Genet* 1989; **82**: 104–8.

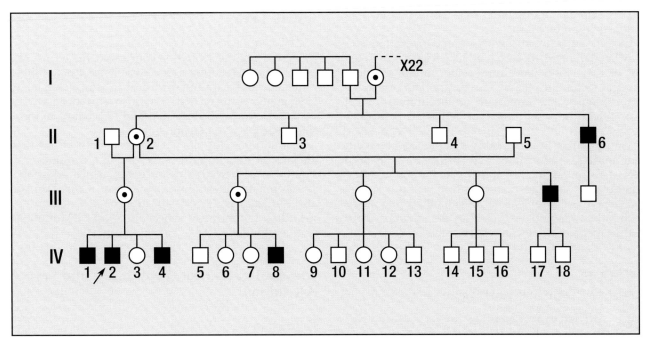

Figure 10.6 *EDS: pedigree of a family with X-linked EDS V. From Beighton P* Br Med J *1968; 3: 409–11*

the EDS phenotype. On this basis it is possible that EDS will turn out to be very heterogeneous indeed.

As diagnostic categorization solely based upon the phenotype is unreliable, genetic counselling hinges upon the perceived mode of transmission within a family. This issue may be confounded by intrafamilial variability, although complete non-penetrance is unusual. As previously mentioned, transmission is AD in the majority of instances.

Antenatal diagnosis is possible by means of bio-molecular techniques in some families with EDS IV [6]. In other forms of EDS, with the possible exception of the rare EDS IV, VI and VII, there are no biomolecular abnormalities which would facilitate prenatal detection of an affected fetus. Ultrasonic recognition of abnormal fetal positioning and articular hypermobility is theoretically possible, but the situation is far from clear-cut and there would be little practical value in this approach.

Differential diagnosis

The diagnosis of EDS is an easy matter if the full diagnostic triad is evident (skin hyperextensibility, articular hypermobility and skin fragility). Problems arise, however, when partial manifestations are present, especially in a sporadic case. In these circumstances it may be impossible to establish a firm diagnosis of EDS.

The EDS must be distinguished from a number of rare disorders in which articular hypermobility is a major feature. In the majority of these conditions the presence of additional syndromic manifestations and

the absence of skin hyperextensibility and fragility readily facilitate recognition.

Familial articular hypermobility syndrome

The EDS is frequently confused with the familial articular hypermobility syndrome, but this heterogeneous condition is differentiated by the fact that the sole manifestation is hypermobility, with secondary derived complications thereof, and that the skin is neither hyperextensible nor fragile. Of the various forms of EDS, the phenotypic features of EDS type III (benign hypermobile form) and EDS type VII (arthrochalasis multiplex congenita) most closely resemble this condition.

Cutis laxa

In early reports EDS was termed 'cutis hyperelastica' and this usage sometimes led to confusion with cutis laxa (CL). This problem was purely semantic and the phenotypes are quite different. Cutis laxa is a rare disorder in which the skin hangs in loose folds, and although the skin can be stretched, it does not spring back into place. The conditions are further differentiated by the fact that the connective tissues are not fragile and the joints are not hypermobile in CL (see below).

Treatment

There is no specific treatment for EDS; management revolves around a multiplicity of complications which are consequent upon connective tissue fragility and articular hypermobility.

Closure of traumatic wounds and operation sites may be made difficult by a tendency for sutures to tear out of the tissues, and appropriate modifications to surgical techniques may be necessary. The connective tissue fragility has important implications in obstetrics, where a wide range of lethal complications necessitate careful antenatal care and delivery.

The articular hypermobility predisposes to recurrent sprains, subluxations and dislocations. In addition, deformities such as spinal malalignment, talipes equinovarus and pes planus may develop. Management of these problems is essentially orthopaedic, within the constraints imposed by the inherent abnormal properties of the connective tissue.

References

1 Beighton P, Grahame R, Bird H. *Hypermobility of Joints.* 2nd ed. Springer, London, 1989.
2 Byers PH. Inherited disorders of collagen gene structure and expression. *Am J Med Genet* 1989; **34**: 72–80.
3 Beighton P. *The Ehlers–Danlos Syndrome.* Heinemann, London, 1970.
4 Beighton P, Curtis D. X-linked Ehlers–Danlos syndrome type V: the next generation. *Clin Genet* 1985; **27**: 472–8.
5 Hollister DW. Clinical features of Ehlers–Danlos syndrome type VII and IX. In: Akeson WH, ed. *Symposium on Heritable Disorders of Connective Tissue.* CV Mosby, St Louis, 1982; 102–13.
6 Pope FM, Narcisi P, Nicholls AC et al. Clinical presentations of Ehlers-Danlos syndrome type IV. *Arch Dis Child* 1988; **63**: 1016–25.

Cutis laxa

There is semantic confusion concerning the term 'cutis laxa'. This designation is used as a name for a number of genetic and acquired disorders in which skin laxity is a major feature, and it is also employed in the general descriptive sense for skin that hangs in loose folds, irrespective of pathogenesis.

In addition to the classical forms of cutis laxa, which are specific genetic entities, lax skin is a component of a number of heritable disorders in which additional syndromic manifestations are present. Cutis laxa can also be acquired. A classification of these disorders, including the mode of inheritance and MIM number, is given in Table 10.5.

Classical cutis laxa (benign AD and severe AR forms)

Definition

The classical form of cutis laxa (CL) is a rare, genetically heterogeneous disorder of elastic tissue, in which the skin hangs in loose folds. Affected persons have a characteristic facies and cardiorespiratory complications may occur.

Clinical features

Skin laxity is usually evident at birth, but some affected neonates are oedematous and laxity of the

Table 10.5 *Classification of the cutis laxa group of disorders*

Disorder	Mode of inheritance	MIM no.
Classical cutis laxa		
Benign form	AD	123700
Severe form	AR	219100
Syndromic cutis laxa		
Cutis laxa with joint hypermobility and developmental delay	AR	219200
Cutis laxa with corneal clouding and mental retardation (progeroid syndrome of De Barsy)	AR	219150
Geroderma osteodysplastica	AR	231070
Occipital horn syndrome (formerly EDS IX; X-linked cutis laxa)	XL	304150
Acquired cutis laxa		
Primary generalized elastolysis		
Postinflammatory (autoimmune?)		
Secondary or localized		

AD, autosomal dominant; AR, autosomal recessive; XL, X-linked.

skin only becomes apparent in the first months of life, when the oedema resolves. The hanging folds of the skin produce a mournful or 'Churchillian' appearance and, together with a hooked nose and long upper lip, constitute the characteristic facies (Figure 10.7). All regions of the body are involved; the loose skin can be stretched for several centimetres but it lacks elastic recoil and does not spring back to resume its former position. The connective tissues in CL are not fragile and the skin does not split. Equally, the joints in the classical form of CL are not hypermobile, and orthopaedic problems do not occur.

The AD form of CL is benign and, apart from the skin involvement, there are few complications (Figure 10.8). There have been a few reports of structural cardiac malformations, emphysema and hernia, but these changes are infrequent in this variety of CL.

In the severe AR type of CL (Figure 10.9) the facies and cutaneous manifestations resemble those of the AD form but in addition pulmonary emphysema is a consistent feature. This problem is progressive and death from cardiorespiratory failure before adulthood is usual. Congenital pulmonary artery stenosis and structural cardiac and vascular abnormalities are important but variable syndromic components. Diverticula of the bladder and gut together with hernias of the diaphragm and abdominal wall are often present.

Pathology

Fragmentation and diminution in number of the elastic fibres is a consistent histological feature of the AD and AR forms of CL. These changes are present in all tissues that contain elastin, notably the skin and the blood vessels. Electron microscopy reveals globular and unstructured elastin, with relatively large amounts of the microfibrillar components of elastic fibres.

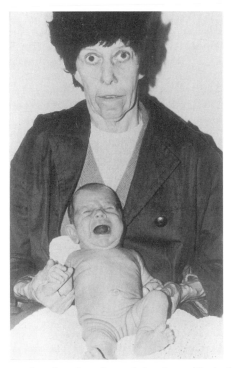

Figure 10.8 *An affected mother and daughter with the benign AD form of CL. From Beighton P J Med Genet 1972; 9: 216–21*

Abnormalities of copper metabolism have been implicated in the pathogenesis of CL, and low serum concentrations with high urinary excretion have been reported. It has been suggested that copper is necessary for the maintenance of serum elastase inhibitor levels and that deficiency leads to excessive activity of elastase, with damage to elastin fibrils. Elevated serum copper levels have also been detected in affected siblings with the AR form of CL, although

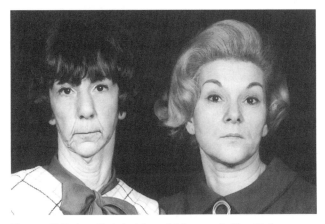

Figure 10.7 *An affected girl aged 16 years (left) with her normal mother (right). The characteristic nasal beaking and long upper lip are evident. From Beighton P, Bull JC, Edgerton MT Br J Plast Surg 1970; 23: 285–90*

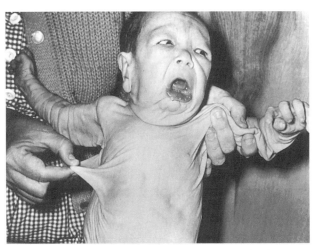

Figure 10.9 *A child with the severe AR form of CL. The skin is hyperextensible and lacks elastic recoil. From Grahame R, Beighton P Br J Dermatol 1971; 84: 326–9, by permission of Blackwell Science Ltd*

uptake of the radioisotope copper 64 was not increased[1]. In other affected persons, copper metabolism has been normal; in view of the inconsistency of these biochemical abnormalities their true pathological significance, if any, is uncertain.

According to Sephel et al[2] fibroblasts from 3 of a series of 6 CL patients produced diminished amounts of trophoelastin compared with normal controls. Elastin-specific messenger RNA levels indicated that this reduced expression of trophoelastin was regulated at a pretranslational level. The authors stated that in other strains diminished production of elastin did not appear to be the primary defect and they concluded that their observations confirmed the biochemical and ultrastructural heterogeneity of CL. In a similar investigation Olsen et al[3] established fibroblast cultures from 6 patients with CL and analysed elastin gene expression by means of RNA hybridization. No qualitative differences between control and CL messenger RNA could be detected, but quantitative reduction of elastin mRNA was consistently present.

Genetics

The AD and AR forms of classical CL have a similar external phenotype, but they are distinguished by the severity of the internal ramifications, especially pulmonary emphysema in the latter entity. It must be emphasized, however, that clinical expression is variable and in the absence of informative pedigree data accurate differentiation is not always possible.

Evidence for genetic heterogeneity was initially presented by Beighton[4]; two families with AD inheritance and two with AR transmission were documented and details of a further 12 affected kindreds in the literature were tabulated. Further reports followed and about 60 affected persons have now been recorded. The ratios of the AD and AR forms are approximately equal. The majority of case descriptions have emanated from Europe and North America and so far no obvious geographic or ethnic predilection has become apparent.

There are no reports of antenatal diagnosis in CL; however, in view of the histopathological changes, fetal skin biopsy would be a possible approach.

Differential diagnosis

Classical CL has been confused in the past with EDS, mainly because of the use of the redundant term 'cutis hyperelastica' for the latter disorder. The absence of connective tissue fragility and articular hypermobility readily distinguishes CL from EDS and there are no real grounds for confusion.

Classical CL must be differentiated from the syndromic and acquired forms of CL, as outlined below.

Syndromic cutis laxa

Cutis laxa with joint hypermobility and developmental delay[5]. Lax skin is syndromically associated with loose joints, mental retardation and developmental delay (Figure 10.10). This AR entity, which has been delineated within the last decade, differs from classical CL by virtue of these additional syndromic components.

De Barsy's syndrome[6]. In De Barsy's syndrome, corneal clouding, mental retardation, a progeroid facies and athetosis are associated with CL. The noncutaneous manifestations of this AR disorder permit differentiation from classical CL.

Geroderma osteodysplastica[7]. Geroderma osteodysplastica is characterized by loose joints, lax skin which is maximal on the face and extremities, mandibular prognathism and generalized osteoporosis. Vertebral collapse and a fracturing tendency are variable features.

Occipital horn syndrome[8]. In the occipital horn syndrome, which was initially termed 'X-linked cutis laxa' and classified as EDS IX, the skin is lax and mildly hyperextensible. Diagnostic features include hypermobile digits, bony protuberances of the occiput, limitation of extension of the elbows and knees, carpal bone coalescences, short clavicles, bladder diverticula and osteomalacia. Chronic diarrhoea and postural hypotension are variable features. Copper metabolism is abnormal in this disorder.

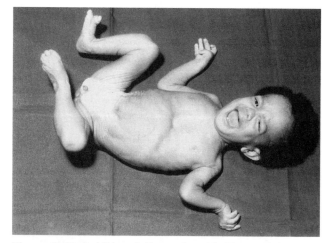

Figure 10.10 *A child aged 11 months with CL, retarded development and joint laxity. Thumb clasping and bilateral inguinal hernias are additional features. From Goldblatt J, Wallis C, Viljoen D et al Dysmorph Clin Genet 1988; **1**: 142–4, by permission of Blackwell Science Inc.*

Acquired cutis laxa

Primary generalized elastolysis[9]. Primary generalized elastolysis is an acquired form of CL of unknown aetiology, in which skin laxity develops insidiously in young adulthood[9] (Figure 10.11). This condition is slowly progressive; elastic tissues throughout the body are involved and vascular complications such as aortic dissection may develop.

Postinflammatory (autoimmune) cutis laxa. In this rare acquired form of CL, pendulous skin lesions develop after an illness characterized by urticarial eruptions and polyserositis. Glomerulonephritis is sometimes a complication and in some instances penicillin therapy has been incriminated as a possible precipitant. The condition may have an autoimmune basis[10].

Secondary or localized cutis laxa. Skin laxity develops in the late stages of pseudoxanthoma elasticum and it is a feature of long-term sun exposure. Sweet's syndrome comprises soft cutaneous plaques which are often associated with underlying malignancy, especially of the lymphatic system. The skin in these affected areas becomes lax when the lesions resolve. These conditions are easily differentiated from classical CL by their appearance and natural history.

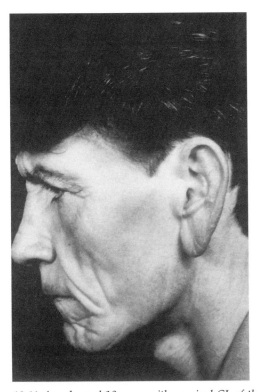

Figure 10.11 *A male aged 18 years with acquired CL of the insidious late-onset type. The facial skin and lobes of the ears are lax. From Reed WB, Horowitz RE, Beighton P* Arch Dermatol *1971;* **103***: 661–9. Copyright 1971, American Medical Association*

Treatment

There is no specific therapy for classical CL but the facial appearance can be improved by cosmetic surgery. There are no problems with tissue fragility or abnormal bleeding, healing is unimpaired and operation scars do not widen[11]. This approach is recommended in autosomal dominant CL, in which general health and lifespan are not compromised. In autosomal recessive CL, decisions concerning cosmetic surgery must be made against a background of cardiopulmonary complications and the poor prognosis for long-term survival.

It is likely that persons with CL are especially liable to acceleration of the normal aging process if the skin is exposed to excessive sunshine. For this reason there are positive indications for avoidance of sunbathing and the use of sunshades and screens.

Hernias and diverticula of the bowel and urinary tract respond to conventional surgical procedures. There are no inherent operative problems, other than those related to underlying cardiorespiratory involvement. The progressive pulmonary emphysema, pulmonary hypertension and cardiorespiratory failure are inexorable. There is no curative therapy and conventional palliative treatment is indicated.

References

1 Van Maldergem L, Vamos E, Liebaers I et al. Severe congenital cutis laxa with pulmonary emphysema: a family with 3 affected sibs. *Am J Med Genet* 1988; **31**: 455–64.

2 Sephel GC, Byers PH, Holbrook KA, Davidson JM. Heterogeneity of elastin expression in cutis laxa fibroblast strains. *J Invest Dermatol* 1989; **93**: 147–53.

3 Olsen DR, Fazio MJ, Shamban AT, Rosenbloom J, Uitto J. Cutis laxa: reduced elastin gene expression in skin fibroblasts cultures as determined by hybridizations with a homologous cDNA and an exon 1-specific oligonucleotide. *J Biol Chem* 1988; **263**: 6465–7.

4 Beighton PH. The dominant and recessive forms of cutis laxa. *J Med Genet* 1972; **9**: 216–21.

5 Goldblatt J, Wallis C, Viljoen D, Beighton P. Cutis laxa, retarded development and joint hypermobility syndrome. *Dys Morph Clin Genet* 1988; **1**: 142–4.

6 Pontz BF, Zepp F, Stoss H. Biochemical, morphological and immunological findings in a patient with a cutis laxa-associated inborn disorder (De Barsy syndrome). *Eur J Pediatr* 1986; **145** (5): 428–34.

7 Hunter AG. Is geroderma osteodysplastica underdiagnosed? *J Med Genet* 1988; **25**: 854–7.

8 Byers PH, Siegel RC, Holbrook KA et al. X-linked cutis laxa. *New Engl J Med* 1980; **303**: 61–5.

9 Reed WB, Horowitz RE, Beighton P. Acquired cutis laxa. *Arch Dermatol* 1971; **103**: 661–9.

10 Tsuji T, Imajo Y, Sawabe M et al. Acquired cutis laxa concomitant with nephrotic syndrome. *Arch Dermatol* 1987; **123**: 1211–16.

11 Beighton PH, Bull JC, Edgerton MT. Plastic surgery in cutis laxa. *Br J Plast Surg* 1970; **23**: 285–90.

Pseudoxanthoma elasticum

Definition

Pseudoxanthoma elasticum (PXE) is a genetically heterogeneous disorder which is characterized by yellowish flexural skin lesions and angioid streaks in the eye. Retinal haemorrhage and neovascularization may lead to significant visual handicap, while vascular occlusion and gastrointestinal tract bleeding are occasional complications. Fragmentation and calcification of elastic fibres is a consistent histological finding but the nature of the basic defect is unknown.

Clinical features

Induration of the skin of the neck, groin, axilla and other flexures produces a characteristic 'cobblestone' appearance (Figure 10.12). The involved areas have a yellowish tinge which may be difficult to discern in poor light. The skin changes commence in adolescence and progress slowly throughout life; in the later stages the affected skin becomes lax and hangs in folds, bearing some resemblance to classical cutis laxa (Figure 10.13). The cutaneous changes may be sufficiently severe to warrant cosmetic surgery.

In the eye, breaks in Bruch's membrane are visible on retinoscopy. These linear lesions resemble dilated blood vessels, hence the term 'angioid streaks' (Figure 10.14). Retinal haemorrhage may occur, and the ocular

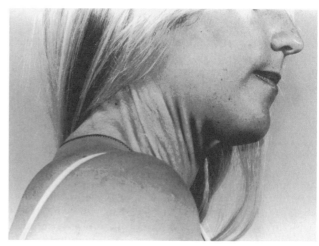

Figure 10.13 *PXE: the affected areas of the skin of the neck eventually become lax and pendulous. From Viljoen D L, Beatty S, Beighton P Br J Obstet Gynaecol 1987; **94**: 884–8, by permission of Blackwell Science Ltd*

complications of neovascularization and sclerosis can lead to blindness. It is noteworthy that there is no direct correlation between the severity of the skin and eye involvement.

The elastin of the tunica media of medium-sized arteries becomes calcified and these vessels may rupture or become blocked. These complications, which are relatively infrequent, can lead to cerebrovascular accidents, angina pectoris, myocardial infarction, intermittent claudication, gastrointestinal haemorrhage and epistaxis.

Pathology

Histopathological studies of the skin reveal calcification, clumping and fragmentation of elastin fibres [1]. Similar changes are evident in other elastin-containing

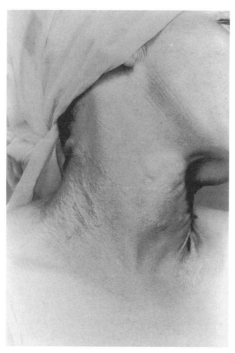

Figure 10.12 *PXE: a young woman with the characteristic indurated 'cobblestone' appearance of the skin of her neck*

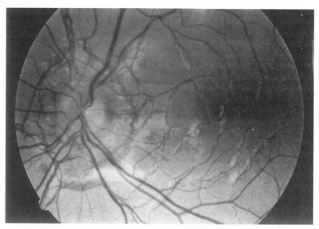

Figure 10.14 *PXE: the fundus of the eye. Angioid streaks, haemorrhage and fibrosis are evident. From Viljoen D J Med Genet 1988; **25**: 488–90, by permission*

tissues, notably the tunica media of small arteries. The histopathological appearances are the same in all forms of PXE. Electron microscopic investigations reveal that the microfibrillar component of the elastin is unchanged[2].

The alteration in the mechanical properties of the elastin of the affected skin eventually leads to laxity. Similarly, involvement of the walls of the small blood vessels leads to vascular rupture or blockage, which underlies the cardiovascular complications.

No consistent biochemical abnormalities have been demonstrated in PXE; in particular, there is no evidence to implicate abnormalities of calcium or copper metabolism. It seems likely that there is a fundamental defect in elastin, but so far no specific biomolecular changes have been reported. The elastin gene is situated on the short arm of chromosome 2, but restriction fragment length polymorphism studies in affected families have not yet yielded positive results.

Genetics

There is good evidence from family studies that PXE is genetically heterogeneous. There have been instances of pseudodominance, which has clouded this issue, but the evidence for distinct AD and AR modes of transmission is overwhelming. Following a survey of 200 patients in the UK, Pope [3–5] postulated that there were two AD and two AR forms of PXE. In a nationwide survey involving 64 affected persons in South Africa and Zimbabwe, Viljoen et al[6] identified an autosomal recessive form of PXE in which ocular problems predominate. The 39 affected persons were all members of the Afrikaans-speaking community, with Dutch and French-Huguenot antecedents. A similar subtype of PXE has been identified in a number of Belgian families[7].

The clinical characteristics of the various forms of PXE, based largely on Pope's investigations, are given below.

1. *AD type I* – severe skin, ocular and cardiovascular manifestations.
2. *AD type II* – localized skin changes with mild cardiovascular and eye involvement. Myopia, loose joints, high palate and scleral blueing are additional features.
3. *AR type I* – moderate skin, ocular and cardiovascular manifestations.
4. *AR type II* – widespread skin changes with few eye or vascular ramifications. Very rare.
5. *AR type III* (Afrikaner type) – moderate cutaneous and cardiovascular manifestations. Severe ocular complications.

Although the independent syndromic status of AD PXE (MIM 177850) and AR PXE (MIM 264800) is accepted, the existence of the subtypes as autonomous entities awaits biomolecular confirmation.

Differential diagnosis

The skin lesions of PXE bear some resemblance to solar elastosis and the normal aging process. Penicillamine therapy and vitamin D toxicity can also produce similar cutaneous changes; however, ocular involvement is not a feature of these disorders.

The lax folds of skin which develop in the later stages of the flexural lesions of PXE can mimic the various forms of cutis laxa; PXE is differentiated by the natural history, residual xanthomatous skin changes and by the presence of retinal angioid streaks.

Angioid retinal streaks occur in Paget's disease; this disorder is differentiated from PXE by the lack of skin involvement and the presence of characteristic skeletal abnormalities. Angioid retinal streaks can also occur in isolation and persons affected in this way have been shown to have histological abnormalities of the elastin in clinically normal skin[8]. The syndromic relationship of this disorder with classical PXE is problematic.

Treatment

There is no specific treatment for PXE but a variety of complications may necessitate specialized management.

Folds of lax skin may become very extensive and produce an unsightly appearance. Cosmetic surgery can provide considerable improvement but the affected skin may eventually deteriorate to its former pendulous condition[9].

Involvement of the eye can cause severe visual handicap and blindness may supervene. Laser therapy has a role in the management of intraocular haemorrhage, fibrosis and neovascularization.

Hypertension due to involvement of renal vessels and coronary and cerebral artery insufficiency warrant treatment on their own merits. Despite the vascular involvement and the multiplicity of potential hazards, pregnancy is unusually uncomplicated. It has been suggested that a low-calcium diet may be beneficial in PXE, but the value of this therapy remains unproved.

References

1 Sandberg LB, Soskel NT, Leslie JG. Elastin structure, biosynthesis and relation to disease states. *New Engl J Med* 1981; **304**: 566–79.
2 Ross R, Fialkow PJ, Altman LK. Fine structure alterations of elastic fibers in pseudoxanthoma elasticum. *Clin Genet* 1978; **13**: 213–23.
3 Pope FM. Two types of autosomal recessive pseudoxanthoma elasticum. *Arch Dermatol* 1974; **110**: 209–12.
4 Pope FM. Autosomal dominant pseudoxanthoma elasticum. *J Med Genet* 1974; **11**: 152–7.
5 Pope FM. Historical evidence for the genetic heterogeneity of pseudoxanthoma elasticum. *Br J Dermatol* 1975; **92**: 493–509.

6 Viljoen DL, Pope FM, Beighton P. Heterogeneity of pseudoxanthoma elasticum: delineation of a new form? *Clin Genet* 1987; **32**: 100–5.

7 De Paepe A, Viljoen DL, Matton M et al. Pseudoxanthoma elasticum: similar autosomal recessive subtype in Belgian and Afrikaner families. *Am J Med Genet* 1991; **38**: 16–20.

8 Lebwohl M, Phelps RG, Yannuzzi L et al. Diagnosis of pseudoxanthoma elasticum by scar biopsy in patients without characteristic skin lesions. *New Engl J Med* 1987; **317**: 347–50.

9 Viljoen DL, Bloch C, Beighton P. Plastic surgery in pseudoxanthoma elasticum. *Plast Reconstr Surg* 1990; **85**: 233–8.

Dermatofibrosis lenticularis disseminata with osteopoikilosis

Synonym: *Buschke–Ollendorff syndrome*

Definition

Dermatofibrosis lenticularis disseminata with osteopoikilosis (DLDO) or Buschke–Ollendorff syndrome is an innocuous AD disorder in which localized cutaneous nodules are associated with radiographically apparent multiple sclerotic foci in the bones (Figure 10.15).

Clinical features

The skin lesions of DLDO consist of one or more patches of indurated, yellowish, lentil-like, sessile naevi (Figure 10.16). Smooth, yellow-white plaques which resemble scars may also be present. These skin abnormalities are inconspicuous and of little clinical importance.

The bone abnormalities, which are usually detected by chance during radiographic investigations for an

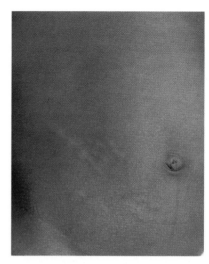

Figure 10.16 *Buschke–Ollendorff syndrome: flesh-coloured papules in a linear configuration (along the lines of Blaschko) (courtesy of Dr J. Harper)*

unrelated purpose, consist of numerous small, discrete patches of sclerosis. These osteopoikilotic foci congregate in the epiphyses and metaphyses of the tubular bones and many hundreds may be present. They do not cause any symptoms, and their major clinical significance lies in differentiation from neoplasia.

There have been isolated reports of affected persons with basal cell naevi and osteosarcoma, but these additional features are extremely rare.

Pathology

The cutaneous lesions have been variously reported as consisting of organized or disorderly masses of elastic or tissue collagen. It seems uncertain whether this histological variation is a reflection of relative maturity of the lesions or whether the different cutaneous abnormalities constitute pleomorphic manifestations of the same faulty gene. The skin in DLDO has been discussed in detail by Verbov and Graham[1].

Genetics

More than 300 cases have been reported. A number of large affected families have been described and AD inheritance is well documented[2,3]. Notable examples are 17 persons in four generations reported by Melnick[4] and 8 persons in three generations studied by Schoenberg[5]. Phenotypic expression is variable and the skin and bone lesions can occur together or separately in members of the same family[6].

Differential diagnosis

The sclerotic bony foci must be differentiated from multiple secondary neoplastic deposits. Their charac-

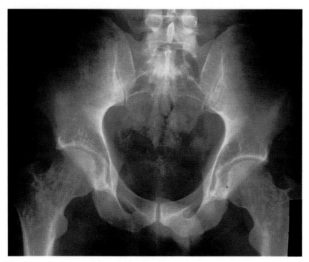

Figure 10.15 *Buschke–Ollendorff syndrome: extensive osteopoikilosis of the pelvis and femoral heads (courtesy of Dr J. Harper)*

teristic appearance and distribution readily permit this distinction. The skin lesions can resemble other connective tissue naevi, notably the shagreen patch in tuberous sclerosis and the familial cutaneous naevus group of disorders. Radiological demonstration of the bone changes of osteopoikilosis facilitates diagnostic confirmation.

Treatment

No treatment is required; DLDO is innocuous.

References

1 Verbov J, Graham R. Buschke–Ollendorf syndrome: disseminated dermatofibrosis with osteopoikilosis. *Clin Exp Derm* 1986; **11**: 17–26.
2 Szabo AD. Osteopoikilosis in a twin. *Clin Orthop* 1971; **79**: 156.
3 Young LW, Gershman I, Simon PR. Osteopoikilosis: familial documentation. *Am J Dis Child* 1980; **134**: 415–16.
4 Melnick JC. Osteopathia condensans disseminata (osteopoikilosis): study of a family of four generations. *Am J Roentgenol* 1959; **82**: 229.
5 Schoenberg H. Osteopoikilia with dermofibrosis lenticularis disseminata (Buschke–Ollendorff syndrome). *Klin Paediatr* 1975; **187**: 123.
6 Berlin R, Hedensio B, Lilja B, Linder L. Osteopoikilosis: a clinical and genetic study. *Acta Med Scand* 1967; **181**: 305.

Wrinkly skin syndrome

Definition

Wrinkly skin syndrome (WSS) is a very rare AR disorder in which wrinkling of the skin of the dorsum of the hands and feet, evident at birth, is associated with an increased number of palmar and plantar creases, microcephaly and mental retardation. About 10 cases have been reported.

Clinical features

As so few affected persons have been documented, the extent of the clinical manifestations is uncertain. Consistent features seem to be wrinkly skin on the abdomen and dorsal surfaces of the extremities, supernumerary creases on the palms of the hands and soles of the feet, microcephaly and low intelligence. Stunted stature, developmental delay, myopia, hip joint dysplasia, hypotonia, prominent venous plexus, atrial septal aneurysm and articular laxity have been present in some patients but not in others. The majority of case reports have concerned affected children and the long-term natural history is unknown.

Pathology

Studies of skin biopsy specimens have yielded conflicting results; Gazit et al[1] and Goodman et al[2] could not demonstrate any abnormalities of cutaneous histology, whereas Casamassima et al[3] noted a decrease in the number and length of elastin fibres from an affected area. There was no fragmentation of elastin, and electron microscopy did not reveal any significant changes. The chromosomes were normal and no biochemical changes have been recorded.

Genetics

Every patient with WSS so far reported has had a Middle Eastern background. The WSS was first described by Gazit et al[1] in affected sisters from an Iraqi Jewish family. An infant brother, aged 3 months, was also thought to be affected but the stigmata were mild and the diagnosis could not be confirmed. Goodman et al[2] subsequently reported affected sisters from an Iranian Jewish family, while Karrar et al[4] documented a Saudi Arabian brother and sister with the condition. Casamassima et al[3] reported a Malaysian girl with WSS. Her parents were Moslems, with antecedents in the Middle East. In each reported family the parents have been unaffected and consanguineous and, although formal segregation analysis has not yet been undertaken, there is little doubt that the WSS is an AR trait.

Differential diagnosis

The diagnosis of WSS is not necessarily an easy matter but, on the other hand, the syndrome is not likely to be confused with other genetic connective tissue disorders. The WSS is differentiated from the various forms of cutis laxa by the limited distribution of lax skin and by the presence of additional features, notably the excessive palmar creases and mental retardation. The EDS and PXE differ by virtue of additional syndromic stigmata.

Treatment

No specific therapy is available. The inconsistent complications warrant management on their own merits.

References

1 Gazit E, Goodman RM, Katznelson MB, Rotem Y. The wrinkly skin syndrome: a new heritable disorder of connective tissue. *Clin Genet* 1973; **4**: 186–92.
2 Goodman RM, Duksin D, Legum C et al. The wrinkly skin syndrome and cartilage hair hypoplasia in sibs of the same family. In: Papadatos CJ, Bartsocas CS, eds. *Progress in Clinical and Biological Research*. 104: *Skeletal Dysplasias*. Alan J. Liss, New York, 1982; 205–14.

3 Casamassima AC, Wesson SK, Conlon CJ, Weiss FH. Wrinkly skin syndrome; phenotype and additional manifestations. *Am J Med Genet* 1987; **27**: 885–93.

4 Karrar ZA, Elidrissy ATH, Al Arabi K, Adam KA. The wrinkly skin syndrome: a report of two siblings from Saudi Arabia. *Clin Genet* 1983; **23**: 308–310.

Connective tissue naevi

The connective tissue naevi are a heterogeneous group of disorders in which nodular skin lesions result from aggregation of collagen or elastin. Collagen naevi may be minor components of pleiotrophic genetic syndromes, as with the shagreen patch of tuberous sclerosis, or occur in isolation, as in familial cutaneous collagenoma and familial reactive collagenosis (see below). Similarly, elastin naevi are a consistent component of pseudoxanthoma elasticum and dermatofibrosis lenticularis disseminata with osteopoikilosis and also occur in isolation or infrequently in association with other connective tissue disorders. The nosology, clinical manifestations and histopathology of the cutaneous connective tissue naevi have been reviewed in detail by Uitto et al[1].

Reference

1 Uitto J, Santa Cruz DJ, Eisen AZ. Connective tissue nevi of the skin. *J Am Acad Dermatol* 1980; **3**: 441–61.

Familial cutaneous collagenoma

Familial cutaneous collagenoma (FCC)[1,2] is characterized by the presence of multiple small skin nodules, composed of dense collagen fibres, which are most often present on the back. The nodules are usually an innocuous AD trait but they may also be syndromically associated with cardiomyopathy and hypogonadism. It is not known whether this condition is an autonomous entity or a more complete phenotypic expression of FCC.

References

1 Sacks HN, Crawley IS, Ward JA, Fine RM. Familial cardiomyopathy, hypogonadism and collagenoma. *Ann Intern Med* 1980; **93**: 813–17.

2 Uitto J, Santa-Cruz DJ, Eisen AZ. Familial cutaneous collagenoma: genetic studies on a family. *Br J Dermatol* 1979; **101**: 185–9.

Familial reactive collagenosis

Familial reactive collagenosis (FRC) [1–3] is a form of connective tissue naevus characterized by recurrent eruptions of umbilicated nodules. These lesions, which result from extrusion of collagen fibres through the dermis, are precipitated by trauma and aggravated by cold weather.

Several sets of affected siblings have been reported and it is likely that the disorder is an AR trait. An inconsistent association with diabetes mellitus and renal failure has been documented.

References

1 Kanan MW. Familial reactive perforating collagenosis and intolerance to cold. *Br J Dermatol* 1974; **91**: 405–14.

2 Mehregan AH, Schwartz OD, Livingood CS. Reactive perforating collagenosis. *Arch Dermatol* 1967; **96**: 277–82.

3 Nair BKH, Sarojini PA, Basheer AM, Nair CHK. Reactive perforating collagenosis. *Br J Dermatol* 1974; **91**: 399–403.

Elastosis perforans serpiginosa

Elastosis perforans serpiginosa (EPS)[1] is an elastic tissue naevus which presents as raised, annular, reddish, indurated skin lesions (Figure 10.17). These nodules can occur in isolation, either sporadically or as an AD trait, and they are occasionally encountered in Down's syndrome, osteogenesis imperfecta and Marfan's syndrome.

There is semantic and nosological confusion concerning the use of the eponymous term 'Miescher's elastoma' as an alternative designation for EPS. This problem has been compounded by the fact that

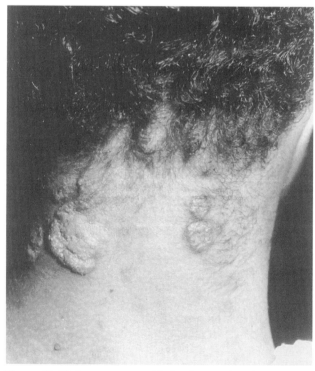

Figure 10.17 *A young man with the characteristic lesions of EPS on the back of his neck*

Miescher's name was also applied to a skin lesion that is now known as actinic granuloma. In order to clarify these issues there is a trend towards discarding the eponym in favour of descriptive designations for these disorders.

Reference

1 Ayala F, Donofrio P. Elastosis perforans serpiginosa: report of a family. *Dermatologica* 1983; **166**: 32–7.

Connective tissue disorders with minor skin involvement

Minor changes are present in the skin in a number of important heritable connective tissue disorders. The dermatological features of the most important of these conditions are briefly outlined in this section.

Marfan's syndrome

Marfan's syndrome[1] is a well-known AD disorder in which the major features are tall stature, limb length disproportion, arachnodactyly, high palate, ectopia lentis, and aortic dilatation and dissection. The phenotype is very variable and in 'partial' cases diagnosis can be difficult. Despite intensive investigations the biomolecular defect in Marfan's syndrome has not yet been elucidated, but there is some evidence to incriminate a connective tissue component, fibrillin.

Striae distensae, maximal over the shoulders, thighs and abdomen, are frequently present in Marfan's syndrome. It is likely that they are a reflection of subtle alterations in the mechanical properties of the skin in the disorder and they are of value in the diagnostic process.

Reference

1 Pyeritz RE, McKusick VA. The Marfan syndrome: diagnosis and management. *New Engl J Med* 1979; **300**: 772–7.

Osteogenesis imperfecta

Osteogenesis imperfecta[1] is a well-known heterogeneous disorder in which bone fragility leads to frequent fractures. Blue sclerae, wormian bones in the cranial sutures and presenile hearing loss are variable features. Abnormalities of type I collagen have been demonstrated in some forms of the disorder.

Affected persons sometimes bruise easily and occasionally skin fragility is present; these features are of minor degree and are overshadowed by the skeletal complications. Elastosis perforans serpiginosa is an infrequent concomitant of osteogenesis imperfecta.

There is genetic heterogeneity with more than one locus involved. Linkage to *COL1A1* (17q21.31–22.05) and *COL1A2* (7q21.3–22.1) has been observed in some forms of osteogenesis imperfecta.

Reference

1 Sykes B, Ogilvie D, Wordsworth P, Anderson J, Jones N. Osteogenesis imperfecta is linked to both type I collagen structural genes. *Lancet* 1986; **ii**: 69–72.

Spondyloepimetaphyseal dysplasia with joint laxity

Spondyloepimetaphyseal dysplasia with joint laxity (SEMDJL) is an AR dwarfing skeletal dysplasia in which gross joint laxity leads to dislocations and spinal malalignment[1,2]. Affected persons have a characteristic facies and the sclerae sometimes have a bluish tinge. The skin in SEMDJL is hyperextensible and, as in EDS, it springs back to its former position following distension. The connective tissues are not fragile, and abnormal splitting and scarring does not occur.

References

1 Beighton P, Gericke G, Kozlowski K, Grobler L. The manifestations and natural history of spondylo-epimetaphyseal dysplasia with joint laxity. *Clin Genet* 1984; **26**: 308–17.
2 Beighton P. Spondyloepimetaphyseal dysplasia with joint laxity (SEMDJL). *J Med Genet* 1994; **31**: 136–40.

Acknowledgements

The author is grateful for expert comment during the preparation of this review from Professor Norma Saxe, Dr Denis Viljoen and Dr Ingrid Winship. Thanks are due to Mrs Gillian Shapley for typing the manuscript with efficiency and dedication. The author is also appreciative of support from the South African Medical Research Council, the Mauerberger Foundation, the Harry Crossley Fund and the University of Cape Town Staff Research Fund.

Chapter 11

Vascular disorders

G. B. Colver and T. J. Ryan

Introduction

The folklore, history and literary aspects of vascular disorders are well described by Mulliken and Young[1]. The classification is discussed by Mulliken[2] and by Pasyk[3].

Some knowledge of embryology and normal anatomy is needed in order to understand the vascular disorders that affect skin. Fetal skin[4] develops its first blood vessels in the second month, but initially there are no connections with deeper vessels. Gradually endothelial proliferation below the epidermis and around sweat glands and hair follicles leads to two layers of capillaries during the third month in utero. Developing adnexal capillaries may provide anastomotic channels. The deeper plexus eventually becomes the site of adipose tissue with its comparatively rich capillary bed[5]. Differentiation into arterioles and venules is modified by anatomical position, surrounding tissue and flow characteristics.

The red skin of the newborn has a huge number of upper dermal capillaries, most of which run horizontally. Slowly papillary loops form tangentially to the overlying epidermis, but it is interesting that some sites (e.g. the cheeks) retain a predominantly horizontal pattern and their redness into adult life.

There is much regional variation; however, the normal adult pattern consists of a subpapillary horizontal plexus connected to deeper periadnexal vessels by vertically oriented capillaries. The papillary loops which arise in the subpapillary plexus often bridge arterioles and venules. Other arteriovenous anastomoses contain glomus structures which can open or close the shunt and control thermoregulation. Pasyk et al[6] estimated the numbers of capillaries independently in the papillary and deeper dermis in different regions of the body. They emphasized that a thin epidermis or dermis is usually correlated with a scant vascular bed – a relationship also emphasized by Ryan[7]. Ryan and Curri[5] have drawn attention to the richest capillary bed of subcutaneous adipose tissue.

In this chapter diseases are classified into four clinical groups according to the nature of the vascular lesion (Table 11.1). Classification of vascular disorders is difficult anyway but it is complicated by a plethora of synonyms on the one hand and a disagreement about the meaning of terms on the other. The *Gould Medical Dictionary* defines telangiectasia as 'dilatation of groups of capillaries forming elevated, dark red, wart-like spots varying in size from 1 to 7 mm'[8]. In this chapter the term 'telangiectasia' is used to refer to permanently dilated small blood vessels, to distinguish them from erythema, flush or blush. They may be punctate, stellate, wiry, in leashes, etc. and are usually described in this way when individual vessels can be identified with the naked eye. They are dilatations in the upper dermis, hence their visibility. These diseases are discussed below. Confusion arises when the telangiectases are seen in densely arranged

Table 11.1 *Classification of genetic vascular disorders of the skin*

I	Telangiectasias
II	Port-wine stains and telangiectatic naevi
III	Cutis marmorata
IV	Palpable haemangiomas

groups and are called a 'salmon patch' or 'port-wine stain'. These conditions are described in the second section of this chapter. The third section deals with diseases associated with the vascular pattern called cutis marmorata, and the last section deals with palpable haemangiomas and venous malformations.

For clinicians this classification is easy to use. In reference the reader need only decide which category a patient's skin lesions fall into and then quickly scan the relevant section. Other classifications often useful for understanding mechanisms are based on endothelial characteristics, growth dynamics, anatomical location or histopathology[3].

In life the cutaneous blood vessels change their size and pattern in response to biological variables. Flushing, healing granulation tissue and the changes of age are all very common. Exaggeration of these processes may be seen in pathological states, e.g. flushing in rosacea, hyperproliferation in a pyogenic granuloma and premature aging in some syndromes. There are other known factors that influence blood vessels; e.g. dilatation may be induced by anoxia, hormones or infection. Some insight has been gained into the pathogenesis of port-wine stains: they were first shown to be due to a progressive ectasia[9] and then the neuronal component of the dermis, in the perivascular zone, was found to be depleted[10]. A complete analysis of all the properties of endothelium and its surrounding connective tissue, pericytes, fibroblasts and mast cells has yet to be applied to the whole spectrum of birthmarks. In spite of a huge expansion in our understanding of the vascular system, we remain ignorant of the causes of vascular dysplasia and hamartoma. Thus the solitary dilated vessels in hereditary haemorrhagic telangiectasia and the multiple cavernous tumours in the blue rubber bleb naevus syndrome appear in normal skin without an obvious trigger factor. Eventually it would be ideal to have a classification based on aetiology, but this seems a long way off.

Some important aspects of treatment of abnormal vasculature can also be dealt with here because they are broadly applicable to many of the diseases to be discussed. Telangiectases may be disfiguring if seen on an exposed body site, particularly the face, and there is a substantial literature on stigmatization and the emotional impact of vascular birthmarks[11]. Cautery, sclerotherapy and laser treatment all have a role[12]. Port-wine stains are now more amenable to treatment than was the case even in the 1980s. There has been a rapid transition from the prelaser era, through an optimistic but not always successful phase using long pulses with argon lasers, into the ultra-short-pulse tunable dye laser era in which we now find ourselves. The flashlamp-pulsed dye laser has proved to be a significant advance in treatment, with especially good results in children[13]. The current management of vascular birthmarks has been reviewed[14].

References

1 Mulliken JB, Young AE. Vascular birthmarks in folklore, history, art and literature. In: Mulliken JB, Young AE, eds. *Vascular Birthmarks, Haemangiomas and Malformations*. WB Saunders, Philadelphia, 1988; 3–23.
2 Mulliken JB. Classification of vascular birthmarks. In: Mulliken JB, Young AE, eds. *Vascular Birthmarks, Haemangiomas and Malformations*. WB Saunders, Philadelphia, 1988; 24–38.
3 Pasyk KA Classification and clinical and histopathological features of haemangiomas and other vascular malformations. In: Ryan TJ, Cherry GW, eds. *Vascular Birthmarks*. Oxford University Press, 1987; 1–7.
4 Johnson CL, Holbrook KA. Development of human embryonic and fetal dermal vasculature. *J Invest Dermatol* 1989; **93**: 2 (suppl.): 10–17S.
5 Ryan TJ, Curri SB. Cutaneous adipose tissue. *Clin Dermatol* 1989; **7**: 87–92.
6 Pasyk KA, Thomas SV, Hassett CA, Cherry GW, Faller R. Regional differences in capillary density of the normal human dermis. *Plast Reconstr Surg* 1989; **83**: 939–45.
7 Ryan TJ. The blood vessels of the skin. In: Jarrett A, ed. *The Physiology and Pathophysiology of the Skin*, vol. 2. Academic Press, London, 1973; 578.
8 *Blakiston's Gould Medical Dictionary*. 4th ed. McGraw-Hill, New York, 1979; 1352.
9 Barsky SH, Rosen S, Geer DE, Noe JM. The nature and evolution of port wine stains: a computer assisted study. *J Invest Dermatol* 1980; **74**: 154–7.
10 Smoller BR, Rosen S. Port wine stains: a disease of altered modulation of blood vessels. *Arch Dermatol* 1986; **122**: 177–9.
11 Harrison AM. The emotional impact of a vascular birthmark. In: Mulliken JB, Young AB, eds. *Vascular Birthmarks, Haemangiomas and Malformations*. WB Saunders, Philadelphia, 1989; 454–62.
12 Goldman MP, Bennett RG. Treatment of telangiectasia. *J Am Acad Dermatol* 1987; **17**: 167–82.
13 Tan OT, Sherwood K, Gilchrest BA. Treatment of children with port wine stains using the flashlamp-pulsed tunable dye laser. *New Engl J Med* 1989; **320**: 416–21.
14 Enjolras O, Mulliken JB. The current management of vascular birthmarks. *Pediatr Dermatol* 1993; **10**: 311–33.

Telangiectasias

The conditions in this group are listed in Table 11.2.

Hereditary haemorrhagic telangiectasia

Synonym: *Rendu–Osler–Weber syndrome*

Definition

Hereditary haemorrhagic telangiectasia (HHT) is a disease affecting blood vessels throughout the body, characterized by the development of telangiectases on skin and mucous membranes. The lesions have a tendency to bleed. Arteriovenous fistulas arising in other organs lead to complications.

Clinical features

Several types of lesion may appear. The most common are punctate (Figure 11.1) and many are wiry. Telangiectatic mats, which are characteristic of the CREST syndrome, are rarely seen. Papular lesions up to several millimetres in height and width are a further variety, and on the lips soft bags of blood resembling venous lakes may occur. Telangiectases can affect any part of the skin but the face, trunk and upper limbs are the most usual sites. The face and hands may be peppered with vessels.

The conjunctivae, nasal and oral or pharyngeal mucosae may reveal visible vessels. Diascopy of lingual lesions often reveals a characteristic single hugely dilated vessel. Any part of the gastrointestinal tract may be involved.

Presentation is usually with epistaxis in childhood or puberty. In early years there may be epistaxis without obvious telangiectasia of the nasal mucosa or

Table 11.2 *The telangiectasias* [1]

Hereditary haemorrhagic telangiectasia
Hereditary benign telangiectasia
Angiokeratoma of Mibelli
Haber's syndrome
Hereditary acrolabial telangiectasia
Angioma serpiginosum
Nieden's syndrome
Telangiectases and glomerulonephritis [2]
Hereditary phlebectasia of the lips [3]
Telangiectasia, spondoepiphyseal dysplasia, etc. [4]

Others
   Photosensitivity disorders: Cockayne's syndrome,
     Bloom's syndrome, etc.
   Atrophic/premature aging syndromes: Werner's
     syndrome, progeria, Goltz's syndrome, etc.
   DNA disorders: ataxia-telangiectasia, Coat's
     disease, etc.
   Metabolic storage diseases: Anderson–Fabry
     syndrome, fucosidosis, mucopolysaccharidosis I
   Ectodermal dysplasias (Berlin)

References

1 Bean WB. *Vascular Spiders and Related Lesions of the Skin.* CC Thomas, Springfield, 1958; 372.
2 Sherwood MC, Pincott JR, Goodwin FJ, Dillon MJ. Dominantly inherited glomerulonephritis and an unusual skin disease. *Arch Dis Child* 1987; **62**: 1278–80.
3 Reed W. Hereditary phlebectasias of the lips. *Arch Dermatol* 1976; **112**: 712–14.
4 Levin MP, Olson JC, Ruttum MS, Esterly NB. Two sisters with telangiectasia, spondyloepiphyseal dysplasia, hypothyroidism, neovascularization, and tractional retinal detachments: a new entity? *Pediatr Dermatol* 1989; **6**: 178–84.

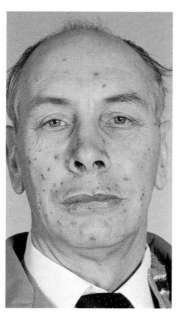

Figure 11.1 *Hereditary haemorrhagic telangiectasia: macular and papular lesions on the face and lips*

elsewhere. The skin lesions lag a little behind and may not appear until the age of 20–30 years. Bleeding from all sites increases with age. Blood loss may be frequent and severe. One-third of patients have mild nasal bleeding, in one-third bleeding is moderate and in one-third it is incapacitating[1]. Both open and occult loss may be life-threatening, but the picture is often of iron deficiency anaemia from chronic loss. When the patient is anaemic the telangiectases may be invisible. It is important to note that whether the clinical presentation is anaemia, bleeding or some complication due to involvement of other organs, there may be only subtle skin changes which are easily missed. The disease is often more prominent in pregnancy.

Pulmonary arteriovenous fistulas (PAVF) occur particularly in some families and may be responsible for round shadows on the chest radiograph, clubbing and dyspnoea with cyanosis. As many as 25% of all patients with HHT may have PAVF[2], and a family history of HHT can be obtained in 50–70% of patients with PAVF. Cerebrovascular malformations are sometimes present, even in the absence of pulmonary lesions, and often lead to neurological symptoms. There is also an increased risk of cerebral abscess due to septic microemboli[2].

Hepatosplenomegaly and cirrhosis may complicate liver arteriovenous malformations; it is also thought that repeated blood transfusions may in some instances have led to cirrhosis as a result of hepatitis B or non-A, non-B hepatitis[3].

Pathology

Dilated vessels are seen in the papillary and subpapillary dermis. The abnormal vessels are probably venules and contain no pericytes. The bleeding tendency may be related to the abnormal surrounding connective tissue, the fibrils of which show a disturbed banding. Alternatively, increased plasminogen activator in the vessels may lead to excessive fibrinolysis. A review of reported dysfunction of the coagulation system and a detailed investigation in 8 related patients has been given by Steel et al[4].

Genetics

The disease is inherited as an autosomal dominant trait with high penetrance and variable expression. Twenty per cent may have no family history. The homozygous form is probably lethal. No definite linkage has been shown between human leucocyte antigens and HHT.

Differential diagnosis

The skin lesions may be confused with those of hereditary benign telangiectasia. Multiple spider angiomata show a different morphology. Dermatomal telangiectasia is usually unilateral but may occasionally be bilateral. The CREST syndrome may be familial and cause mucosal telangiectasia with occasional haemorrhage[5]. The rare concurrence of CREST and HHT leads to a severe vascular dysplasia. Anticentromere antibody may help to differentiate the diseases[6]. Workers using tar may develop widespread telangiectasia on the face, arms, neck and hands, and a similar phenomenon has been seen in workers at an aluminium factory[7]. Finally, it should be remembered that 5% of the population have 3–10 telangiectases of the lips, hands and feet[8].

Treatment

The primary lesions on the skin may be treated by electrodesiccation or cautery. More sophisticated cautery by laser has also been used and topical aminocaproic acid was beneficial in some cases. There is no known treatment for the underlying defect. Oral iron supplementation and hepatitis B vaccination are wise precautions.

Repeated or severe bleeding occasionally requires more drastic surgery such as excision of the entire nasal mucosa, removal of segments of the bowel, liver or lungs.

It is important to exclude a bleeding diathesis because HHT is rarely associated with von Willebrand's disease or hepatic dysfunction. High-dose oestrogen therapy is thought to induce squamous metaplasia of the nasal mucosa and thus have some protective effect. A randomized, double-blind trial with oestrogen in 31 patients showed no significant effect[9].

References

1 Peery WH. Clinical spectrum of hereditary haemorrhagic telangectasia. *Am J Med* 1987; **82**: 989–97.
2 Adams HP, Subbiah B, Bosch EP. Neurologic aspects of hereditary haemorrhagic telangiectasia. *Arch Neurol* 1977; **34**: 101–4.
3 Daly JJ, Schiller AL. The liver in hereditary haemorrhagic telangiectasia (Osler–Weber–Rendu disease). *Am J Med* 1976; **60**: 723.
4 Steel D, Bovill EG, Golden E, Tindle BH. Hereditary haemorrhagic telangiectasia. *Am J Clin Pathol* 1988; **90**: 274–8.
5 Frayha RA, Tabbara KF, Geha RS. Familial CREST syndrome with SICCA complex. *J Rheumatol* 1977; **4**: 53–8.
6 Stolz W, Ring J, Meurer M. Differential diagnosis of Osler's disease and CREST syndrome. *Hautarzt* 1988; **39**: 371–4.
7 Theriault G, Cordier S, Harvey R. Skin telangiectases in workers at an aluminium plant. *New Engl J Med* 1980; **303**: 1278–87.
8 Brown GR. Cutaneous telangiectases on lips and extremities. *Arch Intern Med* 1963; **112**: 889–91.
9 Vase P. Estrogen treatment of hereditary haemorrhagic telangiectasia. A double blind clinical trial. *Acta Med Scand* 1981; **209**: 393.

Hereditary benign telangiectasia

Definition

Hereditary benign telangiectasia[1,2] is a condition whose only feature is the development, early in life, of multiple cutaneous telangiectases.

Clinical features

The major description of this disease was by Ryan and Wells[1]. Seven families were studied, in each of which several individuals had multiple telangiectases on the face, upper limbs and lower chest. Mucosal lesions were rare but one individual had several on the soft palate. The lesions were more numerous in light-exposed areas. None of the affected individuals developed telangiectases in the first year of life, and the onset was generally between 2 and 12 years, the condition being progressive into middle age and exacerbated by pregnancy. In later life the vessels were less readily visible. The vessels were not all punctate telangiectases; some were wiry and others arborizing. The disease was not associated with vessel abnormalities in other organs or a tendency to bleed.

Pathology

Under the capillary microscope there is a decrease in papillary vessels and dilatation of the subpapillary horizontal plexus. The ready visibility of these vessels is due to upper dermal atrophy.

Genetics

Hereditary benign telangiectasia is a rare disease and is probably inherited as an autosomal dominant trait. Every affected person has an affected parent, and the pedigrees are all compatible with a dominant inheritance. Marked interfamily variation is seen. Females are apparently more commonly affected, but it may simply be that men complain less about this relatively trivial condition; another reason why women may notice it more is the exacerbation seen in pregnancy.

Differential diagnosis

The differential diagnosis is the same as for HHT. In some cases it would not be possible to differentiate this disorder from the changes of aging and sun exposure, were it not for the early onset.

Treatment

Local destruction of individual vessels can be undertaken. Cosmetic camouflage may be useful for extensive changes on the face.

References

1 Ryan TJ, Wells RS. Hereditary benign telangiectasia. *Trans St John's Hosp Dermatol Soc* 1971; **57**: 148–56.
2 Gold MH, Eramo L, Prendiville JS. Hereditary benign telangiectasia. *Pediatr Dermatol* 1989; **6**: 194–7.

Angiokeratoma of Mibelli

Definition

Angiokeratoma of Mibelli is a cutaneous disorder characterized by the onset – usually in adolescence – of dark-red, warty papules on predominantly acral sites[1].

Clinical features

Lesions are initially punctate but enlarge into dark-red, warty papules. Girls are more frequently affected. Onset is often in adolescence with the appearance of lesions on the digits, elbows and knees, but sparing volar surfaces. Lesions rarely exceed 0.5 cm in diameter. The common association with chilblains suggests that cold injury plays a part in the induction of angiokeratoma.

Pathology

Hyperkeratosis, acanthosis and dilatation of capillaries in the papillary dermis are the main features.

Genetics

A family with nodular lesions on the leg has been described in which the inheritance was autosomal dominant[2].

Differential diagnosis

Other causes of angiokeratomas must be excluded[3]. In Anderson–Fabry syndrome (Chapter 7) the lesions may be associated with attacks of pain, usually of the extremities. Another type of angiokeratoma affects the scrotum, and the lesions increase in number with age (Figure 11.2).

Treatment

Troublesome lesions can be excised or treated by electrodesiccation, liquid nitrogen or argon laser.

References

1 Mibelli V. Di una nuova forma di cheratosi 'angiocheratoma'. *Gior Stal Mal Ven* 1889; **30**: 285.
2 Smith RBW, Prior IAM, Park RG. Angiokeratoma of Mibelli: a family with nodular lesions of the legs. *Aust J Dermatol* 1968; **9**: 329.
3 Marsden J, Allen Widespread angiokeratomas without evidence of metabolic disease. *Arch Dermatol* 1987; **123**(9): 1125–7.

Haber's syndrome

The first description of Haber's syndrome was of 3 patients in one family with a rosacea-like eruption on the face[1]. Telangiectases were obvious on the face

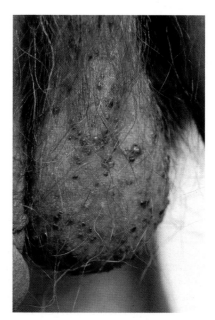

Figure 11.2 *Angiokeratomas of the scrotum*

with small papules, a few pitted scars and prominent follicles. The patients all had multiple intraepidermal carcinomas on the trunk and limbs. Another report[2] of a familial incidence described similar facial lesions, multiple pigmented scaly lesions concentrated particularly in the axillae, and widespread xerosis – there were no lesions of Bowen's disease.

In both families inheritance was as a dominant trait.

There is a report of Haber's syndrome and Dowling–Degos disease[3].

References

1 Sanderson KV, Wilson HTH. Habers syndrome. *Br J Dermatol* 1965; **77**: 1–8.
2 Kikuchi I, Saita B, Inoue S. Habers syndrome. *Arch Dermatol* 1981; **117**: 321–4.
3 Kikuchi I, Crovato F, Rebora A. Haber's syndrome and Dowling–Degos disease. *Int J Dermatol* 1988; **27**: 96–7.

Hereditary acrolabial telangiectasia

One family has been reported with hereditary acrolabial telangiectasia[1]. A mother and 2 daughters had extensive telangiectases causing a blue discolouration of the lips, areolae, nail beds and (to a lesser extent) chest and dorsum of hands. All 3 had severe varicosities of the lower limbs and 2 suffered from migraine.

Reference

1 Millns JL, Dicken CH. Hereditary acrolabial telangiectasia. *Arch Dermatol* 1979; **115**: 474–8.

Angioma serpiginosum

Definition

Angioma sespiginosum is a localized, slowly spreading ectasia of capillaries which form punctate and papular lesions in serpiginous patterns.

Clinical features

Although angioma serpiginosum may appear at any age, it usually appears in adolescence and in females (90%)[1]. It is most common on the lower limbs and usually affects one side only. The first sign is a red blush with minute red to purple puncta. Most of the vessels cannot be fully blanched by pressure. Groups of new lesions appear peripherally with some central resolution. New groups are not always contiguous, but the resulting overall serpiginous pattern is often naevoid. Occasionally a large area may be covered.

With time papular lesions may appear and even develop a degree of lichenification. Areas more like a port-wine stain, with a verrucous surface, were seen in one case[2]. New lesions may appear in adult life. There are no symptoms and no common associations, but ocular and nervous system involvement has been reported[3].

Pathology

One or more dilated capillaries are seen in the dermal papillae and subpapillary venous plexus. The capillary walls are thickened and show ultrastructural abnormalities of the endothelium[4].

Genetics

Most cases are sporadic but families have been reported where several members are affected[5]. The author has seen 2 sisters, 4 years apart in age, who both developed angioma serpiginosum affecting the left lower leg when they were 14 years old. The disease probably has an autosomal dominant inheritance in these families, but penetrance is higher in females.

Differential diagnosis

Angioma serpiginosum must be differentiated from the pigmented purpuras, localized forms of angiokeratoma, and from generalized essential telangiectasia which presents a decade or two later in life and in which the dilatations are less discrete, affecting the full length of many vessels.

Treatment

Camouflage make-up may be used for small areas. Local destruction of vessels, e.g. cryotherapy, electrodesiccation, infrared coagulation and laser therapy, does not give a uniform result, but tends to give patchy improvement to what is already a patchy appearance.

References

1 Frain-Bell W. Angioma serpiginosum. *Br J Dermatol* 1957; **69**: 251–68.
2 Michalowski R, Urban J. Atypical angioma serpiginosum: a case report. *Dermatologica* 1982; **164**: 331–3.
3 Gautier-Smith PC, Sanders MD, Sanderson KV. Ocular and nervous system involvement in angioma serpiginosum. *Br J Ophthalmol* 1971; **55**: 433–43.
4 Kumakiri M, Katoh N, Miura Y. Angioma serpiginosum. *J Cutan Pathol* 1980; **7**: 410–21.
5 Marriott PJ, Munro DD, Ryan TJ. Angioma serpiginosum: familial incidence. *Br J Dermatol* 1975; **93**: 701–6.

Nieden's syndrome

The early development of facial and upper limb telangiectasia may be associated with cataracts. In one example there were familial cases[1]. Associated anomalies included cardiac valve defects and hyper-pigmentation of the neck.

Reference

1 Waardenburg PJ, Franceschetti A, Klein D. *Genetics and Ophthalmology.* CC Thomas, Springfield, 1961; 906.

Port-wine stains and telangiectatic naevi

The conditions in this group are summarized in Table 11.3.

Familial multiple telangiectatic naevi

Merlob and Reisner[1] reported an index case where the patient had a symmetrical naevus on the forehead, shaped like a V, with the point at the glabella; she also had a telangiectatic patch on the nape of the neck. Her sister, brother, mother and grandmother all had forehead lesions and two of them also had a nape lesion. This was concluded to be an autosomal dominant condition. The glabella lesion would normally disappear in the first 4 years of life. There were no associated abnormalities.

In another family a girl, her two non-identical twin siblings, their mother and maternal aunt, all had multiple naevi flammei. There were no other anomalies[2].

Transmission of naevus flammeus through four generations has been reported[3]; the pedigree suggested autosomal dominant inheritance with incomplete penetrance.

References

1 Merlob P, Reisner SH. Familial naevus flammeus and Unna's naevus. *Clin Genet* 1985; **27**: 165–6.
2 Shuper A, Merloss B, Garty B, Varsano I. Familial multiple naevi flammei. *J Med Genet* 1984; **21**: 112–13.
3 Shelley WB, Livingood CS. Familial multiple naevi flammei. *Arch Dermatol Syphilol* 1949; **59**: 343–5.

Sturge–Weber syndrome

Definition

Sturge–Weber syndrome is a complex birth defect characterized by a port-wine stain involving the trigeminal area and angiomatous involvement of the leptomeninges. At least one other of the following must be present: gyriform cortical calcification on the same side, cerebral atrophy, seizures and a degree of hemiparesis or hemiatrophy or mental retardation.

Clinical features

Not all people with a port-wine stain on the face will have Sturge–Weber syndrome. It is important to know the features that carry the greater risk. The facial port-wine stain is usually on the forehead, but may be more extensive, and bilateral (Figure 11.3). Several naevi

Table 11.3 *Port-wine stains and telangiectatic naevi*

Familial multiple telangiectatic naevi
Sturge–Weber syndrome
Bonnet–Dechaume–Blanc/Wyburn-Mason/Bregeat syndromes
Cobb syndrome
Klippel–Trenaunay syndrome
Trisomy 13
Chromosome 4 short arm deletion syndrome
XXYY genotype
Turner's syndrome
Beckwith–Wiedemann syndrome
Proteus syndrome
Rubinstein–Taybi syndrome
Diastrophic dwarfism
Epidermal naevus syndrome
Robert's syndrome
Von Hippel-Lindau disease
Phacomatosis pigmentovascularis
Hereditary neurocutaneous angioma [1]
Neurofibromatosis [2]
Haemangiomatous branchial clefts [3]
Sacral haemangiomas with imperforate anus [4]
Teratogens: alcohol [5], thalidomide [6], trimethadione [7]

References

1 Zaremba J, Stepien M, Jelowicka M, Ostrowska D. Hereditary neurocutaneous angioma: a new genetic entity. *J Med Genet* 1979; **16**: 443–7.
2 Wertelecki W, Superneau DW, Blackburn WR, Varakis JN. Neurofibromatosis, skin haemangiomas and arterial disease. *Birth Def* 1982; **18**: 29–41.
3 Hall BD, De Lorimier A, Forster LH. A new syndrome of haemangiomatous branchial clefts, lip pseudocleft and unusual facial appearance. *Am J Med Genet* 1983; **14**: 135–8.
4 Goldberg NS, Hebert AA, Esterly NB. Sacral haemangiomas and multiple congenital abnormalities. *Arch Dermatol* 1986; **122**: 684–7.
5 Jones KL, Smith DW, Streisguth AP, Myrianthopoulous NC. Outcome of offspring of chronic alcoholic women. *Lancet* 1974; **i**: 1076–8.
6 Mellin GW, Katzenstein M. The saga of thalidomide (concluded): neuropathy to embryopathy, with case reports of congenital anomalies. *New Engl J Med* 1962; **267**: 1238–40.
7 Smith DW. *Recognizable Patterns of Human Malformations.* 3rd ed. WB Saunders, Philadelphia, 1982; 344–5.

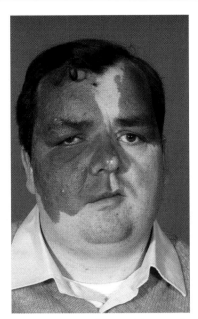

Figure 11.3 *Sturge-Weber syndrome with extensive bilateral facial port-wine stain*

Repeated computed tomographic (CT) scanning and eye examinations are necessary only in the group with extensive V1 involvement. Choroid angioma is common and must also be followed carefully in order to prevent retinal detachment.

Pathology

The flame naevus has a typical histological appearance and the choroidal lesion is cavernous. Involvement of the pia is by a haemangioma. Lateral radiography of the skull may show intracranial calcification.

Genetics

Sturge–Weber syndrome is found in many races[2]. Unlike the other phacomatoses there is no definite genetic pattern. It has an equal sex incidence. Convincing evidence of a genetic factor is lacking, but there is a report of its occurrence in monozygovic twins[3], and one reference to a father and son both with port-wine stain and leptomeningeal involvement[4].

Differential diagnosis

In the past there has been a tendency to subdivide variants of Sturge–Weber syndrome. Jahnke's name has been associated when there is no ocular involvement, and Lawford's name when a flame naevus and late glaucoma are the only signs. Other names that may appear in a literature search are Krabbe, Kalisher, Cushing, Dimitri and Schirmer. These are confusing, and the definition of Sturge–Weber should be adhered to with or without other associated features. Another problem is the place of overlap syndromes, e.g. von Hippel–Lindau disease or Klippel–Trenaunay syndrome occurring in a patient with Sturge–Weber syndrome. Brushfield and Wyatt[5] described 4 patients with a calcifying haemangioma of the cerebral hemisphere, mental retardation, and focal neurological signs with a trigeminal port-wine stain.

may affect both sides of the face and body, but the extent does not correlate with neurological features. If the flame naevus is entirely below the palpebral fissure no intracranial involvement is found. Enjolras et al[1] showed that if the whole area supplied by the fifth cranial nerve was affected there was about a 50% chance of Sturge–Weber syndrome, but if only part of the area was covered the risk was reduced to about 5%.

The risk of glaucoma is also raised in Sturge–Weber syndrome. However, if only the V2 or V3 trigeminal sensory areas are affected by the port-wine stain, the risk of glaucoma is probably zero. In one series of 21 patients with both V1 and V2 areas affected 7 had glaucoma, whereas none of 29 patients with only V2 involvement had glaucoma[1].

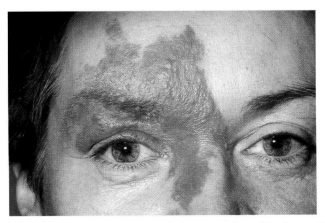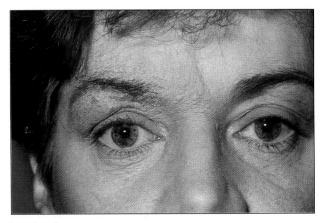

Figure 11.4 *Port-wine-stain (A) before camouflage, (B) after application of make-up*

Treatment

The variable associations and exact localization determine prognosis and management[6,7]. Different components of the syndrome may need attention from the relevant specialist. Until recently, the only treatment for the port-wine stain was camouflage make-up, which can produce an excellent result (Figure 11.4); now the treatment of choice is the flashlamp-pulsed dye laser.

References

1 Enjolras O, Riche MC, Merland JJ. Facial port wine stains and Sturge–Weber syndrome. *Paediatrics* 1985; **76**: 48–51.
2 Yingkun F, Yinchang Y. Sturge–Weber syndrome. A report of 22 cases. *Chinese Med J* 1980; **93**: 697–708.
3 Teller H, Linder B, Gotze W. Konkordanter doppelseitiger Trigeminusnaevus bei eineiigen Zwillingen mit gleichartigen elektroenzephalographischen Befunden. *Dermatol Wochenschr* 1953; **127**: 488–93.
4 Debicka A, Adanezak P. Przypadek dziedziczenia zespoln Sturge'a-Webera. *Klin Oczna* 1979; **81**: 541–2.
5 Brushfield T, Wyatt W. Hemiplegia associated with extensive naevus and mental defect. *Br J Child Dis* 1927; **24**: 98–102.
6 Paller AS. The Sturge–Weber syndrome. *Pediatr Dermatol* 1987; **4**: 300–4.
7 Bebin EM, Gomez MR. Prognosis in Sturge–Weber disease; comparison of unihemispheric and bihemispheric involvement. *J Child Neurol* 1988; **3**: 181–4.

Bonnet–Dechaume–Blanc/Wyburn-Mason/ Bregeat syndromes

There are three rare disorders that share the findings of arteriovenous malformations affecting both the eye and brain. Confusion stems from the fact that early authors did not have access to radiological, angiographic or CT techniques. Also some authors prefer to split off minor variants of one disease into an entirely separate entity – perhaps even in the search of eponymous recognition.

In 1937 Bonnet et al[1] described a 7-year-old girl who developed a right-sided hemiplegia and impairment of speech. She had dilated, tortuous vessels in the left retina. Later an angioma of the left side of her upper lip appeared. Wyburn-Mason[2] described arteriovenous aneurysms of the midbrain and ipsilateral retina. Ipsilateral naevi, either pigmented or of the port-wine type, may also be found. The eponym Wyburn-Mason syndrome has subsequently been used to describe patients without a retinal anomaly[3] and also individuals with the retinal changes alone[4]. A case has also been reported with the retinal changes of Wyburn-Mason but the cutaneous and radiological changes of Sturge–Weber syndrome[5]. The two conditions should be regarded as one, and the variety and severity of neurological symptoms depends on the position and size of the intracranial, ipsilateral arter-

iovenous malformation. Ipsilateral pinkness of the cheek or a naevus flammeus is quite common, but a deeper angioma of the cheek may occur[6].

Bregeat's syndrome is the association of retinal and thalamic angiomatosis on one side with a contralateral naevus flammeus of the face and scalp[6].

Genetics

It is questionable whether these syndromes are genetically transmitted; no distinct pattern of inheritance has been recognized.

Differential diagnosis

The Sturge–Weber syndrome differs by virtue of having a choroidal cavernous haemangioma and a leptomeningeal haemangioma. Other neurocutaneous syndromes should also be differentiated by clinical, ophthalmoscopic and radiological methods.

References

1 Bonnet P, Dechaume J, Blanc E. L'aneurysme cirsoide de la retine (aneurysme racemeux). Ses relations avec l'aneurysme cirsoide de la face et avec l'aneurysme cirsoide du cerveau. *J Med Lyon* 1937; **18**: 163–5.
2 Wyburn-Mason R. Arteriovenous aneurysm of midbrain and retina, facial naevi and mental changes. *Brain* 1943; **66**: 163–203.
3 Brown DG, Hilal SK, Tenner MK. Wyburn-Mason syndrome. Report of 2 cases without retinal involvement. *Arch Neurol* 1973; **28**: 67–8.
4 Archer DB, Deutman A, Ernest T. Arterio-venous communications of the retina. *Am J Ophthalmol* 1973; **75**: 224–41.
5 Ward JB, Katz NNK. Combined phakomatoses: a case report of Sturge–Weber and Wyburn-Mason syndrome occurring in the same individual. *Ann Ophthalmol* 1983; **15**: 1112–16.
6 Brodsky MC, Hoyt WF, Higashide RT, Hieshima GB, Halbach VV. Bonnet-Dechaume-Blanc syndrome with large facial angioma. *Arch Ophthalmol* 1987; **105**: 854–5.

Cobb syndrome

Definition

Cobb syndrome comprises the association of an angioma in the spinal cord, neurological symptoms related to it and a vascular birthmark in the corresponding dermatome.

Clinical features

The clinical features[1] should adhere strictly to the definition, but there has been a tendency to widen the clinical syndrome. Most people accept the term when applied to angioma of the thoracic or lumbar spinal cord, sometimes involving the vertebra with neurological signs of compression of the cord. Dermatomal skin involvement with a naevus flammeus, cavernous angioma, angiolipoma or angiokeratoma is seen at the corresponding level or very close. The symptoms due to pain or weakness and spasticity usually occur in childhood. Sometimes the onset is dramatic and can lead to paraplegia.

Pathology

The spinal lesion is usually intradural and arteriovenous in morphology.

Genetics

Fewer than a hundred cases have been reported. The abnormality appears sporadically. In one family it was suggested that inheritance was autosomal dominant[2], but it seemed to be only the cutaneous component that was handed down.

Differential diagnosis

A vascular stain with or without other neurocutaneous anomalies is often an indication of underlying maldevelopment of the spine, meninges and spinal cord. This has been reviewed by Aminoff[3].

Treatment

Once recognized, the spinal angioma should be fully assessed radiographically and removed whenever possible.

References

1 Jessen RT, Thompson S, Smith EB. Cobb syndrome. *Arch Dermatol* 1977; **113**: 1587–90.
2 Kaplan P, Hollenberg RD, Fraser FC. A spinal arteriovenous malformation with hereditary cutaneous haemangiomas. *Am J Dis Child* 1976; **130**: 1329–31.
3 Aminoff MJ. Vascular malformations of the central nervous system. In: Mulliken JB, Young AE, eds. *Vascular Birthmarks, Haemangiomas and Malformations*. WB Saunders, Philadelphia, 1988; 277–300.

Klippel–Trenaunay syndrome

Definition

Klippel–Trenaunay syndrome is characterized by cutaneous capillary malformation, varicosities and hemihypertrophy, mostly confined to the lower limbs (95%). The vascular naevus stretches the full length of the limb with a metameric distribution.

Clinical features

There is a probable range of disorders which present with vascular anomalies with numerous associations that will eventually be shown to be due to a failure of normal growth early in embryonic development, perhaps triggered by an environmental factor. Many authors have recognized certain constellations of physical signs, and eponymous titles have resulted. For historic and possibly anatomic reasons a distinction is made between the syndromes of Klippel–Trenaunay and Parkes Weber. Parkes Weber described multiple arteriovenous shunts in association with capillary, venous and arterial malformations and hypertrophy, and subsequently these were considered to be cause and effect. Probably, however, as in the original description by Klippel and Trenaunay, arteriovenous shunts are not always obvious, and hypertrophy may be due to non-vascular causes of gigantism in some cases. There is undoubtedly further overlap with syndromes of hemihypertrophy or even atrophy which involve neuronal and pigmentary dysplasia as well as the vascular system. Lymphatic and adipose tissue hypertrophy is commonly associated. In children bradycardia is believed to be a bad sign with respect to the systemic signs of the arteriovenous shunt. Malignant tumours are rare complications or associations, and include reports of nephroblastomas and astrocytomas. Mental retardation and seizures are common but are not due to intracerebral angiomas. Reviewing 20 affected individuals, Viljoen et al[1] gave an excellent description of the skin manifestations and pointed out that episodes of painful, red skin with fever were not uncommon: no bacteria were isolated and they termed the condition 'aseptic cellulitis'. It is a sign of lymphatic malfunction.

Pathology

The diseased calf veins, which are a probable residue of the primitive venous system of the developing limb bud, are grossly incompetent, but the calf muscle pump usually works well. The vein walls are thickened and the soft tissues are hypertrophic. Klippel and Trenaunay did not suggest that the limb hypertrophy was secondary to arteriovenous shunts.

Genetics

Suggestions of a genetic cause are meagre. No pattern of inheritance has emerged. Two siblings are recorded with the syndrome but nearly all cases are sporadic. No trigger factor has been described[2].

Differential diagnosis

Proteus, Sturge–Weber and Maffucci's syndromes must be differentiated[3,4].

Treatment

The naevus flammeus can be improved by cosmetic camouflage but often it can be covered by clothing; it may also be trivial compared to the other disfigurement. Elastic stockings are often required even for minimal disease. Superficial vein surgery can only be undertaken if the deep veins are present. Other procedures have been described by Browse et al[5].

References

1 Viljoen DL, Saxe N, Pearn J, Beighton P. The cutaneous manifestations of the Klippel Trenaunay–Weber syndrome. *Clin Exp Dermatol* 1987; **12**: 12–17.
2 Viljoen DL. Klippel Trenaunay–Weber syndrome. *J Med Gen* 1988; **25**: 250–2.
3 Mahmoud SF, El Benhawi MO, El-Tonsy MH, Kalantar SM. Klippel–Trenaunay syndrome. *J Am Acad Dermatol* 1988; **18**: 1169–72.
4 Ring DS, Mallory SB. Klippel–Trenaunay syndrome. *Pediatr Dermatol* 1992; **9**: 80–2.
5 Browse NL, Burnand KG, Thomas MZ. *Diseases of the Veins*. Edward Arnold, London, 1988; 622.

Trisomy 13

Trisomy 13 is a syndrome of microphthalmia, cleft lip and palate, and polydactyly[1]; 95% of affected individuals do not survive to the age of 3 years.

A telangiectatic naevus of the forehead or nasal ridge is seen in over 50% of patients in all series[2].

References

1 Patau K, Smith DW, Therman E, Inhorn SL, Wagner P. Multiple congenital anomalies caused by an extra chromosome. *Lancet* 1960; **i**: 790–6.
2 Hodes ME, Cole J, Palner CG, Reed T. Clinical experience with trisomies 18 and 13. *J Med Genet* 1978; **15**: 48–60.

Chromosome 4 short arm deletion syndrome

Vascular naevi of the forehead are found, together with low birthweight, microencephaly, hypertelorism, cleft palate and beaked nose[1].

Reference

1 Leao JCV, Bargman GJ, Neu RL, Kajii T, Gardner L. New syndrome associated with partial deletion of short arm of chromosome 4. *J Am Med Assoc* 1967; **202**: 434–7.

Klinefelter's syndrome with XXYY genotype

There are several variants of Klinefelter's syndrome associated with more severe defects than the XXY genotype. Multiple cutaneous vascular naevi may be found[1]. Gupta and Grover reported on an XXXY individual with multiple port-wine stains and telangiectasia of the bladder mucosa which caused haematuria[2].

References

1 Peterson WC, Gorlin RJ, Peagler F, Bruhl H. Cutaneous aspects of the XXYY genotype. *Arch Dermatol* 1966; **94**: 695–8.
2 Gupta MM, Grover DN. XXYY Klinefelters syndrome with bilateral cryptorchidism, obesity, multiple capillary haemangiomas and telangiectasia. *J Urol* 1978; **119**: 103–6.

Turner's syndrome

Definition

Turner's syndrome is the spectrum of clinical features associated with complete or partial monosomy of the X chromosome.

Clinical features

The most common features are gonadal dysgenesis, infantile sexual characteristics, webbed neck, increased carrying angle and cardiovascular anomalies. Degrees of lymphatic hypoplasia may lead to pedal oedema. Telangiectatic veins in the bowel may cause gastrointestinal bleeding. Vascular ectasia of the dorsal foot skin has been described[1,2], and in one case the ectasia persisted[1]. More recently, 2 children have been described with a vascular malformation on the dorsum of the foot composed of thick-walled veins and imperfectly formed muscular walls[3]. The malformations were subcutaneous.

Cardiovascular abnormalities may give rise to cutaneous features[4].

References

1 Paller AS, Esterly NB, Charrow J, Cahan FM. Pedal hemangiomas in Turners syndrome. *J Pediatr* 1983; **103**: 87–90.
2 Bushkell LL, Broughton RA. Pedal haemangiomas versus vascular ectasia in Turner syndrome. *J Paediatr* 1984; **104**: 486.
3 Weiss SW. Pedal haemangioma (venous malformation) occurring in Turners syndrome *Hum Pathol* 1988; **19**: 1015–18.
4 Moore JW, Kirby WC, Rogers WM, Poth MA. Partial anomalous pulmonary venous drainage associated with 45, X Turner's syndrome. *Pediatrics* 1990; **86**: 273–6.

Beckwith–Wiedemann syndrome

Synonym: *Exomphalos–macroglossia–gigantism (EMG) syndrome*

Definition

Beckwith–Wiedemann syndrome is a complex birth defect characterized by visceral and somatic overgrowth and exomphalos.

Clinical features

A great many defects may be present in this complex disorder; those usually found are muscular macroglossia and exomphalos. Many children develop severe hypoglycaemia in the first few weeks of life. There is postnatal gigantism and later in life an increased risk of malignancy. Naevus flammeus, usually on the forehead, is said to occur in up to 80% of cases; it may fade during childhood.

Pathology

There is hyperplasia of the adrenals, kidneys, pancreas and Leydig's cells[1]. Thickening of subcutaneous tissue and enlarged muscle bulk are also prominent. The macroglossia, which is an essential feature of the syndrome, is often histologically normal.

Genetics

Wiedemann's original report concerned 3 affected siblings; however, most cases are sporadic. A review of the literature in 1970 concluded that autosomal recessive inheritance was usual[2]. Other pedigrees have favoured dominant inheritance, or even a delayed mutation requiring two mutational steps to allow expression of the abnormal gene. The finding of discordancy for the syndrome in a pair of monozygotic twins suggests that multifactorial control is more likely[3]. Counselling should be given appropriately; it should be noted that ultrasonographic prenatal diagnosis is possible.

Genetic linkage studies have mapped Beckwith–Wiedemann syndrome to chromosome 11p15[4].

References

1 Beckwith JB. Macroglossia, omphalocele, adrenal cytomegaly, gigantism, and hyperplastic visceromegaly. *Birth Def* 1969; **5**: 188–96.
2 Filippi G, McKusick VA. The Beckwith–Wiedemann syndrome: report of two cases and review of the literature. *Medicine* 1970; **49**: 279–98.
3 Best LG, Hoekstra RE. Wiedemann–Beckwith syndrome: autosomal dominant inheritance in a family. *Am J Med Genet* 1981; **9**: 291–9.
4 Konfos A, Grundy P, Morgan K et al. Familial Wiedemann–Beckwith syndrome and a second Wilms' tumor locus both map to 11p15.5. *Am J Hum Genet* 1989; **44**: 711–19.

Proteus syndrome

Wiedemann[1] described, under the label 'Proteus', 4 boys with gigantism of the hands and/or feet, hemihypertrophy and skull abnormalities: these were subcutaneous nodular, vascular and lipomatous malformations. There is plantar and palmar connective tissue expansion[2]. There is possible overlap with the Riley–Smith and Bannayan syndromes.

There are seven main features of the syndrome[3,4]: macrodactyly; limb hypertrophy; subcutaneous lipomas, lymphangiomas and haemangiomas; linear, verrucous epidermal naevi; scoliosis or kyphosis; skull asymmetry and exostoses; and palmar and plantar connective tissue hyperplasia.

References

1 Wiedemann HR, Burgio GR, Aldenhoff P et al. The Proteus syndrome: partial gigantism of the hands and/or feet, nevi, hemihypertrophy, subcutaneous tumour, macrocephaly or other skull anomalies and possible accelerated growth and visceral affections. *Eur J Pediatr* 1985; **40**: 5.
2 Viljoen DL, Saxe N, Temple-Camp C. Cutaneous manifestations of the Proteus syndrome. *Pediatr Dermatol* 1988; **5**: 14–21.
3 Samlaska CP, Levin SW, James WD, Benson PM, Walker JC, Perik PC. Proteus syndrome. *Arch Dermatol* 1989; **125**: 1109–14.
4 Darmstadt GL, Lane AT. Proteus syndrome. *Pediatr Dermatol* 1994; **11**: 222–226.

Rubinstein–Taybi syndrome

Definition

Rubinstein–Taybi syndrome is characterized by broad thumbs and toes, psychomotor retardation, antimongoloid slant of the eyes and small stature[1].

Clinical features

The initial description was in 1963; over 100 cases have now been described. Mental retardation, microcephaly, downward palpebral slant and a broad terminal phalanx of the thumbs and great toes are characteristic. In half the cases a naevus flammeus was present on the face or neck.

Pathology

Some bones are broad but others are hypoplastic. Growth is limited with delayed bone development.

Genetics

Most reported cases have been sporadic. Relatives occasionally have minor defects typical of the syndrome. Some families have been reported with more than one member affected[2]. In one case 2 siblings were affected and in another the uncle of the index case was affected. Thus there is no clear mode of inheritance. It may have been dominant in the first family but recessive in the other. No chromosomal abnormality has been found.

References

1 Rubinstein JH, Taybi H Broad thumbs and toes and facial abnormalities: a possible mental retardation syndrome. *Am J Dis Child* 1963; **105**: 588–91.
2 Gillies DRN, Roussoúnis D. Rubinstein–Taybi syndrome – further evidence of a genetic aetiology. *Dev Med Child Neurol* 1985; **27**: 751–5.

Diastrophic dwarfism

Midfacial vascular naevi are common in diastrophic dwarfism[1]. Affected babies have an average length at birth of 32.5 cm. They have short, tubular bones, restricted movement of the proximal phalanges, and normal intelligence.

Reference

1 Lamy M, Maroteaux P. Le nanisme diastrophique. *Presse Méd* 1960; **68**: 1977–80.

Epidermal naevus syndrome

Although a linear epidermal naevus is seen from time to time, little emphasis has been placed on associated anomalies. In a study of their own cases and a review of the literature, Solomon et al[1] reported that 18 out of 23 cases had skeletal abnormalities including gigantism, 10 had central nervous system abnormalities, and 9 had both. Vascular anomalies, including widespread vascular naevi, were also seen. The concept of mosaicism has been applied to the syndrome[2]. Neurologic associations are most often described[3,4].

References

1 Solomon LM, Fretzin DF, Dewald RL. The epidermal naevus syndrome. *Arch Dermatol* 1968; **97**: 273–85.
2 Happle R. How many epidermal nevus syndromes exist? *J Am Acad Dermatol* 1991; **25**: 550–6.
3 Baker RS, Ross RA, Baumann RJ. Neurologic complications of the epidermal naevus syndrome. *Arch Neurol* 1987; **44**: 227–32.
4 Goldberg LH, Collins SAB, Siegel DM. The epidermal nevus syndrome: case report and review. *Pediatr Dermatol* 1987; **4**: 27–33.

Robert's syndrome

All children with Robert's syndrome[1] have a naevus flammeus on the midline of the face, hypomelia, silvery hair, hypertelorism and growth retardation. Cleft lip and palate are common. Severely affected children may die in infancy.

The disorder is inherited as an autosomal recessive trait. Chromosomal abnormalities with puffing around the centromeres[2] and premature sister chromatid separation has been reported. Overlap with other forms of phocomelia has been described[3].

References

1 Freeman MVR, Williams DW, Schimke N. The Roberts syndrome. *Clin Genet* 1974; **5**: 1–6.
2 German J. Roberts syndrome. I. Cytological evidence for a disturbance in chromatid pairing. *Clin Genet* 1979; **16**: 441–7.
3 Romke C, Froster-Iskenius U, Heyne K et al. Roberts syndrome and SC phocomelia: a single genetic entity. *Clin Genet* 1987; **31**: 170–7.

Von Hippel–Lindau disease

Definition

Von Hippel–Lindau disease is an inherited disorder with susceptibility to various forms of cancer, including retinal and cerebellar angiomata, phaeochromocytomas, pancreatic malignancies and renal cell carcinomas.

Clinical features

Originally angiomatosis of the retina was described by von Hippel in 1904. At least 20% of these patients also have cerebellar or spinal cord haemangioblastoma (named after Lindau). They are now regarded as components of one syndrome which frequently has other features. Cysts of the gonads, pancreas and kidney may be present[1]. Renal cell carcinoma (often bilateral and multifocal) is found in 25% of cases and is an important cause of death[2]. Phaeochromocytoma is another important complication.

The diagnosis is made if more than one haemangioblastoma of the central nervous system is found, or if one occurs with a visceral manifestation, or if one manifestation is seen in an individual with a positive family history. The importance of screening people with haemangioblastoma has been highlighted[3]. Eight out of 20 patients proved to have the disease. It is proposed that patients and relatives at risk should have regular screening by ophthalmoscopy, vanillylmandelic acid measurement, and abdominal and cranial CT scans.

Telangiectatic naevi of the port-wine stain type occur in 5% of affected individuals.

Genetics

Dominant mendelian inheritance is now generally agreed upon. Shokeii[4] reported three families, in only one of which was inheritance clearly dominant. He believed that one of the other families should be thought of as showing an autosomal recessive trait, but in fact autosomal dominance with incomplete penetrance could equally well explain the pattern. Go et al supported the dominant inheritance pattern[5]; they pointed out that 95% of patients have at least one manifestation by the age of 50 years, so that if the parents of an affected individual have no symptoms by the age of 50 years, it is likely to be a new mutation. The von Hippel–Lindau gene has been mapped to chromosome 3 and to the same region as the oncogene associated with sporadic renal cell carcinoma[6].

References

1 Lamiell JM, Salazar FG, Hsia YE. Von Hippel–Lindau disease. *Medicine* (Baltimore) 1989; **68**: 1–29.
2 Peterson GJ, Codd JE, Cuddihee RE, Newton WT. Renal transplantation in Lindau–Von Hippel disease. *Arch Surg* 1977; **112**: 841–5.
3 Huson SM, Harper PS, Hourihan MD et al. Cerebellar haemangioblastoma and Von Hippel–Lindau disease. *Brain* 1986; **109**: 1297–310.
4 Shokeii MHK. Von Hippel–Lindau syndrome: a report on three kindreds. *J Med Genet* 1970; **7**: 155–7.
5 Go RCF, Lamiell JM, Hsia YE, Yuen JWM, Paik Y. Segregation and linkage analysis of Von Hippel–Lindau disease among 220 descendants from one kindred. *Am J Hum Genet* 1984; **36**: 131–42.
6 Seizinger BR, Rouleau GA, Ozelius LJ et al. Von Hippel–Lindau disease maps to the region of chromosome 3 associated with renal cell carcinoma. *Nature* 1988; **332**: 268–9.

Phacomatosis pigmentovascularis

Definition

Phacomatosis pigmentovascularis (PPV) is a group of diseases in which there is a distinctive association between a cutaneous vascular naevus and a pigmentary naevus.

Clinical features

This group of vascular and pigmented naevi was first reported by Ota et al in 1947[1]. It is often reported in the Japanese literature but has not achieved universal acceptance. In the localized form, only skin lesions are present. There are now thought to be four subtypes, in all of which naevus flammeus is a feature. In type I the association is with a verrucous pigmented naevus, in type II with mongolian blue spots, in type III with naevus spilus and in type IV with blue spots and naevus spilus. In types I to III a naevus anaemicus may be present[2]. In the so-called systemic types of the disease the skin lesions are found in association with Klippel–Trenaunay syndrome[3], Sturge–Weber syndrome or melanosis oculi. It is of note that non-Japanese authors usually omit the term PPV; for example, Noriega-Sanchez et al[4] believed their case to have simply oculocutaneous melanosis with Sturge–Weber syndrome rather than type IIb PPV.

Differential diagnosis

The Japanese cases overlap with other syndromes in which enlargement of a limb or digit is a recognized association, being gigantism rather than the hypertrophy secondary to arteriovenous shunts.

Pathology

Ultrastructural studies comparing the naevus flammeus in PPV and other naevi flammei have shown that only in the former are there obvious peripheral nervous elements in the perivascular region.

Genetics

In a few cases other family members have been found to have a pigmented naevus, but not of the same clinical type. There is no evidence of a distinct pattern of inheritance.

References

1 Ota M, Kowamura T, Ito N. Phacomatosis pigmentovascularis (OTA). *Japan J Dermatol* 1947; **52**: 1–3.
2 Hasegawa Y, Yasuhara M. Phacomatosis pigmentovascularis type IVa. *Arch Dermatol* 1985; **121**: 651–5.
3 Libow LF. Phacomatosis pigmentovascularis type III B. *J Am Acad Dermatol* 1993; **29**: 305–7.
4 Noriega-Sanchez A, Markand ON, Herndon JH. Oculocutaneous melanosis associated with the Sturge-Weber syndrome. *Neurology* 1972; **22**: 256–62.

Cutis marmorata

The different types of cutis marmorata are listed in Table 11.4.

Cutis marmorata telangiectatica congenita

Definition

Cutis marmorata telangiectatica congenita is a widespread or segmental cutaneous pattern of blue-violet reticulated bands that are relatively fixed and readily discernible at rest[1]. Other developmental anomalies may be present.

Clinical features

The marbled appearance (Figure 11.5) of the skin is usually present at birth but may be delayed by a year or two. There is a tendency for the marbling to fade with age, and in a few cases it may disappear entirely. Its extent may range from one limb to the entire body. Varying degrees of telangiectasia and venous engorgement are seen. Other cutaneous changes may involve

Table 11.4 *Cutis marmorata*

Cutis marmorata telangiectatica congenita
Exaggerated physiological cutis marmorata
    Down's syndrome [1]
    Trisomy 18 [2]
    De Lange's syndrome [3]
    Dury–van Bogaert syndrome [4] (X-linked
      recessive, not all cases [5])

References

1 Penrose LS, Smith GF. *Down's Anomaly.* Little, Brown, Boston, 1966.
2 Jones KL. *Smith's Recognizable Patterns of Human Malformation.* WB Saunders, Philadelphia, 1988; 16.
3 Hawley PD, Jackson LG, Kurnit DM. Sixty-five patients with Brachmann–de Lange syndrome: a survey. *Am J Hum Genet* 1985; **20**: 453–61.
4 Dury P, van Bogaert L. Une malade familiale caractérisée par une angiomatose diffuse cortico-méningée calcifiante et une demyelinisation progressive de la substance blanche. *J Neurol Neurochir Psych* 1946; **9**: 41–54.
5 Martin JJ, Navarro C, Roussel JM, Michielssen P. Familial capillaro-venous leptomeningeal angiomatosis. *Eur Neurol* 1973; **9**: 202–15.

hypoplasia or hyperplasia of the affected part, ulceration which is occasionally disabling, focal atrophy and naevus flammeus[2]. The port-wine stain may be part of the Sturge–Weber syndrome and glaucoma must then be sought: however, glaucoma has also occurred when cutis marmorata involved the face. Associated skeletal anomalies may include short stature, syndactyly, asymmetrical skull and spina bifida[3,4].

The morbidity depends firstly on whether there is hyperplasia, ulceration, etc., and in most cases this is not a problem. The second factor is associated anomalies, which have been reported to occur in 27% to over 50% of cases.

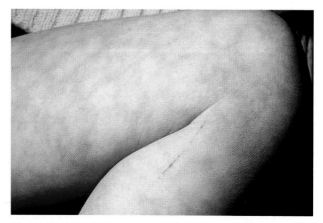

Figure 11.5 *Marbled appearance of cutis marmorata*

Pathology

Histological changes may be minimal with dilatation of capillaries and veins and endothelial swelling. There may be a mononuclear infiltrate, and elastic tissue degeneration has been described[5].

Genetics

Most cases appear to be sporadic. Where several individuals in one family were affected, the inheritance was reported to be autosomal dominant[5] or dominant with low penetrance. Most studies have shown a significant female preponderance. A teratogenic factor was postulated when 4 babies in 18 months developed the disease in the same neighbourhood of Sydney, Australia[6].

Differential diagnosis

Physiological vascular markings of a reticulate pattern cutis marmorata are common in the newborn especially when cool or in shock, but such markings do not persist when the baby is warmed. Somewhat similar markings may be seen in some cases of scarring due to subcutaneous fat necrosis. The differential diagnosis also includes livedo reticularis, Klippel–Trenaunay syndrome, Bockenheimer's syndrome and Adams–Oliver syndrome[7].

Treatment

There is no known treatment for the underlying disorder. Local complications and other anomalies are treated symptomatically. The skin lesions often become less prominent after infancy[8].

References

1 Picascia DD, Esterley NB. Cutis marmorata telangiectatica congenita. *J Am Acad Dermatol* 1989; **20**: 1098–104.
2 Petrozzi JW, Rahn EK, Mafenson H, Greensher J. Cutis marmorata telangiectatica congenita. *Arch Dermatol* 1970; **101**: 74–7.
3 Bjornsdottir US, Laxdal T, Bjornsson J. Cutis marmorata telangiectatica congenita with terminal limb defects. *Acta Paed Scand* 1908; **77**: 780–2.
4 Powell ST, Su WPD. Cutis marmorata telangiectatica congenita: report of nine cases and review of the literature. *Cutis* 1984; **34**: 305–12.
5 Kurczynski TW. Hereditary cutis marmorata telangiectatica congenita. *Paediatrics* 1982; **70**: 52–3.
6 Rogers M, Poyzer KG. Cutis marmorata telangiectatica congenita. *Arch Dermatol* 1982; **18**: 895–9.
7 Bork K, Pfeifle J. Multifocal aplasia cutis congenita, distal limb hemimelia, and cutis marmorata telangiectatica in a patient with Adams–Oliver syndrome. *Br J Dermatol* 1992; **127**: 160–3.
8 Pehr K, Moroz B. Cutis marmorata telangiectatica congenita. Long-term follow up, review of the literature and report of a case in conjunction with congenital hypothyroidism. *Pediatr Dermatol* 1993; **10**: 6–11.

Palpable haemangiomas

Palpable haemangiomas are listed in Table 11.5.

Blue rubber bleb naevus syndrome

Definition

Blue rubber bleb naevus syndrome is an inherited disease characterized by multiple skin and gastro-intestinal angiomas[1].

Clinical features

The skin lesions tend to appear in late childhood and new ones may continue to appear and enlarge for many years; individual lesions persist. They are situated individually or in groups and at various depths so that some protrude while others are just visible as a blue discolouration of the skin. They may simply be of nuisance value, but tenderness on touch or movement can be troublesome. Occasionally large groups on the palms or soles or over a bony prominence can cause significant disability.

Similar lesions may appear at any point in the gastrointestinal tract and may be demonstrated angio-graphically[2]. They may bleed chronically, causing anaemia, or give rise to acute and severe gastro-intestinal bleeding, and intestinal lesions have caused intussusception. Postmortem data suggest that asymptomatic involvement of other organs is not an uncommon condition. Bone and the central nervous system are usual sites. The disease has been seen with Maffucci's syndrome[3] and overlap with Rendu-Osler-Weber syndrome has also been described[4]. Sudoriparous angioma are present at birth and show sweating either spontaneously or when stroked[5]. A non-sweating, spontaneously regressing haeman-gioma of eccrine sweat glands has also been described, which may be mistaken for blue rubber bleb naevus syndrome[6].

Pathology

The vascular tumours are usually cavernous. Post-mortem examination may reveal very widespread tumours, many of which were not apparent in life[7]; indeed, one unfortunate patient had a cardiac hae-mangioma.

Genetics

There are several family studies that prove an autoso-mal dominant pattern of inheritance[8], but in one family only males were affected. Nevertheless, many affected individuals have no family history of the condition and are new mutations.

Differential diagnosis

Multiple glomus tumours can look very similar, but have a characteristic histology. There may be overlap in some pedigrees.

Table 11.5 *Palpable haemangiomas*

Blue rubber bleb naevus syndrome
Multiple glomus tumours
Bannayan's syndrome
Maffucci's syndrome
Favre's disease
Gorham's disease
Eruptive neonatal haemangiomatosis
Riley-Smith syndrome [1]
Von Hippel-Lindau disease [2]
I-cell disease [3]
Klippel-Trenaunay syndrome ⎱ see section on
Cobb syndrome ⎰ port-wine stains
Multiple familial vascular anomalies [4]
Coarctation and haemangiomas [5]
Retinal and cutaneous haemangiomas [6, 7]
Sternal malformation and vascular dysplasia [8]
Neurocutaneous angioma [9]

References

1 Riley HD, Smith WR. Macrocephaly, pseudopapilloedema and multiple haemangiomata: a previously undescribed heredofamilial syndrome. *Paediatrics* 1960; **26**: 293–300.
2 Hall GS. Blood vessel tumours of the brain with particular reference to Lindau syndrome. *J Neurol Psych Pathol* 1935; **15**: 305–8.
3 Leroy JG, Spranger JW, Feingold M, Opitz JM, Crocker AC. I cell disease, a clinical picture. *J Paediatr* 1971; **79**: 360–5.
4 Pasyk KA, Argenta LC, Erickson RP. Familial vascular malformations. Report of 25 members of one family. *Clin Genet* 1984; **26**: 221.
5 Schneeweiss A, Blieden LC, Shem-Tov A et al. Coarctation of the aorta with congenital hemangiomas of the face and neck and aneurysm or dilation of a subclavian or innominate artery. A syndrome? *Chest* 1982; **82**: 194–5.
6 Gass JDM. Cavernous hemangioma of the retina – a neuro-oculo cutaneous syndrome. *Am J Ophthalmol* 1971; **91**: 799–803.
7 Goldberg RE, Pheasant TR, Sheilds JA. Cavernous hae-mangioma of the retina: a four generation pedigree with neurocutaneous manifestations and an example of bilat-eral retinal involvement. *Arch Ophthalmol* 1971; **97**: 2321–8.
8 Hersh JH, Waterfill D, Rutledge J et al. Sternal malforma-tion/vascular dysplasia association. *Am J Hum Genet* 1985; **21**: 177–80.
9 Hurst J, Baraitser M. Hereditary neurocutaneous angio-matous malformation: autosomal dominant inheritance in two families. *Clin Genet* 1988; **33**: 44–8

Treatment

Treatment consists of iron replacement and blood transfusion. Rarely, excision of heavily involved segments of bowel is required, and other surgical treatment may be needed for angiomas in other organs. Skin lesions often recur around the scar.

References

1 Oranje AP. Blue rubber bleb nevus syndrome. *Pediatr Dermatol* 1986; **3**: 304–10.
2 Jennings M, Ward P, Maddocks JL. Blue rubber bleb naevus disease: an uncommon cause of gastrointestinal bleeding. *Gut* 1988; **29**: 1408–12.
3 Hivotada FS, Tetsuro S, Saito T. The association of blue rubber bleb naevus and Maffucci's syndrome. *Arch Dermatol* 1967; **95**: 28.
4 Rosenblum W, Nakoneczna I, Kondering HS. Multiple vascular malformations in the blue bleb naevus syndrome. A case with aneurysm of Galen and vascular lesions suggest a link to Weber–Osler–Rendu syndrome. *Histopathology* 1978; **2**: 301–11.
5 Domonkos AN, Suarez LS. Sudoriparous angioma. *Arch Dermatol* 1967; **96**: 552–3.
6 Rositto A, Ranalletta M, Drut R. Congenital hemangioma of eccrine sweat glands. *Pediatr Dermatol* 1993; **10**: 341–3.
7 Ishii T, Asuwa N, Suzuki S, Suwa H, Shimada K. Blue rubber bleb naevus syndrome. *Virchows Archiv A* 1988; **413**: 485–90.
8 Munkvad M. Blue rubber bleb naevus syndrome. *Dermatologica* 1983; **167**: 307–9.

Multiple glomus tumours

Definition

The sole manifestation of this disorder is the appearance of multiple glomus tumours on the skin.

Clinical features

Some tumours are present at birth or appear in the first or second decade. Normally they are smaller than 1 cm, fewer than 90 in number, and non-tender. The distribution is either localized, the tumours being found over a small area of the body, or generalized. In one patient they were found unilaterally[1].

Pathology

The tumours consist of non-encapsulated, cavernous, blood-filled spaces with a single layer of endothelial cells surrounded by one to several layers of glomus cells. Some believe that they are derived from the arterial segment of the Sucquet-Hoyer canal, others that they are derived from simple cutaneous vessels[2].

Genetics

The condition is inherited as an autosomal dominant trait. Men are affected more often than women. Family pedigrees are consistent with an autosomal dominant inheritance with incomplete penetrance[3,4].

Differential diagnosis

The differential diagnosis includes solitary glomus, cavernous haemangioma and blue rubber bleb naevus syndrome.

Bannayan's syndrome

Definition

Bannayan's syndrome is a complex disorder characterized by macrocephaly and multiple soft-tissue and visceral hamartomas[1].

Clinical features

Multiple, mixed hamartomas are seen with variable elements of lipoma, haemangioma and lymphangiomatous tissue[2]. Angiolipoma and meningioma also occur. One family exhibited mental retardation[3].

Genetics

The pedigrees in reported families support autosomal dominant inheritance. There is considerable variation in expression and some individuals may have only soft-tissue tumours.

Differential diagnosis

Other causes of macrocephaly must be excluded.

Treatment

Intralesional triamcinolone was successful in clearing subcutaneous haemangiomas in 1 patient[4].

References

1 Bannayan GA. Lipomatosis, angiomatosis and macroencephalia – a previously undescribed congenital syndrome. *Arch Pathol* 1971; **92**: 1.
2 Klein JA, Barr RJ. Bannayan–Zonana syndrome associated with lymphangiomatous lesions. *Pediatr Dermatol* 1990; **7**: 48–53.
3 Saul RA, Stevenson RE, Bley R. Mental retardation in the Bannayan syndrome. *Paediatrics* 1982; **69**: 602–44.
4 Jennings WC, Say B. Steroid treatment of soft tissue tumours in Bannayan syndrome. *Plast Reconstr Surg* 1988; **82**: 362–3.

Maffucci's syndrome

Definition

Maffucci's syndrome is a rare disorder characterized by multiple enchondromas and haemangiomas [1–4].

Clinical features

Fewer than 150 cases have been reported. Twenty-five per cent of these individuals were affected at birth and nearly 80% by the age of puberty. Enchondromas and haemangiomas are often widespread and may be very large, leading to functional and growth problems. Pituitary adenoma has been reported. Not only is there a high risk of malignant transformation in the enchondroma, but there is also a high risk of other malignant tumours, e.g. glioma, ovarian tumours. When no haemangiomas are present the condition is called Ollier's disease.

Pathology

All the tumours are of mesodermal origin. The haemangiomas are cavernous.

Genetics

The sexes are affected equally; no pattern of inheritance has been described. There are no reported familial cases.

Differential diagnosis

The syndrome is distinguished from Ollier's disease by the presence of haemangiomas.

Treatment

No time must be lost in investigating new symptoms of pain or growth in a tumour because of the 30% risk of malignant transformation.

References

1 Anderson IF. Maffucci's syndrome – report of a case with a review of the literature. *S Afr Med J* 1965; **39**: 1066.
2 Bean W. Dyschondroplasia and hemangiomata. *Arch Intern Med* 1955; **95**: 767.
3 Carleton A, Elkington JStC, Greenfield JG, Robb-Smith AHT. Maffucci's syndrome (dyschondroplasia and haemangiomata). *Quart J Med* 1942; **11**: 203.
4 Tilsley DA, Burden PW. A case of Maffucci's syndrome. *Br J Dermatol* 1981; **105**: 331–6.

Favre's disease

Although the condition was first described in 1931 by Roueche, the names of Favre and Fiessinger have been associated with this rare disease. Privat et al[1] described another case. Benign-looking telangiectatic lesions appear at the level of the ears in early infancy. Inexorable and rapid spread with ulceration leads to destruction of much of the facial and cervical skin and deeper structures resulting in death. The vessel destruction may affect internal organs. The destructive course of a third case[2] showed some similarities with earlier ones, although it involved a mixed cavernous/capillary haemangioma.

References

1 Privat Y, Satge P, Sanokho A et al. Une forme peu connue d'angiomatose: l'angioscleroplastose de Favre et Fiessinger. *Bull Soc Med Afr Noire* 1967; **12**: 13–15.
2 Rizzo R, Micali G, Incorpora G, Pavono E, Pavone L. A very aggressive form of facial haemangioma. *Pediatr Dermatol* 1988; **5**: 263–5.

Gorham's disease

Multiple cutaneous angiomas are sometimes seen in the rare Gorham's disease. Haemangiomas (or haemolymphangiomas) develop in bone and cause osteolysis which may be severe[1]; this has been termed Haferkamp's syndrome when associated with liver and bone marrow defects. It has also been called disappearing bone disease. Treatment is only indicated if significant loss of bone takes place or if there is damage to vital structures, e.g. the nasal passages. The appropriate use of steroid therapy, radiotherapy and surgery has been reviewed by Atherton[2].

References

1 Halliday DR, Dahlin DC, Pugh DG, Young HH. Massive osteolysis and angiomatosis. *Radiology* 1964; **82**: 637–44.
2 Atherton DJ. Naevi and other developmental defects. In: Champion RH, Burton JL, Ebling FJG, eds. *Textbook of Dermatology*. 5th ed. Blackwell, Oxford, 1992; 503.

Eruptive neonatal haemangiomatosis

The appearance of multiple strawberry naevus-like lesions within the first few weeks of life is called benign eruptive neonatal haemangiomatosis[1,2], if the lesions are restricted to the skin or if no serious complication ensues. The term 'disseminated eruptive neonatal haemangiomatosis' is used if systemic lesions appear and when complications occur (Figure 11.6). The distinction is blurred, and Stern has suggested that high-output cardiac failure and thrombocytopenia may be part of the benign disease provided that the lesions eventually involute[1].

It is easier to diagnose the disseminated form than it is to exclude the benign variety. Systemic lesions may be found in the liver, bone, skeletal muscles, heart, brain and other organs. Although there is probably a tendency to over-report cases with a fatal outcome, there is a high mortality (78%) for infants with visceral

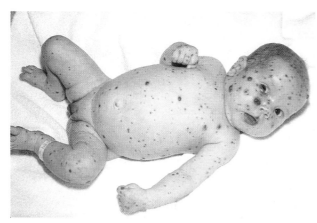

Figure 11.6 *Disseminated eruptive neonatal haemangiomatosis in a baby with liver involvement (courtesy of Dr J. Harper)*

involvement. All infants with multiple, small cutaneous haemangiomas should have detailed radiographic investigations of the brain and abdominal structures.

There is no recognized pattern of inheritance.

Treatment may be medical for cardiac failure or surgical to deal with specific angiomas. Corticosteroids and interferon alfa have been given to reduce the size of hepatic angiomas.

References

1 Stern JK, Wolf JE, Jarratt M. Benign neonatal haemangiomatosis. *J Am Acad Dermatol* 1981; **4**: 442–5.
2 Esterly NB. Cutaneous haemangiomas, vascular stains and associated syndromes. *Curr Probl Paediatr* 1987; **17**: 1–69.

Chapter 12

Photosensitivity diseases

G. M. Murphy

Introduction

Photobiology is the study of ultraviolet and visible non-ionizing radiation on living systems. Ultraviolet radiation (UVR) is arbitrarily divided into UVC (wavelengths less than 280 nm), UVB (280–315 nm) and UVA (315–400 nm); visible light is of wavelength 400–800 nm[1]. Shorter wavelengths are attenuated most effectively by the earth's atmosphere; UVC wavelengths are prevented from reaching the earth's surface by absorption in the atmosphere, particularly the ozone layer[2,3]. Ultraviolet B is likewise attenuated considerably but reaches the earth's surface in significant amounts. Factors increasing the distance traversed through the earth's atmosphere such as time of day, season and altitude influence UVB more than UVA. At midday, when the sun's rays are directly overhead, the UVA content of the solar spectrum is 100 times greater than UVB. However, since UVB is 1000 times more biologically effective than UVA, UVB is ten times more biologically effective than UVA at noon.

Ultraviolet radiation may be absorbed, reflected or scattered in the skin[4]. Transmission of UVR occurs in a wavelength-dependent manner, longer wavelengths penetrating more deeply. In order for a biological effect to occur, radiation must be absorbed by a molecule, known as a chromophore. After absorbing such energy the chromophore is in an excited state, an unstable situation persisting only for a fraction of a second. A chain of events follows: the excited state leads to a photoproduct such as a photochemical reaction in a chromophore such as DNA, RNA, protein or lipid; complex biochemical processes are initiated, leading to enzymatic induction or inhibition culminating in cellular events. The final step may be clinically observable as erythema, hyperplasia or neoplasia, amongst many other results.

A chromophore absorbs only radiation of specific wavelength, its absorption spectrum. Absorption of photons by molecules occurs by interaction of the electric fields of the light wave with the electrons in the molecule. Specific wavelength absorption occurs because molecules have specific energy states determined by their electron orbital distributions. At body temperature, most molecules are in the lowest energy state or ground state. The energy required to lift an electron from the ground state to its excited state is wavelength dependent, varies from molecule to molecule and constitutes the absorption spectrum of the molecule. The colour of compounds likewise is determined by the wavelengths absorbed. Energy absorbed is inversely proportional to wavelength; thus compounds which have large energy separation between ground and excited states absorb short wavelengths. Molecules absorbing UVR of wavelength below 320 nm are colourless, i.e. nucleic acids, some proteins, alcohol and phospholipids. Coloured compounds absorb longer wavelengths (less energy being required to lift them from their ground state): such compounds have double bonds, unsaturated ring structures, nitrogen, sulphur and oxygen atoms as part of their structure. A molecule in its initial excited state is called a singlet (*S), typified by fluorescence of porphyrins. It exists only for a fraction of a second. If *S does not form a photoproduct, it may lose its energy by emitting it as light (fluorescence) or heat, or it may convert into a longer-lasting state called a triplet (*T). The excited triplet may lead to photoproduct formation or may emit its energy as phosphorescence or heat. In human skin, DNA, proteins and other molecules absorb UVR and cause such changes, for example photoproducts in DNA such as pyridimine dimer formation.

In humans the skin and eyes are the organs most affected by ultraviolet radiation. Cutaneous effects of UVR exposure include sunburn, tanning, hyperplasia, skin aging and carcinogenesis. Tanning[5] and hyperplasia[6] are photoprotective mechanisms aimed at limiting the amount of damage caused by UVR exposure. Vitamin D synthesis is the only proved beneficial effect of UVR exposure. Sunburn is an expression of cellular damage; the initial event in the pathogenesis of the sunburn reaction is likely to be absorption of UVB by epidermal cellular DNA, since the action spectrum for human erythema and the absorption spectrum for DNA are so similar[7]. Ultraviolet B is mainly absorbed by the epidermis which consequently bears the brunt of the damage. However, sufficient UVB penetrates to the dermis to cause a dermal inflammatory reaction and endothelial cell swelling[8]. Ultraviolet B exposure, and UVA exposure to a lesser extent, lead to pyrimidine dimer formation in DNA[9,10]; UVA also induces DNA–protein cross-links, a reaction requiring reactive oxygen species. Excision repair mechanisms exist to repair such defects, enabling normal DNA and RNA replication to continue. About 75% of the potential damage induced by UVA may be prevented by endogenous glutathione acting as a free radical scavenger. Photoactivation or visible light-induced repair of pyrimidine dimer formation appears to occur in animals[11] but has not been confirmed in human skin[12]. Failure to repair DNA defects leads ultimately to skin cancer, as evidenced by the increased incidence of skin cancers in xeroderma pigmentosum (XP), in which deficiencies of DNA repair exist at the incisional level in classical XP. The complexity of the repair process is illustrated by the number of subgroups (nine) now identified, suggesting that at least nine different gene products are needed for the incisional step[13]. The DNA repair complex that binds specifically to DNA damaged by UVR is instrumental in DNA repair. Deficiency of this complex leads to defective repair in complementation group E[14].

Most of the skin changes we associate with aging are attributable to the effects of UVR[15]. Ultraviolet A penetrates deeply into the dermis and leads to collagen damage and loss, and a switch from the usual type I to type III synthesis in an effort to repair the damage[16]. Blood vessels are damaged and basement membrane reduplication occurs leading to histologically evident thickened walls. Telangiectasia, loss of small blood vessels and increased dermal glycosaminoglycans deposition are evident[17,18]. These well-known alterations lead to a great variety of cutaneous changes, evident clinically as laxity and sagging of the skin with loss of elasticity, wrinkling

Table 12.1 *Photosensitivity disorders*

The porphyrias
Idiopathic photodermatoses
    Polymorphic light eruption
    Juvenile spring eruption
    Actinic prurigo
    Hydroa vacciniforme
Disorders of tryptophan metabolism
    Hartnup disease
Rothmund–Thomson syndrome
Lupus erythematosus
Disorders of DNA repair
    Xeroderma pigmentosum (see Chapter 17)
    Cockayne's syndrome (see Chapter 17)
    Bloom's syndrome (see Chapter 17)
    Trichothiodystrophy (PIBIDS) (see Chapter 5)

and leatheriness, freckling, mottling, yellowing, scaling and telangiectases. Such changes are commonly noted in the elderly and in some of the premature aging syndromes, such as Bloom's and Rothmund–Thomson syndromes and dyskeratosis congenita. Thus myriads of interacting molecular events consequent to the absorption of ultraviolet radiation by the skin lead to the cutaneous appearances associated with photoaging and disease states.

A list of photosensitivity disorders is given in Table 12.1.

References

1 Commission Internationale d'Eclairage (CIE). *International Lighting Vocabulary.* 3rd ed. Bureau Centrale de la Cie, Paris, 1970.
2 MacKie RM, Rycroft MJ. Health and the ozone layer. *Br Med J* 1988; **297**: 369–70.
3 Editorial. Health in the greenhouse. *Lancet* 1989; **i**: 819–20.
4 Everett MA, Yeargers E, Sayre RM, Olson RL. Penetration of epidermis by ultraviolet rays. *Photochem Photobiol* 1966; **5**: 533.
5 Quevedo WC, Fitzpatrick TB, Pathak MA, Jimbow K. Light and skin color. In: Fitzpatrick TB, Pathak MA, Harber LC, Seiji M, Kukita A, eds. *Sunlight and Man. Normal and Abnormal Photobiological Responses.* University of Tokyo Press, 1974.
6 Blum HF. Hyperplasia induced by ultraviolet light: possible relationship to cancer induction. In: Urbach F, ed. *The Biological Effects of Ultraviolet Radiation (With Emphasis on the Skin).* Pergamon, Oxford, 1974; 83.
7 Setlow RB. The wavelengths in sunlight effective in producing skin cancer: a theoretical analysis. *Proc Nat Acad Sci USA* 1974; **71**: 3363–6.
8 Hawk JLM, Murphy GM, Holden CA. Early histological events in the human sunburn reaction. *Br J Dermatol* 1988; **118**: 27–30.
9 Freeman SE, Gange RW, Sutherland JC, Sutherland BM.

Production of pyrimidine dimers in DNA of human skin exposed to UVA. *J Invest Dermatol* 1987; **88**: 34–6.

10 Freeman SE, Gange RW, Sutherland JC, Sutherland BM. Pyrimidine dimer formation in human skin. *Photochem Photobiol* 1987; **46**: 207–12.

11 Ley RD, Applegate LA, Fry RJM, Stuart RD. UVA/visible light suppression of ultraviolet radiation-induced skin and eye tumours of the marsupial monodelphis domestica. *Photochem Photobiol* 1988; **47**: 45s.

12 Southerland BM, Cimino JS, Dehilas N, Shih AG, Oliver RP. Ultraviolet light-induced transformation of human cells to anchorage-independent growth. *Cancer Res* 1980; **40**: 1934–9.

13 Editorial. Sunlight, DNA repair and skin cancer. *Lancet* 1989; **i**: 1362–3.

14 Chu G, Chang E. Xeroderma pigmentosum group E cells lack a nuclear factor that binds to damaged DNA. *Science* 1988; **242**: 564–7.

15 Kligman LH. Photodamage to dermal connective tissue by UVA. In: Urbach F, Gange RW, eds. *The Biologic Effects of UVA Radiation*. Praeger, New York, 1986; 98–104.

16 Lovell CR, Smolenski KA, Duance VC, Light ND. Type I and III collagen content and fibre distribution in normal human skin during ageing. *Br J Dermatol* 1987; **117**: 419–28.

17 Gilchrest BA. Aging of the skin. In: Fitzpatrick TB, Eisen AZ, Wolff K, Freedberg EM, Austen KF, eds. *Dermatology in General Medicine*. 3rd ed. McGraw-Hill, New York, 1987; 146–53.

18 Kligman LH, Kaidbey KH, Hitchens VM, Miller SA. Long wavelength (>340 nm) ultraviolet-A induced skin damage in hairless mice is dose dependent. In: Passchier WF, Bosnjakovic BF, eds. *Human Exposure to Ultraviolet Radiation: Risks and Regulations*, Elsevier, Amsterdam, 1987; 77–81.

The porphyrias

Porphyrins were first alluded to by Scherer[1] in 1841; the first description of a patient with photosensitivity followed 33 years later under the title *Pemphiques Leprosus*[2]. Hausmann[3] noted in 1908 that porphyrins were photosensitizing. Five years later Meyer-Betz[4] was the first to show that injection of haematoporphyrin (into himself) induced profound photosensitivity. Garrod[5] and Günther[6] explored the metabolic basis of the porphyrias; and Fischer[7] outlined the essentials of porphyrin biochemistry, thereby earning a Nobel Prize. Günther classified the porphyrias in his papers in 1911 and 1922, describing acute and drug-induced porphyria[6,8]. Shemin and Rittenberg used labelled glycine to study the initial phase of haem synthesis which led to the discovery of the role of delta-aminolaevulinic acid as a porphyrin precursor[9]. Westall first identified porphobilinogen[10], and the control of haem synthesis was outlined by Granick[11]. Rimington described brilliantly the chemical pathology of congenital porphyria in South African shorthorn cattle[12]. Description of porphyria variegata by Barnes[13] and Dean[14]

followed. Ten years later erythropoietic protoporphyria was first recognized as a distinct entity by Magnus[15]. More recently mixed and homozygous porphyrias have been described[16,17], enabling categorization of some previously unclassifiable patients. Finally, a new type of porphyria, plumboporphyria, has been described, a consequence of aminolaevulinic acid dehydratase deficiency.

Biochemistry of the porphyrias

Porphyrins are widely distributed in nature, their structure (Figure 12.1) being highly appropriate for oxidation and oxygen transport. They also impart colour to feathers and shells. The initial biosynthetic sequence for synthesis of haem, chlorophylls and corrins is the same. Porphobilinogen is utilized by each separate pathway. Haemoglobin, the end product of the human porphyrin biosynthetic pathway, is red.

The haem biosynthetic pathway (Figure 12.2) begins with simple precursors from the Krebs tricarboxylic acid cycle. Succinyl-CoA combines with glycine in the presence of aminolaevulinic acid (ALA) synthase to form delta-ALA[18]; the pathway then proceeds as outlined in Figure 12.2 to porphobilinogen, a monopyrrole, four molecules of which then link and cyclize to form the first of a series of porphyrins, uroporphyrinogen[19]. A series of decarboxylation and oxidation steps lead to the formation of coproporphyrinogen, protoporphyrinogen and protoporphyrin[20,21]. Finally, with the insertion of iron into the porphyrin ring by haem synthetase[22], haem is formed. The enzyme which controls the pace of this reaction is ALA synthase, a mitochondrial protein, requiring pyridoxal phosphate as a cofactor.

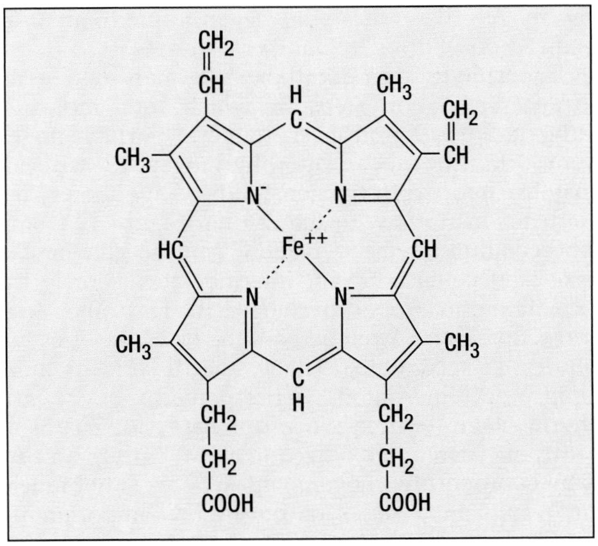

Figure 12.1 *Structure of haem-ferro-protoporphyrin 9*

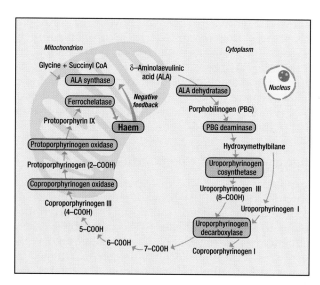

Figure 12.2 *The haem biosynthetic pathway*

The activity of ALA synthase may be affected profoundly by lead and a variety of drugs and chemicals. Aminolaevulinic acid dehydratase is profoundly affected by lead poisoning[23]. Ethanol also affects its activity[24]. To form porphobilinogen, two identical ALA molecules combine in a series of stages. The activity of ALA dehydratase is much higher than that of ALA synthase, and the former enzyme is thought to play only a small role in overall haem regulation. Porphobilinogen deaminase and uroporphyrinogen III synthase are cytoplasmic enzymes which act in concert to condense four molecules of porphobilinogen to hydroxymethylbilane and cyclize them to form the first of the porphyrins, uroporphyrinogen III. Porphobilinogen deaminase, the second rate-limiting step in haem biosynthesis, forms the symmetrical uroporphyrin I; deficiency of uroporphyrinogen III synthase thus leads to predominantly isomer I porphyrins in Günther's disease.

Uroporphyrinogen decarboxylase catalyses a series of decarboxylation steps in which four moles of carboxyl are lost from every mole of porphyrinogen from octacarboxylic uroporphyrinogen to tetracarboxylic coproporphyrinogen. Studies have shown that the reaction starts with the D ring (Figure 12.1) and proceeds through the A, B and C rings to give hepta-, hexa- and pentacarboxylic intermediates prior to the formation of coproporphyrinogen III. The same series of reactions is followed by both the I and III series but because of substrate specificity the III series is more rapidly decarboxylated. At the pentacarboxylic porphyrin stage, one of the propionate side-chains is decarboxylated and oxidized to a vinyl group on ring A by coproporphyrinogen oxidase. This side branching results in a series of porphyrins important in porphyria cutanea tarda[25], the first one being dehydroisocoproporphyrinogen 3. If this sequence of

events is true, it means that uroporphyrinogen decarboxylase, a cytoplasmic enzyme, yields a product that has to return to the mitochondrion to be metabolized by coproporphyrinogen oxidase and then back to the cytoplasm for the next enzyme step. A more likely explanation is that with liver damage coproporphyrinogen oxidase becomes accessible to events in the cytoplasm. In the absence of disease, the path re-enters the mitochondrion catalysed by coproporphyrinogen oxidase, which is not membrane-bound but is situated in the intermitochondrial space[26]. Coproporphyrinogen oxidase requires molecular oxygen, and the end product of the reaction is protoporphyrinogen. This enzyme only oxidizes the III and IV series and not the I or II series. An intermediate is the monovinyl porphyrinogen, isoharderoporphyrinogen[27]. In homozygous hereditary coproporphyria accumulation of harderoporphyrin occurs[28].

Classification

The metabolic defect underlying the porphyrias can in all cases be traced to a specific enzyme in the porphyrin biosynthetic pathway (Figure 12.2). Although the alteration in enzyme activity may be found in numerous tissues, in practice the deficient activity may be expressed mainly in one tissue, for example, by the liver in acute intermittent porphyria, excess amounts of D-ALA and porphobilinogen (PBG) are produced. In the cutaneous porphyrias the enzyme defect lies further down the pathway and therefore overproduction of porphyrins as well as of porphyrin precursors occurs, accounting for the features of photosensitivity.

Traditionally the porphyrias were classified as hepatic or erythropoietic, depending on what was thought to be the primary site of porphyrin overproduction[29]. A clinically based classification dividing porphyrias into acute and non-acute conditions (Table 12.2) is a more useful method of categorizing these disorders. Acute intermittent porphyria, one of the most common porphyrias (particularly in Scandinavia), and the very rare plumboporphyria[30] do not have skin manifestations. Other porphyrias classified as acute include variegate porphyria, hereditary coproporphyria and its homozygous counterpart harderoporphyria[31]. The feature common to this group of porphyrias is the acute attack, in which huge increases in production and excretion of porphyrins and their precursors are associated with neurological and psychiatric symptoms and, less frequently, gastrointestinal disturbances. Photosensitivity is a feature of both acute and non-acute porphyrias, with the exception of acute intermittent and plumboporphyria. Acute attacks do not occur in the non-acute porphyrias, but systemic manifestations may be a feature of both types.

There are two patterns of expression of photosensitivity which occur with the porphyrias. The first

Table 12.2 *Classification of the porphyrias*

Condition	Enzyme deficiency
Non-acute porphyrias	
Günther's disease	Uroporphyrinogen cosynthase
Erythropoietic protoporphyria	Protoporphyrinogen oxidase
Porphyria cutanea tarda	Uroporphyrinogen decarboxylase
Hepatoerythrocytic porphyria	Uroporphyrinogen decarboxylase
Acute porphyrias	
Acute intermittent porphyria	Porphobilinogen deaminase
Variegate porphyria	Protoporphyrinogen oxidase
Homozygous variegate porphyria	Protoporphyrinogen oxidase
Hereditary coproporphyria	Coproporphyrinogen oxidase
Harderoporphyria	Coproporphyrinogen oxidase
Plumboporphyria	ALA dehydratase

ALA, aminolaevulinic acid.

is an immediate, painful phototoxic reaction. The second is a more chronic, painless destruction with skin fragility, blistering, erosions and scarring.

The acute porphyrias in general have their age of onset at or after puberty and are rare in childhood. Although the enzyme activity may be established as deficient prior to puberty by culturing fibroblasts, biochemical manifestations of the diseases may be normal and screening of families is best left until adolescence. By contrast, homozygous porphyrias tend to present in childhood.

References

1 Scherer J. Chemisch-physiologische Untersuchungen. *Leibig's Ann Chem Pharm* 1841; **40**: 1–64.
2 Schultz JH. Ein Fall von Pemphiques Leprosus kompliziert durch Lepra Visceralis. Inaugural dissertation, Greiswald, 1874.
3 Hausmann W. Uber die sensibiliserende Wirkung Tierischer Farbstoffe und ihre physiologische Anwendung. *Biochem Z* 1908; **14**: 275–83.
4 Meyer-Betz F. Untersuchungen uber die biologische (photodynamische) Wirking dees Hamatoporphyrins und anderen derivative des Blut- und Gallenfarbstaffes. *Dtsch Arch Klin Med* 1913 **112**: 476–503.
5 Garrod AE. On hematoporphyrin as a urinary pigment in disease. *J Pathol Bacteriol* 1893; **1**: 187–97.
6 Günther H. Die Hamatoporphyrie. *Dtsch Arch Clin Med* 1911; **105**: 89–146.
7 Fischer H. Beobachtungen am frischen Harn und Kot von Porphyrinpatienten. *Hoppe Seylers Z Rev Physiol Chem* 1916; **97**: 148–70.
8 Günther H. Die Bedeutung der Hamatoporphyrie in Physiologie und pathologie. *Ergeb Allg Pathol Anat* 1922; **20**: 608–764.
9 Shemin D, Rittenberg D. The utilization of glycine for the synthesis of porphyrin. *J Biol Chem* 1945; **159**: 567–8.
10 Westall RG. Isolation of porphobilinogen from the urine of a patient with acute porphyria. *Nature* 1952; **170**: 614–16.
11 Granick S. Porphyrin synthesis in erythrocytes. *J Biol Chem* 1958; **232**: 1101–17.
12 Rimington C. The occurrence of congenital porphyria (Pink Tooth) in cattle in South Africa: chemical studies on the living animals and post-mortem material. *Onderstepoort J Vet Sci Ind* 1936; **7**: 567–609.
13 Barnes AD. Further South African cases of porphyrinuria. *S Afr J Clin Sci* 1951; **2**: 117.
14 Dean G, Barnes HD. The inheritance of porphyria. *Br Med J* 1955; **2**: 89–94.
15 Magnus IA, Jarrett A, Prankerd TAJ et al. Erythropoietic protoporphyria: a new porphyria syndrome with solar urticaria due to protoporphyrinaemia. *Lancet* 1961; **ii**: 448–51.
16 Kordac V, Deybach JC, Martasek P. Homozygous variegate porphyria. *Lancet* 1984; **i**: 851.
17 Murphy GM, Hawk JLM, Magnus IA, Barrett DF, Elder GH, Smith SE. Homozygous variegate porphyria: two similar cases in unrelated families. *J Roy Soc Med* 1986; **79**: 361–4.
18 Granick S, Sassa S. Delta-aminolevulinic acid synthetase and the control of heme and chlorophyll synthesis. In: Vogel HJ, ed. *Metabolic Regulation*, vol. 5. Academic Press, New York, 1971; 77–141.
19 Jordan PM, Shemin D. Delta-aminolevulinic acid synthetase. In: Bover PD, ed. *The Enzymes*, vol. 7. 3rd ed. Academic Press, New York, 1972; 339–56.
20 Battersby AR, Fookes CJR, Matcham GWJ et al. Biosynthesis of the pigments of life. *Nature* 1980; **285**: 17–21.
21 Jackson AG, Elder GH, Smith SG. The metabolism of coproporphyrinogen III into protoporphyrin IX. *Int J Biochem* 1978; **9**: 877–82.

22 Porra RJ, Jones OTG. Studies on ferrochelatase: II. An investigation of the role of ferrochelatase in the biosynthesis of various heme prosthetic groups. *Biochem J* 1963; **87**: 186–92.

23 Moore MR, Meredith PA, Goldberg A. Lead and heme biosynthesis. In: Singhal RD, Thomas JA, eds. *Lead Toxicity*. Urban & Schwartzenberg, Baltimore, 1980; 79–114.

24 Moore MR, McColl KEL, Goldberg A. The effects of alcohol on porphyrin biosynthesis and metabolism. In: Roskali SB, ed. *Clinical Biochemistry of Alcoholism*. Churchill Livingstone, Edinburgh, 1985; 161–87.

25 Elder GH. Differentiation of porphyria cutanea tarda symptomatica from other types of porphyria by measurement of isocoproporphyrin in faeces. *J Clin Pathol* 1975; **28**: 601–7.

26 Grandchamp B, Phung N, Nordmann Y. The mitochondrial localisation of coproporphyrinogen III oxidase. *Biochem J* 1978; **172**: 345.

27 Elder GH, Evans JO, Thomas N et al. The primary enzyme defect in hereditary coproporphyria. *Lancet* 1976; **ii**: 1217–19.

28 Nordmann Y, Grandchamp B, De Verneuil H et al. Harderoporphyria: a variant hereditary coproporphyria. *J Clin Invest* 1983; **72**: 1139–49.

29 Schmidt R, Schwartz S, Watson CJ. Porphyrin content of bone marrow and liver in the various forms of porphyria. *Arch Int Med* 1954; **93**: 167–80.

30 Doss M, Tiepermann RV, Schneider J et al. Porphobilinogen synthase (delta-aminolevulinic acid dehydratase) deficiency in bone marrow cells of two patients with porphobilinogen synthase defect acute porphyria. *Klin Wochenschr* 1983; **61**: 699–702.

31 Moore MR, Disler PB, Biochemical diagnosis of the porphyrias. *Clin Dermatol* 1985; **3**: 7–40.

Günther's disease

Synonym: *Congenital erythropoietic porphyria*

Günther's disease or congenital erythropoietic porphyria is a rare autosomal recessive disorder caused by uroporphyrinogen III synthase deficiency (see Figure 12.2) which may present at birth or in the first year of life[1,2], though milder cases presenting in adult life may rarely occur [3–5] and may be dominated by haematological features such as thrombocytopenia and haemolytic anaemia. Photosensitivity in childhood cases is usually severe and mutilating, accompanied by haemolytic anaemia which may ultimately be the cause of death.

Clinical features

First recognition of this disease may be because of red or pink porphyrin-stained nappies. In sunlight the infant is irritable, and erythema and blisters develop days later in light-exposed sites. Primary teeth are stained a brownish-red colour by deposition of uroporphyrin in the calcium-rich hydroxyapatite dental matrix. The teeth and urine fluoresce red when

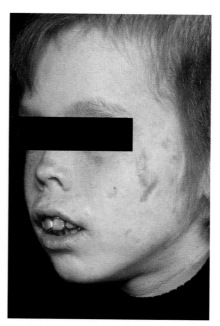

Figure 12.3 *Günther's disease*

illuminated by Wood's light, indicating the creation of singlet-excited porphyrins with subsequent red light energy re-emission from the singlet state. Cumulative exposure to light results in severe mutilating scarring, hypertrichosis, scarring alopecia and pigmentary change. Resorption of the nose and ears, ectropion, eclabium and even scleromalacia perforans may result in significant disfigurement (Figure 12.3) and blindness. Resorption of digital extremities, loss of nails and clawing of hands lead to marked limitation of function.

Diagnosis is established by the pattern of porphyrin excretion in the plasma red cells, urine and faeces (Table 12.3). Wood's light examination of urine and an aqueous suspension of faeces reveals the presence of excess porphyrins. Examination of a blood film (diluted 1:4 with 0.4% NaCl) by a violet light fluorescent microscope allows visualization of stable red fluorescence indicative of congenital porphyria. Table 12.3 summarizes the porphyrin excretion pattern, in which type I uroporphyrin isomer predominates in urine, plasma and red cells and coproporphyrin is predominant in the stool, a pattern which might be anticipated from the deficient activity of uroporphyrinogen III synthase (URO III-S).

Genetics

Isolation and sequencing of a full-length sequence of complementary DNA has enabled study of the enzymatic defect at molecular level[6]. Amplification of DNA from 2 patients with Günther's disease using the polymerase chain reaction showed two distinct point mutations coexisting in one patient and a homozygous defect in the second patient, indicating that the

Table 12.3 *Excretion patterns in the porphyrias*

	Urine				Faeces			Erythrocytes	
	ALA	PBG	Uroporphyrin	Coproporphyrin	Coproporphyrin	Protoporphyrin	X-porphyrin	Coproporphyrin	Protoporphyrin
Acute porphyria									
Acute intermittent porphyria	Raised; very high	Raised; very high	Usually raised	Sometimes raised	Sometimes raised	Sometimes raised	Sometimes raised	Normal	Normal
Variegate porphyria	Raised in attack	Raised in attack	Usually raised in attack	Usually raised in attack	Raised	Raised	Raised very high in attack	Normal	Normal
Hereditary coproporphyria	Raised in attack	Raised in attack	Sometimes raised in attack	Usually raised; always raised in attack	Raised	Usually normal	Sometimes raised; especially with photosensitivity	Sometimes raised in attack	Normal
Plumboporphyria	Raised in attack	Raised in attack	Normal	Normal	Normal	Normal	Normal	Normal	Normal
Non-acute porphyria									
Porphyria cutanea tarda	Normal	Normal	Raised; very high in attack	Slightly raised	Raised in remission	Raised in remission	Raised	Normal	Normal
Erythropoietic protoporphyria	Normal	Normal	Normal	Normal	Normal	Usually raised	Normal	Sometimes slightly raised	Raised; usually very high
Günther's disease	Usually normal	Usually normal	Raised; isomer 1	Raised; isomer 1	Normal	Usually raised	Normal	Usually raised	Usually raised

ALA, aminolaevulinic acid; PBG, porphobilinogen.

primary defect in Günther's disease is a structural alteration of URO III-S gene[7]. Multiple defects have now been identified and correlation between genotype and phenotype is beginning to be possible.

Treatment

In severely affected children careful protection from light exposure is necessary, otherwise debility, growth retardation and haematological crises lead to death before puberty. Splenectomy may prevent haemolytic crises. Protective spectacles with side and top flaps for protection are mandatory. Milder cases are less disabled, and may achieve a normal lifespan with appropriate management of medical problems. Haematin has transient effects on porphyrin synthesis and seems disappointing in its lack of clinical efficacy[5].

References

1 Bhutani LK, Sood SK, Das PK et al. Congenital erythropoietic porphyria. An autopsy report. *Arch Dermatol* 1974; **110**: 427–9.

2 Murphy GM, Hawk JLM, Nicholson DC et al Congenital erythropoietic porphyria (Gunther's disease). *Clin Exp Dermatol* 1987; **12**: 61–5.

3 Murphy A, Gibson G, Elder GH et al. Adult onset congenital erythropoietic porphyria (Günther's disease) presenting with thrombocytopenia. *J Roy Soc Med* 1995; **88**: 357–8.

4 Deybach JC, de Verneuil H, Phung N et al. Congenital erythropoietic porphyria (Gunther's disease): enzymatic studies on two cases of late onset. *J Lab Clin Med* 1981; **97**: 551–8.

5 Rank JM, Straka JG, Weimer MK et al. Haematin therapy in late onset congenital erythropoietic porphyria. *Br J Haematol* 1990; **75**: 617–18.

6 Tsai SF, Bishop DF, Desnick RJ. URO III-S: molecular cloning, nucleotide sequence and expression of a full length cDNA. *Proc Nat Acad Sci USA* 1988; **85**: 7049–51.

7 Deybach JC, de Verneuil H, Boulechfar S et al. Point mutations in the Uroporphyrinogen III Synthase gene in congenital erythropoietic porphyria (Günther's disease). *Curr Probl Dermatol* 1991; **20**: 148–53.

Erythropoietic protoporphyria

Erythropoietic protoporphyria (EPP) is the most common of the childhood porphyrias. As a consequence of defective haem synthetase, lipophilic precursors of haem, the 2-carboxylic protoporphyrins, accumulate in liver, bile, red cells and plasma. Excretion of these compounds is via the hepatobiliary tract and gut.

Clinical features

Photoexcitation of protoporphyrin in the skin leads to cutaneous symptoms and signs. The average age of onset of symptoms is 2 years[1], although presentation as late as the seventh decade has been

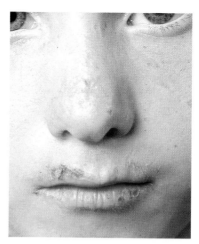

Figure 12.4 *Erythropoietic protoporphyria with crusting and scarring on the nose and lips*

described[2]. Phototoxic symptoms without any visible signs are common. Immediate burning, pain and discomfort of light-exposed skin may occur. With more exposure, swelling of the skin often without accompanying erythema may occur. Purpura may occur with severe attacks but is unusual. More chronic signs include erosions, and crusting leading to shallow, round or oval and linear scarring on the malar areas, nose, chin and forehead (Figure 12.4). Waxy, linear scars are characteristic on the nose. Symptoms vary enormously from patient to patient even within the same family. Thickening of the skin over the knuckles may be pronounced. With continued exposure to sunlight extensive indurated plaques may develop with marked thickening of the skin. Blistering, hypertrichosis and milia are not usually features of EPP. The difference in clinical signs in EPP compared with other porphyrias may be because of lipophilic porphyrins resulting in repeated blood vessel basement membrane damage, leading to reduplication of the basement membrane and large amounts of type IV collagen deposited around the blood vessels[2], an appearance not dissimilar to lipoid proteinosis with which EPP used to be confused.

Systemic manifestations of EPP include a high incidence of cholelithiasis, analysis of which reveals a high protoporphyrin content. Liver dysfunction may be severe [3–5] but is relatively rare. Three cases of progressive liver failure occurred out of 300 cases followed over 5 years[1]. Milder liver dysfunction may occur with slight biochemical abnormalities. Liver biopsy may be normal or reveal deposition of protoporphyrin with periportal and portal fibrosis or severe cirrhosis and liver cell necrosis in liver failure. There appears to be no way of predicting which patients will develop liver disease; it usually supervenes in adult life after many years of symptoms, but childhood cases have also occurred. The level of red cell and plasma porphyrins correlates neither with symptom severity nor liver failure.

Diagnosis of EPP may be made by examination of the red cells, plasma and stool for porphyrins (see Table 12.2). Transient fluorescence of red cells is seen by fluorescent microscopy. Raised free protoporphyrin greater than zinc-bound protoporphyrin is present in red cells. Plasma porphyrin levels are raised, and in stool, protoporphyrin predominates. Porphyrin levels are not abnormally elevated in urine, but in terminal liver failure uroporphyrin and coproporphyrin levels may be raised[6].

Genetics

The human ferrochelatase gene has been mapped to chromosome 18q21.3[7]. Elucidation of the patterns of inheritance in EPP has recently been possible by examining the activity of haem synthetase (ferrochelatase) in lymphocytes from affected patients and their relatives[8]. The competitive action of ferrous ions and the inhibitory effects of *N*-methyl protoporphyrin (a specific inhibitor of haem synthetase) on zinc chelatase demonstrated that ferrochelatase and zinc chelatase activities reside in the same enzyme. Zinc chelatase was shown to be deficient in a pattern suggestive of autosomal dominant inheritance but also in some families in a pattern suggesting autosomal recessive expression of the disease[8]. The DNA sequencing of the EPP gene confirms the heterogeneous nature of genetic defects. Recessive inheritance and homozygous expression may account for some patients with liver failure[9].

Treatment

Although thickly applied reflectant sunscreens, particularly the new microfine preparations, afford some protection against long-wavelength UVR and visible light, the cosmetic acceptability of such an approach is limited. Beta-carotene[10,11] is effective in about one-third of patients, usually given in doses of up to 200–250 mg daily. It causes an orange-brown discolouration of the skin. Canthaxanthin has been incorporated with some beta-carotene preparations to improve the colour, but in view of subtle visual defects induced by retinal deposition of crystalline canthaxanthin[12] pure beta-carotene is preferable. Terfenadine inhibits the flare seen on phototesting patients with EPP[13], suggesting that histamine release is part of the mechanism of porphyrin photosensitivity in addition to generation of reactive oxygen species[14] and complement activation[15]. Liver transplantation should be considered for progressive end-stage liver failure. Protoporphyrin overproduction may remain high after liver transplantation, suggesting predominant erythropoietic origin; thus the long-term prognosis for the transplanted liver with regard to further liver damage remains uncertain, but the procedure offers several years of good-quality life as an alternative to an otherwise fatal outcome[16].

References

1 Murphy GM, Hawk JLM, Corbett MF, Herxheimer A, Magnus IA. The UK erythropoietic protoporphyria register: a progress report. *Br J Dermatol* 1985; **113**: 11.

2 Murphy GM, Hawk JLM, Magnus IA. Late-onset erythropoietic protoporphyria with unusual cutaneous features. *Arch Dermatol* 1985; **121**: 1309.

3 Cripps DJ, Scheuer PJ. Hepatobiliary changes in erythropoietic protoporphyria. *Arch Pathol* 1965; **80**: 500–8.

4 Donaldson EM, McCall AJ, Magnus IA, Simpson JR, Caldwell RA, Hargreaves T. Erythropoietic protoporphyria: two deaths from hepatic cirrhosis. *Br J Dermatol* 1971; **84**: 14–19.

5 Scott AJ, Ansford AJ, Webster BH, Stringer HCW. Erythropoietic protoporphyria with features of sideroblastic anaemia terminating in liver failure. *Am J Med* 1973; **54**: 254–6.

6 Pimstone NR. The hepatic aspects of the porphyrias. In: Read AE, ed. *Modern Trends in Gastroenterology 5*. Butterworth; London, 1975; 373–417.

7 Brenner DA, Didier JM, Fraser F et al. A molecular defect in human protoporphyria. *Am J Hum Genet* 1992; **50**: 1203–10.

8 Norris PG, Nunn AV, Hawk JLM, Cox TM. Analysis of the genetic defect in erythropoietic protoporphyria by measurement of lymphocyte zinc chelatase. *Br J Dermatol* 1989; **120**: 295–6.

9 Sarkany RPE, Alexander GJM, Cox TM. Recessive inheritance of erythropoietic protoporphyria with liver failure. *Lancet* 1994; **343**: 1394–6.

10 Matthews-Roth MM, Pathak MA, Fitzpatrick TB et al. Beta-carotene therapy for erythropoietic protoporphyria and other photosensitivity diseases. *Arch Dermatol* 1977; **113**: 1229–32.

11 Corbett MF, Herxheimer A, Magnus IA et al. The long term treatment with beta-carotene in erythropoietic protoporphyria: a controlled trial. *Br J Dermatol* 1977; **97**: 655–62.

12 Rousseau A. Canthaxanthine deposits in the eye. *J Am Acad Dermatol* 1983; **8**: 123–4.

13 Farr PM, Diffey BL, Matthews JNS. Inhibition of photosensitivity in erythropoietic protoporphyria with terfenadine. *Br J Dermatol* 1990; **122**: 809–15.

14 Weishaupt KR, Gomer CJ, Dogherty TJ. Identification of singlet oxygen as the cytotoxic agent in photoactivation of a murine tumour. *Cancer Res* 1976; **36**: 2326–9.

15 Lim HW, Poh-Fitzpatrick MB, Gigli I. Activation of the complement system in patients with porphyrias after irradiation in vivo. *J Clin Invest* 1984; **74**: 1961–5.

16 Polson RJ, Lim CK, Rolles K. The effect of liver transplantation in a 13 year old boy with erythropoietic protoporphyria. *Transplantation* 1988; **46**: 386–9.

Porphyria cutanea tarda

In most centres in Europe and North America, porphyria cutanea tarda (PCT) is the most common porphyria seen in adults. It is unusual in childhood.

Clinical features

Clinical features of PCT include skin fragility, blistering, erosions and milia formation on light-exposed areas. Facial hypertrichosis, hyperpigmentation, scarring alopecia, and in about 10–15% of cases sclerodermoid plaques (mainly but not exclusively confined to light-exposed areas), cirrhosis of the liver and hepatic tumours may also occasionally occur. Porphyric cutanea tarda may also be a consequence of a hepatic tumour.

Childhood PCT presents similarly, but in some children much more severe manifestations are seen with additional abnormalities of porphyrin excretion. The porphyrin profile of urine, stool and plasma resembles PCT, but in addition the red cells contain increased amounts of free and zinc-bound protoporphyrin. This syndrome, formerly called hepatoerythropoietic porphyria[1], is now thought to represent homozygous PCT[2]. Clinically, erythrodontia may be present, the skin lesions are severe with fragility, bullae and mutilating scarring. In addition anaemia (haemolytic and non-haemolytic) is often a feature. Early cirrhosis and non-specific hepatitis appear to be early features. Measurement of the enzyme uroporphyrinogen decarboxylase (URO-D) indicates profound depression of enzyme activity compared with heterozygous PCT where enzyme activity is approximately 60% of normal, supporting the idea of a homozygous state rather than a recessively inherited disease as was formerly thought. The cDNA and gene for human URO-D have been isolated and sequenced, indicating that a number of different mutations lead to defects of URO-D[3]. Further evidence for genetic heterogeneity derives from demonstration of two patterns of inherited enzyme defect, one in which the enzyme catalytic activity and immunoreactive enzyme are decreased in parallel and a second pattern where catalytic activity is reduced but immunoreactive activity is present[4].

Pathology

Porphyria cutanea tarda is considered to be a hepatic porphyria because porphyrin overproduction occurs in the hepatocytes with normal porphyrin production in the bone marrow. The deficient enzyme, uroporphyrinogen decarboxylase, is responsible for the block in decarboxylation of 4-, 5-, 6-, 7- and 8-carboxylic porphyrins; a characteristic pattern of faecal porphyrin excretion ensues with predominant 8- and 7-carboxylic or uroporphyrins and lesser amounts of the 6-, 5- and 4-carboxylic coproporphyrins with an unusual tetracarboxylic porphyrin isocoproporphyrin, characteristic of PCT, identifiable on thin-layer chromatography or high-pressure liquid chromatography[5]. Since the porphyrins accumulated are predominantly water-soluble, copious amounts of porphyrins are excreted in urine. The ratio of uroporphyrins to coproporphyrins is usually 4:1; if coproporphyrin predominates another diagnosis should be considered. Wood's light fluorescence of urine yields red fluorescence intensified by acidification. Doubtful cases may be clarified by extraction of porphyrins from acidified urine with a few millilitres of ethyl acetate or amyl alcohol, concentrating the porphyrins into a smaller volume, thus intensifying the fluorescence.

Genetics

Porphyria cutanea tarda appears to occur both as an inherited and an acquired disease. Most cases (> 90%) appear to be acquired or sporadic. Others are clearly inherited in an autosomal dominant pattern. It is possible that many of the apparently sporadic cases are in fact inherited tendencies precipitated by exogenous factors. Agents known to precipitate PCT include alcohol, iron overload, oestrogens and polychlorinated aromatic hydrocarbons[6,7]; hepatitis C and human immunodeficiency virus infection have also been implicated.

References

1 Day RS, Strauss PC. Severe cutaneous porphyria in a 12 year old boy. Hepatoerythropoietic or symptomatic porphyria. *Arch Dermatol* 1982; **118**: 663–7.
2 Elder GH, Smith SG, Herrero C et al. Hepatoerythropoietic porphyria: a new uroporphyrinogen decarboxylase defect or homozygous porphyria cutanea tarda. *Lancet* 1980; **i**: 916–19.
3 Garey JR, Harrison LM, Franklin KF et al. Uroporphyrinogen decarboxylase: a splice site mutation causes the deletion of exon 6 in multiple families with porphyria cutanea tarda. *J Clin Invest* 1990; **86**: 1416–22.
4 Koskzo F, Elder GH, Roberts A, Simon N. Uroporphyrinogen decarboxylase deficiency in hepatoerythropoietic porphyria: further evidence for genetic heterogeneity. *Br J Dermatol* 1990; **122**: 365–70.
5 Elder GH. Enzymatic defects in porphyria: an overview. *Semin Liver Dis* 1982; **2**: 87–99.
6 Marks GS. The effects of chemicals on hepatic heme biosynthesis. *Trends Pharm Sci* 1981; **2**: 59–61.
7 Peters HA. Hexachlorobenzene poisoning in Turkey. *Fed Proc* 1974; **35**: 2400–3.

Variegate porphyria

Variegate porphyria is an autosomal dominant porphyria caused by reduced activity of protoporphyrinogen oxidase, leading to the porphyrin excretion pattern indicated in Table 12.2.

Clinical features

The clinical features of variegate porphyria are variable. The latent state is common, with often only minimal biochemical evidence of the underlying enzyme deficiency present. Other patients express photosensitivity to a variable degree. Acute attacks may be unrelated to the severity of cutaneous symptoms and some patients with acute attacks suffer little in the way of photosensitivity. In some patients precipitating causes[1] are of importance, while in others cutaneous symptoms continue despite their avoidance. The cutaneous manifestations are identical to porphyria cutanea tarda. A characteristic finding in the latent state is increased amounts of the lipophilic porphyrins 3-carboxyl porphyrin, coproporphyrin and protoporphyrin in faeces. When disease activity is present the water-soluble porphyrins and precursors (uroporphyrin, coproporphyrin, PBG and ALA) are excreted in urine. A useful screening test in variegate porphyria is the characteristic plasma fluorescence emission spectrum which peaks at 624 nm[2].

Homozygous variegate porphyria is now well described[3,4], though very rare. Porphyrin excretion in urine, stool and plasma is similar to that of variegate porphyria, but in addition levels of erythrocyte protoporphyrin, both free and zinc-bound, are raised[4,5]. Enzyme activity of protoporphyrinogen decarboxylase is profoundly depressed, whereas in variegate porphyria enzyme activity is 50% that of normal controls. This disease has been seen by the author in 4 unrelated patients, all with similar features. Presentation is in childhood; clinical features include blistering, erosions, milia formation and skin fragility. Small stature has been a feature of all cases, with growth in childhood below the third centile. Clinodactyly was a feature of 3 patients. Mental retardation has also been described[5]. Screening of family members indicated variegate porphyria to be present in the parents. One of the female homozygous variegate porphyria patients has had a healthy baby, though the child must be genetically predisposed to develop variegate porphyria. The gene for variegate porphyria has now been mapped to chromosome 1q23[6].

Treatment

Genetic counselling together with advice on the avoidance of porphyrinogenic drugs is essential. Family screening is facilitated by fluorescence emission spectroscopy of plasma[7].

References

1 Moore MR, Disler PB. Drug induction of the acute porphyrias. *Adv Drug React Acute Poison Rev* 1983; **2**: 149–89.
2 Poh-Fitzpatrick MB. A plasma porphyrin fluorescence marker for variegate porphyria. *Arch Dermatol* 1980; **116**: 543–7.
3 Kordac V, Deybach JC, Martasek P. Homozygous variegate porphyria. *Lancet* 1984; **i**: 851.
4 Murphy GM, Hawk JLM, Magnus IA et al. Homozygous variegate porphyria: two similar cases in unrelated families. *J Roy Soc Med* 1986; **79**: 361–4.
5 Kordac V, Martasek P, Zeman J, Rubin A. Increased erythrocyte protoporphyrin in homozygous variegate porphyria. *Photodermatology* 1985; **2**: 257–9.
6 Roberts AG, Whatley SD, Daniels J et al. Partial characterisation and assignment of the gene for protoporphyrinogen oxidase and variegate porphyria to human chromosome 1q23. *Hum Mol Genet* 1995; **4**: 2387–90.
7 Long C, Smyth SJ, Woolf J et al. Detection of latent variegate porphyria by fluorescence emission spectroscopy of plasma. *Br J Dermatol* 1993; **129**: 9–13.

Hereditary coproporphyria

Hereditary coproporphyria is a disease of adults, in which neurovisceral symptoms predominate.

Clinical features

Photosensitivity occurs only in 30% of patients, and the clinical features are identical to variegate porphyria and porphyria cutanea tarda. Very large quantities of coproporphyrin predominate in urine and faeces. Harderoporphyria[1,2] appears to be the homozygous form of coproporphyria; the 3- series of carboxylic porphyrins predominate (60–80%) with 20–40% protoporphyrin excretion. Children are small in stature and acute attacks may occur.

Treatment

Recent advances in treatment of acute attacks include the use of haematin, which is thought to have a selective effect in suppressing porphyrin synthesis in hepatocytes[3]. Haem arginate seems safer with regard to inducing thrombotic events and is successful in the treatment of acute attacks of variegate porphyria but disappointing in its long-term efficacy, and porphyrin levels are not reduced long-term[4]. Enzyme replacement measures remain experimental, but may be more successful in the future[5,6].

References

1 Nordmann Y, Grandchamp B, de Verneuil H et al. Harderoporphyria: a variant hereditary coproporphyria. *J Clin Invest* 1983; **72**: 1139–49.
2 Grandchamp B, Phung N, Nordmann Y. Homozygous case of hereditary coproporphyria. *Lancet* 1977; **ii**: 1348–9.
3 McColl KEL, Moore MR, Thompson GG et al. Treatment with haematin in acute hepatic porphyria. *Quart J Med* 1981; **50**: 161–74.
4 Timonen K, Mustajoki P, Tenhunen R, Lauharanta J. Effects of haem arginate on variegate porphyria. *Br J Dermatol* 1990; **123**: 381–7.
5 Batll AM del C, Bustos N, Stella AM et al. Enzyme replacement therapy in the porphyrias: IV. First successful

human clinical trial of ALA dehydratase: loaded erythrocyte ghosts. *Int J Biochem* 1983; **15**: 1261–5.

6 Espinola LG, Wider EA, Stella AM et al. Enzyme replacement therapy in porphyrias: II. Entrapment of ALA dehydratase in liposomes. *Int J Biochem* 1983; **15**: 439–45.

Idiopathic photodermatoses

Polymorphic light eruption

Polymorphic light eruption (PLE) is the most common of the photodermatoses[1,2] affecting up to 15% of adults in Britain. The usual age of onset is in the second or third decade, but PLE may occur at any age and is not uncommon in childhood.

Clinical features

Symptoms begin in spring or early summer: patients complain of an itching or burning erythematous papular eruption, occurring 1–24 hours after being in sunlight, on exposed skin. With avoidance of further exposure lesions disappear in days. The face is frequently spared, and as summer continues, tolerance builds up in about a third of patients. Polymorphic light eruption is reproduced by broad-band sources of UVA and solar simulated radiation in 75% of cases[3,4] and by UVB in 25%.

Pathology

Histological and immunological features point towards a delayed hypersensitivity mechanism, probably directed against UVR-induced neoallergens [5–7].

Genetics

A family history of the disorder is often obtained[8], but the importance of inheritance is unclear.

Differential diagnosis

Other causes of photosensitivity should be excluded such as lupus erythematosus (LE), particularly subacute cutaneous LE, and allergic contact or photocontact dermatitis which may simulate PLE.

Treatment

Most patients are mildly affected and symptoms may be controlled by frequent application of high-factor sunscreens, now highly effective UVB absorbers. In predominantly UVA-sensitive patients, sunscreens (though increasingly effective at absorbing and reflecting UVA) are not usually effective enough to prevent symptoms. Prophylactic psoralens with UVA (PUVA) or UVB (which is less effective) given each spring before the onset of symptoms induces a state of tolerance[9], possibly by depleting epidermal Langerhans cells[10] and reducing antigen presentation to the immune system. Hydroxychloroquine is a much less effective but occasionally useful treatment[11], given as a short course over the period of maximum exposure and symptoms. With a severe episode of PLE a short course of systemic steroids aborts the attack.

References

1 Morison WL, Stern RS. Polymorphous light eruption: a common reaction uncommonly recognised. *Acta Dermatovenereol* 1982; **62**: 237–40.

2 Ros A, Wennersten G. Current aspects of polymorphous light eruptions in Sweden. *Photodermatology* 1987; **3**: 298–302.

3 Holzle E, Plewig G, Hoffman C, Roser-Maas E. Polymorphous light eruption: experimental reproduction of skin lesions. *J Am Acad Dermatol* 1982; **7**: 111–25.

4 Miyamoto C. Polymorphous light eruption: successful reproduction of skin lesions, including papulovesicular light eruption with ultraviolet B. *Photodermatology* 1989; **6**: 69–79.

5 Muhlbauer JE, Bahn AK, Harris TJ et al. Papular polymorphic light eruption: an immunoperoxidase study using monoclonal antibodies. *Br J Dermatol* 1983; **108**: 153–62.

6 Moncada B, Gonzales-Amaro R, Barcunda ML et al. Immunopathology of polymorphic light eruption. *J Am Acad Dermatol* 1984; **10**: 970–3.

7 Norris PG, Morris J, McGibbon DM, Chu AC, Hawk JLM. Polymorphic light eruption: an immunopathological study of evolving lesions. *Br J Dermatol* 1989; **120**: 173–83.

8 Frain-Bell W, Mason B. The investigation of polymorphic light eruption in identical twins. *Br J Dermatol* 1968; **80**: 314–22.

9 Murphy GM, Logan RA, Lovell CR et al. Prophylactic PUVA and UVB therapy in polymorphic light eruption – a controlled trial. *Br J Dermatol* 1987; **116**: 531–8.

10 Friedmann PS. Disappearance of epidermal Langerhans cells during PUVA therapy. *Br J Dermatol* 1981; **105**: 219–21.

11 Murphy GM, Hawk JLM, Magnus IA. Hydroxychloroquine in polymorphic light eruption: a controlled trial with drug and visual sensitivity monitoring. *Br J Dermatol* 1987; **116**: 379–86.

Juvenile spring eruption

Juvenile spring eruption occurs in spring or early summer, and is characterized by itching papules on the sun-exposed helices of the ears. It is a common disorder frequently unrecognized because it is often mild and transient, thus not presenting to dermatologists. Typically boys are affected, probably because of their shorter hair-styles, but it is frequently seen in girls also. Several members of a family may be affected, some patients also develop typical polymorphic light eruption, or members of the family may have PLE (author's personal observations). The time-course of the reaction and the association with PLE suggest that it is a mild, localized form of PLE. Use of a total sunblock prevents the reaction in most children, and as tolerance usually develops after some weeks of sun exposure, further treatment is not necessary.

Actinic prurigo

Actinic prurigo (AP) is predominantly a disease of childhood in Britain[1]. It is rare by comparison with PLE. The most common age of onset is 5 years, most cases occurring before the age of 11 years. A family history is more frequent (25%) than in PLE, and the male to female ratio is 1:3. It is a chronic disorder tending to improve in adolescence, 25% remitting completely. Some patients develop a clinical picture identical to PLE.

Clinical features

Symptoms are perennial but worse in summer, sun exposure leading to a rash which is sometimes not noticed. Clinical features include erythematous papular and vesicular lesions, predominantly on light-exposed areas including the face. Often there is sparing of the forehead but involvement of the buttocks. Scarring and cheilitis occur, and conjunctivitis with severe involvement.

In Amerindians in North America, Colombia and Mexico, AP is a more clear-cut entity [2–5]. The familial incidence is as high as 75%, which has suggested autosomal dominance with incomplete penetrance, although this has not been confirmed. Human lymphocyte antigens B40 and Cw3 are associated, suggesting both a genetic and an immunological predisposition[6]. The clinical features are similar to those of the UK cases, in whom complete concordance with HLA-DR4 has been demonstrated in all cases investigated[7]. Amerindians are more severely affected, with more frequent cheilitis and conjunctivitis. Seasonal fluctuation may be inapparent because of continued UVR exposure at high altitude in South America.

Differential diagnosis

Actinic prurigo may represent a form of persistent PLE; it has been suggested that PLE and AP may be differentiated by the augmentation rather than suppression of UV erythema by indomethacin in AP[8], but this phenomenon is not specific and may be seen in severe PLE also. Differentiation from atopic eczema may be difficult, but the history, distal light-exposed limb involvement and characteristic excoriated papules may be helpful[9]. Monochromatic irradiation testing is helpful only in the 50% or fewer with abnormal tests. Provocation phototesting with broad-band sources may elicit lesions as in PLE in others. Lupus erythematosus, porphyria and other photogenodermatoses should be excluded.

Treatment

Treatment of AP includes the use of sunscreens, particularly combination UVB and UVA absorbers and reflectants. Topical corticosteroids ease symptoms, and thalidomide may be dramatically effective after an initial slow response[10]. Induction of tolerance with PUVA and UVB may be effective but difficult to administer to small children.

References

1 Calnan CD, Meara RH. Actinic prurigo (Hutchinson's summer prurigo). *Clin Exp Dermatol* 1977; **2**: 365–72.
2 Everett MA, Crockett W, Lamb JH, Minor D. Light sensitive eruptions in American Indians. *Arch Dermatol* 1961; **83**: 243–8.
3 Birt AR, Davis RA. Hereditary polymorphic light eruption of American Indians. *Int J Dermatol* 1974; **14**: 105–11.
4 Birt AR, Hogg GR. The actinic cheilitis of hereditary polymorphic light eruption. *Arch Dermatol* 1979; **115**: 699–702.
5 Dominguez L, Hojyo MT. Actinic prurigo: a variety of polymorphous light eruption. *Int J Dermatol* 1982; **21**: 260–1.
6 Bernal JE, Duran De Rueda MM, de Brigard D. Human lymphocyte antigen in actinic prurigo. *J Am Acad Dermatol* 1988; **18**: 310–12.
7 Menage H duP, Baker C, Proby CM et al. Complete concordance between actinic prurigo and HLA DR4 in Britain. *Br J Dermatol* 1993; suppl. 42: 19.
8 Farr PM, Diffey BL. Augmentation of ultraviolet erythema by indomethacin in actinic prurigo: evidence of mechanism of photosensitivity. *Photochem Photobiol* 1986; **47**: 413–17.
9 Magnus IA. Polymorphic light eruption and summer prurigo. In: *Dermatological Photobiology. Clinical and Experimental Aspects.* Blackwell, Oxford, 1976; 174–88.
10 Lovell CR, Hawk JLM, Calnan CD, Magnus IA. Thalidomide in actinic prurigo. *Br J Dermatol* 1983; **108**: 467–71.

Solar urticaria

Solar urticaria[1] is a rare disease which may occur in childhood. It is an acquired condition with no well-documented familial instances, though it occurs in association with PLE or AP on occasion. Although urticarial wealing has been demonstrated in EPP on phototesting one patient[2], solar urticaria per se is not a feature.

References

1 Magnus IA. Solar urticaria. In: *Dermatological Photobiology. Clinical and Experimental Aspects.* Blackwell, Oxford, 1976; 202–10.

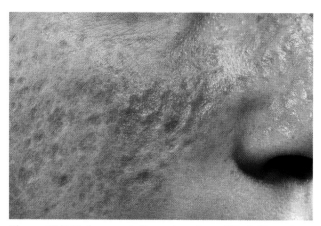

Figure 12.5 *Hydroa vacciniforme (courtesy of Dr J. Harper)*

2 Magnus IA, Jarrett A, Prankerd TAJ et al. Erythropoietic protoporphyria: a new porphyria syndrome with solar urticaria due to protoporphyrinaemia. *Lancet* 1961; **ii**: 448–51.

Hydroa vacciniforme

Hydroa vacciniforme has only rarely been documented as a familial disease[1]. It is a disease of childhood and merits description to distinguish it from porphyria or other childhood photodermatoses. Hartnup disease was associated with lesions indistinguishable from hydroa vacciniforme in one case[2].

Clinical features

The primary skin lesions are vesicles or umbilicated bullae arising on erythematous, sun-exposed skin (Figure 12.5). Lesions heal with scarring[3,4]. Repeated phototesting with UVA broad-band sources reproduce lesions in about half the patients[5,6]. Most patients' symptoms subside when they are in their late teens, though some symptoms continue in adult life.

Treatment

Treatment is difficult[3,4], but regular application of sunscreens incorporating UVA blockers or absorbers tends to be most successful.

References

1 Annamalai R. Hydroa vacciniforme in three alternate siblings. *Arch Dermatol* 1971; **103**: 224–6.
2 Ashurst PJ. Hydroa vacciniforme occurring in association with Hartnup disease. *Br J Dermatol* 1969; **81**: 486–92.
3 Goldgeier MH, Nordlund JJ, Lucky AW et al. Hydroa vacciniforme: diagnosis and therapy. *Arch Dermatol* 1982; **118**: 588–91.
4 Sonnex TS, Hawk JLM. Hydroa vacciniforme: a review of ten cases. *Br J Dermatol* 1988; **118**: 101–8.
5 Goldgeier MH, Nordlund JJ, Lucky AW. Reproduction of hydroa vacciniforme with UVA. *J Am Acad Dermatol* 1983; **9**: 279–80.
6 Halasz LLG, Leach EE, Walther RR et al. Hydroa vacciniforme: induction of lesions with ultraviolet A. *J Am Acad Dermatol* 1983; **8**: 171–6.

Disorders of tryptophan metabolism

Some inherited metabolic diseases may induce niacin deficiency leading to the clinical appearance associated with pellagra, a nutritional disorder due to lack of dietary niacin. Niacin, a non-essential vitamin, is synthesized from the amino acid tryptophan. Disorders of tryptophan metabolism thus may lead to niacin deficiency. The coenzymes nicotinamide adenine dinucleotide and nicotinamide adenine dinucleotide phosphate both incorporate niacin and are critical for intermediate metabolism.

Pellagra-like symptoms include the 'three Ds': dermatitis, dementia and diarrhoea. Erythematous patches and ulceration of mucous membranes and glossitis occur in the early stages. Skin lesions include erythema, pruritus and burning in sun-exposed areas. Acute lesions may be vesicular, and bullous chronic lesions become pigmented, scaly and lichenified; Casal's necklace is a scaling, hyperpigmented appearance involving the neck and 'V' of the chest. Apart from the clinical appearance, the evidence for photosensitivity in pellagra is scanty. Repeated irradiation of 7 pellagrinous Bantu subjects showed very little variation from normal Bantu[1].

Hartnup disease

Hartnup disease[2] is an autosomal recessive disease where defective gut absorption and renal tubular reabsorption of free neutral amino acids leads to tryptophan deficiency. Tryptophan is an important precursor of nicotinamide. In addition, indoles are absorbed from the gut in excess and may exert toxic neurological effects, as may a deficiency of other nicotinamide-dependent neurotransmitters. In some atypical patients, monochromatic irradiation testing has shown photosensitivity to be present[3].

References

1 Findlay GH, Rein L, Mitchell D. Reactions to light on the normal and pellagrous Bantu skin. *Br J Dermatol* 1969; **81**: 345–51.
2 Baron DN, Dent CE, Harris H, Hart EW, Jepson JB. Hereditary pellagra-like skin rash with cerebellar ataxia, constant renal aminoaciduria and other bizarre biochemical features. *Lancet* 1956; **ii**: 421.
3 Fenton DA, Wilkinson JD, Toseland PA. Family exhibiting cerebellar-like ataxia, photosensitivity and shortness of stature – a new inborn error of tryptophan metabolism. *J Roy Soc Med* 1983; **76**: 736–9.

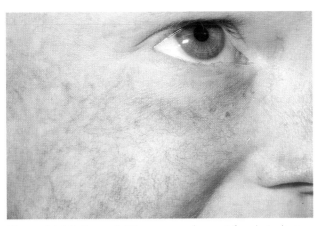

Figure 12.6 *Rothmund–Thomson syndrome: telangiectasia on the cheeks (courtesy of Dr J. Harper)*

Rothmund–Thomson syndrome

Synonym: *Poikiloderma congenitale*

Rothmund–Thomson syndrome[1,2] is a rare autosomal recessive disorder[3], manifesting in infancy or early childhood; 121 patients have been described with this disorder[4].

Clinical features

Diffuse erythema appears on the face and extensor surfaces. Oedematous and vesicular lesions may occur resolving to leave reticulate telangiectasia (Figure 12.6), mottled hyper- and hypopigmentation and atrophy in the first year of life. Skin changes may predominate on (but are not confined to) light-exposed areas, and do not progress after the age of 5 years[5]. One-third of patients have clinical features of photosensitivity[5]. Formal phototesting usually reveals normal minimal erythema doses at 24 hours[5,6]. Berg, however, described a 25-year-old female with clinical photosensitivity to sunlight and to phototesting with UVA[6]. Photosensitivity may be apparent in childhood and resolve by adulthood[4].

Skin cancer including squamous cell carcinoma[7,8] and Bowen's disease may supervene later in life[9]. Other malignancies such as osteosarcoma (reported in 5 patients) and sporadic cases of fibrosarcoma and gastric carcinoma give an impression of susceptibility to malignancy[10]. Reduced DNA repair of gamma-irradiation hypoxic damage in cultured fibroblasts has been described in 2 patients[11].

Terminal hair is sparse and fine with frontal recession. Vellous hair is absent on poikilodermatous areas. Nail and dental defects occur; cataracts develop in childhood in 40% by the age of 7 years, but may occur in the third decade[4]. Dwarfism is a frequent feature, with adult height less than 120 cm in 50% of cases. There are very many associated features[4]: hypogonadism, infertility in 25% of adults, mental retardation in 10%, skeletal abnormalities including absent or hypoplastic metacarpals and phalanges and long-bone deformities, and familial Clq deficiency have been described. Apart from this the prognosis appears to be good, with normal life expectancy. Kindler's syndrome[12] appears to be distinct, with progressive congenital poikiloderma associated with epidermolysis bullosa, macular atrophy, nail dystrophy, palmoplantar keratoderma, eczema and webbing of digits in some patients. In some patients the disorder appears to have autosomal dominant inheritance (hereditary acrokeratotic poikiloderma)[13] and photosensitivity does not appear to be a feature.

References

1 Rothmund A. Uber Kataract in Verbindung mit einer eigentumliche Haut Degeneration 1. *Arch Ophthalmol* 1868; **14**: 159.
2 Thomson MS. Poikiloderma congenitale. *Br J Dermatol* 1938; **48**: 221–34.
3 Hall HG, Pagon RA, Wilson KM. Rothmund Thomson syndrome with severe dwarfism. *Am J Dis Child* 1980; **134**: 165–9.
4 Moss C. Rothmund–Thomson syndrome: a report of two patients and a review of the literature. *Br J Dermatol* 1990; **122**: 821–9.
5 Alexander S. Rothmund–Thomson syndrome: 2 case reports. *Br J Dermatol* 1974; **91** (suppl): 62–4.
6 Berg E, Chuang T, Cripps D. Rothmund-Thomson syndrome. *J Am Acad Dermatol* 1987; **17**: 332–8.
7 Rook W, Whimster G. Congenital cutaneous dystrophy (Thomson's type). *Br J Dermatol* 1949; **61**: 197–205.
8 Taylor W. Rothmund's syndrome – Thomson's syndrome. *Arch Dermatol* 1957; **75**: 236–44.
9 Haneke E, Gutschmidt E. Premature multiple Bowen's disease in poikiloderma congenitale with warty hyperkeratoses. *Dermatologica* 1979; **158**: 384–8.
10 Davies MG. Rothmund-Thomson syndrome and malignant disease. *Clin Exp Dermatol* 1982; **7**: 455–7.
11 Smith PJ, Paterson MC. Enhanced radiosensitivity and defective DNA repair in cultured fibroblasts derived from Rothmund–Thomson syndrome patients. *Mutat Res* 1982; **94**: 213–28.
12 Kindler T. Congenital poikiloderma with traumatic bulla formation and progressive cutaneous atrophy. *Br J Dermatol* 1954; **66**: 104–11.
13 Weary PE, Manley WF, Graham GF. Hereditary acrokeratotic poikiloderma. *Arch Dermatol* 1971; **103**: 409–22.

Lupus erythematosus

Systemic lupus erythematosus (SLE) is a disease of adults and is relatively rare in childhood. Genetic predisposition is important in its pathogenesis[1].

Clinical features

Neonatal lupus

Cutaneous lesions are common, at birth or by 3–4 months of age[2]. The face is most frequently involved, with characteristic periorbital, erythematous, macular lesions. The scalp, trunk and limbs may be affected, with accentuation on light-exposed areas. New lesions may continue to develop for months, but transplacentally acquired neonatal lupus should have resolved by the age of 18 months, though pigmentary and atrophic changes may persist. Systemic manifestations which are transient and generally do not require treatment include lymphadenopathy, thrombocytopenia, Coombs'-positive anaemia and hepatosplenomegaly[3]. Congenital heart block occurs in 10–75% of infants and is potentially fatal if untreated.

Pathology

Inherited complement deficiencies are a major determining factor in the aetiology of SLE[4] and may be associated with discoid lupus erythematosus (DLE)[5]. Neonatal lupus, however, is increasingly recognized[6] in the offspring of mothers with lupus erythematosus and circulating anti-Ro antibodies. Transplacental transfer of these antibodies from mother to fetus appears to be pathogenetic.

Genetics

Though symptoms of neonatal lupus resolve in infancy, some patients have developed SLE in adolescence or adult life, implying a genetic predisposition[7].

Differential diagnosis

Differentiation of polymorphic light eruption from lupus erythematosus may prove difficult occasionally when patients present with a transient photosensitive rash in the absence of other systemic features. The demonstration of positive antinuclear antibodies or Ro antibodies aids diagnosis, and in such patients the disease may evolve into systemic lupus erythematosus, often after many year[8].

Treatment

Insertion of a pacemaker may be required as an emergency in the neonatal period.

References

1 Walport MJ, Black CM, Batchelor JR. The immunogenetics of SLE. *Clin Rheum Dis* 1982; **8**: 3–21.
2 Lane AT, Watson RM. Neonatal lupus erythematosus. *Am J Dis Child* 1984; **138**: 663–6.
3 Spraker MK. Lupus erythematosus in neonates, children and adolescents. *Clin Dermatol* 1985; **3**: 105–12.
4 Fielder AHI, Walport MJ, Batchelor JR et al. Family study of the major histocompatibility complex in patients with systemic lupus erythematosus: importance of null alleles of C4A and C4B in determining disease susceptibility. *Br Med J* 1983; **286**: 425–8.
5 Guenther LC. Inherited disorders of complement. *J Am Acad Dermatol* 1983; **9**: 815–39.
6 Provost PT. Commentary: neonatal lupus erythematosus. *Arch Dermatol* 1983; **119**: 619–22.
7 Fox RJ, McCuistion CH, Schoch EP. Systemic lupus erythematosus: association with previous neonatal lupus erythematosus. *Arch Dermatol* 1979; **115**: 340.
8 Murphy GM, Hawk JLM. The prevalence of antinuclear antibodies in patients presenting with apparent polymorphic light eruption. *Br J Dermatol* 1991; **125**: 448–51.

Chapter 13

Pigmentary disorders

S. S. Bleehen

Introduction

A number of genes are involved in the various biological processes in human melanin pigmentation. The migration and differentiation of melanoblasts in embryonic life from neural crest to the skin is also under genetic control. There are many different and distinct genetic disorders of pigmentation with various modes of inheritance where there is either a partial or complete lack of melanin in the skin, or an increase of melanin. This chapter describes those conditions in which alteration of pigmentation, which may be diffuse or localized, is a major feature.

Table 13.1 *Disorders of hypomelanosis*

Piebaldism
Waardenburg's syndrome
Tietz's syndrome
Piebaldism with deafness (Woolf's syndrome)
Ziprkowski–Margolis syndrome (X-linked albinism–deafness syndrome)
Oculocutaneous albinism
X-linked ocular albinism
Hypomelanosis of Ito
Phenylketonuria (see Chapter 7)
Tuberous sclerosis (see Chapter 9)
Menkes' kinky hair syndrome (see Chapter 15)

Disorders of hypomelanosis

The disorders characterized by hypomelanosis are summarized in Table 13.1

Disorders of hypermelanosis

The classification of disorders in which there is a primary hyperpigmentation of the skin[1] is difficult and often confusing (Table 13.2). Many of the disorders are inherited as autosomal dominant traits, though in some of these the inheritance is unclear. Several, such as incontinentia pigmenti of the Bloch–Sulzberger type, are inherited as X-linked disorders, and some different types of xeroderma pigmentosum are autosomal recessive. A number of disorders, where there is either localized or more systematized hyperpigmentation of the skin, are considered to be naevoid or hamartomatous, and though familial cases have been reported, they are not considered in this chapter.

Reference

1 Fulk CS. Primary disorders of hyperpigmentation. *J Am Acad Dermatol* 1984; **10**: 1–16.

Piebaldism (partial albinism)

Piebaldism is characterized by localized, stable areas of hypomelanosis on the trunk and limbs, and in most

Table 13.2 *Disorders of hypermelanosis*

Lentiginosis
  LEOPARD syndrome
  NAME and LAMB syndromes
  Centrofacial lentiginosis
  Inherited patterned lentiginosis
  Peutz–Jeghers syndrome
  Generalized lentigines with nystagmus
Punctate and reticulate hyperpigmentation
  Reticulate acropigmentation of Kitamura
  Acropigmentation of Dohi
  Dermatopathia pigmentosa reticularis
  Naegeli–Franceschetti–Jadassohn syndrome
  Reticulate pigmented anomaly of the flexures
    (Dowling–Degos disease)
  Dyskeratosis congenita
Hereditary universal melanosis
Dyschromatosis
  Dyschromatosis universalis
  Dyschromatosis symmetrica
  Mendes da Costa syndrome
Fanconi's syndrome (see Chapter 17)
Neurofibromatosis (see Chapter 9)
Albright's syndrome
Incontinentia pigmenti (see Chapter 9)
Xeroderma pigmentosum (see Chapter 17)

cases by a white forelock of hair with hypomelanosis of the adjacent central part of the forehead.

Clinical features

Piebaldism is rare and much less common than oculocutaneous albinism[1]. Males and females are equally affected and no race is spared. Many pedigrees have been described and 80–90% of piebald individuals have a characteristic white forelock[2,3]. Unaffected parents generally do not transmit the condition to their children. The hypomelanotic areas of skin are well circumscribed and symmetrical; they are apparent at birth and remain stable. The chest, abdomen, back and limbs are affected as well as the face and neck. Dark-brown macules are found in the hypomelanotic areas and less often in the normal skin. The hands, feet and central portion of the back are pigmented. Most characteristic is the white forelock or 'white blaze' which is usually midline, triangular in shape and symmetrical. There are no other areas of white hair in the scalp. Associated with the forelock is an area of hypomelanosis of the scalp which extends onto the central part of the forehead and may reach the bridge of the nose. Heterochromia of the irides can occasionally be present[1,4] and neurological abnormalities have been described[5]. The condition has been associated with Hirschsprung's disease[6].

Genetics

Piebaldism is inherited as an autosomal dominant trait with full penetrance. It is likely that a number of gene loci are involved since other abnormalities occur in addition to the pigmentary defects. Studies have shown that in the hypomelanotic areas there is a lack of melanocytes[7,8], and this has been considered to be due to a failure of melanoblast migration to the dermoepidermal junction in early embryonic life. However, melanocytes have been identified in piebald skin[9], and in this type there may be an inhibition of melanogenesis. Piebaldism is seen in animals, and white spotting occurs as an autosomal dominant trait in mice[10]. Mutations of the c-*kit* gene, which encodes the cellular tyrosine kinase receptor for the mast/stem cell factor, has been identified in 3 patients with piebaldism[11].

Treatment

Photoprotection using sunscreen preparations is necessary to prevent the hypomelanotic areas from becoming sunburnt. Mini skin grafts have been used, and psoralen photochemotherapy has been given to pigment the areas[9].

References

1 Comings DE, Odland GF. Partial albinism. *J Am Med Assoc* 1966; **195**: 519–23.
2 Froggatt P. An outline with bibliography of human piebaldism and white forelock. *Irish J Med Sci* 1959; **398**: 86–94.
3 Cooke JV. Familial white skin spotting (piebaldness) ('partial albinism') with white forelock. *J Pediatr* 1952; **41**: 1–2.
4 Cockayne EA. A piebald family. *Biometrika* 1914; **10**: 197–200.
5 Telfer MA, Sugar M, Jaeger EA et al. Dominant piebald trait (white forelock and leukoderma) with neurological impairment. *Am J Hum Genet.* 1971; **23**: 383–9.
6 Mahakrishnann A, Srinavason MS. Piebaldism with Hirschsprung's disease. *Arch Dermatol* 1980; **116**: 1102.
7 Breathnach AS, Fitzpatrick TB, Wyllie LMA. Electron microscopy of melanocytes in human piebaldism. *J Invest Dermatol* 1965; **45**: 28–37.
8 Jimbow K, Fitzpatrick TB, Szabo G et al. Congenital circumscribed hypomelanosis. *J Invest Dermatol* 1975; **64**: 50–62.
9 Hayashibe K, Mishima Y. Tyrosinase-positive melanocyte distribution and induction of pigmentation in human piebald skin. *Arch Dermatol* 1988; **124**: 381–6.
10 Mayer TC. A comparison of pigment cell development in albino, steel and dominant-spotting mutant mouse embryos. *Dev Biol* 1970; **23**: 297–309.
11 Spritz RA, Giebel LB, Holmes SA. Dominant negative and loss of function mutation of the C-*kit* (mast/stem cell growth factor receptor) proto-oncogene in human piebaldism. *Am J Hum Genet* 1992; **50**: 261–9.

Waardenburg's syndrome

Individuals with Waardenburg's syndrome have recognizable facies, partial albinism and congenital deafness.

Clinical features

Waardenburg's syndrome [1–3] is characterized by lateral displacement of the inner canthi and lacrimal ducts, a broad basal root, confluent hyperplastic inner third of eyebrows and, in a quarter of the cases, heterochromia (either partial or total) of the irides. A congenital sensorineural deafness which may be unilateral or bilateral occurs in 20% of cases[4,5]. A white forelock occurs in 17% of cases and can be inconspicuous. Only a few (12%) have lesions of piebaldism. There is an overlap with other disorders and minor expression may be more common. Mental retardation, epilepsy and skeletal abnormalities have also been noted.

Genetics

The condition is inherited as an autosomal dominant with variable penetrance. Within affected families all degrees of severity have been observed. The risk of occurrence is 1 in 4000 live births, and there is a 1 in 2 chance of the child of an affected parent having this syndrome. All races are affected and the incidence in males and females is equal. Apparently unaffected individuals may show slight expression of the mutant gene. An abnormality in the failure of neural crest cells to migrate in early embryonic life to the inner ear and skin has been suggested[2] to account for some of the manifestations of this condition. Several distinct types of Waardenburg's syndrome have been described[6]. Waardenburg's syndrome type I has been mapped to chromosome 2[7].

References

1 Waardenburg PJ. A new syndrome combining developmental anomalies of the eyelids, eyebrows and nose root with pigmentary defects of the iris and head hair and congenital deafness. *Am J Hum Gen* 1951; **3**: 195–253.
2 Fisch L. Deafness as part of an hereditary syndrome. *J Laryng Otol* 1959; **73**: 355–82.
3 DiGeorge AM, Olmsted RW, Harley RD. Waardenburg's syndrome. *J Pediatr* 1960; **57**: 649–69.
4 Reed WB, Shore VM, Boder E et al. Pigmentary disorders in association with congenital deafness. *Arch Dermatol* 1967; **95**: 176–86.
5 Partington MW. Waardenburg's syndrome and heterochromia iridium in a deaf school population. *Canad Med Assoc J* 1964; **90**: 1008–17.
6 Hageman MJ, Delleman JW. Heterogeneity in Waardenburg's syndrome. *Am J Hum Genet* 1977; **29**: 468–85.
7 Foy C, Newton V, Wellesley D et al. Assignment of the locus for Waardenburg's syndrome type 1 to human chromosome 2q37 and possible homology to the splotch mouse. *Am J Hum Genet* 1990; **46**: 1017–23.

Tietz's syndrome

A six-generation pedigree is described with a syndrome of deaf-mutism, blue eyes and hypoplasia of the eyebrows, associated with an absence of pigment in the skin considered to be albinism[1]. The condition in this family appeared to be inherited as an autosomal dominant trait with complete penetrance. A similar disorder is seen in Persian white cats with blue irides[2].

References

1 Tietz W. A syndrome of deaf mutism associated with albinism showing autosomal dominant inheritance. *Am J Hum Genet* 1963; **15**: 259–64.
2 Wolff D. Three generations of deaf white cats. *J Hered* 1942; **33**: 39–43.

Piebaldism with deafness

Synonym: *Woolf's syndrome*

Two Hopi Indian brothers with piebaldism and deafness have been described[1,2] and two similar cases have been reported[3]. These had no other features of Waardenburg's syndrome. This disorder may be transmitted as an autosomal recessive[4] or possibly X-linked recessive trait.

References

1 Woolf CM. Albinism among Indians in Arizona and New Mexico. *Am J Hum Genet* 1965; **17**: 23–35.
2 Woolf CM, Dolowitz, Aldous HE. Congenital deafness associated with piebaldness. *Arch Otolaryngol* 1965; **82**: 244–50.
3 Reed WB, Store VM, Boder E et al. Pigmentary disorders in association with congenital deafness. *Arch Dermatol* 1967; **95**: 176–86.
4 Konigsmark BW. Herediatary childhood hearing loss and integmentary system disease. *J Pediatr* 1972; **80**: 909–19.

Ziprkowski–Margolis syndrome

Synonym: *Albinism–deafness syndrome*

An Egyptian Jewish family with deaf-mutism, heterochromia of the irides, and cutaneous and hair hypomelanosis of a piebald type, has been described[1,2]. Since all the cases were male it is likely that this syndrome is inherited as an X-linked recessive. There is clearly some overlap with piebaldism with deafness, described above, and it is plausible that both syndromes (which have been described separately) fall within the spectrum of the same genetic disorder. Linkage studies indicate the gene locus to be on Xq, probably in the region Xq13–26[3].

References

1 Ziprkowski L, Krakowski A, Adam A et al. Partial albinism and deaf mutism due to a recessive sex-linked gene. *Arch Dermatol* 1962; **86**: 530–9.
2 Margolis E. A new hereditary syndrome – sex-linked deaf-mutism associated with total albinism. *Acta Genet* 1962; **12**: 12–19.
3 Litvak G, Sandknyl L, Ott J et al. Localisation of X-linked albinism–deafness syndrome to Xq by linkage with DNA markers (abstract). *Cytogenet Cell Genet Human Gene Mapping 9*, 1987; **46** (1–4): 652.

Oculocutaneous albinism

There are ten distinct types of oculocutaneous albinism in which there is partial or complete failure to produce melanin in the skin and the eyes[1]. All the forms except one, the rare autosomal dominant type, are inherited as autosomal recessive traits (Table 13.3).

Reference

1 Witkop CJ Jr., White JG, Nance WE et al. *Birth Defects: Original Article Series* 1971; **7** (8): 13–25.

Tyrosinase-negative oculocutaneous albinism

Tyrosinase-negative oculocutaneous albinism is the most severe type, with a failure to produce melanized melanosomes and an absence of tyrosinase activity of the melanocytes. Only stage 1 and 2 melanosomes are produced that are unmelanized[1].

Table 13.3 *Types of oculocutaneous albinism*

Tyrosinase-negative oculocutaneous albinism
Tyrosinase-positive oculocutaneous albinism
Yellow mutant albinism
Hermansky–Pudlak syndrome
Chédiak–Higashi syndrome
Cross syndrome
Brown albinism
Rufous (red) albinism
Minimal pigment albinism
Autosomal dominant oculocutaneous albinism

Clinical features

The incidence in the USA for Caucasians is 1 in 39 000 and for Afro-Caribbeans it is 1 in 28 000. All races are affected and in some countries the incidence is much higher. These patients have snow-white hair and pink-coloured skin, whatever their race, and have grey irides with a prominent red reflex[1]. They have a severe and coarse rotatory nystagmus, strabismus, photophobia and almost invariably poor visual acuity which can deteriorate with age. Incubation of the bulbs of plucked hairs in L-tyrosine or levodopa[2] shows no darkening and no formation of melanin. Ultrastructural studies on the skin and hair bulbs show the presence of melanocytes that only contain stage 1 and 2 melanosomes[1]. Transillumination of the iris and fundoscopy show no pigment. Patients have a marked susceptibility for skin neoplasm, including squamous and basal cell carcinomas and malignant melanoma, and some may die from these malignant tumours at an early age, particularly in the sunny countries[3].

Genetics

The risks of recurrence for a patient's sibling is 1 in 4; for the patient's child there is no risk unless the other parent is a carrier or homozygote for the gene. The human tyrosinase gene has been mapped to chromosome 11[4].

Treatment

There is no treatment apart from sun avoidance and the use of sunscreens. Prenatal diagnosis is possible[5], and the heterozygotic carrier can be detected by the amount of tyrosinase activity in the hair bulbs, using a modification of the Pomerantz assay[6].

References

1 Witkop CJ, Hill CW, Desnick S et al. Ophthalmologic, biochemical, platelet and ultrastructural defects in the various types of oculocutaneous albinism. *J Invest Dermatol* 1973; **60**: 443–56.
2 Kugelman TP, Van Scott E. Tyrosinase activity in melanocytes in human albinos. *J Invest Dermatol* 1971; **37**: 73–6.
3 Okoro AN. Albinism in Nigeria. *Br J Dermatol* 1975; **92**: 485–92.
4 Barton DE, Kwon BS, Francke U. Human tyrosinase gene, mapped to chromosome 11 (q14-q21), defines second region of homology with mouse chromosome 7. *Genomics* 1988; **3**: 17–24.
5 Eady RAJ, Gunner DB, Garner A et al. Prenatal diagnosis of oculocutaneous albinism by electron microscopy of fetal skin. *J Invest Dermatol* 1983; **80**: 210–12.
6 King RA, Witkop CJ. Detection of heterozygotes for tyrosinase-negative oculocutaneous albinism by hair bulb tyrosinase assay. *Am J Hum Genet* 1977; **29**: 164.

Tyrosinase-positive oculocutaneous albinism

Some pigment is formed in the tyrosinase-positive type of oculocutaneous albinism; this type is more common in Afro-Caribbean people, being 1 in 15 000 in American blacks and 1 in 1000 in Nigerians. The amount of pigment in this type of albinism varies with race and age[1]. There is usually darkening of the hair which often becomes flaxen-yellow in colour, and the skin develops dark-brown freckles, particularly in the sun-exposed areas. These changes occur in adult life. The hair bulb test is positive, with some tyrosinase activity[2]. As with the tyrosinase-negative type there are ocular abnormalities, but these are less severe and can improve with age. Patients also have abnormalities of the optic pathways and (like the tyrosinase-negative type) lack binocular vision. There is an increased risk of skin cancers with age, especially in those living in sunny countries. As with other types of oculocutaneous albinism there is accelerated photo-aging of the skin. Sun avoidance and the use of sunscreens are essential, and tinted spectacles or contact lenses should be worn. Heterozygotes as yet cannot be detected.

References

1 Bolognia JL, Pawalek JM. Biology of hypopigmentation. *J Am Acad Dermatol* 1988; **19**: 217–55.
2 Kugelman TP, Van Scott EJ. Tyrosinase activity in melanocytes of human albinos. *J Invest Dermatol* 1971; **37**: 73–6.

Yellow mutant (Amish) albinism

Yellow mutant albinism[1] is most common among the Amish in North America but has been seen in other populations. There is marked pigmentary dilution at birth affecting skin, hair and eyes. During the first few months of life there is some increase in pigment so that by the age of a year the hair is yellow-red in colour. The eye colour also darkens with age. In addition to moderate nystagmus and photophobia, people with this condition have poor visual acuity. The hair bulbs do not darken when incubated in L-tyrosine or levodopa[2], but produce an intensification of yellow-red phaeomelanin when cysteine and tyrosine are added. Treatment is as for the other types of oculocutaneous albinism.

References

1 Nance WE, Jackson CE, Witkop CJ. Amish albinism: a distinctive autosomal recessive phenotype. *Am J Hum Genet* 1971; **22**: 579–86.
2 King RA, Witkop CJ. Hair-bulb tyrosinase activity in oculocutaneous albinism. *Nature* 1976; **263**: 69–71.

Hermansky–Pudlak syndrome

Hermansky–Pudlak syndrome[1,2] is a rare type of oculocutaneous albinism associated with a haemorrhagic diathesis. It was first reported by Hermansky and Pudlak in 1959. So far, only 250 cases have been described. The bleeding tendency is secondary to a platelet storage defect. The platelets have decreased numbers of dense granules and reduced levels of serotonin and ADP[3]. There are also deposits of lipid and ceroid material in the cells of the reticuloendothelial system. The syndrome is more frequent in south Holland and those originating from the Arecibo region of Puerto Rica. Pulmonary fibrosis[3] and granulomatous colitis[4] can occur, as can fatal haemorrhage from ingestion of aspirin.

References

1 Hermansky F, Pudlak P. Albinism associated with a haemorrhagic diathesis and unusual pigmented reticular cells in the bone marrow. *Blood* 1959; **14**: 162–9.
2 White JG, Edson JR, Desnick SJ, Witkop CJ. Studies of platelets in a variant of the Hermansky–Pudlak syndrome. *Am J Pathol* 1971; **63**: 319–29.
3 Garay SM, Gardella JE, Fazzini EP, Goldring RM. Hermansky–Pudlak syndrome. Pulmonary manifestations of a ceroid storage disease. *Am J Med* 1979; **66**: 737–47.
4 Schinella RA, Greco MA, Colbert BL et al. Hermansky–Pudlak syndrome with granulomatous colitis. *Ann Intern Med* 1980; **92**: 20–3.

Chédiak–Higashi syndrome

Chédiak–Higashi syndrome [1–3] is described in detail in Chapter 18. It is inherited as an autosomal recessive trait due to a single defective gene. There is pigmentary dilution of the skin, hair and eyes. Giant cytoplasmic inclusions occur in a variety of cell types owing to a defect in the distribution of normal lysosomal enzymes. Large pigment granules are to be seen in the skin due to fusion of the melanosomes. The skin is fair, and the hair is light-blond to brown and sometimes silver-grey. Patients have a predisposition to recurrent bacterial and viral infections. A similar disorder is found in a number of different animals, including the Aleutian mink. Differential diagnosis includes Griscelli-Prunieras syndrome (Chapter 18).

References

1 Zelickson AS, Windhorst DB, White JG, Good RA. The Chediak–Higashi syndrome: formation of giant melanosomes and the basis of hypopigmentation. *J Invest Dermatol* 1968; **50**: 9–18.
2 Bedoyd V. Pigmentary changes in the Chediak–Higashi syndrome. *Br J Dermatol* 1971; **85**: 336–347.
3 Blume RS, Wolff SM. The Chediak–Higashi syndrome: studies in four patients and a review of the literature. *Medicine* (Baltimore) 1972; **51**: 247–80.

Cross syndrome

The oculocerebral syndrome with hypopigmentation known as Cross syndrome[1] is probably inherited as an autosomal recessive trait, although only a few cases have been described. In addition to hypopigmentation of the skin and hair, there are ocular defects that include cataracts, microphthalmia and nystagmus. Neurological abnormalities include spasticity, athetosis and mental retardation.

Reference

1 Cross HE, McKusick VA, Breen W. A new oculocerebral syndrome with hypopigmentation. *J Pediatr* 1967; **70**: 396–406.

Brown albinism

Brown albinism[1] is a variety of tyrosinase-positive oculocutaneous albinism originally described in Nigerian families and also documented in Puerto Ricans. Albinism in dark-skinned persons is not always obvious because freckled skin and red hair may be present. Red reflex on transillumination of the iris and nystagmus are important clues to the diagnosis.

Reference

1 King RA, Lewis RA, Townsend D et al. Brown oculocutaneous albinism: clinical, ophthalmological and biochemical characterization. *Ophthalmology* 1986; **92**: 1496–1505.

Rufous (red) albinism

Rufous or red albinism[1] is seen in Africans and New Guineans and inherited as an autosomal recessive. The skin colour is red and the hair mahogany red to deep red.

Reference

1 Walsh RJ. A distinctive pigment of the skin in New Guinea indigenes. *Ann Hum Genet* 1971; **34**: 379–85.

Minimal pigment albinism

King et al[1] described a type of oculocutaneous albinism in which affected individuals had no pigment at birth, but minimal amounts of pigment developed in the iris in the first decade. There was no measurable hair bulb tyrosinase activity. In the three families studied, one parent had normal tyrosinase activity and the other abnormally low activity.

Reference

1 King RA, Wirtschafter JD, Olds DP et al. Minimal pigment: a new type of oculocutaneous albinism. *Clin Genet* 1986; **29**: 42–50.

Autosomal dominant oculocutaneous albinism

Several families have been described[1,2] in which the ocular and cutaneous hypopigmentation has been inherited as an autosomal dominant trait. The hair bulb test is positive and slight tanning occurs. Only rarely is there nystagmus or photophobia.

References

1 Bergsma DR, Kaiser-Kupfer M. A new form of albinism. *Am J Ophthalmol* 1974; **77**: 837–44.
2 Fitzpatrick TB, Jimbow K, Donaldson DD. Dominant oculocutaneous albinism. *Br J Dermatol* 1974; **91** (suppl. 10): 23.

X-linked ocular albinism

There are several types of ocular albinism, the most common being inherited as sex-linked conditions. The disorders may be suspected in the patient with congenital nystagmus, poor visual acuity, hypopigmentation of the retina and an absence of foveal reflexes. Macromelanosomes are seen in the skin in this disorder[1,2].

References

1 Garner A, Jay BS. Macromelanosomes in X-linked ocular albinism. *Histopathology* 1980; **4**: 243–54.
2 Yoshika T, Manabe M, Hayakawa M et al. Macromelanosomes in X-linked ocular albinism (XLOA). *Acta Derm Venereol* (Stockholm) 1985; **65**: 66–9.

Hypomelanosis of Ito

Synonym: *Incontinentia pigmenti achromians*

Hypomelanosis of Ito is probably more common than is reported [1–4]. Very characteristic streaks and whorls of hypomelanosis are seen that follow Blaschko's lines (Figure 13.1). Autosomal dominant inheritance has been shown in some but not all cases. Multiple cases within a family have been reported[5]. Chromosomal abnormalities have been found and both diploid/triploid mixoploidy and chromosomal mosaicism occur [6–8]. In addition to the skin hypomelanosis that is apparent at birth, there are associated

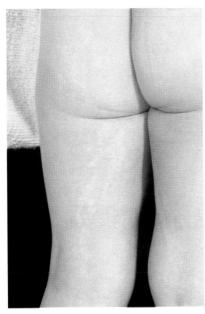

Figure 13.1 *Hypomelanosis of Ito: characteristic linear lesions of hypomelanosis (courtesy of Dr J. Harper)*

neurological and musculoskeletal abnormalities, particularly hypotonia, epilepsy and mental retardation. The teeth and eyes can also be affected.

References

1 Jelinek JE, Bart RS, Schiff GM. Hypomelanosis of Ito (incontinentia pigmenti achromians). *Arch Dermatol* 1973; **107**: 596–601.
2 Glover MT, Brett EM, Atherton DJ. Hypomelanosis of Ito: spectrum of the disease. *J Pediatr* 1989; **115**: 75–80.
3 Takematsu H, Sato S, Igarashi M, Seiji M. Incontinentia pigmenti achromians (Ito). *Arch Dermatol* 1983; **119**: 391–5.
4 Ruiz-Maldonado R, Toussaint S, Tamayo L et al. Hypomelanosis of Ito: diagnostic criteria and report of 41 cases. *Pediatr Dermatol* 1992; **9** (1): 1–10.
5 Rubin MB. Incontinentia pigmenti achromians. Multiple cases within a family. *Arch Dermatol* 1972; **105**: 424–5.
6 Donnai D, Mckeown C, Andrews T et al. Diploid/triploid mixoploidy and hypomelanosis of Ito. *Lancet* 1985; **i**: 1443–4.
7 Rott H-D, Ulmer R, Haneke E et al. Hypomelanosis of Ito and chromosomal mosaicism in fibroblasts. *Lancet* 1986; **ii**: 343.
8 Miller CA, Parker WD Jr. Hypomelanosis of Ito: association with a chromosomal abnormality. *Neurology* 1985; **35**: 607–10.

Lentiginosis

Inherited disorders in which multiple lentigines are a feature are listed in Table 13.2. All of these show autosomal dominant inheritance.

Multiple lentigines (LEOPARD) syndrome

This cardiocutaneous LEOPARD syndrome is characterized by multiple and widespread lentigines and is associated with a wide variety of developmental defects[1,2]. The acronym LEOPARD stands for Lentigines, Electrocardiographic abnormalities (especially conduction defects) Ocular hypertelorism, Pulmonary stenosis, Abnormalities of the genitalia, Retardation of growth and Deafness of the sensineural type. The condition is inherited as an autosomal dominant trait with a high degree of penetrance and variable expression. The lentigines are present at birth and become more numerous by puberty. They are most numerous on the neck and upper trunk and are also found in the axillae. Macromelanosomes have been reported in this syndrome[3]. Multiple granular cell schwannomas have occurred in a child[4].

References

1 Gorlin RJ, Anderson RC, Blaw M. Multiple lentigines syndrome. *Am J Dis Child* 1969; **117**: 652–62.
2 Polani PE, Moynahan EJ. Progressive cardiomyopathic lentiginosis. *Quart J Med* 1972; **41**: 205–25.
3 Weiss LW, Zelickson AJ. Giant melanosomes in multiple lentigines syndrome. *Arch Dermatol* 1977; **113**: 491–4.
4 Apted JH. Multiple granular cell myoblastoma (schwannomas) in a child. *Br J Dermatol* 1968; **80**: 257–60.

Lentiginosis and atrial myxoma (NAME and LAMB syndromes)

Lentiginosis and atrial myxoma were first described in 1973; since then other familial cases have been reported, and various acronyms have been used [1–3]. The inheritance is probably autosomal dominant[4]. In addition to profuse pigmented macules, most marked on the face, neck and upper part of the trunk, myxoid tumours of the left atrium are present as well as cutaneous myxomas. Endocrine disorders may be associated with this syndrome. There may be no previous family history of lentigines[5].

References

1 Rees JR, Ross FGM, Keen G. Lentiginosis and left atrial myxoma. *Br Heart J* 1973; **35**: 874–6.
2 Atherton DJ, Pitcher DW, Wells RS et al. A syndrome of various cutaneous pigmented lesions, myxoid neurofibromata and atrial myxoma: the 'NAME' syndrome. *Br J Dermatol* 1980; **103**: 421–9.
3 Rhodes AR, Silvermann RA, Harrist TJ et al. Mucocutaneous lentigines, cardiomucocutaneous myxomas and multiple blue naevi: the 'LAMB' syndrome. *J Am Acad Dermatol* 1984; **10**: 72–82.
4 Carney JA, Gordon H, Carpenter PG et al. The complex of myomas, spotty pigmentation and endocrine overactivity. *Medicine* 1985; **64**: 270–83.
5 Paterson LL, Serrill WS. Lentiginosis associated with a left atrial myxoma. *J Am Acad Dermatol* 1984; **10**: 337–40.

Centrofacial lentiginosis

Centrofacial lentiginosis[1] is determined by an auto-somal dominant gene. Brown or black macules appear in the first year of life and increase in number with age. The central part of the face is mostly affected, but the mucous membranes are not involved. Associated defects are mental retardation, epilepsy and skeletal abnormalities.

Reference

1 Dociu I, Galaction-Nitelea O, Sirjita N et al. Centrofacial lentiginosis: a survey of 40 cases. *Br J Dermatol* 1976; **94**: 39–43.

Inherited patterned lentiginosis

Inherited patterned lentiginosis occurs only in people of Afro-Caribbean origin[1] and is inherited as an autosomal dominant trait. There are no associated abnormalities other than lentigines found mostly on the central part of the face and lips. Several patients have had lesions on the hands and feet, but in none were the mucosa involved.

Reference

1 O'Neill JF, James WD. Inherited patterned lentiginosis in · blacks. *Arch Dermatol* 1989; **125**: 1231–5.

Peutz–Jeghers syndrome (periorificial lentiginosis)

Clinical features

The pigmented macules may be present at birth but can develop later in life. They are particularly arranged around the mouth, but can involve the palms, soles and the mucosae[1]. The condition is associated with hamartomas of the entire bowel and these polyps can be the cause of intestinal obstruction and bleeding. There are a number of associated abnormalities including clubbing of the fingers and ovarian tumours[2]. There is an increased risk of cancer[3]. Haemangiomas of the small intestine have been described associated with mucocutaneous pigmentation[4].

Genetics

The syndrome is inherited as an autosomal dominant condition with a high degree of penetrance. The risk of occurrence is between 1 in 8300 and 1 in 29 000 live births. All races are affected. In about 40% of cases there is no family history and these represent new mutations.

References

1 Jeghers H, McKusick VA, Katz KH. Generalised intestinal polyposis and melanin spots of the oral mucosa, lips and digits. *New Engl J Med* 1949; **241**: 992–1005, 1031–1036.
2 Dormandy TL. Gastrointestinal polyposis with mucocutaneous pigmentation (Peutz–Jeghers syndrome). *New Engl J Med* 1957; **256**: 1186–90.
3 Giardello FM, Welsh SB, Hamilton SR et al. Increased risk of cancer in Peutz–Jeghers syndrome. *New Engl J Med* 1987; **316**: 1511–14.
4 Bandler M. Haemangiomas of the small intestine associated with mucocutaneous pigmentation. *Gastroenterology* 1960; **38**: 641–5.

Generalized lentigines with nystagmus

A family has been described with generalized lentigines, nystagmus and strabismus[1].

Reference

1 Pipkin AC, Pipkin SB. A pedigree of generalised lentigo. *J Hered* 1950; **41**: 79–82.

Punctate and reticulate hyperpigmentation

Punctate and reticulate hyperpigmentation disorders[1] have been mostly seen in Asian patients and are listed in Table 13.4. These disorders may occur sporadically or be familial, and most are inherited as autosomal dominant traits.

Reticulate acropigmentation of Kitamura

Reticulate acropigmentation of Kitamura[1] is inherited as an autosomal dominant condition. It is characterized by distal reticulated hyperpigmented macules, initially on the backs of the hands and then extending proximally to involve most parts of the body[2]. Pits and breaks in the epidermal ridge patterns are present in the palms and soles. The disorder was originally

Table 13.4 *Punctate and reticulate hyperpigmentation*

Reticulate acropigmentation of Kitamura
Acropigmentation symmetrica of Dohi
Dermatopathia pigmentosa reticularis
Naegeli–Franceschetti–Jadassohn syndrome
Reticulate pigmented anomaly of the flexures
  (Dowling–Degos disease)
Dyskeratosis congenita

described in Japan, but cases have been reported from other countries[3]. A family has been reported from Italy with features of both Kitamura's disease and reticulate pigmented anomaly of the flexures[4].

References

1 Griffiths WAD. Reticulate pigmentary disorders – a review. *Clin Exp Dermatol* 1984; **9**: 439–50.
2 Griffiths WAD. Reticulate acropigmentation of Kitamura. *Br J Dermatol* 1976; **95**: 437–43.
3 Woodley DT, Caro I, Wheeler CE. Reticulate acropigmentation of Kitamura. *Arch Dermatol* 1979; **115**: 760–1.
4 Crovado F, Rebora A. Reticulate pigmentary anomaly of the flexures associating reticulate acropigmentation: one single entity. *J Am Acad Dermatol* 1986; **14**: 359–61.

Acropigmentation of Dohi

Acropigmentation of Dohi[1,2] is inherited as an autosomal dominant condition; most cases have been reported in the Japanese population. Angulated freckle-like lesions appear symmetrically on the dorsa of the hands and feet in the first decade of life. Depigmented macules 1–3 mm in size occur scattered in pigmented areas.

References

1 Gartmann H. Akropigmentation symmetrica Dohi mit angeborenen Fundus Veranderungen bei Mutter und Tochter. *Dermatol Wochenschr* 1952; **125**: 534–5.
2 Kormaya G. Symmetrische Pigmentanomalie der Extremitaten. *Arch Dermatol Syphil* 1924; **147**: 389–93.

Dermatopathia pigmentosa reticularis

Dermatopathia pigmentosa reticularis[1,2] is a rare syndrome characterized by universal reticulate pigmentation with pigmentary incontinence and liquefaction degeneration of the basal layer. It is uncertain whether the inheritance is autosomal dominant. Other features include mild alopecia, nail dystrophy, palmoplantar hyperkeratosis and loss of dermatoglyphics. Most cases have been European, though one case is reported in a man of mixed black, Hispanic and American Indian descent[3].

References

1 Fiegel H. Dermatopathia pigmentosa reticularis. *Hautarzt* 1960; **11**: 262–5.
2 Rycroft RJG, Calnan CD, Allenby CF. Dermatopathia pigmentosa reticularis. *Clin Exp Dermatol* 1977; **2**: 39–44.
3 Maso J, Schwartz RA, Lambert WC. Dermatopathia pigmentosa reticularis. *Arch Dermatol* 1990; **126**: 935–9.

Naegeli–Franceschetti–Jadassohn syndrome

Naegeli–Franceschetti–Jadassohn syndrome was initially described in a Swiss family[1] and is characterized by dark-brown reticulate pigmentation on the trunk and limbs. There is a keratoderma of the palms and soles. Dental defect with enamel hypoplasia can occur and hypohidrosis is common[2]. Inheritance is autosomal dominant.

References

1 Franceschetti A, Jadassohn W. A propos de 'l'incontinentia pigmenti', delimitation de deux syndromes differents figurant sous le même terme. *Dermatologica* 1954; **108**: 1–28.
2 Sparrow GP, Samman PD, Wells RS. Hyperpigmentation and hypohidrosis (the Naegeli–Franceschetti–Jadassohn syndrome): report of a family and review of the literature. *Clin Exp Dermatol* 1976; **1**: 127–40.

Reticulate pigmented anomaly of the flexures

Synonym: *Dowling–Degos disease*

Reticulate pigmented anomaly of the flexures[1,2] affects the axillae, groin, cubital fossae and submammary regions, usually at adolescence. There are dark-brown reticulated areas of pigmentation. Perioral pitting at the angles of the mouth is seen, and other features are dark dots like comedones on the neck[3]. The condition may be sporadic or transmitted as an autosomal dominant trait.

References

1 Dowling GB, Freudenthal W. Acanthosis nigricans. *Br J Dermatol* 1938; **50**: 467–71.
2 Wilson Jones E, Grice K. Reticulate pigmented anomaly of the flexures. *Arch Dermatol* 1978; **114**: 1150–7.

Dyskeratosis congenita

Dyskeratosis congenita[1,2] is very rare, occurring almost exclusively in males, the gene being located on the long arm of the X chromosome. A reticulate hyperpigmentation of the skin develops in childhood preceded by a nail dystrophy. Leucoplakia of the oral, urethral and anal mucosae gradually develops and later the skin has a poikilodermatous appearance. Various haematological disorders have been described. An autosomal dominant form is reported[3]. There is an increased risk of malignant disease[4,5].

References

1 Jansen LH. The so-called dyskeratosis congenita. *Dermato-logica* 1951; **103**: 167–77.
2 Costello MJ, Buncke CM. Dyskeratosis congenita. *Arch Dermatol* 1956; **73**: 123–30.
3 Ping KT, Kohn T. Dyskeratosis congenita: an autosomal dominant disorder. *J Am Acad Dermatol* 1982; **6**: 1034–9.
4 Connor JM, Teague RH. Dyskeratosis congenita. Report of a large kindred. *Br J Dermatol* 1981; **105**: 321–5.
5 Davidson HR, Connor JM. Dyskeratosis congenita. *J Med Genet* 1988; **25**: 843–6.

Hereditary universal melanosis

A number of disorders have been reported in which there is a progressive increase in pigmentation starting in early childhood. One disorder, familial progressive hyperpigmentation, appeared to be inherited as an autosomal dominant trait in a black pedigree[1]. Another disorder was described in a Latin-American boy, who in early infancy became completely black in colour[2]. This case of universal acquired melanosis (carbon baby) is probably not a distinct genetic disorder like acromelanosis[3].

References

1 Chernosky ME, Anderson DE, Chang JP et al. Familial progressive hyperpigmentation. *Arch Dermatol* 1971; **103**: 581–98.
2 Maldonado-Ruiz R, Tamayo L, Fernandez-Diez J. Universal acquired melanosis. *Arch Dermatol* 1978; **114**: 775–8.
3 Gonzalez JR, Botet MV. Acromelanosis. *J Am Acad Dermatol* 1980; **2**: 128–31.

Dyschromatosis

A number of inherited conditions have been described that are characterized by dyschromia of the skin with hypo- and hyperpigmentation and without poikilo-dermatous changes. Some may affect only the extremities, but in others there is universal dyschromia. The conditions are listed in Table 13.5.

Table 13.5 *Inherited dyschromatoses*

Dyschromatosis universalis
Dyschromatosis symmetrica
Mendes da Costa syndrome

Dyschromatosis universalis

Several cases of dyschromatosis universalis have been reported, mostly in Japan[1,2] but also in other countries[3]. One child has been described with universal dyschromatosis and high-tone deafness[4]. The mode of inheritance is uncertain.

References

1 Ichikawa T, Hiraga Y. Uber eine noch nicht beschriebene Pigmentanomatle, Dyschromatosis universalis heredi-taria. *Jap J Dermatol Urol* 1933; **34**: 360–4.
2 Suenaga M. Dyschromatosis universalis hereditaria in 5 generations. *Tohoku J Exp Med* 1952; **55**: 373–6.
3 Findlay G, Whiting DA. Universal dyschromatosis. *Br J Dermatol* 1971; **85** (suppl. 7): 66–70.
4 Rycroft RJG, Calnan CD, Wells RS. Universal dyschroma-tosis, small stature and high-tone deafness. *Clin Exp Dermatol* 1977; **2**: 45–8.

Dyschromatosis symmetrica

In dyschromatosis symmetrica the pattern of the dyschromia affects mainly the extremities[1]. The mode of inheritance is uncertain.

Reference

1 Yoshida Y. Dyschromatosis symmetrica hereditaria. *Ind J Ven Dis Dermatol* 1953; **91**: 151–6.

Mendes da Costa syndrome

Mendes da Costa syndrome is a rare sex-linked condition reported in a single family from Amster-dam[1]. The children are normal at birth but later develop scattered blisters. Soon after there is alopecia and a reticulate dyschromia affects the face and limbs. Some are mentally or physically retarded.

Reference

1 Carol WLL, Kooij R. Typus maculatus der bullosen hereditaren dystrophie. *Acta Derm Venereol* 1937; **18**: 265–83.

Albright's syndrome

Albright's syndrome [1–3] is an autosomal dominant disorder characterized by polyostotic fibrous dyspla-

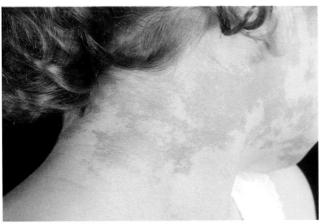

Figure 13.2 *Albright's syndrome: extensive* café au lait *pigmentation (courtesy of Dr J. Harper)*

sia, skin pigmentation (Figure 13.2) and (in females) precocious puberty. It should not be confused with Albright's hereditary osteodystrophy (pseudohypo-parathyroidism). Cutaneous pigmentation usually develops between the ages of 4 months and 2 years; however, it may be present at birth. Extensive light-brown patches occur, mainly on the trunk, buttocks and thighs, and tend to be asymmetrical, often more prominent on the side showing the most severe bone involvement. The differential diagnosis is neurofi-bromatosis, in which bone lesions and endocrine disturbances also occur.

References

1 Albright F, Butler AM, Hampton AO et al. Syndrome characterized by osteitis fibrosa disseminata, area of pigmentation and endocrine dysfunction, with precocious puberty in females: report of five cases. *New Engl J Med* 1937; **21**: 727–46.
2 Delacretaz J, Rutschmann JP. Albright's syndrome and associated disorders. *Dermatologica* 1960; **112**: 107–20.
3 Benedict PH, Szabo G, Fitzpatrick TB et al. Melanotic macules in Albright's syndrome and in neurofibromatosis. *J Am Med Assoc* 1968; **205**: 618–26.

Chapter 14

Premature aging syndromes

D. J. Gawkrodger

Introduction

The process of aging is irreversible. It begins or accelerates at maturity and results in an increased deviation from the ideal state or a reduced rate of return to it[1]. Syndromes of premature aging are only partial copies of normal aging and as such they are a heterogeneous group. Primary growth retardation not infrequently is present. In some conditions skin aging is not present or is mild, whereas in others it is a prominent feature.

Martin[2] attempted to define certain of the stigmata of aging and included the following: increased susceptibility to neoplasia, dementia, deposition of amyloid and lipofuscin, diabetes mellitus, hyperlipidaemia, hypogonadism, autoimmune disease, cataracts, premature greying or loss of hair, osteoporosis, changes in adipose tissue distribution, hypertension and degenerative vascular disease. This list is not comprehensive but it does give a basis with which to compare and contrast the conditions included in this chapter.

In the skin the normal aging process needs to be distinguished from the effects of chronic sun exposure, the influence of age-related internal disease, and age-associated hormonal factors. Aged skin is dry, atrophic, wrinkled, rough, shows loss of elasticity and uneven pigmentation, and is susceptible to the development of a variety of benign and malignant tumours. Chronic sun exposure produces similar skin signs and any differences are mainly in degree of change. Elastosis, telangiectasia and keratoses or tumours are prominent; atrophy and irregular pigmentation are also common. Sun-damaged skin histologically tends to have more tangled elastic fibres and elastotic bodies than non-exposed skin[3].

Temporal hair loss starts during adolescence in males (and to a lesser extent in females), and progresses so that by the seventh decade 60% of men have moderate or advanced hair loss[4]. This process is controlled at least in part by androgens. Melanocytes are lost progressively from the hair bulb. At the age of 50 years, half the body hair is grey in 50% of the population[5].

Several premature aging syndromes have been shown to have hereditary, genetic or chromosomal abnormalities, but others are of unknown aetiology. Certain conditions, e.g. Down's syndrome, have many of the criteria of premature aging[2], although they have not conventionally been thought of as premature aging syndromes. Disorders that show features of generalized aging (including skin changes) are described in the first section of this chapter, while the second section deals with conditions in which the changes of cutaneous aging are prominent although not invariably present (Table 14.1). A comparison of some of the more important premature aging syndromes is summarized in Table 14.2 at the end of this chapter.

References

1 Gilchrest BA. *Skin and Aging Processes*. CRC Press, Boca Raton, 1984.
2 Martin GM. Genetic syndromes in man with potential relevance to the pathobiology of aging. In: Bergsma D, Harrison DE, eds. *Genetic Effects on Aging*. Alan R. Liss, New York, 1978; 5–39.
3 Braverman IM, Fonferko E. Studies in cutaneous aging: I. The elastic fiber network. *J Invest Dermatol* 1982; **78**: 434–43.

4 Burch PRJ, Murray JJ, Jackson D. The age-prevalence of arcus senilis, greying of hair and baldness. *J Gerontol* 1971; **26**: 364–72.

5 Keogh EV, Walsh RJ. Rate of greying of human hair. *Nature* 1965; **207**: 877–8.

Syndromes of premature aging

Acrogeria

Synonym: *Gottron's syndrome*

Definition

Acrogeria is a condition characterized by an aged appearance of the skin of the face and the distal extremities, small stature and various skeletal abnormalities.

Table 14.1 *Syndromes associated with premature aging*

Syndromes of premature aging

Acrogeria (Gottron's syndrome)
Cockayne's syndrome (see Chapter 17)
Congenital generalized lipodystrophy
  (Seip's syndrome)
Down's syndrome
Hallermann–Streiff syndrome
Metageria
Progeria (Hutchinson–Gilford syndrome)
Rothmund–Thomson syndrome (see Chapter 12)
Turner's syndrome
Werner's syndrome

Other syndromes in which premature aging of the skin is often a feature

Ataxia-telangiectasia (Louis-Bar syndrome)
  (see Chapter 17)
Basal cell naevus syndrome (see Chapter 19)
Blepharochalasis
Bloom's syndrome (see Chapter 17)
Cutis laxa (see Chapter 10)
Dyskeratosis congenita (see Chapter 13)
Ehlers–Danlos syndrome (see Chapter 10)
Epidermodysplasia verruciformis (see Chapter 19)
Focal dermal hypoplasia
The porphyrias (see Chapter 12)
Pseudoxanthoma elasticum (see Chapter 10)
Self-healing epithelioma of Ferguson-Smith
  (see Chapter 19)
Xeroderma pigmentosum (see Chapter 17)

Clinical features

The condition is usually manifested in early childhood, with many cases showing signs before the age of 2 years [1–3]. Some individuals have been born prematurely[3]. Features of premature aging are skin atrophy and short stature. The manifestations are as follows.

Skin changes

Skin changes may be present at birth. The skin of the hands, feet and face shows loss of subcutaneous tissue with wrinkling, atrophy, dryness and sometimes hyperpigmentation. Bruising and easy laceration after minor trauma may occur. Typically the blood vessels on the trunk are prominent and the facies is pinched with prominence of the eyes. Various nail abnormalities occur, atrophy and thickening being the most common. Perforating elastoma is reported[4].

Skeletal abnormalities

Short stature is often a feature. Spina bifida, thinning of the long bones, talipes equinovarus and congenital dislocation of the hip are found.

Internal involvement

Cardiac murmurs of aortic sclerosis were recorded in 2 subjects[3], but generally changes in the internal organs are not seen.

Pathology

On skin biopsy the dermis is atrophic with collagen and elastin degeneration. The subcutaneous fat is strikingly reduced. The epidermis may show focal hyperkeratosis, atrophy or basal layer hypermelanosis.

Genetics

In most cases a recessive inheritance seems likely, but there are two reports of mother and offspring involvement which raises the possibility of dominant inheritance[5,6].

Differential diagnosis

Progeria is distinguished by showing prominent growth retardation, hair loss, atherosclerosis and a reduced life expectancy. Ehlers–Danlos syndrome does not show the same degree of mainly acral skin aging as is found in acrogeria.

Treatment

No treatment is currently available. Life expectancy is normal.

References

1 Gottron H. Familiare Akrogerie. *Arch Dermatol Syphil* 1941; **181**: 571–83.
2 Calvert HT. Acrogeria. *Br J Dermatol* 1957; **69**: 69.
3 Gilkes JJH, Sharvill DE, Wells RS. The premature aging syndromes: report of eight cases and description of a new identity named metageria. *Br J Dermatol* 1974; **91**: 243–62.
4 Venencie PY, Powell FC, Winkelmann RK. Acrogeria with perforating elastoma and bony abnormalities. *Acta Derm Venereol* (Stockholm) 1984; **64**: 348–51.
5 De Groot WP, Tafelkruyer J, Woerdeman MJ. Familial acrogeria (Gottron). *Br J Dermatol* 1980; **103**: 213–21.
6 Kaufman I, Thiele B, Mahrle G. Simultaneous occurrence of metageria and Gottron's syndrome in one family. *Z Hautkr* 1985; **60**: 975–84.

Congenital generalized lipodystrophy

Synonym: *Seip's syndrome*

Definition

Congenital generalized lipodystrophy is a rare congenital syndrome with loss of subcutaneous fat, hepatomegaly, hyperlipoproteinaemia and diabetes mellitus.

Clinical features

Changes are evident at birth or during infancy[1,2]. Premature aging features include loss of subcutaneous fat (Figure 14.1), hyperlipoproteinaemia and diabetes mellitus.

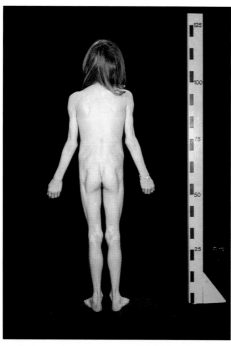

Figure 14.1 *Congenital generalized lipodystrophy (courtesy of Dr J. Harper)*

Complete loss of subcutaneous fat

The loss of subcutaneous fat gives a characteristic gaunt appearance to the facies, and elsewhere the skin appears aged.

Skin changes

Coarse, dry skin, an acanthosis nigricans-like appearance at the axillary and inguinal folds, and hypertrichosis with a low frontal hairline are seen.

Metabolic abnormalities

Hyperlipoproteinaemia is sometimes associated with xanthomata. Insulin-resistant diabetes mellitus develops at the age of about 10 years. Increased bone growth is seen, the hands and feet are often enlarged and the abdomen is protuberant.

Internal organ involvement

Hepatomegaly is characteristic. Occasionally splenomegaly, renal and neurological anomalies are found.

Pathology

The subcutaneous and visceral fat is lost completely.

Genetics

Inheritance is autosomal recessive. Homozygotes may express the full syndrome, with heterozygotes showing hyperlipoproteinaemia only.

Differential diagnosis

Leprechaunism has similar features.

Treatment

No specific treatment is known.

References

1 Seip M. Lipodystrophy and gigantism with associated endocrine manifestations. A new diencephalic syndrome. *Acta Paediatr Scand* 1959; **48**: 555–74.
2 Senior B, Gellis SS. The syndromes of total lipodystrophy and of partial lipodystrophy. *Pediatrics* 1964; **33**: 593–612.

Down's syndrome

Definition

Down's syndrome is the most common major congenital malformation in humans, classically characterized by trisomy of chromosome 21.

Clinical features

Down's syndrome has a prevalence of about 1 in 650 live births. It has been shown in a multifactorial analysis to have more of the characteristics of aging than progeria or Werner's syndrome[1]. Growth retardation is an important finding and adults with Down's syndrome rarely attain their expected height. The craniofacial appearance is readily recognizable. The head is round with flattening of the face and nasal bridge. The ears are small but prominent and often malformed. Eye abnormalities include epicanthic folds, speckling of the iris and fine opacities of the lens. Short, broad hands are typical, with short fingers, curving of the little digit, and a four-finger (simian) crease[2]. The palate is high and arched, the teeth may be hypoplastic and late to erupt, and the lips and the tongue commonly show fissuring. A general laxity of the muscle tone is responsible for the typically sagging mouth. Malformations of the cardiovascular and other systems are frequent.

The skin is often loose, especially over the back of the neck. Scalp hair may grey prematurely and is frequently fine and sparse. Alopecia areata, often of the totalis type, occurs in a high proportion of cases. In early childhood the skin is usually soft, but between the ages of 5 and 10 years it becomes dry and by the middle of the second decade over 70% have a generalized ichthyosis of mild or moderate severity. Patches of lichen simplex on the limbs and neck are seen in the majority of patients. Atopic eczema is thought to be more common than in the general population. Acrocyanosis and livedo reticularis of the limbs may occur.

The features that indicate premature aging are as follows[1]:

1. Growth retardation.
2. Premature greying of hair, and alopecia.
3. Increased incidence of autoimmune disease, including diabetes mellitus.
4. Increased incidence of malignancy (especially leukaemia).
5. Progressive dementia.
6. Cataract formation.
7. Deposition of amyloid and lipofuscin in several organs.
8. Degenerative vascular disease.
9. Hypogonadism.

Pathology

Postmortem examination of the brains of Down's patients with dementia shows senile plaques, Alzheimer's neurofibrillary degeneration and Simcowitz's vacuolar degeneration of nerve cells.

Lymphocytes from patients with Down's syndrome have an increased sensitivity to the induction of chromosomal aberrations by X-rays, and reduced DNA repair synthesis when exposed to ultraviolet irradiation[3]. However, there is no evidence of increased spontaneous chromosomal aberration or sister chromatid exchange in Down's syndrome lymphocytes not exposed to mutagens.

Genetics

In the majority (about 95%) of cases Down's syndrome is due to trisomy of chromosome 21. This usually results from non-dysjunction at meiosis in the mother, both parents having a normal chromosome distribution. The risk of Down's syndrome increases with advancing maternal age and is about 1.6% for women aged over 40 years.

In 2–4% of Down's syndrome cases the cause is translocation rearrangement. The extra 21 chromosome is not free but is attached to another chromosome, usually one of the 13–15 or 21–22 group. The individual's cells may then have 46 chromosomes, but one of them will be disproportionately large since it will in effect consist of two chromosomes. Some translocation cases are inherited. The parent carrier with a translocation of chromosome 21 has only 45 chromosomes but is clinically normal as all the normal chromosome material is represented. Many of the possible chromosomal combinations are lethal to the developing embryo and only a minority of these conceptuses survive to term.

When both parents of a Down's syndrome child have normal chromosomes the chances of a further child being similarly affected are 1–2%. If one of the parents is a carrier of a translocated 21 chromosome, the risk rises to about 1 in 3[2].

Differential diagnosis

The condition is usually obvious; however, when the craniofacial features are not prominent, diagnosis sometimes requires careful assessment of the physical signs and confirmation by examination of the chromosomes.

Treatment

Treatment of the individual is symptomatic and supportive. Investigation of the parents and appropriate counselling is needed. Life expectancy at birth is 16 years; at age 5 years it is 27 years[4]. Only 4% survive to the sixth decade.

References

1 Martin GM. Genetic syndromes in man with potential relevance to the pathobiology of aging. In: Bergsma D, Harrison DE, eds. *Genetic Effects on Aging*. Alan R. Liss, New York, 1978; 5–39.
2 Goldstein S. Human genetic disorders that feature premature onset and accelerated progression of biological aging. In: Schneider EL, ed. *The Genetics of Aging*. Plenum, New York, 1978; 171–224.

3 Lambert B, Hansson K, Bui TH et al. DNA repair and frequency of X-ray and UV light induced chromosome aberrations in leucocytes from patients with Down's syndrome. *Ann Hum Genet* 1976; **39**: 293–303.
4 Salmon MA. *Developmental Defects and Syndromes.* HM & M, Aylesbury, 1978.

Hallermann–Streiff syndrome

Definition

Hallermann–Streiff syndrome is a developmental disorder characterized by dyscephaly, a bird-like profile, cataracts and alopecia.

Clinical features

A combination of mesodermal and ectodermal defects make up the clinical picture [1–3]. Premature aging features include growth retardation, skin atrophy and alopecia.

Facial defects

Brachycephaly with dehiscent sutures, hypoplasia of the mandible and maxilla, a thin, beaked nose and a small mouth give a bird-like profile. Microphthalmia, congenital cataracts and other ocular defects are found. The teeth are malformed or absent.

Growth retardation

Dwarfism is present. Physical and mental development are retarded.

Cutaneous abnormalities

Scalp hair at birth may be normal but subsequently becomes generally thinned with alopecia which characteristically follows the cranial sutures. The eyelashes and eyebrows may be deficient. The skin is atrophic and telangiectatic, especially over the face.

Pathology

The skin is atrophic. The collagen fibres are loosely woven and the elastic fibres are fragmented into short lengths[2].

Genetics

The report of the syndrome occurring in a father and son[4] suggests that the condition is autosomal dominant, with most cases being new mutations.

Differential diagnosis

The complete syndrome is distinctive, but if it is incomplete, progeria and mandibulofacial dysostosis (Treacher Collins syndrome) need to be considered. In progeria, the skin atrophy and alopecia are more widespread. In mandibulofacial dysostosis, general development and the hair are normal, and the face is fish-like with a large mouth.

Treatment

No specific therapy is available. Supportive measures are appropriate.

References

1 Hutchinson D. Oral manifestations of oculomandibulardyscephaly with hypotrichosis. *Oral Surg* 1971; **31**: 234–44.
2 François J, Pierard J. François dyscephalic syndrome and skin manifestations. *Am J Ophthalmol* 1971; **71**: 1241–50.
3 Fitch N, Pinsky L, Lachance RC. A form of bird-headed dwarfism with features of premature senility. *Am J Dis Child* 1970; **120**: 260–4.
4 Golomb RS, Porter PS. A distinctive hair shaft abnormality in the Hallermann–Streiff syndrome. *Cutis* 1975; **16**: 122.

Metageria

Definition

Metageria is a very rare syndrome characterized by a tall, thin habitus, a bird-like facies and loss of subcutaneous tissue[1].

Clinical features

Only 3 patients have been described[1,2]. The subjects were tall and thin with little subcutaneous fat. The face was bird-like with a beaked nose, staring eyes and hollowed cheeks. The skin was atrophic, bound tightly over the extremities, and showed telangiectasia and mottled pigmentation which developed early in the second decade. Scalp hair was fine but there was no canities. Secondary sexual characteristics developed normally. Cataracts and senile arcus were not evident; all 3 individuals developed diabetes mellitus. One subject had peripheral vascular disease: ulceration of the feet and ankles developed at the age of 7 years, continued intermittently and ultimately resulted in bilateral below-knee amputations early in her third decade[1].

Pathology

Skin biopsy showed an atrophic epidermis, hypotrophic appendages and normal subcutaneous fat[1].

Genetics

Inheritance is unclear, because of the small number of cases.

Differential diagnosis

The individuals described did not conform to the recognized pictures of progeria or Werner's syndrome (no growth retardation, normal genitalia, no alopecia), nor to that of acrogeria (atherosclerosis and diabetes mellitus). However, the description of the third case of metageria[2] raised a doubt that it is a distinct entity, as both the mother and sister of this patient had acrogeria.

Treatment

No treatment is known. One subject died at the age of 25 years[1].

References

1 Gilkes JJH, Sharvill DE, Wells RS. The premature ageing syndromes: report of eight new cases and description of a new identity named metageria. *Br J Dermatol* 1974; **91**: 243–62.
2 Kaufman I, Thiele B, Marle G. Simultaneous occurrence of metageria and Gottron's acrogeria in one family. *Z Hautkr* 1985; **60**: 975–84.

Progeria

Synonym: *Hutchinson–Gilford syndrome*

Definition

Progeria is a rare syndrome of growth retardation and specific, progressive, premature senescent changes.

Clinical features

Individuals are normal at birth although they may be of low birthweight[1]. The onset of symptoms is during the first 12 months of life and the diagnosis is usually made in the second year.

Growth retardation

Weight gain after birth is very slow and linear growth is half the normal rate[1]. Failure to thrive is one of the most common presentations[1]. Sexual maturity is not attained and the voice remains high-pitched. Emotionally, individuals with progeria are similar to their peers and are conscious of their different appearance.

Skeletal abnormalities

The cranium is disproportionately large with a small face, the anterior fontanelles remain open and the scalp veins are easily visible (Figure 14.2). The clavicles are short, the gait wide-based and shuffling, the limbs are thin and the joints become prominent and stiff. Osteoporosis is found.

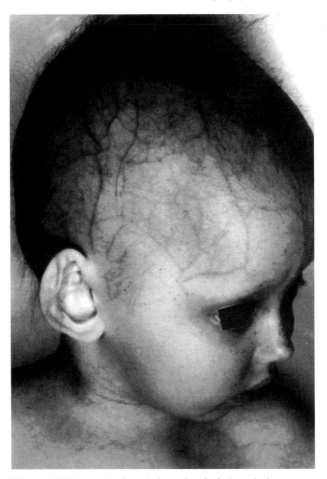

Figure 14.2 *Progeria: there is loss of scalp hair and of eyebrows, with prominent scalp veins, micrognathia, abnormal ears and freckle-like pigmentation (courtesy of Dr A. J. Keay)*

Skin changes

Skin changes are prominent and may be the presenting feature[1]. By the age of 2 years, the skin has become thin, dry, taut and shiny in certain areas but lax and wrinkled in others (most commonly over the fingers and toes). The subcutaneous fat is reduced and the veins visible. Scleroderma-like areas over the hips and trunk are seen[2]. Sweating is sometimes diminished. Irregular pigmentation subsequently develops, notably in light-exposed sites.

Hair and nails

Scalp alopecia is invariable and starts during the first 2 years of life. It is total except for a few white or blond, fine, downy hairs. The eyebrows and eyelashes are often absent and body hair is sparse. The fingernails and toenails are usually short and thin but may be dystrophic, with koilonychia and onychogryphosis.

Abnormal facies

The cranium is disproportionately large, the eyes are prominent, the lips thin, the ears protrude and the nose is beaked with a sculptured tip. Micrognathia is found and primary and secondary dentition is delayed and incomplete.

Internal organ involvement

Atherosclerotic cardiovascular disease is usually progressive. Diabetes mellitus is not a feature, nor is neoplasia.

Pathology

At autopsy, atherosclerotic plaques are found uniformly in several vessels, including the aorta and coronary arteries. The aortic and mitral valves may be calcified, and myocardial fibrosis may be present[3]. Bone lesions show osteolysis, osteoporosis and avascular hip necrosis. Histologically, the epidermis is atrophic with increased melanin in the basal layer, and the dermis shows thickened collagen bundles with areas of hyalinization. Sebaceous glands and hair follicles are decreased in number and subcutaneous fat is reduced. Urinary excretion of hyaluronic acid is increased[4].

Genetics

Progeria occurs about once in every 8 million births[1]. Males outnumber females by 1.5 to 1. A sporadic autosomal mutation of the fertilizing sperm or ovum is most likely, related to advanced paternal age[1,5]. Some have argued that the inheritance is autosomal recessive, but this seems unlikely as the rate for affected siblings is much less than the 25% that this would predict and consanguinity is rare. The mode of inheritance cannot be proved since progeria patients do not reproduce.

Skin fibroblasts from progeria patients have a reduced growth capacity in vitro, but there is conflicting evidence on whether progeric cells can repair single-strand DNA breaks induced by X- or gamma-irradiation[6]. The increased hyaluronic acid production by progeric fibroblasts (related to a defect in degradation) is postulated as the underlying metabolic abnormality in progeria[6], although this has yet to be confirmed.

Differential diagnosis

Progeria in its full manifestation at the age of 2 years is characteristic, but differentiation from Werner's syndrome, acrogeria, metageria, Rothmund–Thomson syndrome and Cockayne's syndrome may be required.

Treatment

No effective treatment is known. In reported cases, death has occurred between the ages of 7 years and 27 years, with an average life expectancy of 13 years[1]. Death usually results from myocardial infarction or cardiac failure.

References

1 DeBusk FL. The Hutchinson–Gilford progeria syndrome. *J Pediatr* 1972; **90**: 697–724.
2 Moynahan EJ. Progeria presenting as scleroderma in early infancy. *Proc R Soc Med* 1962; **55**: 233–4.
3 Baker PB, Baba N, Boesel CP. Cardiovascular abnormalities in progeria: case report and a review of the literature. *Arch Pathol Lab Med* 1981; **105**: 384–6.
4 Brown WT, Zebrower M, Kieras FJ. Progeria, a model disease for the study of accelerated aging. *Basic Life Sci* 1985; **35**: 375–96.
5 Brown WT, Kieras FJ, Houck GE Jr, Dutkowski R, Jenkins EC. A comparison of adult and childhood progerias: Werner syndrome and Hutchinson–Gilford progeria syndrome. *Adv Exp Med Biol* 1985; **190**: 229–44.
6 Badame AJ. Progeria. *Arch Dermatol* 1989; **135**: 540–4.

Turner's syndrome

Definition

Turner's syndrome is a sex chromosome abnormality (45,XO) in which affected females have some features of premature aging.

Clinical features

Turner's syndrome is not one of the classic progeroid conditions, but has several features in common with them[1]. Phenotypic abnormalities vary considerably and may be mild. Affected individuals may show the following features.

Growth retardation

Growth retardation is one of the most consistent features. Secondary sexual characteristics are often poorly developed and primary amenorrhoea is frequent. Intelligence is usually normal.

Habitus

A short, webbed neck, shield chest, cubitus valgus, short fourth metacarpal, micrognathia, high palate, low-set ears and ocular abnormalities are seen[2].

Internal organ involvement

The ovaries are small. Congenital heart disease (notably aortic coarctation) and renal anomalies occur. Autoimmune thyroid disease, diabetes mellitus, hypertension and osteoporosis are more common in individuals with Turner's syndrome[3].

Skin abnormalities

Lymphoedema of the hands and feet may be present at birth and is sometimes the only detectable abnormality. The scalp hair may thin prematurely. Cutis laxa of the neck and buttocks is seen. The nails may be hypoplastic. Multiple melanocytic naevi are often present.

Features of Turner's syndrome that correspond to premature aging include primary growth retardation and an increased incidence of autoimmune disease, diabetes mellitus, osteoporosis, hypertension, alopecia and atherosclerosis[1].

Pathology

The ovaries are smaller than normal. The cutaneous and subcutaneous lymphatics are hypoplastic.

Genetics

About 80% of cases have a 45,XO karyotype. Most of the remaining 20% are mosaics with partial deletion of one X chromosome. Turner's syndrome has an incidence of 0.4 per 1000 live female infants.

Differential diagnosis

The full phenotypic expression is characteristic, but the diagnosis may be difficult if abnormalities are mild.

Treatment

Androgens or growth hormone can be used to stimulate growth. Oestrogen replacement therapy is needed for puberty development. The prognosis is good.

References

1 Martin GM. Genetic syndromes in man with potential relevance to the pathobiology of aging. In: Bergsma D, Harrison DE, eds. *Genetic Effects on Aging*. Alan R. Liss, New York, 1978; 5–39.
2 Engel E, Forbes AP. Cytogenetic and clinical findings in 48 patients with congenitally defective or absent ovaries. *Medicine* (Baltimore) 1965; **44**: 177–221.
3 Goldstein S. Human genetic disorders that feature premature onset and accelerated progression of biological aging. In: Schneider EL, ed. *The Genetics of Aging*. Plenum, New York, 1978; 171–224.

Werner's syndrome

Definition

Werner's syndrome is a disorder of primary growth retardation with features of premature aging and an increased prevalence of malignancy.

Clinical features

The diagnosis is often not made until the fourth decade, although the initial symptoms may have appeared several years previously. The approximate worldwide prevalence is 1–2 per million population[1], although the syndrome is more common in Japan[2]. An outline of the clinical manifestations is as follows [1–3].

Primary growth retardation

Affected individuals are shorter than expected (average height 1.57 m for males and 1.46 m for women[1] and have a stocky trunk and spindly limbs. Growth stops at about 13 years of age.

Facies

The face is often rounded, with a thin, beaked nose, loss of periorbital fat and sometimes radial furrowing of the skin around the mouth.

Skin changes

Skin changes are often prominent. One of the earliest changes is greying of the scalp hair, which often begins in the second decade. Alopecia develops in the third decade. The skin is atrophic with loss of subcutaneous fat, and over the lower legs and forearms may have a shiny, scleroderma-like appearance. Hyperpigmentation and telangiectasia may also occur. Hyperkeratotic patches develop over bony prominences such as the ankle, and these can ulcerate.

Eye and laryngeal changes

Cataracts are found. A high-pitched, hoarse voice is present in 50% of cases and tends to be noticed in the second decade.

Endocrine abnormalities

Secondary sexual characteristics are frequently underdeveloped. Diabetes mellitus (often mild) or biochemical glucose intolerance is found in half of all subjects[1]. Soft-tissue calcification is seen and osteoporosis may develop. Pituitary, adrenal and thyroid functions are usually normal.

Atherosclerosis

Atherosclerosis may cause vascular calcification and result in ulceration of the feet or lower legs. Amputation is sometimes required. In subjects with concomitant diabetes mellitus, vascular changes may be a consequence of this or of primary atherosclerosis.

Malignant neoplasia

Between 6% and 10% of cases develop a malignancy[1,2]. Sarcomas and meningiomas are reported as well as carcinomas.

Pathology

Skin fibroblasts from patients with Werner's syndrome are more difficult to culture, proliferate more slowly, and produce less glycosaminoglycans (GAG) in comparison with normal controls[3,4]. Evidence of a GAG abnormality is conflicting: the amount of GAG may be increased in the sclerodermatous-like skin but reduced in normal-looking skin[4]. Urinary hyaluronic acid levels may be increased[3,4]. Electron microscopy of scleroderma-like skin reveals amorphous material lying between collagen bundles[3], but collagen synthesis by fibroblasts is qualitatively normal[3].

Genetics

Inheritance is autosomal recessive. Parental consanguinity was reported in two-thirds of a large Japanese series[2] and in one-third of another large series[1]. Affected siblings are seen in a quarter of cases and the sex incidence is equal.

Chromosomal rearrangements have been reported in cultured lymphocytes and fibroblasts from patients with Werner's syndrome[4,5]. Changes range from deletion of a single chromosome to variable multiple rearrangements, which are stable and clonal. These findings suggest that Werner's syndrome may belong to the group of 'chromosomal instability syndromes' that also includes Bloom's syndrome, ataxia-telangiectasia and Fanconi's anaemia[4]. The gene for Werner's syndrome has recently been mapped to chromosome 8p[6].

Treatment

No treatment is known. Death usually occurs in the fourth, fifth or sixth decade, and mainly results from myocardial infarction, cerebrovascular disease or malignancy.

References

1 Epstein CJ, Martin GM, Schultz AL. Werner's syndrome: a review of its symptomatology, natural history, pathologic features, genetics, and relationship to the natural aging process. *Medicine* (Baltimore) 1966: **45**: 177–221.

2 Murata K, Nakashima H. Werner's syndrome: twenty-four cases with a review of the Japanese medical literature. *J Am Geriatr Soc* 1982; **30**: 303–8.

3 Gawkrodger DJ, Priestley GC, Vijayalaxmi et al. Werner's syndrome: biochemical and cytogenetic studies. *Arch Dermatol* 1985; **121**: 636–41.

4 Salk D. Werner's syndrome: a review of recent research with an analysis of connective tissue metabolism, growth control of cells, and chromosomal aberrations. *Hum Genet* 1982; **62**: 1–15.

5 Scappaticci S, Cerimele D, Fraccaro M. Clonal structural chromosomal rearrangements in primary fibroblast cultures and in lymphocytes of patients with Werner's syndrome. *Hum Genet* 1982; **62**: 16–24.

6 Goto M, Rubenstein M, Weber J et al. Genetic linkage of Werner's syndrome to five markers on chromosome 8. *Nature* 1992; **355**: 735–7.

Syndromes in which premature aging of the skin is often a feature

Blepharochalasis

Definition

Blepharochalasis is a condition characterized by atrophy, wrinkling and sagging of the eyelids.

Clinical features

Atrophy, telangiectasia and fine wrinkling of the upper eyelids may be noticed at birth or in infancy but usually appear between the ages of 10 years and 18 years[1,2]. Progression is slow until puberty when it accelerates for a year or so and the changes then persist throughout life. Recurrent attacks of oedema of the eyelids often precede these changes. The skin of

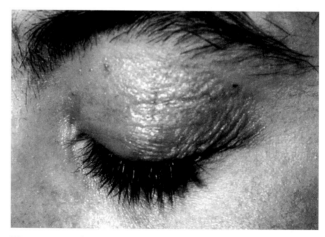

Figure 14.3 *Blepharochalasis: the atrophy and telangiectasia in this 16-year-old girl followed episodes of oedema (reproduced with permission from Blackwell Scientific Publications Ltd)*

the upper eyelid has a prematurely aged appearance (Figure 14.3) and may become baggy and sag down over the eye. Occasionally the lower lids are also affected. Reduplication of the upper lid mucous membrane is seen in 10% of cases. A late-onset variant is recognized.

Pathology

The elastic tissue of the eyelid is diminished and fragmented [2].

Genetics

Pedigrees show autosomal dominant inheritance. Sporadic cases seem to occur but minor involvement is easily overlooked.

Differential diagnosis

In cutis laxa, blepharochalasis is associated with more widespread changes. Blepharochalasis forms part of Ascher's syndrome in which it is associated with a progressive enlargement of the upper lip.

Treatment

Surgical correction of the baggy eyelids may help the cosmetic appearance but recurrence is not uncommon.

References

1 Klauder JV. The interrelationship of some cutaneous and ocular diseases. *Arch Dermatol* 1959; **80**: 515–28.
2 Tapaszto I, Liszkay L, Vass Z. Some data on the pathogenesis of blepharochalasis. *Acta Ophthalmol* 1963; **41**: 167–75.

Focal dermal hypoplasia

Definition

Focal dermal hypoplasia is a syndrome of mesodermal and ectodermal dysplasia featuring underdevelopment of the dermis with skeletal and ocular defects.

Clinical features

Abnormalities are usually evident at birth although they may progress in extent and severity through childhood. The following features are seen [1–3].

Cutaneous abnormalities

Areas of underdevelopment and thinness of the skin in a reticular, cribriform and often linear distribution are seen (Figure 14.4), mostly on the limbs or trunk.

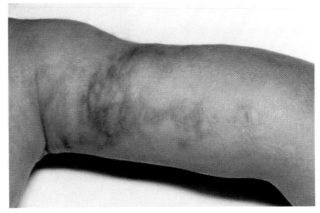

Figure 14.4 *Focal dermal hypoplasia: linear skin atrophy (courtesy of Dr J. Harper)*

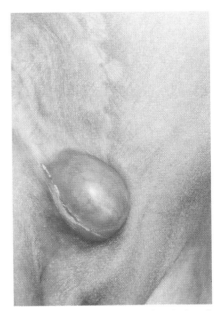

Figure 14.5 *Focal dermal hypoplasia: herniation through an area of skin atrophy (courtesy of Dr J. Harper)*

Linear or reticular areas of hyper- or hypopigmentation are found and telangiectatic lesions are seen. An initial inflammatory or bullous phase is recognized. Reddish-yellow nodules of subcutaneous fat may herniate through the attenuated dermis (Figure 14.5). Occasionally the skin may be totally absent from various sites at birth: the scalp seems to be most commonly affected. Papillomatous lesions are present on or around the lips, inside the mouth, at the anus and vagina, and sometimes in the axilla or inguinal areas. Palmar or plantar hyperkeratosis may occur.

Hair and nails

The scalp hair is often sparse and brittle; it may be totally lacking from circumscribed areas of the scalp. The fingernails or toenails may be dystrophic or completely absent.

Skeletal abnormalities

A large number of anomalies have been described [2]. The facies is usually pointed with prognathism. Kyphosis, scoliosis, spina bifida occulta and other vertebral anomalies are seen, along with asymmetrical development of the face, trunk or limbs. Deformity of the radius or clavicle, absence of part of an extremity, and anomalies of the hands and feet (including hypoplasia of digits, syndactyly, and abnormalities of the metacarpals and metatarsals) are reported.

Ocular anomalies

Ocular anomalies include coloboma iridis, microphthalmia, strabismus and nystagmus.

Dental anomalies

Dysplasia of teeth, microdontia and other anomalies occur.

Pathology

Skin biopsy from lesional areas shows a normal epidermis, but the dermis is hypoplastic and the collagen is largely replaced by adipose tissue. Indeed, subcutaneous fat may in some places approach close to the epidermis. Capillaries may be increased in number, and sweat glands reduced in number.

Genetics

The majority of reported cases have been female although the syndrome has been recorded in males [2]. Evidence from family histories suggests that the condition is caused by a single mutant gene whose inheritance may be X-linked dominant, or autosomal dominant but sex-limited [2]. The trait may be lethal in its fullest expression in males.

Differential diagnosis

The syndrome may need to be distinguished from Rothmund–Thomson syndrome, incontinentia pigmenti and connective tissue naevus. The Rothmund–Thomson syndrome differs in that the skin signs develop in a photodermatitis distribution and show poikiloderma: short stature and cataracts are also found. In incontinentia pigmenti linear areas of atrophy and pigmentation occur but dermal hypoplasia is not a feature. Connective tissue naevus is normally more localized and does not have the same array of associated ectodermal and mesodermal changes.

Treatment

No treatment is known.

References

1 Goltz RW, Peterson WC, Gorlin RJ, Ravits HG. Focal dermal hypoplasia. *Arch Dermatol* 1962; **86**: 708–17.
2 Goltz RW, Henderson RR, Hitch JM, Ott JE. Focal dermal hypoplasia syndrome. *Arch Dermatol* 1970; **101**: 1–11.
3 Temple IK, MacDowell, Baraister M et al. Focal dermal hypoplasia (Goltz syndrome). *J Med Genet* 1990; **27**: 180–7.

Table 14.2 *A comparison of syndromes with features of premature aging*

Syndrome	Mode of inheritance	Sex incidence	Age of onset	Skeletal anomalies	Skin changes	Neurological abnormalities	Systemic complications
Acrogeria	Recessive	M = F	Before 2 years	Dwarfism, spina bifida, equinovarus	Atrophy, wrinkling, pigmentation	None	Not usual
Ataxia-telangiectasia	Recessive	M = F	Second year	Some have growth retardation	Atrophy, eczema, canities	Cerebellar ataxia	Infections, lymphomas (immune deficient)
Bloom's syndrome	Recessive	M > F	First year	Growth-retarded, slender features, narrow face	Photosensitivity, telangiectasia, atrophy	None	Many develop leukaemia
Cockayne's syndrome	Recessive	M = F	Second year	Dwarfism, kyphosis, micrognathia	Photosensitivity, telangiectasia, pigmentation	Ataxia, cerebral atrophy, deafness	Optic atrophy, hypogonadism
Congenital generalized lipodystrophy	Recessive	M = F	Birth or early infancy	Increased bone growth	Loss of subcutaneous fat, coarse dry skin, hypertrichosis	Neurological impairment may be seen	Hyperlipidaemia, diabetes, hepatomegaly
Down's syndrome	Trisomy 21 usually	M = F	Birth	Growth retardation, skeletal malformations	Lax soft skin, ichthyosis, alopecia, canities	Progressive dementia	Cataract, atherosclerosis, malignancy, diabetes
Dyskeratosis congenita	Sex-linked recessive	M	5–15 years	None	Dystrophic nails, poikiloderma	None	Pancytopenia, carcinomas of mucous membrane
Hallermann–Streiff syndrome	Unknown (possibly dominant)	M = F	Early life	Dwarfism, brachycephaly, micrognathia	Atrophy on face, scalp alopecia	Mental retardation	Cataract, dental abnormalities
Progeria	Unknown (? sporadic autosomal mutation)	M > F	First 12 months	Small stature, cranium large, face small, osteoporosis	Atrophic, scleroderma-like areas, severe alopecia	Not prominent	Progressive atherosclerotic cardiovascular disease
Rothmund–Thomson syndrome	Recessive	M = F	3–6 months	Growth-retarded, forearm deformity	Photosensitivity, telangiectasia, poikiloderma	Not prominent	Cataract, malignancy, hypogonadism
Turner's syndrome	45,XO	F	Birth to adolescence	Growth-retarded, shield chest, cubitus valgus	Lymphoedema, cutis laxa, alopecia	Not prominent	Small ovaries, coarctation
Werner's syndrome	Recessive	M = F	Second to third decade	Growth-retarded, thin extremities	Atrophy, canities, alopecia, scleroderma-like areas	Not prominent	Cataracts, hypogonadism, diabetes, malignancy

Chapter 15

The hair and scalp

R. P. R. Dawber

Introduction

The specific hereditary and congenital abnormalities described in this chapter can be grouped into the three categories shown in Table 15.1. The historical background and evaluation of the nomenclature of the various disease have been described in great detail by Rook and Dawber[1] and are not outlined here.

Table 15.1 *Classification of hereditary and congenital hair disorders*

Defects of the hair shaft
Hereditary alopecia and hypotrichosis
Hypertrichosis

Reference

1 Rook A, Dawber RPR. *Diseases of the Hair and Scalp.* 2nd ed. Blackwell, Oxford, 1991.

Defects of the hair shaft

Structural defects of the hair shaft may be sufficient in degree to cause significant cosmetic disability, or they may render the hair abnormally susceptible to injury by minor degrees of trauma. They may also be the result of hereditary metabolic disorders, to which they afford valuable diagnostic clues.

Price[1] classified anomalies of the shaft into those associated with increased fragility, and those that are not (Table 15.2); this distinction is useful because only the former present clinically as patchy or diffuse alopecia. Price's classification is followed in this section. Whiting[2,3] has published a detailed and authoritative outline of all the major structural defects. Birnhaum and Baden[4] have also carefully reviewed the rarer structural abnormalities.

Table 15.2 *Defects of the hair shaft*

Structural defects of the shaft with increased fragility
    Monilethrix
    Pseudomonilethrix
    Pili torti
    Menkes' syndrome
    Netherton's syndrome (bamboo hair)
      (see also Chapter 5)
    Trichorrhexis nodosa
    Trichothiodystrophy (see also Chapters 5 and 17)
    Marinesco–Sjögren syndrome
Structural defects of the shaft without increased fragility
    Ringed hair (pili annulati)
    Woolly hair
    Uncombable hair syndrome
    Straight hair naevus
Other abnormalities of the shaft
    Weathering of the hair shaft

References

1 Price VH. Strukturanomalien des Haarschaftes. In: Orfanos CE, ed. *Haar und Haarkrankheiten*. Fischer, Stuttgart, 1979; 387.
2 Whiting DA. Structural abnormalities of the hair shaft. *J Am Acad Dermatol* 1987; **16**: 1–25.
3 Whiting DA. Hair shaft defects. In: Olsen EA ed. *Disorders of Hair Growth, Diagnosis and Treatment*. McGraw-Hill, New York, 1994; 91–138.
4 Birnhaum PS, Baden HP. Hereditable disorders of hair. *Dermatol Clin* 1987; **5**: 137–53.

Monilethrix

Monilethrix shows considerable variation in age of onset, severity and course. There is not yet sufficient information to establish whether these variations are in part consistently correlated with different genotypes. There is, however, much variation even within the more commonly reported autosomal dominant form, but some of it is merely apparent: vigorous hair brushing may reveal a defect, the presence of which would otherwise have been overlooked.

Clinical features

The hair may be obviously abnormal at birth but is most commonly normal, and is progressively replaced by abnormal hair during the first months of life: in other cases the normal hair is succeeded by horny follicular papules, from the summit of which emerge brittle, beaded hairs. The follicular keratosis and the abnormal hairs are most frequent on the nape and occiput, but may involve the entire scalp (Figures 15.1 and 15.2). However, the keratosis is not directly related to the beading; either change may precede the other and the keratosis is sometimes absent. In a typical case the short stubble of broken hairs and rough, horny plugs gives a distinctive appearance. However, the apparent onset of monilethrix may occur in early childhood or even as late as adolescence. Severe alopecia may develop or only a few affected hairs may be present, which may be overlooked unless they are carefully sought. In some cases, the eyebrows and eyelashes, pubic and axillary hair and general body hair may be affected, or one or more of these sites may show few or many abnormal hairs, when the scalp is normal.

In cases of early onset, the degree of baldness tends to increase during childhood, but only to a limited extent if trauma is avoided. In many patients the condition persists with little change throughout life, though spontaneous improvement or complete recovery have occurred. Temporary improvement has followed an epilating dose of X-rays and has been reported during pregnancy.

Associated defects

Only 1 of 134 patients with monilethrix had oligophrenia and schizophrenia: genetic linkage is improbable[1]. However, other investigators[2] thought the association with oligophrenia and with nail and tooth defects was significant. It is possible that such associations may be a feature of the recessive phenotype, since oligophrenia and poor physical development were noted also in 2 siblings with monilethrix[3]. In another family in which the authors suggested that

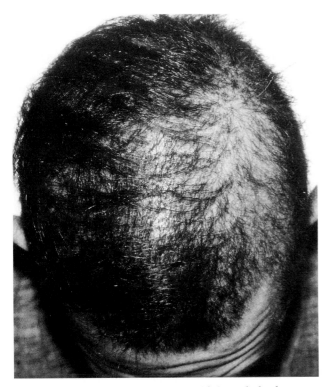

Figure 15.1 *Monilethrix: gross view with irregularly short, broken hair*

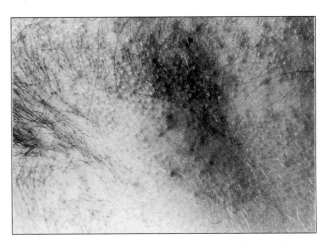

Figure 15.2 *Nape of neck of same patient as in Figure 15.1, showing obvious follicular keratosis. Close inspection of individual hairs reveals the noding*

inheritance was of the autosomal recessive type, 2 of the 5 affected individuals were oligophrenic and 1 was epileptic[4]. An association with juvenile cataract has been reported on a number of occasions[5].

Reports on abnormalities in amino acid metabolism are conflicting. Argininosuccinicaciduria has been reported in a number of cases, but a technical error was subsequently detected in some of these. An apparent excess of aspartic acid and of arginine in the urine of an affected mother and daughter remains unexplained.

Pathology

The hair shaft is beaded and brittle as the result of a developmental defect. Elliptical nodes 0.7–1.0 mm apart are separated by narrower internodes at which the medulla is lacking (Figure 15.3). The width of the nodes and the distance between them show some variation within a single family but interfamily variation is probably not significant. In the scanning electron microscope, the nodes and some of the internodes show a normal imbricated scale pattern, but most internodes show longitudinal ridging [6–8]. This ridging is acquired and progressive as internodes move away from the scalp. Studies using X-ray diffraction techniques show parallel keratin less well accentuated than in normal hair.

Histologically the follicle shows wide and narrow zones corresponding to the nodes and internodes, but the general structure of the follicle is traditionally said to be otherwise normal. However, the follicles are abnormally distributed and there is no whorl formation. Gummer et al[9] in a detailed electron microscopic study noted that changes were visible in the zone of keratinization; the cell membranes of the deeper hair-shaft cuticular cells were thrown into folds, particularly at the narrower internodes where breakage occurs; the adjacent inner root sheath was also abnormal[10].

Attempts have been made to investigate the mechanism of node formation and to relate it to the diurnal rate of hair growth, without any success[11]. Studies in the electron microscope [6–8] have shown that increased susceptibility of the hair shaft to the effects of trauma – premature weathering – is an important factor in the failure of the hair to attain a normal length.

Genetics

The hereditary nature of monilethrix was recognized soon after the condition was first identified. Autosomal dominant transmission has been demonstrated in numerous large pedigrees[4,12]. The gene for monilethrix has recently been mapped to the keratin gene cluster on chromosome 12q.

The alleged occurrence of normal carriers of the dominant gene has not been proved, for a parent with only 5% abnormal follicles easily passes as normal[13]. The gene appears to have high penetrance but variable expressivity.

Cockayne[14] reviewed the evidence that monilethrix may be determined also by an autosomal recessive gene; several pedigrees have suggested this possibility[15]. If the existence of a second genotype is established, it is likely that phenotypic differences can be shown to be present[16].

Treatment

No specific treatment is available, but Tamayo suggested that oral retinoids can induce some hair regrowth[17,18] – this may, however, relate to effects on the associated keratosis pilaris. Reduction of hairdressing trauma may be followed by some improvement in the less severely affected cases.

References

1 Korn-Heydt GE. Uber einem Fall von Monilethrix mit Schwadsinen und Achizophrenia. *Arch Klin Exp Dermatol* 1967; **228**: 445.
2 Salamon T, Scheyder UW. Uber die Monilethrix. *Arch Klin Exp Dermatol* 1962; **215**: 105.
3 Sfaello Z, Hariga J. Monilethrix associé à la débilité mentale: étude d'une famille. *Arch Belges Derm Syphil* 1967; **23**: 363.
4 Bartosova K, Jorda V. Monilethrix. *Ceskoslov Dermatol* 1973; **48**: 232.
5 Thiel E. Monilethrix und Frühstar. *Hautarzt* 1959; **10**: 271.

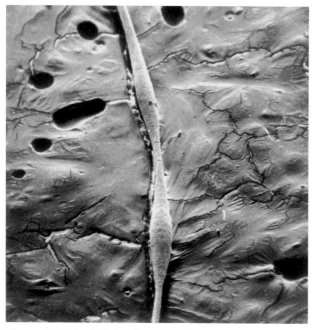

Figure 15.3 *Monilethrix: alternate wide and narrow parts of hair shaft are abnormal (scanning electron micrograph × 100)*

6 Dawber RPR. Weathering of hair in monilethrix and pili torti. *Clin Exp Dermatol* 1977; **2**: 271.
7 Dawber RPR. Weathering of hair in some genetic hair shaft abnormalities. In: Brown A, Cronin RG, eds. *Hair: Trace Elements and Human Illness*. Praeger, New York, 1980.
8 De Berker DAR, Ferguson DJP, Dawber RPR. Monilethrix: a clinico-pathological illustration of the cortical defect. *Br J Dermatol* 1993; **128**: 327–31.
9 Gummer CL, Dawber RPR, Swift JA. Monilethrix: an electron microscopic and electron histochemical study. *Br J Dermatol* 1981; **105**: 529–41.
10 Ito M, Hashimoto K, Yorder FW. Monilethrix: an ultrastructural study. *J Cutan Pathol* 1984; **11**: 513–21.
11 Comaish S. Autoradiographic studies of hair growth and rhythm in monilethrix. *Br J Dermatol* 1969; **81**: 443.
12 Alexander J O'D, Grant PW. Monilethrix. *Scot Med J* 1958; **3**: 351.
13 Deraemaeker R. Monilethrix: report of a family with special reference to some problems concerning inheritance. *Am J Hum Genet* 1957; **9**: 195.
14 Cockayne EA. *Inherited Abnormalities of The Skin and Its Appendages*. Oxford University Press, 1933; 144.
15 Hanhart E. Erstmaliger Hinweis auf das Vorkommen iners Monohybrid-rezessivere Erbbangs bei Monilethrix (Moniletrichosis) *Arch Julius-Klaus Stift Verebungsforsch* 1955; **30**: 1.
16 Finley EM, Ertle JO, Marschal SF. Alopecia in a 19-month-old boy. *Arch Dermatol* 1994; **130** (8): 451–2.
17 Tamayo L. Monilethrix treated with the oral retinoid Ro-109359 (Tigason). *Clin Exp Dermatol* 1973; **8**: 393–6.
18 De Berker DAR, Dawber RPR. Monilethrix treated with oral retinoids. *Clin Exp Dermatol* 1991; **16**: 226–8.

Pseudomonilethrix

It is not uncommon to see patients who complain that their hair is of poor quality or brittle, and if the patient in question is a young child, microscopy of the hair to exclude shaft defects is a routine procedure. It should be a routine procedure also in the older child or adult. Bentley-Phillips and Bayles[1] found a syndrome which they named 'pseudomonilethrix' and which was relatively frequent in South Africans of European or Indian descent. The status of the syndrome is uncertain; some of the shaft deformities may be artefactual.

Clinical features

The patients present with alopecia from the age of 8 years onwards, and their lack of hair can be shown to be the result of a defect, the inheritance of which is determined by an autosomal dominant gene, which renders the hair so fragile that it readily breaks with the trauma of brushing, combing or other hairdressing procedures.

Pathology

On microscopy one, or occasionally two, of three abnormalities can be seen.

1. Pseudomonilethrix – irregular nodes, which on electron microscopy prove to be the protruding edges of depressions in the shaft.
2. Irregular twists of 25–200 degrees without flattening of the shaft.
3. Breaks with brush-like ends in apparently normal shafts.

There is no keratosis pilaris. Most authorities now believe that pseudomonilethrix microscopic changes are artefactual; they can be produced in normal hairs by trauma from tweezers or forceps, or from compressing overlapping hairs between two glass slides, when the indentation in one shaft caused by another overlying hair exactly mimics the appearance of pseudomonilethrix. It would seem reasonable to suggest that this artefact may be more common in genetic abnormalities that 'soften' hair structure, e.g. sulphur deficiency syndromes[2,3].

Genetics

The condition is inherited as an autosomal dominant trait.

Treatment

The reduction of hairdressing trauma may be followed by a marked improvement in the condition.

References

1 Bentley-Phillips B, Bayles MAH. Pseudomonilethrix. *Br J Dermatol* 1975; **92**: 113.
2 Zitelli JA. Pseudomonilethrix: an artefact. *Arch Dermatol* 1986; **122**: 688–90.
3 Ferrando J, Fontarnau R, Haussman G. Is pseudomonilethrix an artifact. *Int J Dermatol* 1990; **29**: 380–1.

Pili torti

Definition

The term 'pili torti' was first suggested by Galewsky[1]. In pili torti, the hairs are flattened and at irregular intervals they are rotated through 180 degrees around their long axis. This may be regarded as a definition of classical pili torti. The widespread use of the scanning electron microscope has made it clear that twisted hairs occur in many distinct forms, and that the twisting may be associated with a number of other shaft defects. Many more studies will be needed before the significance and specificity of minor variations can be established. As new syndromes are characterized a residue of cases remains in which twisted hair is apparently the sole defect; many reported cases cannot be classified retrospectively since even the known syndromes cannot be excluded on the inadequate data. Occasional twists of varying angle should not be taken to be this distinctive, genetically 'fixed' abnormality of pili torti. Many dystrophies and distortions of the follicular zone of keratinization will vary the hair shaft 'bore' – sometimes showing irregular twists of less than 180 degrees.

Clinical features

The hair is usually normal at birth, but is gradually replaced by abnormal hair which becomes clinically evident as early as the third month, or not until the second or third year. There is wide variation from case to case in the fragility of the hair, and hence in the clinical picture.

Affected hairs are brittle and may break off at a length of 5 cm or less, or grow longer in areas of the scalp least subject to trauma (Figure 15.4). There may therefore be only a short, coarse stubble over the whole scalp, or there may be circumscribed baldness, irregularly patchy or occipital. Affected hairs have a 'spangled' appearance in reflected light. In mild cases the abnormal hairs have to be carefully sought, for there may be few and the hair may appear generally normal. Such is sometimes the case after puberty, as normal hairs may replace most of the pili torti during the later years of childhood. However, some patients remain severely affected throughout life. One patient first diagnosed in early childhood retained the microscopic appearance of pili torti into adolescence, but the hair darkened, ceased to weather badly and grew to a cosmetically acceptable length[2]. The involvement of sites other than the scalp has often been reported, but is an inconstant feature, most often seen in the more severe cases.

Other ectodermal defects may be associated with pili torti. Keratosis pilaris is the most frequent of them, but nail dystrophies, dental abnormalities, corneal opacities and mental retardation have all been reported, though not simultaneously. The syndrome described by Whiting et al as 'corkscrew hair'[3,4] is usually classified with pili torti, although microscopically it is strictly a twisting dystrophy.

Pathology

Early reports emphasized that affected hairs were flattened and twisted through 180 degrees around their long axis, at irregular intervals along the shaft. Electron microscopic studies have shown that structural defects other than flattening may accompany and indeed probably determine the development of twists. Histologically, the only abnormality is some curvature of the hair follicles. With the scanning electron microscope, the cuticle of the hair shaft appears normal[6], though severe weathering changes and trichorrhexis nodes are not uncommon.

Genetics

In cases where classical pili torti of early onset appears to have occurred as an isolated defect, inheritance has usually been determined by an autosomal dominant gene[7]. No explanation is available for the apparently high incidence in females. There are many reports of apparently sporadic cases[8]. Some of these could be explained if one parent was affected so mildly that the diagnosis was overlooked. However, there are also cases in which the siblings of normal but consanguineous parents have been affected, and in which recessive inheritance must be suspected[9]. There is at present insufficient evidence to allow any dogmatic statements as to possible differences between the two phenotypes.

Pili torti of postpubertal onset is genetically distinct[10]. The inheritance of this form is apparently also of autosomal dominant type.

Differential diagnosis

The diagnosis should be suspected if the hair is brittle and dry. The typical 'spangled' appearance in reflected light is present only if the hair is at least moderately severely affected, yet is not so brittle that it breaks to leave only a sparse stubble. Microscopical examination of several hairs must be made to confirm the diagnosis. The associated defects of other syndromes with twisted hair should be sought.

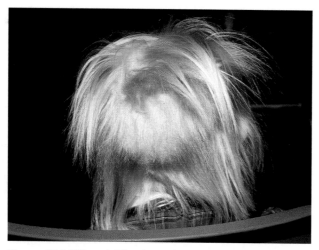

Figure 15.4 *Pili torti. The obviously unruly hair is irregularly broken and 'weathered' at sites of friction and pressure*

Syndromes of which twisted hair is a feature

Menkes' syndrome: light-coloured twisted hair is a manifestation of a hereditary defect of intestinal copper transport: the inheritance is sex-linked recessive.

Björnstad's syndrome: twisted hair with sensorineural deafness: probably autosomal dominant inheritance.

Bazex's syndrome: twisted hair, with basal carcinomas of the face and follicular atrophoderma.

Crandall's syndrome: twisted hair and deafness are associated with hypogonadism; probable sex-linked recessive inheritance.

Hypohidrotic ectodermal dysplasia: twisted hairs associated with characteristic facies and dental defects.

Pseudomonilethrix: twisted hair is associated in the individual or the family with apparently beaded hairs of autosomal dominant inheritance.

When these syndromes are excluded, only pili torti remains, but there is evidence that the condition is not a homogeneous entity; the hairs show considerable variation from patient to patient in their ability to withstand breaking and pulling forces; in other words, the hairs in some patients weather badly, but in others they do not.

A syndrome has been reported[5] in which siblings with mental retardation had pili torti and trichorrhexis nodosa; their hair keratin was deficient in cystine. However, dystrophic pili torti may occur with a normal cystine content; in this case the patient developed less weathered hair after puberty, but the twists remained – possibly due to hair sebum 'protecting' the hair shafts from weathering[2].

Treatment

There is no effective treatment, but reduction of the physical and chemical trauma of hairdressing procedures may allow a considerable increase in length of the hair to take place.

References

1 Galewsky E. Pili torti. *Arch Derm Syph* 1932; **167**: 659.
2 Telfer N, Cutler TP, Dawber RPR. The natural history of pili torti. *Br J Dermatol* 1989; **120**: 323–5.
3 Whiting DA, Jenkins T, Witcomb MJ. Corkscrew hair – a unique type of congenital alopecia in pili torti. In: Brown AC, Cronin RG, eds. *Hair, Trace Elements and Human Illness*. Praeger, New York, 1980; 238.
4 Trueb R, Burg G, Bottani A, Schinzel A. Ectodermal dysplasia with corkscrew hairs. *J Am Acad Dermatol* 1994; **29**: 289–90.
5 Pollitt RJ, Jenner FA, Davies M. Sibs with mental and physical retardation, with abnormal amino-acid composition of the hair. *Arch Dis Child* 1968; **43**: 211.
6 Dawber RPR, Comaish S. Scanning electron microscopy of normal and abnormal hair shafts. *Arch Dermatol* 1970; **101**: 316.
7 Gedda L, Cavalieri R. Relievi genetici delle distrofie congenita dei capilli. *Cron Inst Derm Immac* 1962; **17**: 3.
8 Laub D, Horan RF, Yaffe H et al. A child with hair loss: pili torti, apparently unassociated with other abnormalities. *Arch Dermatol* 1987; **123**: 1071–4.
9 Pierini LE, Borda JMC. Pili torti. *Rev Arg Dermatosifil* 1947; **31**: 75.
10 Beare JM. Congenital pilar defect showing features of pili torti. *Br J Dermatol* 1952; **64**: 366.

Björnstad's syndrome/Crandall's syndrome

In 1935, Björnstad[1] reported 5 patients in whom pili torti was associated with sensorineural hearing loss. Four of the 5 were female; members of their families appear not to have been examined, but the aunt of one patient is said to have had pili torti and hearing loss, and the brother of another probably had pili torti. A brother of the male patient had both pili torti and deafness. The loss of hair usually began in infancy but in one case it was not noticed until the age of 8 years. There was a correlation between the severity of the hair defect and the degree of hearing loss. On microscopy, the hair shafts showed longitudinal ridging and irregular twisting. A report of a further affected brother and sister suggests that the mode of inheritance is probably autosomal recessive[2].

Three brothers were reported with this same association of deafness and pili torti. Two of the brothers were reinvestigated after they had reached puberty and were found to have secondary hypogonadism with deficiency of luteinizing hormone and growth hormone[3]. The pedigree suggests that inheritance of this syndrome is determined by an autosomal recessive gene.

Although they have two features in common, these syndromes must be regarded as distinct.

References

1 Björnstad RT. Pili torti and sensorineural loss of hearing. *Proceedings of the Fennoscandinavian Association of Dermatologists*, Copenhagen, 1935; 3.
2 Voigtlander V. Pili torti with deafness (Björnstad's syndrome). *Dermatologica* 1979; **159**: 50.
3 Crandall BF, Samec L, Sparkes RS, Wright SW. A familial syndrome of deafness, alopecia and hypogonadism. *J Pediatr* 1973; **82**: 461.

Menkes' syndrome

Synonym: *Trichopoliodystrophy*

Although Menkes' syndrome was not recognized until 1962[1], it is estimated to occur in 1 in 35000 live births. The biological defect of this syndrome affects the skin, hair and central nervous system, reflecting the fact that many enzyme systems are copper-dependent[2]. A partial blocking in the intestinal absorption of copper[3] leads to gross copper deficiency, to which the pathological changes are believed to be attributable[4].

Analysis of the abnormal hair showed a ninefold increase in the free sulphydryl content compared with normal control subjects[4]. Similar but less marked changes have been found in the wool of copper-deficient sheep[5].

Clinical features

Hair present at birth may appear normal[6,7]. As it is shed it is replaced by short, brittle, light-coloured, twisted hair, which has the microscopic features of pili torti. Trichorrhexis nodosa has also been observed[1], but this is a non-specific abnormality which occurs readily in structurally defective hair shafts.

The skin generally is pale; the pallor was strikingly evident in an affected child of Afro-Caribbean parentage[8]. The facies is recognizable: the cheeks are plump, the expression lacks emotive mobility, and the eyebrows are horizontal and twisted[6].

During the first 2 months the child may appear normal. There is progressive psychomotor retardation from the third month associated with drowsiness and lethargy. Temperature regulation is impaired and there is a high susceptibility to infection. Convulsions, usually myoclonic jerking movements, are frequent. Survival for more than a year or two is unusual.

Pathology

The internal elastic lamina of arteries is fragmented, resulting in tortuosity and wide variation in their calibre. The brain shows gliosis and cystic degeneration. The metaphyses of the long bones show changes resembling those of scurvy[1,9].

The serum levels of copper and of caeruloplasmin are low, as is the copper content of the hair[10].

Study of the hairs shows several different patterns of hair-twisting[11]. There may be multiple loose twists in a single direction; close twists in a single direction; two or three twists in one direction, followed by two or three in the opposite direction; or a single twist of 180 degrees in one direction followed by a single twist in the other.

Genetics

The inheritance of Menkes' syndrome is determined by a sex-linked recessive gene.

Differential diagnosis

Before the characteristic hair changes become overt at about 3 months the diagnosis may be suspected on the basis of the systemic symptoms and the facies. The suspicion may be strengthened by the radiological findings[12] and confirmed by the estimation of the serum copper concentration.

The obligate heterozygote may have pili torti but her hair may be clinically normal[6]. The serum copper is normal. Skin fibroblasts from heterozygotes show metachromasia in primary culture, and this test may prove to be valuable in detecting carriers amongst the female relatives of a patient.

Treatment

Treatment with parenteral copper may become feasible as detailed knowledge of the metabolic defect accumulates; prenatal therapy has not so far shown any success.

References

1 Menkes JH, Alter M, Steigleder GK, Weakley DR, Sung JH. A sex-linked recessive disorder with retardation of growth, peculiar hair and focal cerebral and cerebellar degeneration. *Pediatrics* 1962; **29**: 764.
2 Peltonen L, Kuivaniemi H, Palotie A et al. Alterations in copper and copper metabolism in Menkes' syndrome. *Biochemistry* 1983; **22**: 6156–63.
3 Lott IT, Di Paolo R, Schwartz D, Janonska S, Kaufer JN. Copper metabolism in the steely-hair syndrome. *New Engl J Med* 1975; **292**: 197.
4 Danks DM, Stevens BJ, Campbell PE et al. Menkes' kinky-hair syndrome. *Lancet* 1972; **i**: 1100.
5 Gillespie JM. The isolation and properties of some soluble proteins from wool. VIII. The proteins of copper deficient wool. *Austr J Biol Sci* 1964; **17**: 282.
6 Danks DM, Campbell PE, Stevens BJ, Mayne V, Cartwright E. Menkes's kinky hair syndrome; an inherited defect in copper absorption with widespread effect. *Pediatrics* 1972; **50**: 188.
7 Collie WR, Goka TJ, Moore CN, Howell RR. Hair in Menkes disease. A comprehensive review. In: Brown AC, Cronin RG, eds. *Hair, Trace Elements and Human Illness.* Praeger, New York, 1980; 197.
8 Volpintesta EJ. Menkes kinky hair syndrome in a black infant. *Am J Dis Child* 1974; **128**: 244.
9 Mollekaer AM. Kinky hair syndrome. *Acta Paed Scand* 1974; **63**: 289.
10 Singh S, Bresnan MJ. Menkes kinky hair syndrome. *Am J Dis Child* 1973; **125**: 572.
11 Dupré A, Enjobras O. Syndrom de Menkes an Polorten alternant. *Ann Derm Vénéréol* (Paris) 1980; **102**: 269.
12 Wesenberg RL, Gwinn JL, Barnes GR. Radiological findings in the kinky-hair syndrome. *Radiology* 1969; **92**: 500.

Netherton's syndrome

Netherton's syndrome represents the association of an ichthyosiform erythroderma with hair shaft defects. These are often seen as 'bamboo' hairs (trichorrhexis invaginata) (Figure 15.5). This syndrome is discussed in more detail in Chapter 5.

Trichorrhexis nodosa

The defect of the hair shaft known as trichorrhexis nodosa [1–4] was first described in 1857 after a variety of terms had been considered such as 'trichoclasis' and 'fragilitas crinium'.

The literature of past years constantly questioned whether trichorrhexis nodosa was a primary developmental defect (sometimes hereditary), the result of acquired, nutritional or metabolic disturbance, or solely a reaction to physical or chemical trauma (or both)[4]. All these factors may be specifically or collectively important in individual cases. Indeed, distal trichorrhexis nodosa mainly from 'cosmetic

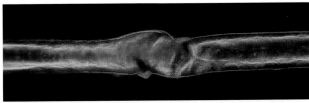

(a)

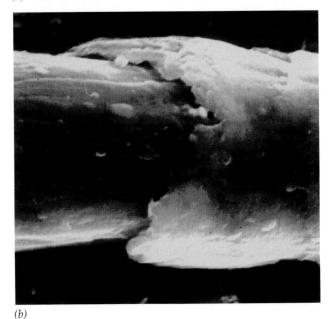

(b)

Figure 15.5 *Hair in Netherton's syndrome: (a) light micrograph showing 'bamboo' nodes; (b) scanning electron micrograph showing an 'invaginate' node*

insult' [5] is probably the most common defect of the hair shaft.

Trichorrhexis nodosa is best regarded as a distinctive response of the hair shaft to injury, i.e. a sign rather than a disease entity[2,3]. If the degree or frequency of the injury is sufficient the disorder can be induced in normal hair. The cuticular cells become disrupted allowing the cortical cells to splay out to form nodes[6]. If, however, the hair is abnormally fragile, trichorrhexis may follow relatively trivial injury. The trauma of hairdressing procedures has often been incriminated. Trichorrhexis nodosa is one sign of hair weathering. The severity of experimentally induced trichorrhexis nodosa was related to the degree of trauma in patients without pre-existing trichorrhexis[4].

That congenital and hereditary defects of the hair shaft can predispose to trichorrhexis nodosa is well established. It may occur in pseudomonilethrix, in Netherton's syndrome or with pili annulati[7].

Trichorrhexis nodosa is a feature of the rare metabolic defect arginosuccinic aciduria in which it is associated with mental retardation. There is deficiency of the enzyme argininosuccidase. Some 20 patients have been reported[8]. The patients can be classified in three groups, according to the age of the onset of the symptoms[9]. Where symptoms begin at birth, early death is usual: gradual onset during the first months of life is characterized by physical and mental retardation and enlargement of the liver. Onset from the second year onwards is characterized by psychomotor retardation and also by episodes of ataxia. The hair tends to be dry, brittle and lustreless; it may show trichorrhexis nodosa, but not all patients with this metabolic disorder develop it[10]. As soon as the diagnosis is established, a special diet should be provided[9].

Trichorrhexis nodosa may occur in certain families as an apparently isolated defect of the hair; node formation and fracture are induced by minimal trauma and develop during the early months of life. Such a defect associated with abnormalities of teeth and nails was determined by an autosomal dominant gene in one family[11]. Wolff et al described as trichorrhexis congenita the presence from birth of trichorrhexis nodosa confined to the scalp, in a boy with normal teeth and nails[12].

Clinical features

In trichorrhexis nodosa complicating a congenital defect of the hair shafts, the hair breaks so easily that large or small portions of the scalp show only broken stumps and alopecia may be gross.

In the much more common conditions in which trauma plays a proportionately larger role and the predisposing inadequacy of the shaft a proportionately smaller one, there are three principal clinical presentations[5]:

1. Proximal trichorrhexis nodosa occurs in blacks. The hair is short in areas subjected to the greatest trauma, and trichorrhexis, trichoptilosis and trichoclasis are seen on microscopy.
2. Distal trichorrhexis nodosa occurs in other races. Often it is discovered incidentally and only a few whitish nodules are seen near the ends of scattered hairs. If many hairs are affected the patient may complain that the hair is dry, dull or brittle. On examination, hairs with white nodules are seen among others which have fractured through the nodes.
3. The third clinical form now appears to be rare. In a localized area of scalp, moustache or beard, some hairs are broken, and others show from one to five or six nodules[13]. It is said that trauma of any sort can be excluded, and that spontaneous recovery eventually occurs. Some type of primary hair 'weakness' is postulated to underlie this type.

Pathology

In simple trichorrhexis nodosa the shaft between nodes may appear normal with the light or electron microscope except at the nodes; or the shaft, apart from the proximal 1 cm may show signs of abnormal wear and tear[6]. At the nodes the cortex bulges and is split by longitudinal fissures. If fracture occurs transversely through a node, i.e. trichoclasis, the end of the hair resembles a small paint-brush.

Diagnosis

The congenital forms must be differentiated from other shaft defects. The distal acquired form may simulate dandruff or even pediculosis. In all cases diagnosis depends on careful microscopy.

Treatment

The avoidance of all unnecessary cosmetic trauma may be followed by marked improvement.

References

1 Rook A, Dawber RPR. *Diseases of the Hair and Scalp.* 2nd ed. Blackwell, Oxford, 1991.
2 Whiting DA. Structural abnormalities of the hair shaft. *J Am Acad Dermatol* 1987; **16**: 1–25.
3 Whiting DA. Hair shaft defects. In: Olsen EA, ed. *Disorders of Hair Growth, Diagnosis and Treatment.* McGraw-Hill, New York, 1994; 91–138.
4 Owens DW, Chernosky ME. Trichorrhexis nodosa. *Arch Dermatol* 1966; **94**: 568.
5 Price V. Office diagnosis of structural hair anomalies. *Cutis* 1975; **15**: 231.
6 Dawber RPR, Comaish S. Scanning electron microscopy of normal and abnormal hair shafts. *Arch Dermatol* 1970; **101**: 316.
7 Leider M. Multiple simultaneous anomalies of the hair. *Arch Derm Syph* 1950; **62**: 510.
8 Brenton DP, Cudsworth DC, Harthy S, Lundy S, Kuzembo JA. Argininosuccinicaciduria; clinical, metabolic and dietary study. *J Mental Def Res* 1974; **18**: 1.
9 Shih VE. Early dietary management in an infant with argininosuccinase deficiency: preliminary report. *Journal of Pediatrics* 1972; **80**: 645.
10 Cederbaum SD, Shaw KNF, Valente M, Cotton ME. Argininosuccinic aciduria. *Am J Mental Def* 1973; **77**: 395.
11 Rousset MJ. Génodermatose difficilement classable (trichorrhexis nodosa) prédominant chez les mâles dans quatre générations. *Bull Soc Fr Dermat Syphil* 1952; **59**: 298.
12 Wolff HH, Vigl E, Braun-Falco O. Trichorrhexis congenita. *Hautarzt* 1975; **26**: 576.
13 Camacho-Martinez F. Localised trichorrhexis nodosa. *J Am Acad Dermatol* 1989; **20**: 696–7.

The trichothiodystrophies

The term 'trichothiodystrophy'[1,2] was coined to describe brittle hair with an abnormally low sulphur content[3–6]. Various syndrome complexes have been reported, some of which have been shown to have a DNA repair defect (see Chapter 17). The trichothiodystrophies are described in more detail in Chapter 5.

The hair is brittle and weathers badly[7]. With the polarizing microscope the hairs show alternating bright and dark zones (Figure 15.6a). With trauma the hair may break cleanly (trichoschisis) or may form nodes somewhat resembling trichorrhexis nodosa (Figure 15.6b), but without conspicuous release of individual spindle cells[1,2]. The hairs are flattened and can be twisted into various appearances – rather like a flat ribbon or shoe-lace. In the scanning electron microscope the hairs are seen to be flattened and sometimes folded over themselves with a ribbon-like appearance (Figure 15.6c). The shaft is irregular with ridging and fluting and the cuticular scales are patchily absent. Gummer and Dawber[8], using transmission electron microscopic methods, showed a decrease in the amount of high-sulphur protein in the hair shaft and a failure of this protein to migrate to the exocuticular part of the cuticle cells. Gillespie and Marshall[9] showed that the low sulphur and cystine levels were related to a decrease in concentrations of high-sulphur protein.

References

1 Price VH, Odom RB, Jones FT, Ward WH Trichothiodystrophy: sulphur-deficient brittle hair. In: Brown AC, Cronin RG, eds. *Hair, Trace Elements and Human Illness.* Praeger, New York, 1980; 220.
2 Price VH, Odom RB, Ward WH, Jones FT. Trichothyodystrophy: sulphur-deficient brittle hair as a marker for a neuroectodermal symptom complex. *Arch Dermatol* 1980; **116**: 1375.
3 Van Neste D, Degreef H, Van Haute N et al. High sulphur protein deficient hair. In: *Trends in Human Hair Growth and Alopecia Research.* Kluwer, Dordrecht, 1989; 195–206.

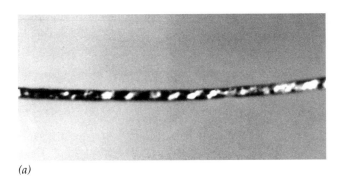

(a)

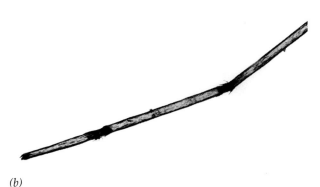

(b)

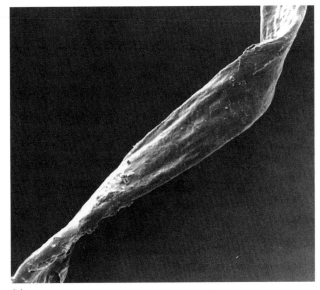

(c)

Figure 15.6 *Trichothiodystrophy: (a) abnormal 'striped' pattern under polarized light; (b) severe weathering – trichorrhexis nodosa appearance; (c) flat, ribbon-like hairs with surface cuticle lost (scanning electron micrograph)*

4 Van Neste D, Miller X, Bohnert E. Clinical symptoms associated with trichothiodystrophy. In: *Trends in Human Hair Growth and Alopecia Research.* Kluwer, Dordrecht, 1989; 183–93.

5 Feier V, Solovan C. Trichothiodystriophie et syndrome d'hyperéosinophilie. *Ann Dermatol Venereol* 1994; **121**: 151–5.

6 McCuaig C, Marcoux D, Rasmussen JE, Werner MM, Geatner NE. Trichothiodystrophy associated with photosensitivity, gonadal failure and striking osteosclerosis. *J Am Acad Dermatol* 1993; **28**: 820–6.

7 Venning VA, Dawber RPR, Ferguson DJP, Kanan MW. Weathering of hair in trichothiodystrophy. *Br J Dermatol* 1986; **114**: 591–5.

8 Gummer CL, Dawber RPR. Trichothyodystrophy: an ultrastructural study of the hair follicle. *Br J Dermatol* 1985; **113**: 273–80.

9 Gillespie JM, Marshall RC. Comparison of the proteins of normal and trichothiodystrophic human hair. *J Invest Dermatol* 1983; **80**: 195–202.

Marinesco–Sjögren syndrome

Marinesco–Sjögren syndrome is a rare syndrome of autosomal recessive inheritance, which has as its principal features cerebellar ataxia, dysarthria, retarded physical and mental development and congenital cataracts. The teeth are abnormally formed and the lateral incisors may be absent. The nails are flat, thin and fragile.

The hair is sparse, fine, light in colour, short and brittle. On microscopy, transverse fractures – trichosis – can be seen at the sites of impending fractures. In polarized light the hair is irregularly birefringent. Scalp biopsy shows normal anagen follicles but with incomplete keratinization of the internal root sheath[1].

Reference

1 Porter PS. The genetics of human hair growth. *Birth Defects Orig Art Ser* 1971; **7**: 69.

Ringed hair

Synonyms: *Pili annulati, leucotrichia annularis*

The first description of ringed hair is often ascribed to Karsch of Münster[1], but the pigmentary defect in his patient was more complex, with rings of irregular width as only one of several abnormal features. Erasmus Wilson[2] presented to the Royal Society an account of the condition now known as ringed hair, pili annulati or leucotrichia annularis.

Clinical features

Ringed hair is associated with a very variable degree of fragility. When the fragility is slight and relatively few hairs are affected, the condition may be discovered only when deliberately sought. If many hairs are affected and fragility is great, then short hair may attract attention in early life and the 'spangled' appearance of the shafts in reflected light can be readily detected. The axillary hair is occasionally

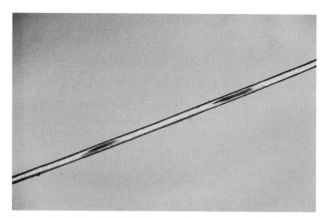

Figure 15.7 *Ringed hair (pili annulati): a single hair shaft showing alternate light (normal) and dark (abnormal) bands*

affected. The fractures in some brittle hairs take the form of trichorrhexis nodosa.

Pathology

When the hair is seen under the light microscope, abnormal dark bands alternate with normal light bands (Figure 15.7); in reflected light the colours of normal and abnormal bands are reversed. The light appearance of the abnormal bands in reflected light is due to air spaces in the cortex. The rate of growth has been measured in one case[3] and found to be 0.16 mm per day, which is less than half the average normal rate. Breaking stress analysis showed no significant abnormality in ringed hair, but fractures always occurred in the abnormal bands.

Electron microscopic studies[4] showed that the clusters of air-filled cavities, randomly distributed throughout the cortex in the abnormal bands, lie partly within cortical cells and between macrofibrils, or in case of larger cavities, appear to replace cortical cells. There is perhaps a defect in the formation of the microfibril matrix complex. Recent work has indicated that both these suggestions are correct. Hairs from the family described by Dawber[3] showed an abnormal surface cuticle which had a 'cobblestone' appearance on scanning electron microscopy. The work of Gummer and Dawber using electron histochemical methods confirmed this; cuticular cells are thrown into folds[4].

On biochemical analysis[3] the cystine content of affected hair was low, but its sulphur content was normal. The pathogenesis of ringed hair remains uncertain. The abnormal bands appear to be produced at random and not cyclically in relation to specific periods of growth[3].

In Ebbing's patients[5], in whom recessive inheritance of the trait seemed probable, the bands were regularly spaced. It remains to be seen whether this will prove to be a constant feature of a recessive form.

Genetics

The inheritance of ringed hair has been shown in many extensive pedigrees to be determined by an autosomal dominant gene[6]. One pedigree[5] is compatible with autosomal recessive inheritance; there are reports of apparently sporadic cases[7]. However, the expression of the dominant gene is variable, and mild cases without any great increase in hair fragility are easily overlooked. Blue naevus and ringed hair were associated in some members of a family, but the two conditions segregated[3].

Differential diagnosis

The diagnosis is readily established on microscopy of affected hair. A defect in which partially twisted shafts have an elliptical cross-section has been named pseudo-pili annulati because such hair may give an impression of alternating light and dark bands [8–10].

Treatment

If the hair can be spared chemical and physical trauma, including unnecessary brushing, it may grow to an acceptable length. The prognosis is good in the sense that the severity of the defect does not increase with age, but the cosmetic appearance depends largely on restraint in the use of hair-dressing procedures.

References

1 Karsch A. De Capillitili humani colorbus quaidan (1846). Cited by Landois L. Das plötzliche Ergrauer der Haupthaare. *Arch Path Anat Physiol* 1866; **35**: 575.
2 Wilson E. A remarkable alteration of appearance and structure of human hair. *Proc Roy Soc* 1867; **15**: 406.
3 Dawber R. Investigation of a family with pili annulati associated with blue naevus. *Trans St John's Hosp Derm Soc* 1972; **58**: 51.
4 Gummer CL, Dawber RPR. Pili annulati: electron histochemical studies on affected hairs. *Br J Dermatol* 1981; **105**: 303.
5 Ebbing HC. Gibt es auch bei Ringelhaaren (Pili annulati) einen einfach-rezessiven Erbgang. *Homo* 1957; **8**: 35.
6 Tomedei M, Ghetti P, Puiatti P et al. Pili annulati: family study. *Giord Ital Dermatol-Venereol* 1987; **122**: 427–30.
7 Dini G, Casigliani R, Rinöli L et al. Pili annulati. *Int J Dermatol* 1988; **27**: 256–7.
8 Price VH, Thomas RS, Jones FT. Pseudopili annulati. *Arch Dermatol* 1970; **102**: 54.
9 Price VH, Thomas RS, Jones FT. Pili annulati. *Arch Dermatol* 1968; **98**: 640.
10 Whiting DA. Hair shaft defects. In: Olsen EA, ed. *Disorders of Hair Growth, Diagnosis and Treatment.* McGraw-Hill, New York, 1994; 91–138.

Woolly hair

Woolly hair is more or less tightly coiled hair occurring over the entire scalp or part of it, in an individual not of Negroid origin. The clinical syndromes of which woolly hair is a feature have been much confused by many authors. The investigation by Hutchinson et al[1] has done much to clarify the position; the classification proposed by these authors is followed here. It remains possible, however, that woolly hair is a feature also of other syndromes not yet characterized.

Clinical features

Excessively curly hair is evident at birth or in early infancy; it has sometimes been described as Negroid in appearance[2], but tending to become less so in adult life. Anderson[3] considered that the hair, though tightly coiled, was not Negroid. The degree of variation in severity within a family is inconstant[1]. There is no consistent association with any hair colour. The hair shaft may be twisted[4].

In some cases the hair is brittle and breaks readily, probably as a result of trichorrhexis nodosa. The hair in sites other than the scalp is usually normal, but Hoffmann[2] found it to be sparse and thin.

Familial woolly hair

So few cases have been reported that generalizations are unwarranted. In three cases[1] fine, tightly curled, poorly pigmented hair was present from birth; in two of them the hair never achieved a length of more than 2–3 cm. Eyebrows and body hair were sparse.

Symmetrical circumscribed allotrichia

Among cases reported as woolly hair naevus are some for which Norwood[5] proposed the term 'whisker hair', but which are identical with the cases reported by Knierer[6] as 'symmetrical circumscribed allotrichia'.

From adolescence onwards the hair in an irregular band extending around the edge of the scalp from above the ears towards the occipital region becomes coarse and whisker-like. Many people believe that whisker hair is synonymous with acquired progressive kinking.

Woolly hair naevus

The hair in a circumscribed area of the scalp is tightly curled from birth or from early infancy. The size of the affected areas usually increases only proportionately with general growth, but it may extend for 3–4 years. The abnormal hair may be slightly paler in colour than that of the rest of the scalp.

In over half of the reported cases a pigmented or epidermal naevus has been present, but not in the same site.

Pathology

In some pedigrees the shaft diameter in affected individuals is reduced[1]; the hair is fragile and may show trichorrhexis nodosa. Pili torti and pili annulati have been reported as associated defects, but in different families.

Familial woolly hair

There is a marked reduction in the diameter of hair shafts, which may be poorly pigmented. The hair is brittle and on scanning electron microscopy shows signs of cuticular wear and tear[1].

Woolly hair naevus

The hair in the affected region of the scalp is finer than elsewhere. Electron microscopy of the abnormal hair shows the absence of cuticle; trichorrhexis nodosa was present [7–9].

Genetics

Hereditary woolly hair

The inheritance of hereditary woolly hair is determined by an autosomal dominant gene. It has been reported in six generations of a Rhineland family[2].

Familial woolly hair

The genetic evidence is inconclusive, but familial woolly hair has occurred in siblings whose parents were normal. Autosomal recessive inheritance is probable[10].

Symmetrical circumscribed allotrichia

Symmetrical circumscribed allotrichia appears to be a distinct syndrome[6].

Woolly hair naevus

Woolly hair naevus is a circumscribed developmental defect, present at birth, and apparently not genetically determined.

References

1 Hutchinson PE, Cairns RJ, Wells RS. Woolly hair. *Trans St John's Hosp Derm Soc* 1974; **60**: 160.
2 Hoffmann E. Über einen Kräuselanevus innerhalb sonst glatten Kopfhaares im Vergleich zum erblichen Kraushaar und zur Lockenbildung nach Röntgenepilation. *Dermatologica* 1953; **197**: 281.

2 Robinson VNE. A study of damaged hair. *J Soc Cosmet Chem* 1976; **27**: 155.
3 Dawber RPR. Weathering of hair in some genetic hair shaft abnormalities. In: Brown A, Cronin RG, eds. *Hair: Trace Elements and Human Illness*. Praeger, New York; 1980.

Hereditary and congenital alopecia and hypotrichosis

Case reports of individuals who have been almost or totally hairless throughout life can be found in the early literature, but these reports and some more recent ones are of limited value, because they include no histological information and an inadequate account of associated defects; there is at the most a note to the effect that the nails and teeth were or were not normal.

Table 15.3 is a list of disorders characterized by congenital alopecia or hypotrichosis. There have been numerous attempts to classify these conditions. In 1892 Bonnet[1] proposed a classification which was widely used for 40 years, and which was said to be based on embryological principles, as follows:

1. Congenital absence of hair with associated defects of teeth and nails.

2. Congenital absence of hair with normal teeth and nails.

3. Congenital absence of hair with partial or complete recovery at puberty.

Ideally, one would like a complete logical classification of hair abnormalities and any associated changes based on dysmorphology – with clear-cut malformations, disruptions, deformations, etc – together with the specific follicular, scalp and hair shaft faults worked out to biochemical level[2]. In practice, one is confronted by often unique, sporadic and ill-studied entities with little detailed mechanistic investigation for many moral and ethical reasons.

Cockayne[3] attempted a more critical analysis of the literature. Each of the Bonnet's groups can be shown to contain a number of genetically distinct entities as well as many cases which cannot yet be categorized. Although there are now many conditions which are so well defined that they can be diagnosed on clinical features alone, there are many more which are still of questionable status, and will remain so until adequate histological studies of the scalp and electron microscopic studies of shafts of any hairs that may be present have been combined with analysis of the chemical and physical properties of such hairs, and the detailed examination of the patient for structural and metabolic defects involving other organs.

Table 15.3 *Hereditary and congenital alopecia and hypotrichosis*

The ectodermal dysplasias
Hereditary alopecia without associated defects
   Recessive forms
   Dominant forms
Hereditary hypotrichosis: Unna type
Hallermann–Streiff syndrome
Atrichia with papular lesions
Hair loss in the premature aging syndromes
Hair defects and skeletal abnormalities
   Cartilage-hair hypoplasia
   Chondrodysplasia punctata
   Focal dermal hypoplasia
   Hypomelia–hypotrichosis–facial haemangioma
     syndrome
Hypotrichosis in other hereditary syndromes
   Dyskeratosis congenita
   Pachyonychia congenita
   Xeroderma pigmentosum
   Bazex's syndrome
   Hypomelanosis of Ito
   Dubowitz's syndrome
   Hypotrichosis, nail, retinal angioma syndrome
Hypotrichosis in chromosomal abnormalities
   Down's syndrome
   Klinefelter's syndrome

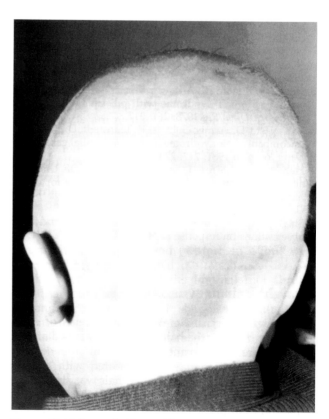

Figure 15.10 *Congenital hypotrichosis. Almost total atrichia, in this case permanent*

As a working classification which allows the known syndromes to be identified, and provides a provisional status for those not yet characterized, the following modification of Muller's proposals has been found useful[4]:

1. Congenital alopecia or hypotrichosis without associated defects (Figure 15.10).
2. Congenital alopecia or hypotrichosis as a major feature of well-defined hereditary syndromes.
3. Congenital alopecia or hypotrichosis as a major feature of uncharacterized syndromes.
4. Congenital alopecia or hypotrichosis as a minor or inconstant feature of hereditary syndromes.

Bertolinó and Freedberg[5] used these subsections to produce charts outlining most of the syndromes described up to 1987.

Any classification of congenital and hereditary alopecias must be tentative. However, the work of Baden and Kubilus[6] suggested that it may eventually be possible to differentiate congenital alopecias which are due to an abnormality in the formation of the follicles, from those due to an abnormality in some component of hair differentiation, e.g. defects of keratinocyte migration and keratins produced.

References

1 Bonnet R. Ueber Hypotrichosis congenita universalis. *Anat Hefte* 1892; **1**: 233.
2 Kingston HM. Dysmorphology and teratogenesis. *Br J Dermatol* 1989 **298**: 1235–9.
3 Cockayne EA. *Inherited Abnormalities of the Skin and Its Appendages*. Oxford University Press, 1933; 144.
4 Muller SA. Alopecia: syndromes of genetic significance. *J Invest Dermatol* 1973; **60**: 475.
5 Bertolinó AP, Freedberg IM. Disorders of epidermal appendages and related disorders. In: Fitzpatrick TB, Eisen AZ, Wolff K et al, eds. *Dermatology in General Medicine*. 3rd ed. McGraw-Hill, New York, 1987; 636–8.
6 Baden HP, Kubilus J. Analysis of hair from alopecia congenita. *J Am Acad Dermatol* 1980; **3**: 623.

Ectodermal dysplasias

The ectodermal dysplasias are described in Chapter 8; those in which hair abnormalities are typically found are listed in Table 15.4.

Hereditary alopecia without associated defects

Recessive forms

There are several apparently distinctive genotypes. Most commonly reported is a total and permanent absence of hair, probably determined by an autosomal recessive gene. Two brothers[1], whose parents were

Table 15.4 *Ectodermal dysplasias associated with hair abnormality*

Anhidrotic ectodermal dysplasia
Ankyloblepharon–ectodermal defects–cleft lip and palate (AEC) syndrome
Basab's syndrome
Clouston's hidrotic ectodermal dysplasia
Curly hair–ankyloblepharon–nail dysplasia (CHAND) syndrome
Dubowitz syndrome
Ectrodactyly–ectodermal dysplasia–cleft lip and palate (EEC) syndrome
Ellis–van Creveld syndrome
Moynahan's syndrome
Onychotrichodysplasia with neutropenia
Orofaciodigital syndrome
Popliteal web syndrome
Rapp–Hodgkin hypohidrotic ectodermal dysplasia
Sensenbrenner syndrome
Tooth–nail syndrome
Trichodental syndrome
Trichodento-osseous syndrome
Trichorhinophalangeal syndromes I and II
Xeroderma–talipes–enamel defect (XTE) syndrome

consanguineous, came of a family in which 261 individuals could be traced through over a century: 3.04% were affected. Lundbäck[2] reported 9 cases in two families. The hair was normal at birth, but was soon shed and never replaced. Hair follicles were absent, but sebaceous glands were normal in number, but small. In the family reported by Birke[3], 2 of 3 children of consanguineous parents were bald from birth; a third child was born with some head hair, which was soon lost. A biopsy showed short follicles containing horny plugs; there were no milia or papules. Other authors have reported cases of what appears to be the same condition[4]. The siblings reported by Porter[5] probably had the same syndrome; histological and histochemical investigations suggested that the essential defect was dyskeratosis of the hair shaft.

Dominant forms

Several pedigrees have been published showing autosomal dominant inheritance of hypotrichosis as an apparently isolated defect. There are differences in the clinical features and more than one genotype is involved[6,7].

References

1 Calco Melendro J. Atriquia congenita total y permanente. *Med Clin* 1955; **24**: 253.

2 Lundbäck H. Total congenital hereditary alopecia. *Acta Derm Venereol* 1944; **25**: 189.
3 Birke G. Uber Atrichia congenita und ihren Erbgang. *Arch Derm Syph* 1954; **197**: 322.
4 Cantu JM, Sanchez-Corona J, Gonzalez-Mendoza A, Martinez RM, Garcia-Crez D. Autosomal recessive inheritance of atrichia congenita. *Clin Genet* 1980; **17**: 209.
5 Porter PS. Genetic disorders of hair growth. *J Invest Dermatol* 1973; **60**: 493.
6 Toribio J, Quiñones PA. Hereditary hypotrichosis simplex of the scalp. *Br J Dermatol* 1974; **91**: 687.
7 Bentley-Phillips B, Grace HJ. Hereditary hypotrichosis. *Br J Dermatol* 1979; **101**: 331.

Hereditary hypotrichosis: Unna type

Marie Unna of Hamburg[1] published in 1925 an account of a family in which 27 individuals in seven generations were affected by a previously unreported type of hypotrichosis. The syndrome is distinctive and most subsequent authors have associated it eponymously with Marie Unna [2–6].

Clinical features

The hair may be normal at birth and be shed during infancy, but more frequently is sparse or absent at birth, and remains fine and sparse for the first years of life. During the third year, coarse, twisted hair grows on the scalp, but with the approach of puberty (Figure 15.11) is progressively lost from the vertex and scalp margins. The ultimate extent of the scarring alopecia shows some variation, and it tends to be more severe in males. It is often patchy. Rijzewijk[7] noted that if individual hairs are pulled gently, they develop kinks similar to those produced by stretching an iron wire.

Eyebrows, eyelashes and body hair are typically absent or scanty from birth, and after puberty, axillary,

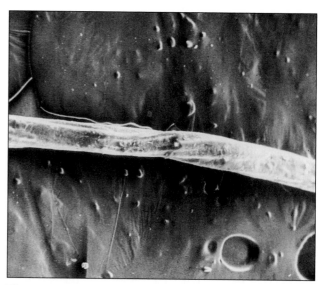

Figure 15.12 *Unna syndrome: hair showing characteristic irregular shaft bore and slight twisting (scanning electron micrograph)*

pubic and beard hair is also sparse. Affected individuals are usually otherwise normal; facial milia were present at birth in all of 8 cases in one family[6].

Pathology

The histological changes in the balding scalp are not pathognomonic. The number of follicles is markedly reduced; granulomatous reactions may be seen around partially destroyed follicles. Solomon et al[6] found proliferation of the internal root sheath and horn cyst formation in the lower third of some follicles; also noted was proliferation of the external root sheath in the region of the keratogenous zone, with a tendency for it to bulge into the internal root sheath. Viewed with the light microscope the hairs are coarse and twisted at irregular intervals[2]. The shaft diameter may be up to 100 μm as compared with 65–75 μm in normal relations.

In the scanning electron microscope, the hair shafts are ridged and the scale pattern is lost, particularly in the valleys between the ridges[4] (Figure 15.12). On routine electron microscopy[6] there are intracellular fractures of cuticular cells and an increase in interfibrillar matrix. On chemical analysis a small decrease in cysteine-cystine and an increase in methionine levels are found.

Genetics

The inheritance of this form of hypotrichosis is determined by an autosomal dominant gene[7]. This mode of inheritance has been noted in all pedigrees in which the diagnosis is beyond question. There may be minor differences between families, but the main

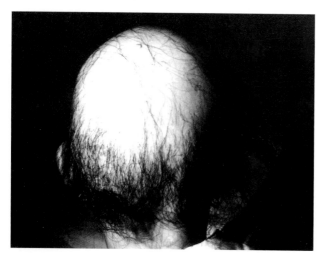

Figure 15.11 *Unna syndrome: a late stage showing permanent hypotrichosis. The remaining hairs are coarse, wiry and irregularly twisted*

features of the syndrome are remarkably consistent[4].

Differential diagnosis

Despite the reported variations in the age of onset and degree of severity of the alopecia, the growth of coarse, twisted hair in early childhood and its subsequent destruction with scarring on the vertex and the scalp margins cannot be confused with any other syndrome. The histopathological changes are not diagnostic. The defects in the structure of the hair shaft support the clinical diagnosis.

Treatment

There is no effective treatment, but avoidance of trauma may bring some cosmetic benefit as the abnormal hairs may be brittle and are also easily extracted. When folliculitis is troublesome, long-term antibiotic treatment may be useful[4]. The author has personally treated 4 cases with topical minoxidil (Regaine, Upjohn Ltd, Crawley, UK) for more than 6 months without benefit.

References

1 Unna M. Uber hypotrichosis congenita hereditaria. *Dermatol Wochenschr* 1925; **81**: 1167.
2 Ludwig E. Hypotrichosis congenita hereditaria. Type M. Unna. *AMA Arch Dermatol Syph* 1953; **196**: 261.
3 Borelli S. Hypotrichosis congenita hereditaria Marie-Unna. *Hautarzt* 1954; **5**: 18.
4 Peachey RDG, Wells RS. Hereditary hypotrichosis (Marie-Unna type). *Trans St John's Hosp Derm Soc* 1971; **57**: 157.
5 Lalevic-Vasic BM, Polic D, Nikolic MM. Hypertrichose héréditaire de Marie Unna. *Ann Dermatol Venereol* 1992; **119**: 25–9.
6 Solomon LM, Esterly MB, Medenica M. Hereditary trichodysplasia: Marie-Unna's hypotrichosis. *J Invest Dermatol* 1971; **57**: 387.
7 Rijzewijk J. Congenital hereditary hypotrichosis of the Marie-Unna type. *Br J Dermatol* 1988; **119**: 129.

Atrichia with papular lesions

Atrichia with papular lesions is a descriptive term for a distinctive association of atrichia with numerous follicular keratinous cysts; many familial groups of cases have been described during the last 35 years[1,2].

Clinical features

The first of the three cases of Damsté and Prakken[3] was a woman aged 26 years. She had been born with normal hair which was soon shed and never replaced. She had sparse eyebrows, normal lashes and no body hair. She began to develop horny papules on her face at the age of 18 years, and these gradually spread to other parts of the body. In the 2 other patients described by these authors, the hair loss was similar but the papules began to appear at the age of 5 or 6 years. In some cases the papules developed as early as the second year[1]. The papules are pinhead-sized, smooth and white.

The 3 patients reported by Czarnecki and Stiegl[2] were hairless from birth, and developed follicular cysts from the age of 7 years; they also showed retarded ossification and abnormal dental implantation. Physical and mental development were normal, except in 2 sisters[1] who were mentally retarded. A Japanese patient also had extensive polyposis throughout the gastrointestinal tract[4].

Pathology

The papules are keratin-filled follicular cysts. The scalp shows normal sebaceous glands and horn plugs in the follicular orifices[1].

Genetics

Although all cases show lack of hair in association with keratinous cysts, there is considerable variation between them and it cannot yet be established whether one or more genotypes are concerned. Since the cases described are few and infrequent, the exact mode of inheritance is not known, though autosomal recessive transmission was suggested by del Castillo et al[1].

References

1 Del Castillo V, Ruiz-Maldonado R, Carvale A. Atrichia with papular lesions and mental retardation in two sisters. *Int J Dermatol* 1974; **13**: 261.
2 Czarnecki N, Stiegl S. Atrichia congenita mit Hornzysten – Variante einer partiellen ektodermalen Dysplaasia. *Z Hautkrankh* 1980; **55**: 210.
3 Damsté C, Prakken JR. Atrichia with papular lesions; a variant of congenital ectodermal dysplasia. *Dermatologica* 1954; **108**: 14.
4 Ishii Y, Kremhara T, Nagata T. Atrichia with papular lesions associated with gastrointestinal polyposis. *J Dermatol* (Tokyo) 1979; **6**: 111.

Hypertrichosis

Hypertrichosis (Table 15.5) is the term used to describe all forms of hair growth that are excessive for the site and age of an individual and which do not conform to the pattern of androgen-mediated hirsutism. Hypertrichosis may occur as a manifestation of, or sequel to, a wide range of circumstances. In some cases, the hair growth is conspicuous and persistent; in others it may be faint and transitory, and included only in the most

Table 15.5 *Hypertrichosis*

Congenital generalized hypertrichosis
    Hypertrichosis lanuginosa
    Hypertrichosis with gingival fibromatosis
    Hypertrichosis with osteochondrodysplasia
    X-linked hypertrichosis
    Prepubertal hypertrichosis

Congenital circumscribed hypertrichosis
    Congenital melanocytic naevi
    Becker's naevus
    Spinal dysraphism
    Naevoid hypertrichosis
    Hypertrichosis overlying benign tumours
    Congenital hemihypertrophy with hypertrichosis
    Transient thickening of the skin with
       hypertrichosis

Congenital syndromes of hypertrichosis and mental
      retardation
    Coffin–Siris syndrome
    De Lange's syndrome
    Gorlin–Chaudhry–Moss syndrome
    Leprechaunism
    Lissencephaly
    Rubinstein–Taybi syndrome
    Schinzel–Giedion syndrome
    Fetal alcohol syndrome

complete descriptions of the disorder. There are a number of difficulties in establishing a classification for the conditions associated with hypertrichosis. Firstly, clinical descriptions of the pattern of hair growth are often incomplete and vague; secondly; the terms 'hirsuties' and 'hypertrichosis' are often used interchangeably; and thirdly, the mechanisms controlling hair growth are still poorly understood.

There exists much confusion in the literature concerning congenital generalized hypertrichosis owing to the plethora of names which have been applied to this state; Felgenhauer reviewed the literature[1] and found no fewer than 29 names such as 'ape-man', 'bear-man', 'dog-man', 'man-lion' and 'wild-man'. Many of these unfortunate subjects were paraded in circuses and show grounds, as techniques for hair removal were either not available or not considered. It is probable that many of these conditions would now be diagnosed as the following congenital and metabolic disorders or as androgen-mediated hirsuties.

Reference

1 Felgenhauer WR. Hypertrichosis lanuginosa universalis. *J Genet Hum* 1969; **17**: 1.

Hypertrichosis lanuginosa

Hypertrichosis lanuginosa (HL) is a rare disorder characterized by the retention and continued growth of fetal lanugo hair[1]. There have not, however, been any studies to determine whether there are differences in lanugo compared with vellus or terminal hair, nor has there been any confirmation that the hair roots are synchronized (as in utero). It is transmitted by an autosomal dominant gene, but about a third of cases are sporadic[2] and there has been a single pedigree reported with a possible autosomal recessive inheritance[3].

Clinical features

The infants are born with a thick coat of fine silky hair, which may be as long as 5 cm, covering the entire non-glabrous surface (Figure 15.13). The scalp hair may be easily distinguished from the body hair. The degree of hair growth may increase in severity during infancy but in some cases tends to decrease during early childhood[4,5]. At the age of 3–4 years, the cheeks, back and the proximal aspects of the limbs are most prominently affected. A heavy growth on the eyebrows may occur. Profuse growth in the ear may lead to difficulty with hearing and the external auditory canal may need to be surgically cleared. At puberty, there is the usual growth of sexual hair but without the usual conversion to terminal hair, and therefore, long, fine lanugo hairs grow in the beard and the pubic and axillary regions.

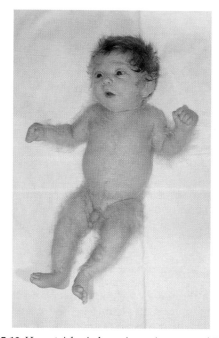

Figure 15.13 *Hypertrichosis lanuginosa (courtesy of Dr J. Harper)*

There may be an associated delay or a deficiency in dental development or retention of the deciduous teeth[6]. Individuals are otherwise entirely healthy and have a normal intellect.

There is presumably a degree of variability in the overall course. Many of the cases reported from the eighteenth to the twentieth century remained hairy throughout their lives. The author examined the 28-year-old father of a case of HL[5]. The father carried the gene and was extremely hypertrichotic as a child, but as an adult had only sparse body and facial hair. Individual pedigrees exhibit variations from the norm, such as bushy eyebrows or neonatal teeth and pyloric stenosis[5].

References

1 Flesch P. Hair growth. In: Rothman S, ed. *Physiology and Biochemistry of the Skin*. University of Chicago Press, 1954; 619.
2 Felgenhauer WR. Hypertrichosis lanuginosa universalis. *J Genet Hum* 1969; **17**: 1.
3 Janssen TAE, de Lange C. Hypertrichosis (trichostasis) lanuginosa. *Ned Tijdschr Geneesk* 1946; **90**: 198.
4 Berres HH, Nitschke R. Vergleichende klinische und morphologische Untersuchungen zwischen einem Neugeborenen mit Hypertrichosis universalis. *Zeitschrift für Kinderheilkunde* 1968; **102** (4): 327–40.
5 Partridge JW. Congenital hypertrichosis lanuginosa: neonatal shaving. *Arch Dis Child* 1987; **62**: 623.
6 Freire-Maia M, Felizail J, Figueredo AC. Hypertrichosis lanuginosa in a mother and son. *Clin Genet* (Copenhagen) 1976; **10**: 303.

Hypertrichosis with gingival fibromatosis

Hypertrichosis may develop in association with gingival fibromatosis and epilepsy. This association was recognized before the introduction of the hydantoins, and therefore the side-effect of these drugs represents a phenocopy. Eighty per cent of cases are familial and the condition has only been reported in Caucasian and Mongoloid races[1].

Hypertrichosis is noted at or soon after birth; the face, upper limbs and the middle of the back are most prominently affected[2]. The gingival abnormality usually presents after 10 years; however, in the more severe cases in which epilepsy is associated, there is gingival enlargement in infancy.

Hypertrichosis with gingival fibromatosis may be associated with multiple hamartomas and peripubertal or postpubertal giant fibroadenomas of the breasts[3]. The hypertrichosis is usually present at birth but may be delayed until the age of 4–5 years; and it may increase in severity at the menarche. The hair may be uncharacteristically coarse and pigmented for the family.

References

1 Witkop CJ Jr, Gentry WC Jr. Heterogeneity in gingival fibromatosis. *Birth Def Orig Art Ser* 1971; **7**: 210.
2 Winter GB, Simpkiss MJ. Hypertrichosis with hereditary gingival hyperplasia. *Arch Dis Child* 1974; **49**: 394.
3 Witkop CJ Jr, Gentry WC Jr. Gingival fibromatosis, Cowden type. In: Bergasma D, ed. *Birth Defects Compendium*. 2nd ed. Macmillan, New York, 1979; 464.

Hypertrichosis with osteochondrodysplasia

An association of congenital hypertrichosis with a distinct abnormality of the skeleton has been described[1]. The physical characteristics include a narrow thorax and cardiomegaly, with radiological abnormalities of the ribs, vertebrae and ischiopubic rami, and generalized osteopenia. The mode of inheritance is thought to be autosomal recessive.

Reference

1 Cantu JM, Garcia-Cruz D, Sanchez-Corona J, Hernandez A, Nazara Z. A distinct osteochondrodysplasia with hypertrichosis – individualisation of a probable autosomal recessive entity. *Hum Genet* 1982; **60**: 36.

X-linked hypertrichosis

A pedigree with an apparent X-linked dominant mode of transmission has been described[1]. There is generalized hypertrichosis at birth which increases in severity during the first year. The hair growth is generalized but is particularly dense over the face, back, upper chest and pubic area. The facial growth obscures the eyebrow margins; only the eyes and lips may be visible beneath the dense growth of hair. There is a mild reduction in hair growth on the trunk and limbs after puberty.

Reference

1 Macias-Flores MA, Garcia-Cruz D, Rivera H et al. A new form of hypertrichosis inherited as an X-linked dominant trait. *Hum Genet* 1984; **66**: 66.

Prepubertal hypertrichosis

The author has described a series of healthy children with generalized hypertrichosis which had been noted at birth but which increased in severity in early childhood[1]. It occurred in both Asian and European children and in none of the cases was there a family history of hypertrichosis.

There is hair growth on the temples spreading across the forehead, bushy eyebrows, and marked growth on the upper back and proximal limbs. This form of hypertrichosis differs from hypertrichosis lanuginosa as the hair is terminal and root studies have revealed asynchronous growth, whereas lanugo hair roots are synchronized.

This hypertrichosis may represent the condition often described as 'racial hirsuties'. The latter nomenclature is misleading, as this form of hypertrichosis is not limited to a specific race nor is it androgen-mediated (suggested by the term 'hirsuties'). However, it may be a form of hypertrichosis seen in postpubertal females which is assumed to be androgen-dependent but which does not respond to anti-androgen therapy.

Reference

1 Barth JH, Wilkinson JD, Dawber RPR. Prepubertal hypertrichosis: normal or abnormal? *Arch Dis Child* 1988; **63**: 666.

Congenital melanocytic naevi

Coarse hair often accompanies melanocytic naevi present at birth. Such naevi may be extensive and grossly disfiguring. The German term *Tierfellnevus* (animal skin naevus) is graphically descriptive. The naevus may be flat with a more or less dense covering of hair, but is often raised and is sometimes irregularly nodular. Nodule formation is not necessarily evidence of malignant change[1] but should raise this suspicion, for malignant melanoma develops in a significant proportion of these lesions. Early excision, if necessary in stages, is advisable on both prophylactic and cosmetic grounds, if it is technically practicable.

Reference

1 Krinitz K, Wozniak KD. Malignesa Melanom und Tierfellnevus. *Dermatol Medizinschr* 1972; **158**: 130.

Becker's naevus

Becker's naevus, as originally described[1], is a localized, unilateral area of hyperpigmentation and hypertrichosis. It has subsequently been widely reported, and an incidence of 0.5% has been reported in French army recruits[2]. It occurs predominantly in males and has been described in families[3] and in most races[4].

The aetiology of this naevus is unclear. The original cases and others described [2, 4, 5] followed sun exposure, However, the author believes that it represents a functional androgen-dependent naevus for the following reasons: firstly, this disorder occurs in a male to female ratio of 10:1[4]; secondly, the lesion develops at puberty; thirdly, acneiform lesions and terminal hairs are present within the lesion, and both are considered to occur in the skin in response to androgen stimulation; and fourthly, affected skin contains androgen receptors[6].

Clinical features

Most cases of Becker's naevus probably develop about the time of puberty, although most series have defined the onset by age[2,4]. The appearance of the naevus is characterized by variable pigmentation, hypertrichosis and acneiform papules and pustules. The lesion is usually a well-defined, irregularly shaped patch of brown pigmentation, often with smaller islands of pigmentation beyond its margin. Hypertrichosis (which develops in only 50%) occurs after puberty, but is often not uniformly distributed over the pigmented area and some hairs may grow on normal skin. Both pigmentation and hypertrichosis extend irregularly for several years, but do not cross the midline. The pigmentation is said to decrease slowly in some cases.

Becker's naevus is unilateral: 30–50% occur on the shoulder, most of the remainder are on the trunk and a few are on the limbs or face.

Many associated abnormalities have been described with Becker's naevus, including hypoplasia of the ipsilateral breast and/or arm, bony abnormalities of the spine and thoracic cage, enlargement of the ipsilateral foot, and morphoea[5,7].

Pathology

Histologically there may be little to differentiate lesional from perilesional skin. There are no naevus cells[4]. There may be increased basal pigmentation of a somewhat acanthotic epidermis. The dermis may be thickened and contain bundles of smooth muscle[8]. Ultrastructural examination reveals giant melanosomes and multiple layers of basement membrane surrounding the dermal venules. There are increased numbers of melanin-laden melanophores in the dermis.

Differential diagnosis

Hypertrichosis extending onto the face beyond the edge of the pigmented areas may cause diagnostic problems unless the characteristic pattern of the pigmentation is recognized.

Treatment

Either the hypertrichosis or the pigmentation may present the greater cosmetic problem. A good result has been obtained with electrolysis in unilateral facial hypertrichosis. The pigmentation is very difficult to treat.

References

1 Becker WS. Concurrent melanosis and hypertrichosis in the distribution of nevus unius lateris. *Arch Derm Syph* 1949; **60**: 155.
2 Tymen R, Forestier J-F, Boutet B, Colomb D. Naevus tardif de Becker. *Ann Derm Vénéréol* 1981; **108**: 41.
3 Pannizon R, Schnyder UW. Familial Becker's naevus. *Dermatologica* 1988; **176**: 275.
4 Copeman PCM, Wilson-Jones E. Pigmented epidermal hairy naevus (Becker). *Arch Dermatol* 1965; **92**: 249.
5 Ruffli T. Melanosis Becker mit lokalisierter Sklerodermie. *Dermatologica* 1972; **145**: 222.
6 Person JR, Longcope C. Becker's nevus: an androgen-mediated hyperplasia with increase in androgen receptors. *J Am Acad Dermatol* 1984; **10**: 235.
7 Glinick SE, Alper JC, Bogaars H, Brown JA. Becker's melanosis: associated abnormalities. *J Am Acad Dermatol* 1983; **9**: 509.
8 Haneke E. The dermal component in melanosis neviformis Becker. *J Cutan Pathol* 1979; **6**: 53.

Spinal dysraphism

Lumbosacral hypertrichosis occurs in spinal dysraphism[1,2]. Dysraphism – failure of spinal fusion – occurs four times more frequently in girls than in boys. Transfixation of the cord by a bony spicule – diastematomyelia – or tethering of cord or cauda by fibrous cords, may result in serious damage to the cord as differential growth of vertebra and cord exerts traction on the latter. The defect is usually in the sacral region, but may be lumbar, thoracic or cervical. There may be no overlying cutaneous abnormality, but usually there is a tuft of long, soft, silky hair (a 'fauntail'), a capillary naevus, a lipoma or a dimple or sinus. In the presence of cord traction, progressive neurological signs develop from early childhood: weakness of the legs, sensory loss and a sphincter impairment.

In every case, full neurological and radiological investigation is essential. Diastematomyelia is an indication for surgical intervention. In the absence of conclusive radiological findings, prolonged observation is essential so that surgery may be undertaken at the first sign of cord damage.

Bony abnormalities of other types[3] and tumours such as meningioma[4] may be associated with overlying focal hypertrichosis.

References

1 Harris HW, Miller OF. Midline cutaneous and spinal defects. *Arch Dermatol* 1976; **112**: 1724.
2 James CCM, Lassman LP. Spinal dysraphism. *Arch Dis Child* 1960; **35**: 315.
3 Reed OM, Mellette JR, Fitzpatrick JE. Familial cervical hypertrichosis with underlying kyphoscoliosis. *J Am Acad Dermatol* 1989; **20**: 1069–72.
4 Peñas PF, Jones-Caballero M, Amigo A. Cutaneous meningioma underlying congenital localized hypertrichosis. *J Am Acad Dermatol* 1994; **30**: 363–6.

Naevoid hypertrichosis

Hypertrichosis of limited extent may occur as a developmental defect in the absence of any other cutaneous abnormality.

Hypertrichosis overlying benign tumours

Plexiform neurofibromas in von Recklinghausen's disease may be covered by an area of hypertrichosis and hyperpigmentation. When these occur over the spine, abnormal hair whorls may be seen[1].

Congenital smooth muscle hamartomas usually present as asymptomatic swellings. They normally occur on the trunk. The majority of lesions are associated with overlying hypertrichosis and hyperpigmentation[2,3]. Transient piloerection may be induced by stroking the skin if there are associated smooth muscle elements[4].

References

1 Riccardi VM. Neurofibromatosis and Albright's disease. *Dermatol Clin* 1987; **5**: 193.
2 Berberian BJ, Burnett JW. Congenital smooth muscle hamartoma: a case report. *Br J Dermatol* 1986; **115**: 711.
3 Goldman MP, Kaplan RP, Heng MCY. Congenital smooth-muscle hamartoma. *Int J Dermatol* 1987; **26**: 448.
4 Gvosden AB, Barnett NK, Schron DS. Congenital pilar and smooth muscle nevus. *Pediatrics* 1987; **79**: 1021.

Congenital hemihypertrophy with hypertrichosis

Hemihypertrophy is usually present at birth but may become more noticeable at puberty. It is often associated with mental retardation and cutaneous abnormalities. These may include naevi, telangiectases and hypertrichosis[1]. Seemingly appropriate increases in the activity of the adnexal secretory glands have not been apparent to clinical observation[2]. There may be associated internal abnormalities and tumours; children with this disorder should therefore be carefully evaluated.

References

1 Hurwitz S, Klaus SN. Congenital hemihypertrophy with hypertrichosis. *Arch Dermatol* 1971; **103**: 98.
2 Scott AJ. Hemihypertrophy. *J Pediatr* 1935; **6**: 650.

Transient thickening of the skin with hypertrichosis

Unexplained hypertrichosis was present on the limbs at birth in a full-term male infant. The hairy skin appeared somewhat thickened and parchment-like.

The hair was shed after 4 months and the texture of the skin returned to normal[1].

Reference

1 Van der Meeiren L, Achten G, Pierard P. Hypertrichose chez un nouveau-ne. *Arch Belges derm Syphil* 1960; **16**: 206.

Coffin–Siris syndrome

Coffin–Siris syndrome is characterized by profound mental and growth retardation with congenital absence of the distal phalanges and nails of the fifth fingers and toes. There is usually a generalized hypertrichosis with bushy eyebrows and eyelashes, but paradoxically the scalp hair is often sparse[1,2].

References

1 Coffin GS, Siris E. Mental retardation with absent fifth fingernail and terminal phalanx. *Am J Dis Child* 1970; **119**: 433.
2 Carey JC, Hall BD. The Coffin–Siris syndrome. *Am J Dis Child* 1978; **132**: 667.

De Lange's syndrome

Hypertrichosis is a constant and distinctive feature of de Lange's syndrome, which is not excessively rare. The cause is unknown, and most cases are sporadic. In some cases siblings have been affected, and some features of the syndrome have been identified in other relatives[1,2].

The birthweight is low and there is both physical and mental retardation. There is a mild, generalized hypertrichosis, and abundant head hair with low frontal and nuchal hairlines. The eyebrows are bushy and confluent, and the eyelashes are long and curved. The palpebral fissure has a downward slant. Marbling of the skin is conspicuous and often persistent. One or more fingers may be short. The nose is upturned, but downturned labial commissures result in a 'carp mouth'.

There are a variable range of other defects which may occur in addition to the above abnormalities. These are predominantly ocular[3] and skeletal, but also involve other systems.

References

1 Daniel WL, Higgins JV. Biochemical and genetic investigation of the de Lange syndrome. *Am J Dis Child* 1971; **121**: 401.
2 Beck B. Familial occurrence of Cornelia de Lange's syndrome. *Acta Paed Scand* 1974; **63**: 225.
3 Milot J, Demay F. Ocular anomalies in de Lange syndrome. *Am J Ophthalmol* 1972; **74**: 394.

Gorlin–Chaudhry–Moss syndrome

The following collection of abnormalities has been reported only in two siblings: marked generalized hypertrichosis with mid-facial flattening, patent ductus arteriosus and hypoplasia of the teeth, eyes and labia majora[1].

Reference

1 Gorlin RJ, Chaudhry AP, Moss MI. Craniofacial dysostosis, patent ductus arteriosus, hypertrichosis, hypoplasia of the labia majora, dental and eye anomalies – a new syndrome? *J Pediatr* 1960; **56**: 778.

Leprechaunism

Leprechaunism is an entity characterized by a grotesque, elfin-like face with thick lips, large, low-set ears, breast enlargement and prominent genitalia. Absence of subcutaneous tissue gives rise to excessive folding of the skin. Generalized hypertrichosis occurs in three-quarters of cases[1].

Reference

1 Summitt RL. Leprechaunism. In: Bergasma D, ed. *Birth Defects Compendium*. 2nd ed. Macmillan, New York, 1979; 644.

Lissencephaly

Lissencephaly[1] is a form of arrested brain development in which no sulci or gyri develop, rendering the surface of the brain smooth. There is severe mental and growth retardation and affected children rarely survive more than a year. Hypertrichosis may be localized to the face or back but may be extensive.

Reference

1 Dieker H, Edwards RH, ZuRhein G et al. The lissencephaly syndrome. *Birth Def Orig Art Ser* 1969; **5**: 53.

Rubinstein–Taybi syndrome

The broad thumbs syndrome[1], as its original describers modestly prefer to call it, is also a collection of many clinical signs. Hypertrichosis occurs in 64% of cases and affects the trunk, limbs and face. The more important diagnostic features are growth and mental retardation, beaked nose with low septum, high-arched palate, hypertelorism, broad first (and other) digits, cryptorchidism and piebaldism[2].

References

1 Rubinstein H. The broad thumbs syndrome – progress report 1968. *Birth Def Orig Art Ser* 1969; **5**: 25.
2 Herranz P, Borbujo J, Martinez W. Rubinstein–Taybi syndrome with piebaldism. *Clin Exp Dermatol* 1994; **19**: 170–2.

Schinzel–Giedion syndrome

Schinzel–Giedion syndrome has been described in two reports of unrelated children. The cutaneous features are generalized hypertrichosis and abundant folds of skin overlying a short neck. The face is characterized by mid-face retraction. The nose is short with a saddle, a short bridge and upturned tip. There are also club feet, hypoplasia of dermal ridges, and radiological bony abnormalities which particularly affect the skull, ribs and terminal phalanges[1,2].

References

1 Donnai D, Harris RA. A further case of a new syndrome including mid-face retraction, hypertrichosis and skeletal anomalies. *J Med Genet* 1979; **16**: 483.
2 Schinzel A, Giedion A. A syndrome of severe mid-face retraction, multiple skull anomalies, club feet and cardiac and renal malformations in sibs. *Am J Med Genet* 1978; **1**: 361.

Fetal alcohol syndrome

The fetal alcohol syndrome is not uncommon: 60% of the infants of chronic alcoholic women are either stillborn or severely diseased[1].

Such infants are small and microcephalic, with mental and physical retardation and defects of the heart and of the joints. The facies is unusual and may be distinctive with short palpebral fissures, a prominent nose and maxillary hypoplasia. Numerous other defects may include hypertrichosis, which may be very conspicuous, and capillary haemangiomatosis[2].

References

1 Jones KL, Smith DW. The fetal alcohol syndrome. *Teratology* 1975; **12**: 1.
2 Hanson JW, Jones KL, Smith DW. Fetal alcohol syndrome experience with 41 patients. *J Am Med Assoc* 1976; **235**: 1458.

Chapter 16

Hereditary and congenital nail disorders

L. Juhlin and R. Baran

Introduction

The human nail develops between the ninth and twentieth weeks of intrauterine life. Nail defects occurring during this period are called embryopathies and those appearing later are called fetopathies. The embryopathies are often hereditary, whereas the fetopathies as a rule are caused by vascular or mechanical factors. After birth, hereditary disorders with epidermal manifestations such as blisters and hypertrophic or atrophic changes can cause secondary nail abnormalities. A defect in the nail matrix is the most common cause of abnormal nails. The matrix can have an abnormal position, size or function. In some disorders the nail bed is also involved, and these have therefore been called nail field defects[1]. The defects of the nails can be isolated but often they are combined with disturbances of other organs. The nail changes can then be an important sign to identify the disorder. In this chapter the hereditary and congenital nail disorders are classified according to the underlying embryological defects (Tables 16.1–16.3).

Reference

1 Telfer NR, Barth JH, Dawber RPR. Congenital and hereditary nail dystrophies – an embryological approach to classification. *Clin Exp Dermatol* 1988; **13**: 160–3.

Anonychia

Congenital absence of nails (anonychia) without other symptoms occurs sporadically or may exhibit either dominant or recessive inheritance. The anonychia can be total, or partial with dysplastic nails. If radiography is undertaken an underlying bone abnormality is generally found[1]. There will be no nail if the distal phalanx is lacking, and when it is hypoplastic the nails may be absent, dystrophic or normal. Often there are other skeletal or dental abnormalities associated with anonychia[2].

References

1 Baran R, Juhlin L. Bone dependent nail formation. *Br J Dermatol* 1986; **114**: 371–5.
2 Juhlin L, Baran R. Hereditary and congenital nail disorder. In: Baran R, Dawber RPR, eds. *Diseases of the Nails and Their Management*. 2nd ed. Blackwell, Oxford, 1994.

Nail–patella syndrome

Synonym: *Hereditary onycho-osteodysplasia*

The best-known syndrome where the nails may be missing (especially on the thumbs) is the nail–patella syndrome (Figure 16.1). The severity of the defects decreases from the thumb to the little finger. Where fingernails are present they may be short, narrow and fragile, and the lunula can be triangular or missing. The patella is aplastic or luxated in 90% of patients, the head of the radius bone is small and there are iliac crest exostoses. The kidneys are involved in 42% of cases with various degree of dysfunction[1,2].

The hallmark of the renal lesion is the presence of collagen-like fibrins in the glomerular basement membrane as revealed by electron microscopy. Radiography of the knees and a search for protein and blood

Table 16.1 *Embryopathies: hereditary and congenital nail disorders occurring between 9 weeks and 20 weeks of gestation*

Absence, reduction or changed form of nail matrix

Anonychia
   Nail–patella syndrome
   DOO syndrome
   DOOR syndrome
Hypoplastic nails with hereditary ectodermal
   dysplasia
   Tricho-oculovertebral syndrome
   Focal dermal hypoplasia syndrome
   Trichorhinophalangeal syndromes I and II
   Coffin–Siris syndrome
   Chondroectodermal dysplasia (Ellis–van Creveld
     syndrome)
   Anhidrotic and hypohidrotic ectodermal
     dysplasias
   Odonto-onychotic syndromes
Broad nails
   Racket thumbnail
   Rubinstein–Taybi syndrome
   Cartilage–hair hypoplasia syndrome
   Acrodysostosis
   Heart–hand syndromes
   Robinow's syndrome
   Larsen's syndrome
   Otopalatodigital syndrome

Change in nail matrix position

Ectopic nails
Congenital malalignment of the great toenail
Congenital onychodysplasia of the index fingers
   (Iso–Kikuchi syndrome)

Change in nail matrix function

Hyperonychia
Onychogryphosis
Clubbing
Koilonychia
Dyskeratosis congenita (Zinsser–Cole–Engman
   syndrome)
Leuconychia

Embryopathies affecting both nail matrix and nail bed

Hereditary partial onycholysis
Hidrotic ectodermal dysplasia
Pachyonychia congenita types I and II

Table 16.2 *Fetopathies: hereditary and congenital nail disorders occurring after 20 weeks of gestation*

Ainhum – amniotic constriction bands
Malformations due to drugs

Table 16.3 *Hereditary disorders causing secondary nail changes*

Epidermolysis bullosa
Acrodermatitis enteropathica
Tuberous sclerosis
Incontinentia pigmenti

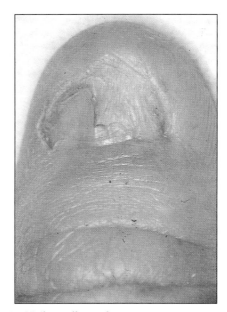

Figure 16.1 *Nail–patella syndrome*

in urine is therefore indicated in this disorder. Heterochromia of the iris with hyperpigmentation of the papillary margin is common, and webs on fingers or popliteal areas have also been described.

The syndrome is autosomal dominant and the gene is found on the long arm of chromosome 9[3]. The locus is linked to that of the ABO group[4].

References

1 Carbonara P, Albert M. Hereditary osteo-onychodysplasia (HOOD). *Am J Med Sci* 1964; **248**: 139–51.
2 Croock AD, Kahaleh MB, Powers JM. Vasculitis and renal disease in nail-patella syndrome: case report and literature review. *Ann Rheum Dis* 1987; **46**: 562–5.
3 Westerveld A, Jongsma APM, Meera Khan P, Van Someren

H, Bootsma D. Assignment of the AK (1): NP: ABO linkage group to human chromosome 9. *Proc Nat Acad Sci* 1976; **73**: 895–9.

4 Renwick JH, Lawler SD. Genetical linkage between the ABO and nail-patella loci. *Ann Hum Genet* 1955; **19**: 312–31.

Deafness–onycho-osteodystrophy with or without mental retardation

Anonychia can be seen in the syndromes of deafness and onycho-osteodystrophy (DOO) and of deafness and onycho-osteodystrophy and mental retardation (DOOR). The existing nails do not grow and are dystrophic. Feinmesser and Zelig first described the syndrome with onychodystrophy and deafness which has an autosomal dominant inheritance[1]. Wallbaum et al described a similar syndrome where the patients in addition had mental retardation and seizures[2]. The acronym DOOR was coined by Cantwell[3] for the latter syndrome; DOO was suggested for the former syndrome and the literature was reviewed by Patton et al[4].

In the DOOR syndrome, which has an autosomal recessive inheritance, there is an inborn metabolic error with an increase of 2-oxyglutarate in plasma and urine. Phalangeal malformations, spiny hyperkeratosis, abnormal dermatoglyphics, alopecia and erythroderma may also occur in both syndromes.

References

1 Feinmesser M, Zelig S. Congenital deafness associated with onychodystrophy. *Arch Otolaryngol* 1961; **74**: 507–8.
2 Wallbaum R, Fountain G, Lieuhardt J, Piquet JJ. Surdité familiale avec osteo-onycho-dysplasie. *J Genet Hum* 1970; **18**: 101–8.
3 Cantwell RJ. Congenital sensori-neural deafness associated with onycho-osteo dystrophy and mental retardation (DOOR syndrome). *Humangenetik* 1975; **26**: 261–5.
4 Patton MA, Krywawych S, Winter RM, Brenton DP, Baraitser M. DOOR syndrome (deafness, onycho-osteodystrophy and mental retardation): elevated plasma and urinary 2-oxyglutamate in three unrelated patients. *Am J Med Genet* 1987; **26**: 207–15.

Hypoplastic nails with hereditary ectodermal dysplasia (HED)

Hypoplastic nails (Figure 16.2) are a feature of a number of syndromes.

Tricho-oculovertebral syndrome

In tricho-oculovertebral syndrome[1] the fingernails are thin and brittle, and the toenails short and wide with paronychia. The patients have hypotrichosis;

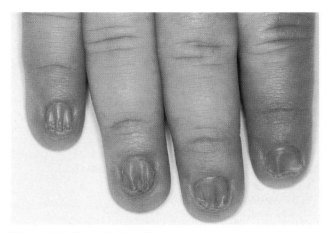

Figure 16.2 *Hypoplastic nails*

bilateral nuclear cataracts; entropion; palpebral fissures; dry, often infected, scaling skin with hyperkeratotic spots; and webbing of fingers. Skeletal anomalies occur such as spina bifida occulta; kyphoscoliosis; genu valgum; enlarged interphalangeal joints; small lower jaw and wide nasal bridge. The syndrome has an autosomal recessive inheritance.

Reference

1 Alves AFP, dos Santos PAB, Castelo-Branco-Neto E, Freire-Maia N. An autosomal recessive ectodermal dysplasia syndrome of hypotrichosis, onychodysplasia, hyperkeratosis, dwarfism, kyphoscoliosis; cataract and other manifestations. *Am J Med Genet* 1981; **10**: 213–18.

Focal dermal hypoplasia

In focal dermal hypoplasia syndrome[1] the nails are thin and spoon-shaped, or they can be absent. The hair is sparse on focal areas of the scalp or pubis, and bone anomalies such as syndactyly, polydactyly or hypoplasia and a striated pattern of the metaphyseal regions of the long bones[2] are reported. The skin changes are characteristic, with focal thinning, herniation of fat and linear hypo- and hyperpigmentation.

The syndrome is an X-linked dominant disorder.

Focal hypoplasia of skin also occurs in a heterogeneous group of disorders now often called aplasia cutis congenita (ACC). Sybert[3] divided ACC in four types, of which types II and III could have limb defects as described by Goltz et al[1] and type IV was associated with epidermolysis bullosa.

References

1 Goltz RW, Henderson RR, Hitch JM, Ott JF. Focal dermal hypoplasia syndrome – a review of the literature and report of two cases. *Arch Dermatol* 1970; **101**: 1–11.
2 Larrègue M, Duterque M. Striated osteopathy in focal dermal hypoplasia. *Arch Dermatol* 1975; **11**: 1365.

3 Sybert VP. Aplasia cutis congenita: a report of 12 new families and review of the literature. *Pediatr Dermatol* 1985; **3**: 1–14.

Other tricho-onychotic syndromes

Two other tricho-onychotic syndromes with hypoplastic nails have been reported, one associated with trichorrhexis nodosa, neutropenia and repeated infections[1], and the other with curly hair, fused eyelids and ankyloblepharon at birth[2]. They both have an autosomal recessive inheritance.

References

1 Verhage J, Habema L, Vrensen GFJM, Roord JJ, Blecker-Wagemakers EM. A patient with onychotrichodysplasia, neutropenia and normal intelligence. *Clin Genet* 1987; **31**: 374–80.
2 Toriello HV, Lindstrom JA, Waterman DF, Bangham FA. Reevaluation of CHANDS. *J Med Genet* 1979; **16**: 316–17.

Trichorhinophalangeal syndrome

Trichorhinophalangeal (TRP) syndrome[1] has two forms. In type I the nails are thin, short, striated and often with koilonychia. The hair is sparse, blond, fine and slow-growing. The teeth are peg-shaped and supernumerary. The nose is pear-shaped, the philtrum is long and wide and the palate is high-arched. Prominent or cleft lip and brachial cyst can occur. The type II TRP syndrome or Langer–Giedion syndrome is a similar disorder but also includes multiple exostoses, loose skin with naevi, hypermobility of joints and mental deficiency with delayed onset of speech[2].

The transmission is autosomal dominant in most cases. There is a smaller deleted segment (8q24.12) in type I than in type II (8q24.11–13)[3].

References

1 Parizel PM, Dumon J, Vossen P, Rigaux A, De Scheppes AM. The tricho-rhino-phalangeal syndrome revisited. *Eur J Radiol* 1987; **7**: 154–6.
2 Langer LO Jr, Krassikoff N, Laxova R et al. The tricho-rhino-phalangeal syndrome with exostoses (or Langer–Giedion syndrome): four additional patients without mental retardation and review of the literature. *Am J Med Genet* 1984; **19**: 81–111.
3 Bühler EM, Bühler UK, Bentler C, Fessler R. A final word on the tricho-rhino-phalangeal syndromes. *Clin Genet* 1987; **31**: 273–5.

Coffin–Siris syndrome

The characteristic feature of Coffin–Siris syndrome[1,2] is the hypoplastic or absent nails on the little fingers and toes. Sparse scalp hair, microdontia with delayed eruption, thick lips, and psychomotor and growth retardation are other features of the syndrome.

The inheritance is assumed to be autosomal recessive, but a possible autosomal dominant phenotype cannot be excluded.

References

1 Coffin GS, Siris E. Mental retardation with absent fifth fingernail and terminal phalanx. *Am J Dis Child* 1970; **119**: 433–9.
2 Carey JC, Hall BD. The Coffin–Siris syndrome. Five new cases including two siblings. *Am J Dis Child* 1978; **132**: 667–71.

Chondroectodermal dysplasia

Synonym: *Ellis–van Creveld syndrome*

Chondroectodermal dysplasia[1,2] is a combination of dystrophic, spoon-shaped nails, sparse, brittle, hypochromic hair, hypodontia, broad nose, and chondrodysplasia of the long bones, resulting in acromelic dwarfism with short limbs and hypoplastic genitalia. Respiratory difficulties due to thoracic abnormalities and congenital heart disease are other important signs.

The inheritance is autosomal recessive. It has been speculated that the syndrome is determined by genes on the long arm of chromosome 9[3].

References

1 Ellis RWB, van Creveld S. A syndrome characterized by ectodermal dysplasia, polydactyly, chondro-dysplasia and congenital morbus cordis. Report of three cases. *Arch Dis Child* 1940; **15**: 63–84.
2 McKusick VA, Egeland JA, Eldridge R, Krusen DE. Dwarfism in the Amish. I. The Ellis–van Creveld syndrome. *Bull Johns Hopkins Hosp* 1964; **115**: 306–36.
3 Christian JC, Dexter RN, Palmer CG, Muller J. A family with three recessive traits and homozygosity for a long 9qh+ chromosome segment. *Am J Med Genet* 1980; **6**: 301–8.

Anhidrotic and hypohidrotic ectodermal dysplasias

Anhidrotic and hypohidrotic ectodermal dysplasias are included in this group since in many of the syndromes the sweat glands often have been investigated poorly or not at all. One anhidrotic or hypohidrotic type of ectodermal dysplasia (Christ–Siemens–Touraine syndrome) is X-linked[1,2] and another is autosomal recessive[3]. The hair of scalp and body is fine, dry and hypochromic, with scanty eyebrows and lashes but usually normal beard growth. There is hypodontia, reduced sweating and decreased function of lacrimal ducts. The nails can be normal, fragile, dystrophic or absent at birth. Saddle-shaped nose and prominent lips are seen in severely affected patients. A special type combined with hypothyroidism and ciliary dyskinesia has been described[4]. The anhidrotic dysplasia can be combined with cleft lip and palate (Rapp–Hodgkin syndrome)[5] and also with ectrodactyly (ectrodactyly–ectodermal dysplasia–cleft lip/palate or EEC syndrome)[6] as well as with genitourinary anomalies[7] which have an autosomal dominant inheritance. Hay–Wells syndrome or the ankyloblepharon–ectodermal defects–cleft lip and palate (AEC) syndrome is another of these autosomal dominant constellations of ectodermal defects with dystrophic and hypoplastic nails[8,9].

References

1 Reed WB, Lopez A, Landing B. Clinical spectrum of anhidrotic ectodermal dysplasia. *Arch Dermatol* 1970; **102**: 134–43.
2 Norval EJG, van Wyk CW, Bassan NJ, Coldrey J. Hypohidrotic ectodermal dysplasia: a genealogic, stereomicroscope, and scanning electron microscope study. *Pediatr Dermatol* 1988; **5**: 159–66.
3 Passarge E, Fries E. Autosomal recessive hypohidrotic ectodermal dysplasia with subclinical manifestations in the heterozygote. *Birth Defects* 1977; **13**: 95–100.
4 Pabst HF, Groth O, McCoy EE. Hypohidrotic ectodermal dysplasia with hypothyroidism. *J Pediatr* 1981; **98**: 223–7.
5 Schroeder HW Jr, Sybert VP. Rapp–Hodgkin ectodermal dysplasia. *J Pediatr* 1987; **110**: 72–5.
6 Freire-Maria N, Pinheiro M. *Ectodermal Dysplasias: A Clinical and Genetic Study.* Alan R. Liss, New York, 1984.
7 Rollnick BR, Hoo JJ. Genitourinary anomalies as a component manifestation in the ectodermal dysplasia, ectrodactyly, cleft lip/palate (EEC) syndrome. *Am J Med Genet* 1988; **29**: 131–6.
8 Schwayder TA, Lane AT, Miller ME. Hay–Wells syndrome. *Pediatr Dermatol* 1986; **3**: 399–402.
9 Greene SL, Michels VV, Doyle JA. Variable expression in ankyloblepharon–ectodermal defects–cleft lip and palate syndrome. *Am J Med Genet* 1987; **27**: 207–12.

Odonto-onychotic syndromes

Autosomal dominant inherited syndromes have been reported with hypoplastic nails, tooth abnormalities and other features such as deafness[1], big ears and everted lips[2].

References

1 Robinson GC, Miller JR, Bensimon JR. Familial ectodermal dysplasia with sensorineural deafness and other anomalies. *Pediatrics* 1962; **30**: 797–802.
2 Ellis J, Dawber RPR. Ectodermal dysplasia syndrome: a familial study. *Clin Exp Dermatol* 1980; **5**: 295–304.

Broad nails

The differential diagnosis of broad thumbs and broad great toes includes clubbing and pseudoclubbing which can be isolated or part of syndromes. One should also consider acquired racket nails such as potter's thumb, and broad nails from tertiary hyperparathyroidism and the consequent erosion of terminal phalanges[1].

Reference

1 Fairris GM, Rowel NR. Acquired racket nails. *Clin Exp Dermatol* 1983; **9**: 267–9.

Racket thumbnail

In racket thumbnail[1] the distal phalanx is about two-thirds the usual length (Figure 16.3). Since shortening occurs in the distal half of the terminal phalanx, the thumbnail is only about a half or a third of its usual length. The distal phalanx and the nail are both broadened, giving the thumb a paddle or spatula shape with a thickened tip. The nail also appears wider than normal because its transverse curvature is diminished making the nail seem flat. The wider the nail, the narrower are the lateral nail folds which may appear to be almost absent. Because of its resemblance to a tennis racket it has been named racket thumbnail. Bilateral involvement occurs in about half the cases.

An X-ray view of the abnormal thumb shows that the first phalanx is of normal size in every respect, while the second phalanx is short and broad – thus the base is often considerably broader than the distal articular surface of the first phalanx. This, together with some general distal hyperplasia, is the reason for the 'racket' or 'drumstick' appearance of the thumb. The epiphyses of the terminal phalanx of the thumbs normally close at the age of 13–14 years in girls, and a year later in boys. In individuals with this hereditary

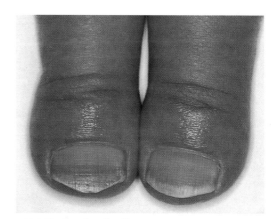

Figure 16.3 *Racket thumbnails*

defect, the epiphyseal line is obliterated on the side where the anomaly has its seat at the age of 7–10 years while it is still present according to age in the normal thumb. Since the periosteal growth continues the result will be the deformed racket-like thumb.

The disorder shows an autosomal dominant inheritance with a variability in expression, lack of penetrance, and more affected females than males.

Reference

1 Ronchese F. The racket thumb-nail. *Dermatologica* 1973; **146**: 199–202.

Rubinstein–Taybi syndrome

Rubinstein–Taybi syndrome[1] is characterized by microcephaly and psychomotor retardation, typical facies, certain eye abnormalities and broad terminal phalanges of the thumbs and great toes. The distal phalanges of these digits are broad, flattened and shortened. Increased soft tissues add to the width of the terminal phalanges. The inheritance is autosomal dominant.

Reference

1 Berry AC. Rubinstein–Taybi syndrome. *J Med Genet* 1987; **24**: 562–6.

Cartilage–hair hypoplasia syndrome

The characteristic features of cartilage–hair hypoplasia syndrome[1,2] are small stature, and abnormalities of the skeleton, hair and immune system. The hands are pudgy with loose joints and foreshortened fingernails.

When dwarfism is taken as the phenotype for diagnosis the inheritance is autosomal recessive with reduced penetrance.

References

1 McKusick VA, Eldridge R, Hostetler JA, Egeland JA, Ruangwit U. Dwarfism in the Amish. II. Cartilage–hair hypoplasia. *Bull Johns Hopkins Hosp* 1965; **116**: 285–326.
2 Polmar SH, Pierce GF. Cartilage hair dysplasia: immunological aspects and their clinical implications. *Clin Immunol Immunopathol* 1986; **40**: 87–93.

Acrodysostosis

Synonym: *Peripheral dysostosis*

In acrodysostosis[1] the hands of the patients are small, with short, stubby fingers which taper toward their tips. The distal phalanges and their nails are short.

The inheritance is autosomal dominant.

Reference

1 Robinow M, Pfeiffer RA, Gorlin RJ et al. Acrodysostosis: a syndrome of peripheral dysostosis, nasal hypoplasia and mental retardation. *Am J Dis Child* 1971; **121**: 195–203.

Heart–hand syndromes

In the Tabatznik type of heart–hand syndrome[1] the main features are cardiac arrhythmias and dysplasia of the radius and in the Holt–Oram syndrome there are brachytelephalangy of thumbs, electrocardiographic conduction abnormalities and atrial septal defects[2]. It is possible that the syndromes are a variant of the same disease[3].

The inheritance is autosomal dominant with variable expression.

References

1 Tentamy S, McKusick V. The genetics of hand malformation. *Birth Defects* 1978; **14** (3): 241.
2 Zhang K-Z, Sun Q-B, Cheng TO. Holt–Oram syndrome in China: a collective review of 18 cases. *Am Heart J* 1986; **111**: 572–7.
3 Lin AF, Perloff JK. Upper limb malformations associated with congenital heart disease. *Am J Cardiol* 1985; **55**: 1576–83.

Robinow's syndrome

The patients affected by Robinow's syndrome[1] present with mental deficiency, distinctive facies and variable degrees of broad thumbs, fingers and toes.

Both autosomal dominant and recessive types of inheritance have been reported.

Reference

1 Butler MG, Wadlington WB. Robinow syndrome: report of two patients and review of literature. *Clin Genet* 1987; **31**: 77–85.

Larsen's syndrome

The main features of Larsen's syndrome[1,2] are multiple congenital dislocations, flat facies, dislocations of multiple major joints and cylindric non-tapering fingers with short distal phalanges, creating pseudoclubbing. The thumbs are broad and spatulated with short nails.

The syndrome is usually autosomal recessive, but patients with autosomal dominant inheritance have been reported. No phenotypic difference between the two types have been delineated.

References

1 Marques MDNT. Larsen's syndrome: clinical and genetic aspects. *J Genet Hum* 1980; **28**: 83–8.
2 Larsen LJ, Schottstaedt ER, Bost FC. Multiple congenital dislocations associated with characteristic facial abnormality. *J Pediatr* 1950; **37**: 574–81.

Otopalatodigital syndrome

The main features of otopalatodigital syndrome[1] are short stature, characteristic facies, deformities of hands and feet, cleft palate and conductive deafness. Distal digits are broad with short nails.

The mode of transmission can be X-linked with intermediate expression in the female, or autosomal dominant with sex limitation of expression.

Reference

1 Pizzaglia UE, Beluff G. Oto-palato-digital syndrome in four generations of a large family. *Clin Genet* 1986; **30**: 338–44.

Embryopathies with change in nail matrix position

Ectopic nails

Except in cases of trauma to the nail matrix, where a portion of the matrix can produce a nail outside the nail fold, the rare ectopic nails are usually congenital. They are located on the terminal phalanx, on the palmar or dorsal side, sometimes a centimetre from the normal nail. The abnormalities usually involve the ulnar portion of the hand, especially the ring and little fingers. The ectopic nail may be located ventrally in parallel with a normal nail, vertically to the skin near a normal nail, or may even be circumferential. Ectopic nails can be divided into three categories:

1. Isolated cases with, usually, an additional nail (polyonychia) or small nails (micronychia) usually affecting the little finger[1]. This type is not associated with any specific pathology.
2. Familial onychoheterotopia where several digits are involved with just annular nails[2].
3. Onychoheterotopia associated with multiple malformations, such as in the Pierre Robin syndrome[2].

Ectopic nails should be differentiated from rudimentary polydactyly and from Iso–Kikuchi syndrome where the polyonychia is a central anonychia with a small nail on the ulnar aspect and a still smaller nail on the radial aspect of the index fingers.

References

1 Kikuchi J. Congenital polyonychias: reduction versus duplication digit malformation. *Int J Dermatol* 1985; **24**: 211–15.
2 Roger H, Souteyrand P, Collin JP, Vanneuville G, Teinturier P. Onychohétérotopie avec polyonychie associée a un syndrome de Pierre Robin: a propos d'une nouvelle observation. *Ann Dermatol Venereol* 1986; **113**: 235–42.

Congenital malalignment of the great toenail

Congenital malalignment of the great toenail was called 'great toenail dystrophy' by Samman[1]. The authors have renamed it, because the essential underlying abnormality is the lateral deviation of the long axis of nail growth relative to the distal phalanx[2] (Figure 16.4). A medial deviation is rare. The nail is discoloured, thickened with prominent transverse ridging, and is unable to grow to normal length. There is insufficient forward thrust to allow the nail plate to mount the heaped-up proximal pulp tissue in front of it. This may in infancy produce an ingrowing toenail from distal embedding which is superimposed by postnatal trauma, from walking or crawling. In adulthood the dysplasia may result in hemionychogryphosis with lateral deviation of the nail plate.

Congenital malalignment of the great toenail is probably an inherited condition, as identical twins have been observed with similar changes of their great toes.

Some cases have demonstrated a tendency to spontaneous improvement and even disappearance of the disorder. In all cases where the dystrophy cleared it did so before the patient was 10 years old.

Dawson reviewed 42 cases of which 19 patients with bilateral and 2 with unilateral dystrophic great toenails healed[3]. It is important to assess accurately the degree of the malalignment and the associated changes to ascertain how frequently spontaneous realignment really does occur.

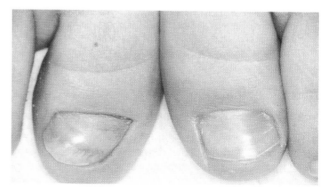

Figure 16.4 *Congenital malalignment of the great toenails*

If the deviation is mild and there are no other complications, the nail may when it hardens overcome the initial slight distal embedding, allowing sufficient normal nail to grow to the tip of the digit, which prevents further secondary traumatic changes.

If the deviation is marked and the nail is buried in the distolateral tissues, disabling changes may occur in childhood and in adult life. Surgical rotation of the misdirected matrix before the age of 2 years prevents permanent nail dystrophy and is therefore better than relying on spontaneous healing.

References

1 Samman PD. Great toenail dystrophy. *Clin Exp Dermatol* 1978; **3**: 81–2.
2 Baran R. The treatment of ingrowing toenails. *J Derm Treat* 1989; **1**: 55–7.
3 Dawson TAJ. Great toenail dystrophy. *Br J Dermatol* 1989; **120**: 139.

Congenital onychodysplasia of the index fingers

Synonym: *Iso–Kikuchi syndrome*

Congenital onychodysplasia of the index fingers (COIF) or Iso–Kikuchi syndrome[1] was originally characterized by five criteria:

1. Congenital occurrence.
2. Unilateral or bilateral index finger involvement.
3. Variability in nail appearance.
4. Possible hereditary involvement.
5. Frequently associated bone anomalies.

The syndrome has now been broadened to include second and third toe involvement and renamed 'congenital onychodysplasia'[2].

The following types of nail dysplasia can be seen: polyonychia, micronychia, anonychia, hemionychogryphosis and malalignment. The radial side of the nail is more involved than the ulnar side, especially on fingers with polyonychia and micronychia. In case of rolled micronychia, however, the small, curved nails are located more mid-dorsally. In curved nails the lunula may have an abnormal shape[3].

The distal phalanx of the index finger may be narrowed, but more often it is enlarged with a Y-shaped bifurcation in the lateral radiographic view. One index finger may, however, have a normal nail but show bone changes typical of COIF. Digits other than the index fingers may also show developmental and roentgenographic abnormalities. An autosomal dominant inheritance seems most probable from the families reported[4].

References

1 Kikuchi J. Congenital polyonychias: reduction versus duplication digit malformation. *Int J Dermatol* 1985; **24**: 211–15.
2 Biedermann T, Schirren CG, Schirren H, Plewig G. Kongenitale onychodysplasie (Iso–Kikuchi syndrome). *Hautarzt* 1995; **46**: 53–6.
3 Baran R, Stroud JD. Congenital onychodysplasia of the index finger (Iso and Kikuchi syndrome). *Arch Dermatol* 1984; **120**: 243–4.
4 Harper KJ, Beer WE. Pattern of inheritance in Iso and Kikuchi syndrome. *Clin Exp Dermatol* 1985; **10**: 476–8.

Embryopathies with change in matrix function

The clinical features such as hyponychia, onychogryphosis, clubbing, koilonychia and leuconychia may appear in isolation or combined with other defects.

Hyperonychia

Hyperonychia or thick nails are common in patients with hyperkeratosis palmoplantaris and hereditary ectodermal dysplasias such as trichothiodystrophy, ED–ADHD syndrome (Ectodermal Dysplasia–Alopecia, Onychodysplasia, Hyperkeratosis, Deafness), KID syndrome (Keratitis, Ichthyosis and Deafness), keratoderma palmoplantare (Thost–Unna), and keratoderma palmoplantare with clubbing of nails and lamellar ichthyosis[1].

Reference

1 Juhlin L, Baran R. Hereditary and congenital nail disorder. In: Baran R, Dawber RPR, eds. *Diseases of the Nails and Their Management*. 2nd ed. Blackwell, Oxford, 1994.

Onychogryphosis

Onychogryphosis has been described as an isolated occurrence and with autosomal dominant inheritance. It often first becomes evident in early childhood. It can occur with ectodermal dysplasias with growth retardation and keratoderma palmoplantare of the progressive Meleda type, the type with periodontosis and the Buschke–Fischer type[1].

Reference

1 Juhlin L, Baran R. Hereditary and congenital nail disorder. In: Baran R, Dawber RPR, eds. *Diseases of the Nails and Their Management*. 2nd ed. Blackwell, Oxford, 1994.

Clubbing

Clubbing of curved and thick nails is mainly acquired in association with pulmonary and other systemic diseases, but an autosomal dominantly inherited form of clubbing has been described[1]. Clubbing can be associated with keratoderma (as mentioned above) or pachydermoperiostosis with thickening and furrowing of face and scalp[2].

References

1 Juhlin L, Baran R. Hereditary and congenital nail disorder. In: Baran R, Dawber RPR, eds. *Diseases of the Nails and Their Management.* 2nd ed. Blackwell, Oxford, 1994.
2 Pramatarow K, Daskarev L, Schurliev L, Tonev S. Pachy-dermoperiostose (Touraine-Solente-Golé Syndrom). *Z Hautkrankh* 1988; **63**: 55–6.

Koilonychia

Koilonychia or spoon nail with a concave form of the nails is often acquired and is associated with anaemia, thyroid dysfunction or trauma. An autosomal dominantly transmitted form of koilonychia without other defects has been reported[1]. Koilonychia has also been described in combination with keratoderma palmoplantare of the Meleda type, with knuckle pads and deafness[2]. Koilonychia can also be seen in the earlier mentioned trichorhinophalangeal syndrome[3], trichothiodystrophy, nail–patella syndrome, onychogryphosis, incontinentia pigmenti, trichoepithelioma multiplex and monilethrix[2].

References

1 Almagor G, Haim S. Familial koilonychia. *Dermatologica* 1981; **162**: 400–3.
2 Juhlin L, Baran R. Hereditary and congenital nail disorder. In: Baran R, Dawber RPR, eds. *Diseases of the Nails and Their Management.* 2nd ed. Blackwell, Oxford, 1994.
3 Parizel PM, Dumon J, Vossen P, Rigaux A, De Scheppes AM. The tricho-rhino-phalangeal syndrome revisited. *Eur J Radiol* 1987; **7**: 154–6.

Dyskeratosis congenita

Synonym: *Zinsser–Cole–Engman syndrome*

In dyskeratosis congenita the nails after late childhood become short and atrophic, especially on the fingers where the nails later may be lost[1]. There is palmar hyperkeratosis and hyperhidrosis, and the skin of the face, neck and chest can have a reticulated pigmentation. Deafness, blepharitis, patchy leucoplakia on the conjunctiva, lacrimal duct obstruction, oral leucoplakia and abnormal immunology with subsequent aplastic anaemia and pancytopenia are the main characteristics. The inheritance is X-linked recessive and the gene has been assigned to Xq28[2].

References

1 Ogden GR, Connor E, Chisholm DM. Dyskeratosis congenita. A case and review of literature. *Oral Surg Oral Med Oral Pathol* 1988; **65**: 586–91.
2 Connor JM, Gatherer D, Gray JC, Pirrit LA, Affara NA. Assignment of the gene for dyskeratosis congenita to Xq28. *Hum Genet* 1986; **72**: 348–51.

Leuconychia

Leuconychia can occur alone as milky or porcelain white nails, and can be either total, partial or striated[1]. The inheritance is autosomal dominant. The leuconychia can also be combined with koilonychia alone or koilonychia with keratoderma palmoplantare, deafness and knuckle pads. Leuconychia has also been described in combination with other syndromes such as multiple sebaceous cysts and renal calculi, onychorrhexis and hypoparathyroidism, the LEOPARD syndrome with lentigines and various abnormalities, acrokeratosis verruciformis[1] and the FLOTCH syndrome (Familial LeucOnychia, Tricholemmous cysts and Ciliary dystrophy with autosomal dominant Heredity)[2].

References

1 Juhlin L, Baran R. Hereditary and congenital nail disorder. In: Baran R, Dawber RPR, eds. *Diseases of the Nails and Their Management.* 2nd ed. Blackwell, Oxford, 1994.
2 Friedel J, Heid E, Grosshans E. Le syndrome 'Flotch' survenue Familiale d'une LeucOnychie totale, de kystes Trichilemmaux et d'une dystrophie Ciliaire à Hérédité autosomique dominante. *Ann Derm Venereol* 1986; **113**: 549–53.

Embryopathies affecting both matrix and nail bed

Hereditary partial onycholysis

Hereditary partial onycholysis with autosomal dominant transmission has been reported[1,2]. The clinical features include, beside distal onycholysis, decreased rate of nail growth, scleronychia, palmoplantar hyperhidrosis and subungual paraesthesia especially when exposed to cold.

References

1 Schultze HD. Hereditäre Onycholysis partialis mit Scleronychie. *Dermatol Wochensch* 1966; **30**: 766–75.
2 Bazex J, Baran R, Monbrun F et al. Hereditary distal onycholysis: a case report. *Clin Exp Dermatol* 1990; **15**: 146–8.

Hidrotic epidermal dysplasia

Hidrotic epidermal dysplasia (Clouston) is an autosomal dominant inherited disorder with hyperkeratosis palmoplantaris where the nails show onycholysis and grow slowly[1]. The nails are thick, especially on the toes, and often are small and conical with pits and ridges. Hair can be sparse and thin.

Reference

1 Ando Y, Tanaka T, Horionchi Y, Ikai K, Tomono H. Hidrotic ectodermal dysplasia: a clinical and ultrastructural observation. *Dermatologica* 1988; **176**: 205–11.

Pachyonychia congenita

Pachyonychia congenita has been classified into four types with increasing clinical symptoms[1]. In type I – which is most common – the yellow-brown nails show subungual hyperkeratosis and become progressively thicker. The patients also have palmoplantar hyperkeratosis, follicular hyperkeratosis and oral leucokeratosis. Type II has the same findings and also bullae and hyperhidrosis of palms and soles, teeth at birth and steatocystoma multiplex. Type III has in addition angular cheilosis, corneal dyskeratosis and cataracts; and type IV has these features plus hoarseness, mental retardation and hair anomalies. For the treatment of the condition retinoids have been tried, with as a rule only moderate improvement of skin and nail lesions.

It is considered to be a disease of an autosomal dominant inheritance with a high degree of penetration. However, 3 cases of autosomal recessive pachyonychia have been described[2]. Two of them were clinically different, with epidermolysis bullosa-like blisters since birth and proximal leuconychia with obliteration of the lunula as in 'half and half' nails. Pachyonychia congenita is discussed in Chapter 6.

References

1 Feinstein A, Feinstein J, Schewach-Millet M. Pachyonychia congenita. *J Am Acad Dermatol* 1988; **19**: 705–11.
2 Haber RM, Rose TH. Autosomal recessive pachyonychia congenita. *Arch Dermatol* 1986; **122**: 919–23.

Fetopathies

Ainhum

Ainhum or amniotic constriction bands encircling a digit or limb may result in swelling, vascular obstruction and gangrene. Amputations, brachydactyly and nail dysplasia may take place in utero. The cause of the constriction is probably that parts of the limb become entangled in chorion or a ruptured amnion[1].

Reference

1 Feingold M. Amniotic constriction bands (Streeter dysplasia, ring constrictions). *Am J Dis Child* 1984; **138**: 199–200.

Iatrogenic causes of nail dystrophy

Drugs ingested during pregnancy can also cause malformations ranging from changes in growth rate and pigmentation abnormalities to onycholysis and hypoplasia[1]. Hydantoin, trimethadione, paramethadione and warfarin have all been reported to induce such changes. Alcohol and contamination in food can also induce similar changes[2,3].

References

1 Verdeguer JM, Ramon D, Moragon M et al. Onychopathy in a patient with fetal hydantoin syndrome. *Pediatr Dermatol* 1988; **5**: 56–7.
2 Crain LS, Fitzmaurice NE, Mondry C. Nail dysplasia and fetal alcohol syndrome. Case report of a heteropaternal sibship. *Am J Dis Child* 1983; **137**: 1069.
3 Taylor JS. Congenital Yucheng – dermatological findings. *The American Dermatological Association Program of the 108th Annual Meeting* 1988; 30.

Hereditary disorders causing secondary nail changes

Epidermolysis bullosa

Nail changes in epidermolysis bullosa are characteristic and sometimes highly suggestive of the condition, but are not pathognomonic[1]. Patients with this condition have fragile skin which easily forms blisters even on slight pressure. At least 17 subtypes with different clinical features have now been described[2]. The classification is usually based on the site of the split in the skin into simplex (epidermal), junctional and dermolytic (dystrophic) types. The simplex type with mainly autosomal dominant inheritance can show loss of nails with regeneration, which in some can cause dystrophic nails with peculiar curving or onychogryphosis of the great toe in adulthood. The junctional types have deformed, heaped-up, onychogryphotic or hypoplastic nails. The dystrophic types have various changes such as thick, short, split or absent nails[3].

References

1 Bruckner-Tuderman L, Schnyder U, Baran R. Nail changes in epidermolysis bullosa: clinical and pathogenetic considerations. *Br J Dermatol* 1995; **132**: 339–44.
2 Lin A, Carter DM. Epidermolysis bullosa: when the skin falls apart. *J Pediatr* 1989; **114**: 349–55.
3 Juhlin L, Baran R. Hereditary and congenital nail disorders. In: Baran R, Dawber RPR, eds. *Diseases of the Nails and Their Management*. 2nd ed. Blackwell, Oxford, 1994.

Acrodermatitis enteropathica

Acrodermatitis enteropathica is an autosomal recessively inherited disorder characterized by the inability to absorb sufficient zinc from the diet. Acral dermatitis, alopecia and diarrhoea form a triad of important clinical markers. There is periungual eczema, candidal infections causing Beau's lines, and sometimes dystrophic nails[1].

Reference

1 Neldner KH, Hambridge KM, Walravens PA. Acrodermatitis enteropathica. *Int J Dermatol* 1978; **17**: 380–7.

Tuberous sclerosis

Koenen's periungual fibromas (Figure 16.5) are seen in 50% of patients with tuberous sclerosis[1]: the lesions usually first appear at age 12–14 years and then increase in size until they distort the nail and cause longitudinal depressions.

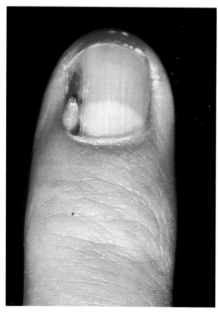

Figure 16.5 *Periungual fibroma in tuberous sclerosis (courtesy of Dr J. Harper)*

The inheritance is autosomal dominant with variable expression.

Reference

1 Kint A, Baran R. Histopathologic study of Koenen tumors. *J Am Acad Dermatol* 1988; **18**: 369–72.

Incontinentia pigmenti

Incontinentia pigmenti (IP) or Bloch–Sulzberger syndrome is a multiorgan disease with an X-linked dominant inheritance which affects females and usually is lethal in males.

There are three clinical stages of skin changes. First, a linear erythematovesicular and bullous reaction is present at birth. It is followed by a second stage of verrucous lesions which gradually disappear. The third stage is characterized by a splashed or whorled pigmentation in a pattern which follows Blaschko's lines. From 15 to 26 years of age painful subungual keratotic tumours[1] or warty periungual tumours[2] can appear as a manifestation of IP. It is usually the fingers that are involved. The keratotic subungual mass produces dystrophy or simple onycholysis of the nail which is displaced from its bed. Erythema and swelling of the fingertip are found at the border of the lesion. The tumour may be sited only on the subungual proximal nail area leading to the destruction of a portion of the nail plate, or on the fold with tender swellings which are smooth proximally and warty distally[2]. The tumours destroy the distal bony phalanx. They may disappear spontaneously after several months leaving a 2 mm scar on the pulp just under the free edge of the nail at the site of a warty lesion[2]. Hartman[3] reported the case of a 30-year-old woman with painful subungual tumours from the age of 20 years. The keratotic lesions resulted in nail dystrophy and scalloped bone deformities of the terminal phalanges of the fingers. Twice regression followed pregnancy.

Histological examination of the tumours shows a verrucous or pseudoepitheliomatous hyperplasia of the epidermis where dyskeratotic cells are found at all levels. Differential diagnoses include warts, epidermoid cyst, subungual fibroma, squamous cell epithelioma and, above all, keratoacanthoma which is clinically and histologically indistinguishable.

Despite the possibility of spontaneous healing, patients often ask for treatment because of pain and disability. Management by desiccation and curettage or surgical excision is usually successful, but permanent nail atrophy may occur. A course of etretinate or acitretin therapy should therefore be encouraged, despite possible recurrence[4].

References

1 Mascaro JM, Palou J, Vives P. Painful subungual keratotic tumors in incontinentia pigmenti. *J Am Acad Dermatol* 1985; **13**: 913–18.

2 Moss C, Ince P. Anhidrotic and achromians lesions in incontinentia pigmenti. *Br J Dermatol* 1987; **116**: 839–49.

3 Hartman DL, Danville PA. Incontinentia pigmenti associated with subungual tumours. *Arch Dermatol* 1976; **112**: 535–42.

4 Bessems PJMH, Jagtman BA, van de Staak WJB et al. Progressive, persistent, hyperkeratotic lesions in incontinentia pigmenti. *Arch Dermatol* 1988; **124**: 29–30.

Chapter 17

Disorders of DNA and chromosomal instability

W. C. Lambert and M. W. Lambert

Introduction

All of the inherited diseases currently believed to be associated with defective DNA repair and/or chromosomal instability [1–6] are quite rare. The main conditions are listed in Table 17.1. This is probably due to the extremely complex nature of chromatin structure, with different proteins playing more than one role, interacting with each other, and partially compensating for any loss or deficiency of each other, so that specific diseases can be traced only to very severe – or combined – deficiencies. It is likely that a number of more common diseases are related aetiopathologically to less extreme defects in chromatin proteins and nuclear enzymes, but this has yet to be conclusively proved. It is also probable that the genetics of some of these rare diseases is much more complex than the simple phrase 'autosomal recessive' would imply, with perhaps some of them requiring combinations of recessively transmitted genes, at different loci, for the disease to become manifest. There is convincing evidence for genetic heterogeneity within several of these diseases. Thus, different involved loci or combinations of involved loci may produce different genetic subtypes of the same disease. However, from the standpoint of patient management, considering these disorders to be autosomal recessive conditions is usually adequate.

References

1 Friedberg EC. *DNA Repair*. 2nd ed. WH Freeman, New York 1994.
2 Lambert WC. Genetic diseases associated with DNA and chromosomal instability. *Dermatol Clin* 1987; **5**: 85–108.
3 Lambert MW, Laval J, eds. *DNA Repair Mechanisms and their Biologic Implications in Mammalian Cells*. Plenum, New York, 1989.
4 Lambert WC, Hanawalt PC. DNA repair mechanisms and their biological implications in mammalian cells. *J Am Acad Dermatol* 1990; **22**: 299–308.
5 Lambert WC, Lambert MW. Diseases associated with DNA and chromosomal instability. In: Alper J, ed. *Genetic Diseases of the Skin*. Mosby/Year Book, St Louis, 1991.
6 Lambert WC, Kuo H-R, Lambert MW. Xeroderma pigmentosum. *Dermatol Clin* 1995; **13**: 169–209.

Table 17.1 *The main skin disorders associated with defective DNA repair and/or chromosomal instability*

Xeroderma pigmentosum
Cockayne's syndrome
Ataxia-telangiectasia (see also Chapter 18)
Fanconi's anaemia
Bloom's syndrome
The trichothiodystrophies (see also Chapters 5 and 15)

Xeroderma pigmentosum

Xeroderma pigmentosum (XP)[1,2] is a rare autosomal recessive disorder, estimated to present in approximately 2 out of each million live births, with a significantly higher incidence in Egypt, North Africa and Japan. There are two components to XP, both extremely variable in degree of manifestation, each of which occurs independent of the other. These are (1) increased sensitivity to ultraviolet (UV) radiation, including those wavelengths (especially UVB, 290–320 nm) found in sunlight, and (2) progressive neurodegenerative disease. The latter does not occur in all patients.

Clinical features

Except for the very unusual cases in which the neurodegenerative component of the disease is severe, the hypersensitivity to UV radiation in sunlight almost always accounts for the presenting signs of the disease. The term 'xeroderma pigmentosum' refers to dry, oddly pigmented skin, which is precisely the usual appearance when the patient first presents (Figure 17.1). Typically, the patient at presentation is an infant or small child. The parents may be unaware that the cutaneous changes are related to sun exposure, or they may be very aware of it, depending on whether the child cries or otherwise complains while in the sun. Rarely, the child is brought to the physician with a complaint of sun sensitivity before skin manifestations are evident. On the other hand, if considerable sun exposure has taken place, the skin may be indurated and leathery, as well as dry and pigmented. A fine, uniform scale may be present. Often, but not always, the bulbar conjunctivae are injected. At this point the diagnosis may be difficult, especially if this is the first affected sibling and the family history is negative. In the majority of cases, the parents are not related.

As the disease progresses, the mottled pigment changes and dry skin become more prominent and tumours begin to appear on the areas most exposed to sun, usually first on the face (see Figure 19.5) or sometimes on the hands. Actinic (solar) keratoses, keratoacanthomas, basal cell carcinomas, squamous cell carcinomas, and – much less commonly – melanoma (usually of the superficial spreading type) or a lentigo maligna may appear. If any of these neoplasms appears before the age of 12 years in the above clinical context, the diagnosis should be strongly suspected.

The skin of XP patients shows the same changes seen in chronically sun-exposed skin of the elderly, but at a much earlier age. One sees mottled pigmentary

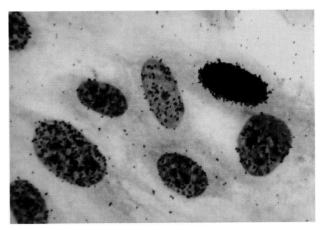

Figure 17.2 *Unscheduled DNA synthesis occurring on cultured normal fibroblasts following ultraviolet irradiation. The darkly labelled cell on the right is in S phase (reproduced from Lambert and Lambert [3], with permission)*

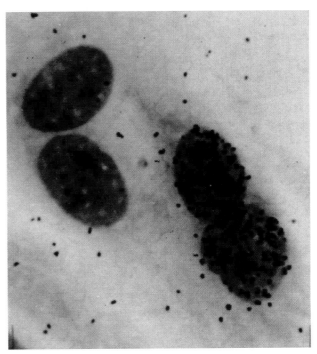

Figure 17.3 *Unscheduled DNA synthesis occurring in two fused cultured fibroblasts from two different XP patients (heterokaryons) following ultraviolet irradiation. Unfused cells showing no UDS are seen on the left (reproduced from Lambert and Lambert [3], with permission)*

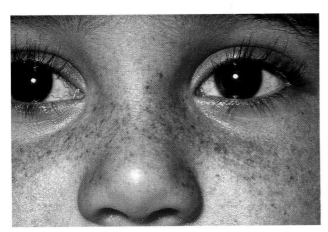

Figure 17.1 *Xeroderma pigmentosum: early freckling and actinic conjunctivitis (courtesy of Dr J. Harper)*

changes, irregularly shaped freckles, epidermal atrophy, xerosis, mottled erythema and focal scarring. However, the dermal elastosis observed in sun-exposed skin is not seen or is very slight in XP patients. The degree to which these changes occur is very variable, and depends upon the severity of the sun sensitivity and the degree to which the patient is protected from sunlight. Thus a 50-year-old patient may show only mild changes, and a 3-year-old may show severe changes.

In addition to skin changes, eye disease is often severe, with pingueculae and carcinomas arising on the bulbar conjunctivae, and other changes requiring enucleation in many cases. Entropion, exotropia and other changes of the lids are common. Tumours of the inferior lip, anterior mouth and anterior tongue are also seen.

The neurological changes are only seen in a minority of patients with XP, and in many cases are rather mild. They are always progressive. The first manifestation is usually hearing loss of high-frequency sounds. Hyporeflexia of deep tendons may also occur early. The De Sanctis–Cacchione syndrome refers to patients with XP and neurodegenerative disease, but some authors feel that this term should only apply to severely affected individuals who manifest severe neurodegenerative disease in infancy. Such cases usually also show growth retardation, especially microcephaly.

Routine laboratory studies are initially of no value in establishing a diagnosis of XP, although tests for porphyrins may help to rule out porphyria in the differential diagnosis. An important non-routine laboratory test, which should be performed whenever there is any question regarding the diagnosis, is the unscheduled DNA synthesis (UDS) test, which is carried out on living cells derived from the patient, usually either skin fibroblasts or peripheral blood lymphocytes (Figures 17.2 and 17.3).

DNA repair studies and complementation groups

Biochemical studies on XP performed in a large number of laboratories have shown conclusively that in most cases there is a defect in the first step, mediated by a DNA endonuclease (an endonuclease is an enzyme that cuts a DNA strand at a phosphodiester bond, either on one strand, as in the present case, or on both strands of the DNA double helix) of the nucleotide excision pathway for removal of ultraviolet light-induced adducts in cellular DNA (Figure 17.4). Xeroderma pigmentosum cells also show deficiencies in repair of adducts produced in DNA by UV-mimetic drugs, such as nitroquinoline-1-oxide or *N*-acetoxy-2-acetylaminofluorene. These UV-induced adducts are mainly covalent linkages between adjacent pyrimidines, especially adjacent thymines, both of them on the same strand of the DNA double helix. They are of two types, cyclobutane thymine (or pyrimidine)

dimers, in which two covalent bonds join the two pyrimidines, and 6–4 pyrimidine-pyrimidones, also called 6–4 photoproducts, joined by a single covalent bond. The nucleotide excision systems for repairing these two types of lesions are *not* identical, accounting for some of the genetic heterogeneity of XP (see below), but they are similar. The first step is a single strand cleavage at or near the site of the adduct, and on the same strand as the adduct, by an endonuclease (this is the step defective in most cases of XP), followed by removal of the affected segment containing the adduct, replacement (via a polymerase) of the removed segment with new DNA, using the opposite strand as a template, and finally re-sealing the phosphodiester backbone of the repaired strand by a ligase. The polymerase-mediated replacement step, above, requires insertion of new nucleotides into the DNA. If the cell is growing in medium containing radiolabelled nucleotides, this leads to labelling of the cellular DNA. If the cell is not in the S phase of the cell cycle, in which replicative (i.e. scheduled) DNA synthesis occurs, then this non-replicative (i.e. unscheduled) DNA synthesis produces radiolabel in a cell that otherwise would not become labelled. If the cells are then placed on an autoradiographic slide, on which photographic emulsion is placed over the cells so as to produce precipitation of silver grains over nuclei from which radioactive emissions are occurring, grains overlying non-S-phase cells are seen whenever nucleotide excision repair has occurred. The nuclei of S-phase cells are clearly identified by their very dense radiolabel and are eliminated from consideration.

The UDS assay also detects UDS occurring in the base excision repair pathway, in which a glycosylase cleaves the affected base from an associated sugar moiety. The abasic site so generated is then cleaved by an endonuclease, followed by the same steps as for nucleotide excision repair. The base excision repair pathway is less important in XP, but is important in some other diseases. Use of the UDS assay in those other disorders, using a number of DNA damaging agents, is at present a research technique only.

Using the above UDS assay, or some modification of it, cells are exposed to ultraviolet light or some other agent in culture, followed by radiolabelled nucleotides (usually thymidine) and then subjected to autoradiography or some other method of determining degree of radiolabel per cell. The label in XP cells is diminished compared with similarly treated control cells, allowing a diagnosis to be made. Studies of viability and cloning ability (colony-forming ability) are also performed on these cells. Viability is markedly reduced in XP cells following UV irradiation.

In a minority (about 20%) of XP patients, referred to as the variant group, the above UDS assay following UV irradiation is normal, even though unequivocal clinical XP is present and viability of the cells following UV irradiation is reduced. The biochemical defect in the variant group is unknown. In some

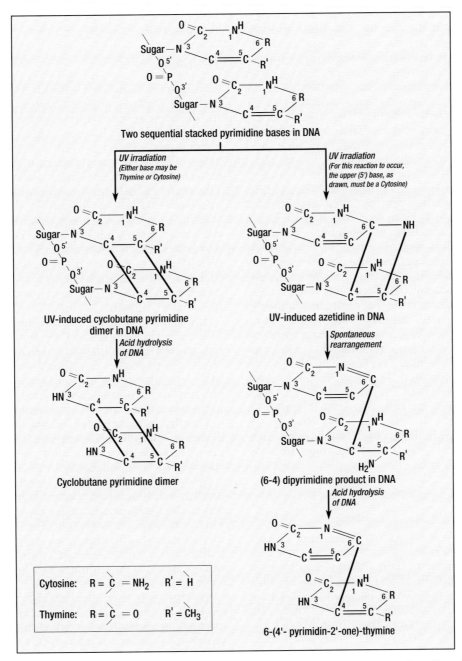

Figure 17.4 *Generation of photoadducts in DNA by ultraviolet irradiation. These adducts create a tertiary distortion (not shown) in the DNA structure which is recognized by the DNA repair enzymes, assisted by histone proteins (redrawn from Lambert and Lambert [3], with permission)*

laboratories, altered responses of variant cells to UV radiation in the presence of caffeine is used as a test for the variant group. This is by no means a standard test in all laboratories.

Decreased UDS following UV radiation is not unique to XP; it has been found in several other rare diseases (e.g. some trichothiodystrophies), as well as in at least one unaffected first-degree relative of a patient with XP. However, in a clinical context

suggestive of XP, the UDS assay is an important diagnostic test.

The UDS test may be performed on fetally derived cells, allowing a prenatal diagnosis of XP to be established in families at risk. This procedure is now routine in several laboratories and should be carried out, where appropriate, on siblings of XP patients.

An important modification of the UDS assay is a complementation assay for XP in which cells from different patients are fused in culture and UDS is examined in each of the two (or more) nuclei of the resulting heteropolykaryons after UV irradiation. In many cases, the two nuclei show normal or near-normal UDS even though UDS was depressed in both cell lines individually. This indicates that the genetic defects in the two cell lines, and thus in the patients with XP from whom they were derived, are different. On this basis seven different complementation groups of excision-deficient XP have now been established, labelled A through G (groups H and I are now thought to belong to groups D and C respectively, and have been withdrawn). Fused cells within complementation groups fail to complement each other in the UDS assay; fusion of cells in different complementation groups leads to complementation of UDS to normal or nearly normal levels following UV irradiation. Thus the complementation assay has established that a large amount of genetic heterogeneity is present in XP. Patients within complementation groups tend to have similar manifestations of XP. In most areas of the world, complementation groups A, C and the variant type are most common, with group D somewhat less common, and the remainder very rare with only a handful of cases reported. However, in Japan most cases are either group A or the variant type. Sun sensitivity is greatest in group A, least in group D. Neurodegenerative disease is found mainly in groups A, D and E. Late onset, mild, often sub-clinical neurological disease may be found in other groups.

Genetics

Five of these genes have been reported to be cloned. Many are called 'excision repair cross-complementing' (ERCC) genes because of their ability to complement DNA repair in mutant rodent cells. Some of these genes have been proposed to be DNA helicases; at least one is a DNA endonuclease. Two or more also play a role in the initiation of transcription[4,5].

Differential diagnosis

In the basal cell naevus syndrome, numerous small basal cell carcinomas appear, usually after puberty, together with palmar pitted lesions and mandibular cysts evident on X-ray. The multiple keratoacanthomas seen in the Ferguson-Smith syndrome similarly occur later and without the pigmentary changes seen in XP (see Chapter 19). In the dysplastic naevus syndrome, a common autosomal dominant condition with partial penetrance, numerous dysplastic naevi of clinically and histologically irregular appearance arise in childhood or later. Each of these has the potential to develop into a melanoma, and patients must be closely followed up so that changing lesions can be excised early.

Treatment

Management of patients with XP consists most importantly of *avoidance of bright light*, especially of all but the dimmest of *sunlight*. It is important that erythema be avoided. Most patients with XP can live quite comfortably avoiding light sufficiently to prevent acute effects, yet not sufficiently to prevent chronic skin changes leading to large numbers of skin cancers. The need for extreme avoidance of light places an enormous burden on the family of affected children, leading to numerous management problems. Often the family simply makes the decision that so much and only so much can be done. Since the child with XP usually does not show the devastating skin changes that appear later, the physician may be seen as a 'false prophet of doom' by the family, and compliance may be a major problem.

The second important management tool is surgery to remove skin cancers as they arise. It is critical that the patient be evaluated at frequent intervals for development of skin, mouth and eye cancers, and that each neoplasm be treated as conservatively as possible, conserving normal tissue, since repeated excisions in the same sites are often necessary.

Thirdly, in patients in whom neurodegenerative disease is present or is expected, it is necessary to provide supportive care and (when appropriate) special education facilities.

Retinoids – isotretinoin, etretinate and more recently acitretin – have been given to XP patients to retard the development and growth of skin cancers. There have been some reports of modest success using this treatment, although it has also been suggested that tumours tend to arise in 'crops' when the drug is discontinued. Topical fluorouracil may be helpful for early or premalignant lesions.

In some centres, removal of the epidermis from sun-exposed areas of skin and replacement with less sun-exposed epidermal cells either taken from adnexal structures or from cultures of skin from sites that are not sun-exposed, is being attempted as an experimental treatment for XP. Dermabrasion and special lasers are among the methods for removing sun-damaged epidermis. A modification of this technique is introduction of cloned DNA repair genes into the cells used for replacing the epidermis. Attempts to introduce DNA repair genes into sun-exposed cells in situ are also under way. All of these approaches should be considered experimental.

Patients with moderately severe XP usually die of metastatic melanoma or other cancer at an early age. A few cases have developed internal cancers, with a slight propensity to develop primary brain tumours.

There is a registry for xeroderma pigmentosum, care of the authors.

References

1 Kraemer KH, Lee MM, Scotto J. Xeroderma pigmentosum. *Arch Dermatol* 1987; **123**: 241–50.
2 Lambert WC, Lambert MW. Xeroderma pigmentosum. *Cancer Rev* 1987; **7**: 27–50.
3 Lambert WC, Lambert MW. Diseases associated with DNA and chromosomal instability. In: Alper J, ed. *Genetic Diseases of the Skin*. Mosby/Year Book, St Louis, 1991.
4 Bortsma D. The genetic defect in DNA repair deficiency syndromes. *Eur J Cancer* 1993; **29A**: 1482–8.
5 Lambert WC, Lambert MW. DNA repair deficiency and skin cancer in xeroderma pigmentosum. In: Mukhtar H, ed. *Skin Cancer: Mechanisms and Human Relevance*. CRC Press, Boca Raton 1995, pp. 39–70.

Cockayne's syndrome

Cockayne's syndrome (CS) is a rare autosomal recessive condition, in which patients are small and show altered facies in some ways resembling premature aging[1]. The face is often thin and angular, giving the patient a bird-like appearance. Mental deficiency, deafness, optic atrophy, intracranial calcification, large ears and nose, sunken eyes, overly long arms and legs for body size and photosensitivity are characteristic. A type II lipoproteinaemia is also seen. Patients with CS do *not* have an increased incidence of neoplasia of any type.

Hyper-reflexia, rather than hyporeflexia, of deep tendons is a useful diagnostic feature in distinguishing between CS and xeroderma pigmentosum. Several cases of CS have also had concurrent xeroderma pigmentosum, however, demonstrated on both clinical and laboratory grounds. Except for these cases, UDS in CS cells in culture following UV irradiation is usually normal, although depression of S phase, replicative DNA synthesis in CS is markedly prolonged following UV exposure. Synthesis of RNA is also depressed. Cockayne's syndrome clinically resembles progeria of the Hutchinson–Gilford type, but is distinguished from that disorder by the presence of microcephaly, mental retardation, nerve deafness and retinal degeneration.

Management of these severely affected patients is essentially supportive.

The clinical appearance is so striking that the diagnosis is seldom in doubt.

Three complementation groups of CS have been identified.

Reference

1 Lehmann AR, Thompson AF, Harcourt SA et al. Cockayne's syndrome: correlation of clinical features with cellular sensitivity of RNA synthesis to ultraviolet irradiation. *J Med Genet* 1993; **30**: 679–82.

Ataxia-telangiectasia

Synonym: *Louis-Bar syndrome*

Ataxia-telangiectasia[1,2] is an autosomal recessive disorder characterized by fusiform dilatations of small vessels of the skin, particularly on the ears and around the eyes, as well as on the bulbar conjunctivae; cerebellar ataxia; mental retardation; immunodeficiency, and a susceptibility to neoplasms of the lymphoreticular system. A more detailed account is given in Chapter 18. Cells from ataxia-telangiectasia (AT) patients show a high frequency of spontaneous chromosomal abnormalities. Cells containing polypoid or endoreduplicated chromosomes have been found to be 10–20 times more common in peripheral blood lymphocytes and other cells derived from AT patients, than in cells from normal persons.

Cells in culture derived from AT patients also show an increased incidence of chromosomal abnormalities. These alterations, as well as decreased viability, are seen following X-irradiation or treatment with X-ray-mimetic chemicals such as bleomycin or neocarzinostatin. Cells from AT patients in culture show a continuation of replicative DNA synthesis at near-control levels, whereas normal cells show a marked inhibition of this DNA synthesis, following X-ray irradiation. These AT cells do not characteristically show an increase in chromosomal abnormalities, reduced viability or diminished UDS following ultraviolet irradiation.

Cancer therapy, particularly radiation therapy, should be undertaken with great caution, owing to the extreme sensitivity of the patients to X-rays, gamma rays and certain antimetabolites (such as bleomycin or neocarzinostatin). Treatment with these agents may be possible, since the tumour cells also show the increased susceptibility to these agents, but may require that markedly reduced doses be employed.

Four different complementation groups of AT have been identified, a fifth having been withdrawn. However, as many as eight or nine have been proposed.

References

1 Taylor AM, Byrd PJ, McConville CM et al. Genetic and cellular features of ataxia-telangiectasia. *Int J Rad Biol* 1994; **64**: 65–70.
2 Gatti RA. Ataxia-telangiectasia. *Dermatol Clin* 1995; **13**: 1–6.

Fanconi's anaemia

Fanconi's anaemia (FA) is a rare autosomal recessive condition, probably about as prevalent as xeroderma pigmentosum[1]. Patients present in childhood with widespread, more or less mottled skin pigmentation, petechiae, microcephaly, genital hypoplasia, generalized hyper-reflexia, internal strabismus and normal intelligence[2]. Low birthweight, growth retardation, skeletal deformities (especially dystrophy of the thumb and radius), micro-ophthalmia, renal malformations and endocrinopathies are seen. A progressive pancytopenia is present, usually causing death in childhood. Patients who survive to adulthood have a markedly increased incidence of leukaemia, hepatocellular carcinoma and squamous cell carcinoma. The clinical features are extremely variable, often making diagnosis difficult. Fanconi's anaemia may occur without any of the above congenital malformations; this condition has been referred to as the Diamond–Blackfan syndrome or as the Estren–Dameshek variant of FA.

Multiple chromosomal breaks are observed. Cells in culture derived from patients with FA show an increased susceptibility to DNA damaging agents which create interstrand cross-links in DNA. There are now five complementation groups recognized – A to E[3]. Defective DNA endonucleases found in chromatin which selectively attack DNA containing DNA interstrand cross-links have been identified in FA cells by the authors' laboratory[4].

Linkage has been demonstrated between FA and loci on chromosome 20q12–13.3, but with evidence of possible heterogeneity[5].

Diagnosis is made on clinical grounds and by haematologic evaluation.

Management consists primarily of anticipating the anaemia and cancers, and treating them as they arise. The standard treatment for bone marrow failure – transfusion and long-term androgen therapy – places these patients at risk from complications of this therapy, which may be a contributing factor in the development of malignancy. Patients with FA are generally hypersensitive to cyclophosphamide. However, by reducing the standard dose given prior to bone marrow transplantation, successful engraftment is possible.

Prenatal diagnosis has been achieved by demonstrating increased spontaneous and induced chromosome breakage in fetal cells (cultured amniocytes or chorionic villus cells)[6].

There is a registry for cases of Fanconi's anaemia c/o The Laboratory for Investigative Dermatology, Rockefeller University, New York, NY 10021, USA.

References

1 Auerbach AD. Fanconi's anemia. *Dermatol Clin* 1995; **13**: 41–9.
2 Butturini A, Gale RP, Verlander PC et al. Hematologic abnormalities in Fanconi anemia: an international Fanconi anemia registry study. *Blood* 1994; **84**: 1650–5.
3 Strathdee CA, Gavish H, Shannon WR et al. Cloning of cDNAs for Fanconi's anaemia by functional complementation. *Nature* 1992; **356**: 763–7.
4 Lambert MW, Tsongelis GJ, Lambert WC et al. Defective DNA endonucleases in Fanconi's anaemia cells, complementation groups A and B. *Mutat Res* 1992; **273**: 57–71.
5 Mann WR, Venkatraj VS, Allen RG et al. Fanconi anaemia: evidence of linkage heterogeneity on chromosome 20q. *Genomics* 1991; **9**: 329–37.
6 Auerbach AD, Sagi M, Adler B. Fanconi anaemia: prenatal diagnosis in 30 fetuses at risk. *Paediatrics* 1985; **76**: 794–800.

Bloom's syndrome

Bloom's syndrome (BS) is a rare autosomal recessive disease, presenting as small but proportionate body size and a sun-sensitive telangiectatic skin rash over the face[1,2]. The cutaneous manifestation usually occurs in a 'butterfly' distribution over the malar eminences and around the eyes. It often also involves the lower lip, which may ulcerate and be a source of discomfort. Bloom's syndrome occurs mainly in Ashkenazic Jews and is more common in males than in females. The head is elongated and the facial appearance is typical, although sometimes these latter characteristics are rather subtle. *Café au lait* macules are almost always present; some patients also have minor anatomic changes.

Diagnosis is made primarily on clinical grounds. Plasma levels of both IgA and IgM are characteristically low and bacterial infections are often present. The incidence of leukaemia and of gastric cancer is markedly increased in BS patients. Cells in culture derived from BS patients show, in addition to increased numbers of chromosome breaks and rearrangements, increased sister chromatid exchanges during mitotic division. A defective DNA ligase has been reported. Other DNA repair defects have also been suggested.

Management consists mainly of monitoring patients for infections and for early detection and treatment of neoplasms.

No evidence for genetic heterogeneity in BS has been found on either clinical or laboratory grounds.

There is a registry for cases of Bloom's syndrome c/o The Laboratory of Human Genetics, The New York Blood Center, New York, NY 10021, USA.

References

1 German J. Bloom's syndrome. *Dermatol Clin* 1995; **13**: 7–18.
2 German J. Bloom's syndrome: a Mendelian prototype of somatic mutational disease. *Medicine (Baltimore)* 1993; **72**: 397–406.

The trichothiodystrophies

The trichothiodystrophies[1,2] are a group of autosomal recessive disorders in which hair is brittle and deficient in sulphur content. They are described in more detail in Chapter 5. Some, but not all, cases also have photosensitivity and defective repair of adducts introduced into cellular DNA by ultraviolet irradiation, particularly with short wavelength UVB (290–320 nm) or UVC (200–290 nm) radiation. Thus, the DNA repair deficiency resembles that seen in xeroderma pigmentosum, with reduced UDS in UV-irradiated cells in culture derived from these patients. Those cases that have been studied by complementation analysis fall either into group D of XP, or into one of the two complementation groups of trichothiodystrophy (A or B) identified to date. Trichothiodystrophy is not associated with a risk of skin cancer or other malignancy, regardless of photosensitivity or defective DNA repair.

References

1 Itin PH, Pittelkow MR. Trichothiodystrophy: review of sulfur-deficient brittle hair syndromes and association with the ectodermal dysplasias. *J Am Acad Dermatol* 1990; **22**: 705–17.
2 Lehmann AR, Arlett CF, Broughton BC et al. Trichothiodystrophy: a human DNA repair disorder with heterogeneity in the cellular response to ultraviolet light. *Cancer Res* 1988; **48**: 6090–6

Chapter 18

Primary immunodeficiency diseases

M. Lacour, T. Duvanel and J.-H. Saurat

Introduction

The human body enjoys a very sophisticated system able to detect and destroy any 'non-self' intruder, whether chemical, infectious or tumoral. Although infectious agents are the primary target of immune defences, the other aspects should be kept in mind in order to understand the wide variety of pathological manifestations of immunodeficiencies. Four components of the immune system can be distinguished:

1. *Antibody-mediated immunity* or 'humoral immunity'. Through a very complex process of gene rearrangements and cell maturation, bone marrow precursors give rise to pre-B lymphocytes, mature B lymphocytes and finally plasma cells that secrete immunoglobulins of one class (IgM, IgG_1, IgG_2, IgG_3, IgG_4, IgA_1, IgA_2 or IgE). The very complexity of this differentiation process makes it prone to errors at any stage.
2. *Cellular immunity*. Cellular immunity is mediated by lymphocytes that have undergone differentiation in the thymus, namely T lymphocytes. This differentiation process enables subsets of these lymphocytes to fight altered cells, especially cells infected with viruses or parasites; other infectious agents such as fungi are also controlled by these T lymphocytes, which in addition display aspecific toxicity against transformed cells as well as regulatory functions in the immune system itself.
3. *Phagocytosis by inflammatory cells*. Although this is basically an effector mechanism, the very intricacy of the immune system is shown by the fact that macrophages are also important in processing and presenting antigens (in conjunction with HLA membrane proteins) to lymphocytes in order to elicit the immune reaction.
4. *The complement system*. Its plasmatic factors amplify inflammatory and immune reactions.

Each of these components of the immune system may come into play alone, but more often the protection of the host against infections requires the coordinated activation of all components of the immune system.

The role of skin

The skin, along with mucous membranes of the respiratory and the digestive tracts, constitutes the interface between the environment and the organism. One of its functions is protection against environmental aggression, not only by its non-specific structural characteristics, but also by setting the stage for the first interaction between the immune defences of the organism and potential invaders. As a result, defects in immunity often result in recurrent bacterial, viral or mycotic infections. Other cutaneous alterations that emphasize the role of skin as a constituent of the immune system include autoimmune or dysimmune skin changes which frequently occur in association with primary immunodeficiencies. This provides models for the understanding of these disorders and of the relationship between the skin and other organs of the immune system[1,2].

Cutaneous manifestations of primary immunodeficiencies can be classified into six different groups (Table 18.1).

Table 18.1 *Cutaneous manifestations of primary immunodeficiencies*

Chronic and recurrent infections
Eczema
Graft-versus-host reactions
Collagen-vascular syndromes
Independent cutaneous markers
Other skin symptoms associated with primary
   immunodeficiencies

Adapted from Saurat et al [1].

Infections

Infectious manifestations in primary immunodeficiencies can be differentiated from those occurring in immunocompetent patients by the presence of the following features:

1. Increased incidence and recurrence of common primary skin infections, such as cellulitis and carbuncles.
2. Dissemination of normally localized infections, such as warts, herpes simplex and herpes zoster.
3. Cutaneous metastatic dissemination of systemic infections due to *Pseudomonas aeruginosa* or opportunistic fungi (*Aspergillus, Cryptococcus, Candida, Mucoraceae*).
4. Primary skin infections due to opportunistic agents, such as mycobacteria, *Prototheca* and fungi (*Alternaria, Fusarium, Trichosporon, Rhizopus, Aspergillus*).
5. Recurrence and/or dissemination of specific organisms associated with specific immune disorders, such as neisserial infections in complement deficiencies.

Eczema

The relationship between eczema and primary immunodeficiencies presents special interest to the dermatologist, in so far as atopic dermatitis itself can be viewed as an immune dysfunction, and analysis of the eczematiform eruptions of immunodeficiencies is likely to help in uncovering the pathogenesis of atopic dermatitis[3]. For this reason, in this chapter the term 'atopic dermatitis' is used only when the eruption associated with a particular immunodeficiency meets the criteria proposed by Hanifin and Rajka[4] for the diagnosis of that dermatosis. Otherwise, the expression 'eczematoid eruption' describes less specific dermatoses.

Graft-versus-host reaction

Graft-versus-host reaction may occur whenever cellular immunity is defective, either spontaneously following transplacental passage of maternal cells, or as an iatrogenic disease complicating transfusion of non-irradiated blood products or treatment of the underlying disorder by bone marrow graft. Symptoms progress from an acute phase with maculopapular rashes, alopecia and even (rarely) toxic epidermal necrolysis, to a chronic phase marked by lichenoid plaques that may evolve into a scleroderma-like state[5].

Collagen-vascular syndromes

Collagen-vascular syndromes usually occur long-term in primary immunodeficiencies. Lupus erythematosus may be found in patients with complement deficiencies, IgA deficiency or common variable immunodeficiency, and in mothers and sisters of patients with chronic granulomatous disease. Dermatomyositis may be found in patients with C2 deficiency, X-linked agammaglobulinaemia, and common variable immunodeficiency. Scleroderma has been associated with C7 deficiency. Lastly, vasculitis is usually typical of complement deficiency.

Independent cutaneous markers

The group of independent cutaneous markers of primary immunodeficiencies is composed of symptoms specific for one type of immunodeficiency. They include pigment dilution in Chédiak–Higashi and Griscelli–Prunieras syndromes; thrombocytopenic purpura in Wiskott–Aldrich syndrome; telangiectasia and progeric changes in ataxia-telangiectasia; abnormal facies in DiGeorge's syndrome; and redundant skin folds and hair hypoplasia in primary immunodeficiency with short-limbed dwarfism.

Other skin symptoms

The last group of manifestations is composed of skin symptoms that have been found in association with primary immune disorders but are not characteristic markers of an underlying immune deficit. Typical examples include urticaria in hyper-IgE syndromes and complement deficiencies (C2, C3 inhibitor); cutaneous cancers in ataxia-telangiectasia; non-caseating granulomas in common variable immunodeficiency; or 'cold' abscesses in hyper-IgE syndrome and chronic granulomatous disease.

Burgio and Ugazio[6] distinguished 'immunodeficiency syndromes', where all symptoms (e.g. infections) are the result of the immune defect, from 'syndromes with immunodeficiency', defined by the occurrence of many features that cannot be explained by the immune defect. Many primary immunodeficiencies with prominent cutaneous manifestations would fall into the latter group. However, in this chapter the conventional classification is kept, and primary immunodeficiencies are reviewed under the four headings of antibody deficiency disorders, T-cell immunodeficiencies, phagocytic and granulocytic disorders and complement deficiencies[7].

References

1 Saurat J-H, Woodley D, Helfer N. Cutaneous symptoms in primary immunodeficiencies. *Curr Probl Dermatol* 1985; **13**: 50–91.
2 Norris DA, ed. *Immune Mechanisms in Cutaneous Disease.* Marcel Dekker, New York, 1989.
3 Saurat J-H. Atopic dermatitis-like eruptions in primary immunodeficiencies. In: Happle R, Grosshans E, eds. *Pediatric Dermatology.* Springer, Berlin, 1987; 96–100.
4 Hanifin JM, Rajka G. Diagnostic features of atopic dermatitis. *Acta Derm Venereol* 1980; **92** (suppl.): 44–7.
5 Saurat J-H. Cutaneous manifestations of graft-versus-host disease. *Int J Dermatol* 1981; **20**: 249–56.
6 Burgio GR, Ugazio AG. Immunodeficiency and syndromes: a nosographic approach. *Eur J Pediatr* 1982; **138**: 288–92.
7 Rosen FS, Cooper MD, Wedgewood RJP. The primary immunodeficiencies. *New Engl J Med* 1984; **311**: 235–44, 300–10 (two parts).

Antibody (B-cell) immune deficiency disorders

Transient hypogammaglobulinaemia of infancy

Definition

In transient hypogammaglobulinaemia of infancy an unexplained delay in the maturation of the immunoglobulin-producing system takes place, resulting in a fall of the serum concentrations of one or more of the three major immunoglobulin classes below the 95% confidence interval for age, with subsequent analyses showing a definite rise of these values towards normal; IgG is usually more affected than IgM and IgA.

Clinical features

The manifestations are usually benign and include sinopulmonary infections, recurrent diarrhoea and recurrent skin infections such as cellulitis and pyodermas. These may be identified in both sexes at 3–6 months of age, when maternal antibodies disappear from the child's serum.

Pathology

Tiller and Buckley[1] described 11 cases and distinguished a symptomatic group of patients, detected because they have recurrent infections, in whom the immunoglobulin levels do rise with age but remain abnormally low, and an asymptomatic group, detected because they have immunodeficient relatives. In the latter group, the condition might be a manifestation of genetic heterozygosity for some other immunodeficient state.

Genetics

The genetic basis, if any, of this heterogeneous disorder remains unknown.

Differential diagnosis

Other forms of primary immunodeficiency should be ruled out. By definition, all patients recover, usually by the second year of life. Affected children may be at higher risk for developing persistent IgA deficiency[2].

Treatment

There is no specific treatment.

References

1 Tiller TL, Buckley RH. Transient hypogammaglobulinemia of infancy: review of the literature, clinical and immunologic features of 11 new cases, and long term follow-up. *J Pediatr* 1978; **92**: 347–53.
2 McGready SJ. Transient hypogammaglobulinemia of infancy: need to reconsider name and definition. *J Pediatr* 1987; **110**: 47–50.

X-linked agammaglobulinaemia

Definition

Also referred to as Bruton's or congenital agammaglobulinaemia, X-linked agammaglobulinaemia (XLA) is defined by the absence of B cells in the blood as well as in the lymphoid organs, associated with a global agammaglobulinaemia. Only boys are affected. Levels of IgG are well below 1 g/l, and IgA, IgM and IgD are undetectable; IgE may be present in detectable levels. Antigenic stimulation does not result in antibody production. Cellular immunity is unimpaired[1].

Clinical features

Clinical manifestations begin 5–6 months after birth, when placentally transferred maternal antibodies no longer protect the infant. Affected boys have recurrent pyogenic infections, such as otitis, rhinopharyngitis and bronchitis. Skin infections consist of impetigo and furunculosis, particularly severe around body orifices. Ecthyma gangrenosum due to *Pseudomonas aeruginosa* can be a presenting feature. Chronic cutaneous herpes simplex and caseating cutaneous granulomas have been described during the course of the disease (granulomas are discussed below in the section on common variable immunodeficiency). Diarrhoea due to rotavirus or enterovirus infection is also common, as well as *Giardia lamblia* infestation. An important risk is the development of vaccine-associated polio-myelitis if a live vaccine is inadvertently used. Patients are at risk of developing a chronic dermato-myositis-like syndrome[2], often accompanied by encephalitis and caused by persistent echovirus infec-tion[3]. It has been claimed that these children also develop atopic eczema, which is unresponsive to gamma-globulin replacement therapy, but in a com-prehensive review of 96 patients with X-linked agam-maglobulinaemia, Lederman and Winkelstein[4] found no case of eczematous skin lesions. Thus, atopic dermatitis is not an obligate feature of X-linked agammaglobulinaemia. In older children a syndrome resembling rheumatoid arthritis can also be seen, which seems not to be related to the echovirus-induced dermatomyositis[5].

Pathology

The responsible defect is restricted to the B-cell lineage, causing a block in the clonal expansion of B cells from pre-B cells.

Genetics

Mutations of the gene *btk*, member of the *src* family of protein kinases, are responsible for the disorder[6]. This gene also colocalizes with the X-linked immuno-deficiency gene (*xid*) in mice. Introduction of new XLA mutations is due to the occurrence of X-chromosomal mosaicisms[7]. Heterozygotic female carriers (pheno-typically normal) can now be detected[8].

Differential diagnosis

The diagnosis of XLA relies on the existence of familial antecedents (not obligatory), on the absence of circu-lating B lymphocytes demonstrated by immunostain-ing (CD19, CD20), and on the absence of plasma cells in lymphoid tissues. Two other disorders have been described with the same laboratory findings and clinical course: one occurs in males who present an associated growth hormone deficiency (XLA with growth hormone deficiency); the second one affects both sexes and is indistinguishable from XLA. The latter condition has been named autosomal recessive agammaglobulinaemia[9].

Treatment

The mainstay of the management of affected children is the intravenous injection of immunoglobulins, the average dose to achieve an effective plasma level being 200 mg/kg every 3 weeks[10]. Aggressive anti-microbial therapy is also needed. Previously, about 15% of patients died from chronic pulmonary disease, viral meningoencephalitis or reticular malignancy; however the outcome has now improved.

References

1 Wedgewood RJP. X-linked agammaglobulinemia. In: Sellgeon D, ed. *CRC Handbook Series in Clinical Laboratory Science*. CRC Press, West Palm Beach, 1978; 41–50.
2 Thyss A, El Baze P, Lefebvre JC, Schneider M, Ortonne JP. Dermatomyositis-like syndrome in X-linked hypogam-maglobulinemia. *Acta Dermatol Venereol* 1990; **70**: 309–13.
3 McKinney RE, Katz S, Wilfert M. Chronic enteroviral meningoencephalitis in agammaglobulinemic patients. *Rev Infect Dis* 1987; **9**: 334–56.
4 Lederman HM, Winkelstein JA. X-linked agammaglobu-linemia: an analysis of 96 patients. *Medicine* 1985; **64**: 145–56.
5 Rosen FS. The primary immunodeficiencies: dermato-logic manifestations. *J Invest Dermatol* 1976; **6**: 402–11.
6 Kinnon C, Hinshelwood S, Levinsky RJ, Lovering RC. X-linked agammaglobulinemia – gene cloning and future prospects. *Immunol Today* 1993; **14**: 554–8.
7 Hendricks RW, Schuurman RB. Genetics of human X-linked immunodeficiency diseases. *Clin Exp Immunol* 1991; **85**: 182–92.
8 Conley ME, Puck JM. Carrier detection in typical and atypical X-linked agammaglobulinemia. *J Pediatr* 1988; **122**: 688–94.
9 Rosen FS, Cooper MD, Wedgewood RJP. The primary immunodeficiencies. *New Engl J Med* 1984; **311**: 235–44, 300–10 (two parts).
10 Ammann AJ, Ashman RF, Buckley RH et al. Use of intravenous gamma-globulin in antibody immunodefi-ciency: results of a multicenter controlled trial. *Clin Immunol Immunopath* 1982; **22**: 60–7.

Common variable immunodeficiency

Definition

Common variable immunodeficiency (CVID) is a heterogeneous group composed of different syn-dromes. The characteristic these syndromes share is hypogammaglobulinaemia with a normal number of B lymphocytes[1]. This indicates a block in the differentiation of antigen-stimulated B lymphocytes into antigen-secreting plasma cells. Since various T-cell disorders may be associated, the term 'common variable immunodeficiency' is better than another frequently used term, 'common variable hypogam-maglobulinaemia'.

Clinical features

Onset of the disease is often delayed to the second or third decade (hence the often-used term 'acquired hypogammaglobulinaemia'), but also frequently occurs in childhood[2]. The degree of hypogammaglobulinaemia varies from one patient to another. The capacity to synthesize antibodies is variable too, and usually dissociated (normal for certain antigens, low or non-existent for others). Prominent clinical features are pyogenic recurrent respiratory tract infections, always present and usually leading to bronchiectasis, and persistent secretory diarrhoea, often due to *Giardia lamblia* infestation. Pyodermas do occur. Eczematoid eruptions are commonly seen; they may be linked to the nutritional state because of chronic diarrhoea, but sensitization to poison ivy has been documented as well. Angioedema and drug eruption have been described. Autoimmune disorders are common, including lupus erythematosus, dermatomyositis, alopecia, vitiligo, rheumatoid arthritis, haemolytic anaemia and idiopathic thrombocytopenic purpura[3]. In children, secondary growth failure and failure to complete puberty are frequent[4]. Another distinguishing feature of common variable immunodeficiency is the occurrence of non-caseating granulomas of the skin, lungs, spleen and liver; their presence should be suspected when hepatosplenomegaly is found. Nodular lymphoid hyperplasia is a common finding in the gut of these patients, and may predispose them to gastrointestinal lymphoreticular malignancy[5].

Cutaneous granulomas

The occurrence of cutaneous granulomas in a child with immunodeficiency is a difficult problem that needs further research. Granulomatous lesions may be a presenting feature of an underlying combined immunodeficiency, occurring as erythematous papules or disseminated plaques with scaling, progressive scarring and central atrophy. When non-infectious, these lesions may resemble granuloma annulare, or tend to have a facial and acral distribution[6].

Infectious causes in an immunodeficient patient are likely and should be thoroughly investigated. Mycobacteria, atypical mycobacteria and fungi are the usual causative organisms, and usually respond to specific treatment and immunoglobulin therapy.

Non-infectious cutaneous granulomas have been described in X-linked hypogammaglobulinaemia, common variable immunodeficiency, severe combined immunodeficiency (SCID) and Griscelli–Prunieras syndrome (personal observation). In chronic granulomatous disease (the most common deficiency associated with granulomas) cutaneous granulomas are unusual and occur much less frequently than in the liver, lung and gastrointestinal tract. Immunodeficient patients with granulomas are difficult to differentiate from patients with sarcoidosis[7], because they share many similarities such as lymphadenopathy, hepatosplenomegaly, pulmonary infiltrates, anaemia,

eosinophilia, elevated levels of angiotensin converting enzyme (ACE) and cutaneous anergy. However, children with sarcoidosis are prone to eye involvement, arthritis and hypergammaglobulinaemia, and they do not have a predisposition to infections.

The mechanism of granuloma formation in combined immunodeficiencies is not understood. In other granulomatous disorders, T-cell derived cytokines (interferon gamma, interleukins 2, 4 and 5) have been shown to play a major role, and it is likely that T-cell subsets imbalance or abnormal T-cell response to stimuli is responsible. This may explain why corticosteroid treatment often results in clinical improvement[6]. Much care, however, should be taken before giving corticosteroids to a child with immunodeficiency.

Genetics

Although the disorder is often familial, no mode of inheritance has been defined and males and females are equally affected. This is due to the fact that there are at least five subgroups of CVID based on B-cell function as well as numerous T-cell associated defects[8]. There is a high incidence of connective diseases like lupus erythematosus, haemolytic anaemia and idiopathic thrombocytopenic purpura in first-degree relatives[9]. HLA association, as in IgA deficiency, has been described.

Differential diagnosis

Acquired cases following viral infection such as congenital rubella or hepatitis B have been described.

Treatment

The treatment of common variable immunodeficiency is similar to that of X-linked agammaglobulinaemia, i.e. intravenous gamma-globulins. Adverse reactions during infusions are more common than in the latter, presumably because of the formation of isoantibodies[10].

References

1 Preud'homme JL, Griscelli C, Seligmann M. Immunoglobulins on the surface of lymphocytes in fifty patients with primary immuno-deficiency disease. *Clin Immunol Immunopath* 1973; **1**: 241–56.

2 Hausser c, Virelizier JL, Burlot D, Griscelli C. Common variable hypogammaglobulinemia in children. *Am J Dis Child* 1983; **137**: 833–7.

3 Cunningham-Rundles C. Clinical and immunogical analysis of 103 patients with common variable immunodeficiency. *J Clin Immunol* 1989; **9**: 22–33.

4 Conley ME, Park CL, Douglas SD. Childhood common variable immunodeficiency with autoimmune disease. *J Pediatr* 1986; **108**: 915–22.

5 Rosen FS. The primary immunodeficiencies: dermatologic manifestations. *J Invest Dermatol* 1976; **67**: 402–11.
6 Siegfried EC, Prose NS, Friedman NJ, Paller AS. Cutaneous granulomas in children with combined immunodeficiency. *J Am Acad Dermatol* 1991; **25**: 761–6.
7 Clark SK. Sarcoidosis in children. *Pediatr Dermatol* 1987; **4**: 291–9.
8 Spickett GP, Webster ADB, Farrant J. Cellular abnormalities in common variable immunodeficiency. *Immunodef Rev* 1990; **2**: 199–213.
9 Rosen FS, Cooper MD, Wedgewood RJP. The primary immunodeficiencies. *New Engl J Med* 1984; **311**: 235–44, 300–10 (two parts).
10 Ammann AJ, Ashman RF, Buckley RH et al. Use of intravenous gamma-globulin in antibody immunodeficiency: results of a multicenter controlled trial. *Clin Immunol Immunopath* 1982; **22**: 60–7.

Selective immunoglobulin deficiencies

Selective immunoglobulin deficiencies are characterized by a deficiency of one or several immunoglobulin classes, while the others remain normal or are even elevated.

Deficiency of IgA

Definition

Deficiency of IgA, the most common primary immunodeficiency, is a very heterogeneous clinical disorder which may be associated with a variety of infections, allergies, autoimmune disorders, gastrointestinal disorders and genetic disorders. Its frequency varies greatly in different population groups, being found in 1 in every 500–700 Caucasians, which is more than 20 times the frequency in Japan. The disease is usually defined as a serum IgA concentration of less than 0.05 g/l, and in most cases there is a lack of the two subclasses (IgA1 and IgA2) in both the serum and the secretory fluids[1].

Clinical features

The clinical expression of IgA deficiency is highly variable. Many affected individuals have no obvious health problems, while others may have severe disease. Infections do occur in IgA deficiency, but are much more frequent when there is an associated deficiency of the IgG subclasses 2 and/or 4. The most common sites of infections are the upper and lower respiratory tract, and the urinary tract[2]. Other clinical features of IgA deficiency include coeliac disease with an increased risk of cancer, atopy and autoimmune disorders. The last two complications are of interest to the dermatologist. In the atopic population the prevalence of IgA deficiency is 1 in 200–400, i.e. twice that in the normal population. This association may reflect an associated T-cell dysregulation and

seems unrelated to the absence of secretory IgA[3]. The cutaneous findings of the IgA deficiency-associated collagen-vascular diseases are indistinguishable from those of lupus erythematosus[4].

Pathology

In most IgA-deficient patients, there is an arrest in the B-cell differentiation pathway. Plasma IgA-producing cells are absent from the circulation, whereas immature IgA-bearing B cells are normally present. On this basis, it has been proposed that IgA deficiency and CVID may represent opposite ends of a disease spectrum caused by a single underlying genetic defect. In rare cases, the defect lies in the absence of the secretory component of the immunoglobulin.

Genetics

There is a clear linkage of genetic susceptibility to IgA deficiency with particular major histocompatibility complex (MHC) haplotypes, but the putative IgA deficiency gene remains to be located. Environmental factors do play a role[1].

Differential diagnosis

An IgA deficiency may precede by several years the development of a global immunoglobulin deficiency. A reversible, selective IgA deficiency can be induced by phenytoin and penicillamine[5].

Treatment

Intravenous infusions of immunoglobulins lead to the formation of anti-IgA antibodies and severe reactions. Only selected cases of associated IgA and IgG$_2$ deficiencies may benefit from such treatment[6]. Patients with associated autoimmune, gastrointestinal or allergic diseases should be treated in the same manner as patients with normal IgA levels.

References

1 Schaffer FM, Monteiro RC, Volanakis JE, Cooper MD. Iga deficiency. *Immunodef Rev* 1991; **3**: 15–44.
2 Ugazio AG, Out TA, Plebani A et al. Recurrent infections in children with 'selective' IgA deficiency: association with IgG$_2$ and IgG$_4$ deficiency. *Birth Defects* 1983; **19**: 169–71.
3 Plebani A, Ugazio AG, Monafo V. Selective IgA deficiency: an update. *Curr Probl Dermatol* 1989; **18**: 66–78.
4 Weston WL. Cutaneous manifestations of defective host defenses. *Pediatr Clin North Am* 1977; **24**: 395–407.
5 Cooper MD, Buckley RH. Developmental immunology and the immunodeficiency diseases. *J Am Med Assoc* 1982; **248**: 2658–69.
6 Rosen FS, Cooper MD, Wedgewood RJP. The primary immunodeficiencies. *New Engl J Med* 1984; **311**: 235–44, 300–10 (two parts).

Selective deficiencies of IgG subclasses

Definition

One or more immunoglobulin G subclasses (e.g. IgG2 and IgG4) are missing in patients with selective IgG deficiencies. Selective IgG subclass deficiencies can be isolated or combined with other immune deficiencies, such as IgA deficiency, ataxia-telangiectasia, CVID, SCID, DiGeorge's syndrome or chronic mucocutaneous candidiasis.

Clinical features

Generally, affected patients present with infections commonly encountered in other defined humoral immunodeficiencies. Deficiency of IgG2 is associated mainly with respiratory tract infections due to encapsulated bacteria such as *Pneumococcus* and *Haemophilus influenzae*, and with lymphadenopathy. There is also a high frequency (12.5%) of skin and/or visceral vasculitis. Deficiency of IgG3 may lead to various infections, frequently enteral and usually milder than in IgG2 deficiency.

Pathology

The defects involve the gene rearrangement process required for the terminal differentiation of the B-cell line. There is some evidence that the expression of subclasses whose genes are located downstream in the CH locus (IgG2 and IgG4) requires more T-cell help than the upstream isotypes (IgG1–IgG3), hence the more common finding of IgG2–4 deficiency in defects characterized by a predominant T-cell defect[1].

Genetics

The genetic background of this group of conditions remains unclear.

Differential diagnosis

It should be pointed out that hypergammaglobulinaemia does not preclude the presence of a subclass deficiency, and that investigation of children with high levels of IgG and features of immunodeficiency should include IgG subclass analysis[2]. The finding of an IgG subclass deficiency in a patient also requires further immunological studies in the search for an associated defect.

Treatment

The management of these patients does not differ from the management of other patients with selective immunoglobulin deficiencies[3].

References

1 Preud'homme JL, Hanson LA. IgG subclass deficiency. *Immunodef Rev* 1990; **2**: 129–49.
2 Shield JPH, Strobel S, Levinsky RJ, Morgan G. Immunodeficiency presenting as hypergammaglobulinemia with IgG2 subclass deficiency. *Lancet* 1992; **340**: 448–50.
3 Oxelius VA. IgG subclass levels in infancy and childhood. *Acta Paed Scand* 1979; **68**: 23–7.

Selective IgM deficiency

Definition

Selective IgM deficiency is an extremely rare disease characterized by very low serum IgM levels and normal levels of the other serum immunoglobulins[1].

Clinical features

Infections such as otitis media, sinusitis, bronchitis, pneumonia, meningitis, septicaemia and periorbital cellulitis are prominent. The most common causative micro-organisms are pneumococci, *Haemophilus influenzae*, meningococci and staphylococci; but tuberculosis and disseminated molluscum contagiosum have been described in this setting. An eczematoid eruption may occur.

Pathology

The immunological defect is considered to be at the plasma cell differentiation stage; T-cell factors or dysfunction may also be involved.

Genetics

Various types of dysgammaglobulinaemia in the relatives of patients with deficient IgM have been reported, suggesting the existence of inherited mechanisms in IgM deficiency.

Differential diagnosis

Patients with gluten enteropathy may develop secondary IgM deficiency that resolves with the introduction of a gluten-free diet[2].

Treatment

Early and vigorous antibiotic treatment is recommended to avoid fatal septicaemia[3].

References

1 Hobbs JR. Selective IgM deficiency. *Birth Defects* 1975; **11**: 112–16.
2 Hobbs JR, Hepner GW. Deficiency of γM-globulin in coeliac disease. *Lancet* 1976; **i**: 217–20.
3 Buckley RH. Immunodeficiency. *J Allerg Clin Immunol* 1983; **72**: 627–41.

Immunoglobulin deficiency with increased IgM

Definition

Immunoglobulin deficiency with increased IgM is characterized by low IgG and IgA levels, and normal to increased levels of polyclonal IgM. Cellular immunity is altered in the X-linked form.

Clinical features

Affected children have a high prevalence of recurrent upper respiratory tract infections, pneumonia, otitis, stomatitis, diarrhoea and neoplasms. Major dermatological features are atopic dermatitis, recurrent pyodermas and intractable viral warts. Lymphoid hyperplasia and neutropenia are common. In contrast to X-linked agammaglobulinaemia, patients with immunodeficiency with increased IgM levels are not prone to severe enteroviral infections nor to severe dissemination of live attenuated vaccines, but they present an increased frequency of opportunistic infections, including *Pneumocystis carinii* pneumonia.

Pathology

The defect originates from an impairment of the immunoglobulin heavy-chain class switch of B lymphocytes, from IgM to IgG or IgA production. Whether the deficit is intrinsic to the heavy-chain class switch mechanism or dependent on a switch-inducing factor produced by T lymphocytes is controversial[1].

Genetics

The X-linked form of the disorder has been linked to mutations of the CD40 ligand on T cells[2]. Autosomal recessive and autosomal dominant traits occur, indicating a genetic heterogeneity. Carrier detection by analysis of X-chromosome inactivation or by linkage analysis is insufficiently reliable for genetic counselling. Mutation analysis is, however, reliable.

Differential diagnosis

Acquired forms of the syndrome have been described, allegedly caused by congenital rubella.

Treatment

Because patients do not secrete IgG antibodies, replacement therapy with intravenous immunoglobulins is possible, and may correct to some extent the lymphoid hyperplasia and serum IgM levels[3].

References

1 Notarangelo LD, Duse M, Ugazio AG. Immunodeficiency with hyper-IgM (HIM). *Immunodef Rev* 1992; **3**: 101–22.
2 Callard RE, Armitage RJ, Fanslow WC, Spriggs MK. CD40 ligand and its role in X-linked hyper IgM syndrome. *Immunol Today* 1993; **14**: 559–64.
3 Buckley RH. Immunodeficiency. *J Allerg Clin Immunol* 1983; **72**: 627–41.

Cellular (T-cell) immune deficiency disorders

DiGeorge's anomaly

Definition

The DiGeorge's anomaly (DGA) is known to be a developmental field defect in which pharyngeal pouch derivatives do not arise, leading to congenital hypoplasia or aplasia of the thymus and parathyroid glands, with resulting immunodeficiency and hypoparathyroidism. It is commonly separated into partial (75%) and complete (25%) DGA; the complete form requires correction of the immunodeficiency.

Clinical features

Hypocalcaemia, facial malformations and conotruncal heart malformations (interrupted aortic arch type B or truncus arteriosus) are frequently found in the neonatal period, followed by development of a syndrome that ranges from mildly abnormal susceptibility to infections to full-blown severe combined immunodeficiency. The severity of the immune defect parallels the degree of hypoplasia of affected tissues. Thus, some children never suffer life-threatening infections (incomplete DiGeorge's syndrome) while others are readily infected by low-grade pathogens or opportunistic agents such as fungi and *Pneumocystis carinii*, and develop graft-versus-host disease as a result of non-irradiated blood product transfusions.

Pathology

DiGeorge's anomaly is an embryopathy, caused by dysmorphogenesis of the pharyngeal pouches because of inadequate neural crest contributions. The anomaly may result from teratogens, mendelian disorders, cytogenetic abnormalities or rare syndromes such as Kallmann's syndrome or CHARGE association (Coloboma, Heart defect, Atresia of the choanae, Retardation of growth, Genital anomalies, Ear abnormalities)[1].

Genetics

Most cases of DGA are sporadic. However, autosomal dominant transmission seems more frequent than previously thought, with or without chromosomal abnormalities (usually involving chromosome 22)[2].

Differential diagnosis

A high degree of diagnostic certainty can be achieved with a criteria scale[1]. Specific tests required are parathyroid, cardiac, chromosome and immune system assessments. Numbers of T cells are decreased in the peripheral blood as well as in lymphoid tissues. In contrast, there is an increased number of B cells. The T-cell functions are absent or diminished, depending on the gravity of the thymic abnormalities. These functions should be assessed by non-specific T-cell mitogenic stimulation tests and by intradermal delayed hypersensitivity response. As a general rule, levels of serum immunoglobulins are normal for age, but low levels of IgA may be present and IgE levels may be elevated.

Treatment

Hypoparathyroidism is managed with calcium supplements, vitamin D administration and a low-phosphorus diet. Life-threatening cardiac malformations should be corrected surgically prior to correction of the immune deficit. Patients should receive trimethoprim–sulphamethoxazole (co-trimoxazole) prophylaxis and live vaccines should not be given. In complete DGA, thymus transplantation and bone marrow transplantation from an HLA-matched sibling are the two alternatives for therapy.

References

1 Hong R. The Di George anomaly. *Immunodef Rev* 1991; **3**: 1–14.
2 Keppen LD, Fasules JW, Burks AW et al. Confirmation of autosomal dominant transmission of the Di George malformation complex. *J Pediatr* 1988; **113**: 506–8.

Severe combined immunodeficiencies

Definition

Severe combined immunodeficiencies (SCID) represent a heterogeneous group of diseases characterized by a profound defect in either T-cell differentiation or function. Classical SCID syndromes include adenosine deaminase (ADA) deficiency, reticular dysgenesis, X-linked SCID and alymphocytosis. By extension, various qualitative T-cell deficiencies have been described as SCID; these include Omenn's syndrome, immunodeficiency with short-limbed dwarfism, purine nucleoside phosphorylase (PNP) deficiency, and T-cell deficiencies with defective membrane receptor expression. More recently, several activation disorders have been added to the list. Classification of SCID disorders is likely to be modified with the increasing characterization of new variants[1].

This chapter describes the common features of typical SCID disorders and particular aspects of the best-defined forms of the syndrome, with emphasis on genetic and pathological mechanisms.

Clinical features

Infants with severe combined immunodeficiency usually become ill during the first few months of life. Failure to thrive is a prominent feature, accompanied by a characteristic triad of extensive mucocutaneous candidiasis, *Pneumocystis carinii* pneumonia and intractable diarrhoea. It should be noted, however, that the association of erythroderma, failure to thrive and diarrhoea in infancy is not specific to any particular type of immune defect[2] (see Omenn's syndrome, below).

Graft-versus-host disease, due to transplacental passage of maternal lymphocytes, is commonly seen. More frequently, graft-versus-host disease represents an accidental complication of the therapeutic transfusion of non-irradiated blood products. In some instances, its manifestations are limited to a morbilliform exanthem with an onset in the few weeks following birth, which resolves leaving hyperpigmentation. In other cases, the skin manifestations can be more severe, acute (toxic epidermal necrolysis) or chronic with widespread lesions resembling lichen planus or erythroderma (see Omenn's syndrome, below). The relationship between SCID and graft-versus-host disease is a complex one, since according to Pollack et al[3] certain features of the autosomal recessive form of the syndrome might be the result of early intra-uterine non-lethal graft-versus-host disease.

Affected infants are very susceptible to infections due to viruses of the herpes group, such as varicella, herpes simplex and cytomegalovirus. Measles also has a high mortality, because of the occurrence of Hecht's pneumonia.

Vaccination with live material has catastrophic results – BCG vaccination invariably leads to fatal disseminated infection.

Pathology

The SCID syndromes are characterized histologically by a profound hypoplasia of secondary lymphoid organs. The thymus gland displays endodermal cells that have not become lymphoid, and no Hassall's corpuscles are found. The bone marrow is also devoid of lymphoid cells, and lymph node biopsy (when feasible) reveals only an uninhabited stroma. These changes are present in all forms of SCID and are helpful in the diagnosis of this syndrome, but not in differentiating its various aetiologies.

Genetics

About 50% of SCID patients have the X-linked form. All other deficiencies have an autosomal recessive inheritance. Overall, 70–80% of patients with SCID are male. Specific known genetic abnormalities are discussed below. Prenatal diagnosis by means of enzymatic, immunological or genetic determination is currently available for ADA/PNP deficiencies, alymphocytosis, reticular dysgenesis, SCID with B cells, MHC class II deficiency and X-linked SCID[1,4].

Differential diagnosis

Where SCID is suspected, its characterization is usually achieved by a combination of immunological, enzymatic and genetic studies.

Treatment

Neither antibiotic therapy nor gamma-globulin administration is of any help in severe combined immunodeficiency. Successful treatment in more than 75% of SCID patients is currently achieved by bone marrow grafting[5]. It must be remembered that if transfusion of blood products is needed, these must be irradiated in order to avoid the development of graft-versus-host disease.

References

1 Fisher A. Severe combined immunodeficiencies. *Immunodef Rev* 1992; **3**: 82–100.
2 Glover MT, Atherton DJ, Levinsky RJ. Syndrome of erythroderma, failure to thrive, and diarrhea in infancy: a manifestation of immunodeficiency. *Pediatrics* 1988; **81**: 66–72.
3 Pollack MS, Kirkpatrick D, Kapoor N, Dupont B, O'Reilly RG. Identification by HLA typing of intra-uterine-derived maternal T cells in four patients with severe combined immunodeficiency. *New Engl J Med* 1982; **307**: 662–6.
4 Durandy A, Dumez Y, Guy-Grand D et al. Prenatal diagnosis of severe combined immunodeficiency. *J Pediatr* 1982; **101**: 995–7.
5 Thomas ED. Marrow transplantation for nonmalignant disorders. *New Engl J Med* 1985; **312**: 46–8.

Adenosine deaminase deficiency

Definition

Severe combined immunodeficiency caused by a deficiency of adenosine deaminase was described in 1972 by Giblett et al[1]. Adenosine deaminase is a major enzyme of the salvage pathway for purine synthesis.

Clinical features

Although cellular immunity is more deeply impaired than humoral immunity (immunoglobulins may be absent or present in reduced levels), the clinical manifestations are similar to those of other forms of severe combined immunodeficiency. In addition, a non-specific pseudochondrodysplasia may be present.

Pathology

Florid pathological changes are primarily restricted to the immune system and appear to result from the accumulation of substrates (deoxyadenosine) and metabolites (deoxy-ATP)[2]. The direct interaction between ADA and the T-cell activation antigen CD26 may also be disturbed[3].

Genetics

Adenosine deaminase deficiency is responsible for half the cases of autosomal recessive SCID. Patients are homozygous for a mutant adenosine deaminase gene, located on chromosome 20. The gene has been sequenced and cloned. The activity of the enzyme is diminished in the red cells of heterozygotes, who can therefore be readily detected.

Differential diagnosis

No adenosine deaminase activity can be detected in patients' red cells. Chronic villous sampling (CVS) permits prenatal diagnosis of the disorder. Deficiency of ADA can also result in a much later onset and milder immunodeficiency.

Treatment

The treatment of choice is bone marrow transplantation from a histocompatible donor. Enzyme replacement, using polyethylene glycol, has been successful, but long-term efficacy remains to be evaluated[4]. Finally, the most exciting alternative treatment is gene therapy, which was first tried in two ADA patients[5].

References

1 Giblett ER, Anderson JE, Cohen F, Pollara B, Meuwissen HJ. Adenosine-deaminase deficiency in two patients with severely impaired cellular immunity. *Lancet* 1982; **ii**: 1067–9.
2 Hischhorn R. Adenosine deaminase deficiency. *Immunol Rev* 1990; **2**: 153–98.
3 Kameoka J, Tanaka T, Nojima Y, Schlossman SF, Morimoto C. Direct association of adenosine deaminase with a T cell activation antigen, CD 26. *Science* 1993; **261**: 466–9.

4 Hershfield MS, Buckley RH, Greenberg MI et al. Treatment of adenosine deaminase deficiency with polyethylene glycol-modified adenosine deaminase. *New Engl J Med* 1987; **316**: 589–96.
5 Culver KW, Osborne WRA, Miller AD et al. Correction of ADA deficiency in human T lymphocytes using retroviral-mediated gene transfer. *Transpl Proc* 1991; **23**: 170–1.

Reticular dysgenesis

Definition

Reticular dysgenesis is a rare disorder, considered to be the most severe form of SCID. Patients completely lack both cellular and humoral immunity (alymphocytosis) as well as myeloid cells. The underlying abnormality remains to be elucidated. Many cases may in fact represent severe maternal graft–versus–host disease.

Genetics

Transmission is autosomal recessive[1].

Differential diagnosis

Reticular dysgenesis should be distinguished from alymphocytosis with neutropenia (due to infection or drug toxicity).

Reference

1 Fisher A. Severe combined immunodeficiencies. *Immunodef Rev* 1992; **3**: 82–100.

X-Linked severe combined immunodeficiency

Definition

This disease is the most frequent phenotype (50%) in classical SCID, and is characterized by an absence of mature T cells, while B cells are present in the blood.

Genetics

The X-linked SCID gene has been localized on the Xq13 region and corresponds to the interleukin-2 receptor gamma-chain. Mutation of this gene dramatically interferes with the thymic maturation of T cells[1].

Reference

1 Noguchi M, Yi H, Rosenblatt HM et al. Interleukin-2 receptor γ chain mutation results in X-linked severe combined immunodeficiency in humans. *Cell* 1993; **73**: 147–57.

Alymphocytosis

Definition

Twenty-five per cent of patients with typical SCID show the absence of T and B lymphocytes, although ADA activity is detectable.

Pathology

Lymphopenia is present but not total since natural killer (NK) cells are present and functional. This phenotype seems to correspond closely to the mouse model of SCID, and tentative explanation of the defect involves the recombinase system.

Genetics

Transmission is autosomal recessive; the molecular basis of this disorder involves defects in the recombination activating genes (RAG).

Omenn's syndrome

Definition

In 1965, Omenn reported an 'extraordinary kindred in which 12 infants, in 6 sibships, have died from disease of the reticuloendothelial system with eosinophilia'[1]. The syndrome is now considered to be an autosomal recessive form of combined immunodeficiency.

Clinical features

Omenn reported that 'in these children, a widespread skin eruption, followed by hepatosplenomegaly, generalized lymphadenopathy, eosinophilia, and a febrile illness, has developed in the first weeks of life, with poor growth, progressing inexorably to a fatal outcome within two to six months'[1]. Since the original description, more than 20 infants with SCID have been reported to have Omenn's or an Omenn-like syndrome. It is important to point out that the cutaneous lesions, mainly erythroderma, represent the initial sign of the disease (Figure 18.1).

Erythroderma, as a presenting feature of combined immunodeficiency, is highly heterogeneous in its clinical aspect, as described below.

1. In Omenn-like cases, erythroderma has been depicted as a widespread desquamative erythematous rash that may resemble seborrhoeic dermatitis or atopic dermatitis, but is usually typical of neither[2]. The rash may stay erythematous and scaly, or progress to an infiltrated skin, which then takes on a pachydermal aspect. Alopecia is commonly associated.

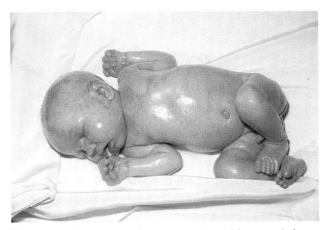

Figure 18.1 *Omenn's syndrome presenting with congenital erythroderma (courtesy of Dr J. Harper)*

2. Leiner's syndrome represents the association of generalized erythroderma, failure to thrive and diarrhoea in an infant. Here, the cutaneous lesions resemble seborrhoeic dermatitis. The disorder was originally attributed to nutritional factors in fully breast-fed infants, and then to C5 dysfunction associated with a yeast opsonization defect. It is now considered to be a common presentation of various underlying immunodeficiencies[3], and most authors therefore prefer to abandon the term 'Leiner's syndrome' (for references on this syndrome, see under complement deficiencies, page 306).

Pathology

Omenn's syndrome is a manifestation of a combined immunodeficiency in all described patients, but the immunodeficiencies involved are heterogeneous, as are the histopathological findings[2]. In the same way, several mechanisms have been suggested to be responsible for the syndrome. They include (maternal) graft-versus-host disease[4], infiltration of a population of T cells with either a unique phenotype[5] or a small clonality[6], and lack of T-helper cell factor[7]. Being the clinical manifestation of various underlying immunodeficiencies, the erythroderma in Omenn-like syndromes may hypothetically represent the result of the accumulation of cytotoxic T cells, whether the latter are of maternal (allogenic), autoimmune or proliferative origin.

Genetics

The disorder is autosomal recessive. Association with typical alymphocytosis has been described in a family, and with cartilage–hair hypoplasia in a patient.

References

1 Omenn GS. Familial reticuloendotheliosis with eosinophilia. *New Engl J Med* 1965; **273**: 427–32.
2 Liorente CP, Amoros JI, Ortiz de Frutos FJ et al. Cutaneous lesions in severe combined immunodeficiency: two case reports and a review of the literature. *Pediatr Dermatol* 1991; **8**: 314–21.
3 Glover MT, Atherton DJ, Levinsky RJ. Syndrome of erythroderma, failure to thrive, and diarrhea in infancy: a manifestation of immunodeficiency. *Pediatrics* 1988; **81**: 66–72.
4 Jouan H, Le Deist F, Nezelof C. Omenn's syndrome: pathologic arguments in favor of a graft-versus-host pathogenesis. *Hum Pathol* 1987; **18**: 1101–8.
5 Pupo RA, Tyring SK, Raimer SS et al. Omenn's syndrome and related combined immunodeficiency syndromes: diagnostic considerations in infants with persistent erythroderma and failure to thrive. *J Am Acad Dermatol* 1991; **25**: 442–6.
6 De St Basile G, Le Deist F, de Villartay JP et al. Restricted heterogeneity of T lymphocytes in combined immunodeficiency with hypereosinophilia (Omenn's syndrome). *J Clin Invest* 1991; **87**: 1352–9.
7 Wyss M, von Fliedner V, Jacot-des-Combes E et al. A lymphoproliferative syndrome 'cutaneous dystrophy' and combined immunodeficiency with lack of Helper T-cell factor. *Clin Immunol Immunopath* 1982; **23**: 34–49.

Immunodeficiency with short-limbed dwarfism

Synonym: *Cartilage–hair dysplasia*

Definition

This extremely rare syndrome consists of the association of short-limbed dwarfism, a dermatosis described as ichthyosiform erythroderma with redundant skin folds, and a severe combined immune deficiency. This syndrome is also known as cartilage–hair hypoplasia[1].

Clinical features

The dwarfism is present at delivery. It involves mostly the proximal segments of the limbs. There are typical alterations of the pelvic bones, while the skull, vertebrae, hands and feet are normal. The cutaneous manifestations are skin infections (due to the immunodeficiency) and abnormalities in skin, hair and nails. Redundant skin folds are characteristic. Ichthyosiform erythroderma was present in at least two patients. The hair, eyelashes and eyebrows are sparse, fine and clear. Under the microscope, the diameter of the hair shaft is reduced and the central core is absent. With age, alopecia often ensues. The nails are abnormally short but have normal width. Anaemia is also frequent[2].

The classic complications of severe combined immunodeficiency are present, but less severe immunodeficiencies, predominating in either humoral or cellular immunity, occur in attenuated forms of the syndrome.

Pathology

The defect underlying all aspects of the syndrome may be a disturbance of the cell cycle involving the G_1 phase, but this remains hypothetical. Histologically, a gross disorganization of growth plates explains the micromelic dwarfism. The skin lesions seem to be related to a degeneration of elastin in the connective tissue. The immune system shows the pathologic findings typical of severe combined immune deficiency.

Genetics

Owing to the rarity of the disease, most reports concern sporadic cases. The initial cases, however, were described in the endogamous Amish community, where the existence of attenuated forms of the disease has been described. Therefore, the mode of inheritance is believed to be autosomal recessive with variable penetrance[3].

Differential diagnosis

Achondroplasia is often considered; its inheritance as a dominant trait and the different radiologic appearance of the pelvis rule out this diagnosis. Skeletal abnormalities and severe combined immune deficiency are suggestive of adenosine deaminase deficiency; again, the radiological lesions are different in this disorder. The ADA activity was assessed in one case of short-limbed dwarfism, and was found to be normal.

Treatment

The occurrence of autoimmune disorders may worsen the prognosis. Supportive treatment may be sufficient. Bone marrow transplantation, as the treatment of choice, is ethically problematic since the dwarfism is persistent[4].

References

1 Lux SE, Johnston RB, August CS et al. Chronic neutropenia and abnormal cellular immunity in cartilage hair hypoplasia. *New Engl J Med* 1970; **282**: 234–6.
2 Mäkitie O, Kaitila I. Cartilage-hair hypoplasia – clinical manifestations in 108 Finnish patients. *Eur J Pediatr* 1993; **152**: 211–17.
3 Brennan TE, Pearson RW. Abnormal elastic tissue in cartilage-hair hypoplasia. *Arch Dermatol* 1988; **124**: 1411–14.
4 Rubie H, Graber D, Fisher A et al. Hypoplasie du cartilage et des cheveux avec déficit immunitaire complet. *Ann Pédiatr* 1989; **36**: 390–2.

Purine nucleoside phosphorylase deficiency

Definition

Purine nucleoside phosphorylase is the enzyme distal to adenosine deaminase in the purine salvage pathway. Its defect also causes immunodeficiency[1].

Clinical features

Apart from infections, two-thirds of the patients have evidence of neurological disorders, and one-third develop autoimmune disorders, mainly haemolytic anaemia[2].

Pathology

The T cells seem to be more sensitive than B cells to deoxyguanosine, a metabolite that particularly accumulates in purine nucleoside phosphorylase deficiency.

Genetics

This enzymatic defect is an autosomal recessive disease. Heterozygotes display abnormally low activity of the enzyme in their red cells.

The gene has been cloned and is localized on chromosome 14.

Differential diagnosis

The number of T cells is extremely low, whereas the number of B cells as well as the immunoglobulin levels are within the normal range. There is no measurable PNP activity in the patients' red blood cells. Adenosine deaminase activity is normal. Other very rare metabolic disturbances may cause a similar syndrome and should be ruled out. These are hereditary orotic aciduria[3] and hereditary transcobalamin II deficiency[4].

Treatment

Bone marrow transplantation has been successful in treating this disorder.

References

1 Giblett ER, Ammann AJ, Wara DW, Sandman R, Diamond LK. Nucleoside phosphorylase deficiency in a child with severely defective T-cell immunity and normal B-cell immunity. *Lancet* 1975; **i**: 1010–13.
2 Markert ML. Purine nucleoside phosphorylase deficiency. *Immunodef Rev* 1992; **3**: 45–81.
3 Girot R, Hamet M, Perignon J-L. Cellular immune deficiency in two siblings with hereditary orotic aciduria. *New Engl J Med* 1983; **308**: 700–4.

4 Hitzig WH, Dohmann U, Pluss J, Vischer D. Hereditary transcobalamin II deficiency: clinical findings in a new family. *J Pediatr* 1974; **85**: 622–8.

T-Cell deficiencies with defective membrane receptor expression

Definition

The deficiencies described here are characterized by deficient expression of membrane proteins. Typical of this group is the bare lymphocyte syndrome. Other defects include low TCR/CD3 complex expression and depletion of CD8+ or CD4+ T cells.

Pathology

In the bare lymphocyte syndrome, the class II HLA antigens (HLA-DP, DQ and DR) may be the only defective proteins, or in addition the class I HLA antigens (HLA-A and HLA-B) and the beta-2-microglobulin are also defective. The HLA genes are present on chromosome 6, but corresponding mRNA is found in greatly reduced amounts. Thus, the basic anomaly in this disease appears to be defective regulation of HLA gene transcription[1].

Genetics

Severe combined immunodeficiency syndrome with defective expression of HLA is an autosomal recessive disorder. Although the cause of the disorder lies in abnormal regulation of HLA gene expression, the complex mechanisms of this regulation still remain to be elucidated.

Differential diagnosis

The presence of severe immunodeficiency with HLA-negative lymphocytes, using the usual immunofluorescence techniques to determine the HLA phenotype, defines the bare lymphocyte syndrome[2].

Treatment

Bone marrow transplantation presents more difficulties than in other forms of severe combined immunodeficiencies, owing to the absence of expression of HLA antigens. This makes classic HLA typing uninformative. Instead, molecular biology techniques must be applied to perform HLA genotyping, in order to make therapeutic decisions regarding bone marrow transplantation[3].

References

1 De Préval C, Hadam MR, Mach B. Regulation of genes for HLA class II antigens in cell lines from patients with severe combined immunodeficiency. *New Engl J Med* 1988; **318**: 1295–1300.

2 Griscelli C, Lisowska-Grospierre B, Le Deist F et al. Combined immunodeficiency with abnormal expression of MHC class II genes. *Clin Immunol Immunopath* 1989; **50** (suppl.): 140–8.

3 Marcadet A, Cohen D, Dausset J et al. Genotyping with DNA probes in combined immunodeficiency syndrome with defective expression of HLA. *New Engl J Med* 1985; **312**: 1287–92.

T-Cell immunodeficiency due to defective T-cell activation

Definition

As our understanding of the pathophysiology of the immune system is increasing, new disorders are characterized. They include defective production of interleukin 1 and interleukin 2, and NF-AT disorders[1,2].

References

1 Fisher A. Severe combined immunodeficiencies. *Immunodef Rev* 1992; **3**: 82–100.

2 Matsumoto S, Sakiyama Y, Ariga T, Gallagher R, Taguchi Y. Progress in primary immunodeficiency. *Immunol Today* 1992; **13**: 4–5.

Ataxia-telangiectasia

Definition

Three types of apparently unrelated abnormalities are associated in ataxia-telangiectasia: cerebellar ataxia, mucocutaneous telangiectasias and combined immunodeficiency.

Clinical features

The first symptoms of cerebellar ataxia appear in the second or third year of life. They parallel an important decrease in the number of Purkinje cells. Later, other neurological defects may appear such as choreoathetosis, nystagmus, extrapyramidal signs, posterior columns involvement and mental retardation.

Telangiectasias are especially prominent on the bulbar conjunctivae (Figure 18.2), which deserve close examination when the diagnosis is considered. Other mucosal telangiectasias do occur, and epistaxis is then a feature. Cutaneous lesions are more prominent on areas of skin exposed to sun and wind, with a 'butterfly' distribution on the face and a predilection for the dorsal aspects of the hands and feet, but the antecubital and popliteal fossae are also often involved. These lesions consist of fine, star-shaped clusters of vessels that usually develop later than the ataxia. Progeric skin changes are a significant clinical

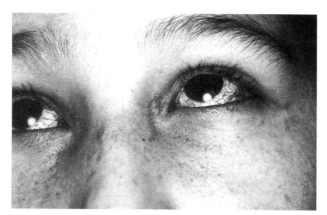

Figure 18.2 *Telangiectasia on the conjunctivae in a child with ataxia-telangiectasia*

Genetics

Ataxia-telangiectasia is transmitted as an autosomal recessive trait. Mapping with DNA polymorphisms has localized the predominant mutation to chromosome 11q22–23 and the gene responsible has recently been identified [4]. Designated *ATM*(*AT* mutated), the gene encodes a product similar to several yeast and mammalian phosphatidylinositol-3-prime kinases that are involved in mitogenic signal transduction, meiotic recombination, and cell cycle control. An abnormal chromosomal instability following ionizing radiation is also found in heterozygotes, who represent as much as 1% of the population. These people have an increased risk of cancer, particularly breast cancer in women [5]. Cloning of the involved alleles will assist prenatal diagnosis and carrier detection.

finding and are related to undue sensitivity to ultra-violet radiation. These changes consist of a poikilodermatous appearance, initially described by Louis-Bar as *café au lait* spots. In addition, some patients develop an eczematoid dermatitis and cutaneous granulomatous lesions [1].

The combined immunodeficiency is partial but progressive. Low serum levels of IgA are observed in 50% of cases, often accompanied by a defect in the IgG2 and IgG4 subclasses. In a small percentage of cases, total IgG deficiency is observed. Levels of IgM are normal or elevated [2]. The cellular defect is characterized by progressive lymphopenia and lymphoid hypoplasia. This immunodeficiency accounts for the recurrent bacterial infections in the respiratory tract and the ear, nose and throat, with the secondary development of bronchiectasia. Pneumonia is the leading cause of death. The digestive tract is relatively spared in ataxia-telangiectasia. Severe impetigo and treatment-resistant forms of mucosal and cutaneous candidiasis are common. Autoimmune manifestations are frequent. An important feature of the syndrome is the high incidence of cancers, especially lymphomas. Cancers are the immediate cause of death in up to 10% of affected patients. Other disorders may be present, e.g. gonadic hypoplasia and a peculiar form of insulin-resistant diabetes mellitus.

Pathology

There is a high incidence of cancers as well as an increased sensitivity of lymphoid and undifferentiated mesenchymal cells to ionizing radiations in ataxia-telangiectasia. These observations point to a defect in the DNA repair mechanism as the basis of the multisystem abnormalities that characterize the disease [3]. The increased ratio of γ/δ-bearing T cells to α/β-bearing T cells may reflect an added recombinational defect.

Differential diagnosis

Ataxia-telangiectasia may be difficult to diagnose before the syndrome complex becomes complete, and this may take years. Careful ophthalmologic examination, thorough screening of the immune functions and a karyotype or, if available, study of the chromosomal sensitivity of cultured skin fibroblasts to ionizing radiations are warranted. An elevated level of alpha-fetoprotein argues in favour of the diagnosis.

Treatment

Only symptomatic treatment can be offered to affected patients, and in most cases they do not survive to adulthood [6].

References

1 Paller AS, Massey RB, Curtis MA et al. Cutaneous granulomatous lesions in patients with ataxia-telangiectasia. *J Pediatr* 1991; **119**: 917–22.

2 Rivat-Pérant L, Buriot D, Salier JP et al. Immunoglobulins in ataxia-telangiectasia: evidence for IgG₄ and IgA₂ subclass deficiencies. *Clin Immunol Immunopath* 1981; **20**: 99–110.

3 Hischhorn R. Metabolic defects and immunodeficiency disorders. *New Engl J Med* 1983; **308**: 714–16.

4 Savitsky K, Bar-Shira A, Gilad S et al. A single ataxia-telangiectasia gene with a product similar to P1-3 kinase. *Science* 1995; **268**: 1749–53.

5 Swift M, Morell D, Massey RB, Chase CL. Incidence of cancer in 161 families affected by ataxia-telangiectasia. *New Engl J Med* 1991; **325**: 1831–6.

6 Smith LL, Conerly SL. Ataxia-telangiectasia or Louis-Bar syndrome. *J Am Acad Dermatol* 1985; **12**: 681–96.

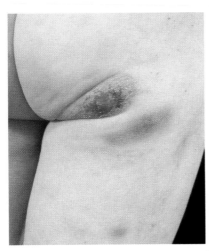

Figure 18.3 *Wiskott–Aldrich syndrome in a young child with eczema and bruising*

Wiskott–Aldrich syndrome

Definition

The triad of atopic dermatitis, thrombocytopenic purpura and undue susceptibility to infections clinically characterizes the Wiskott–Aldrich syndrome.

Clinical features

A haemorrhagic diathesis (usually manifesting clinically as bloody diarrhoea, as well as skin and mucosal petechial haemorrhages), eczematous dermatitis identical to atopic eczema[1] and infections develop during the first year of life (Figure 18.3). Younger patients are especially prone to infections caused by pneumococci and other bacteria that have a polysaccharide capsule. Later, agents such as *Pneumocystis carinii* and herpesviruses can be the cause of infections. Extensive warts may develop, but candidiasis is rare. Autoimmune disorders are more frequent than in the general population, Coombs' positive haemolytic anaemia and arteritis being the most common complications of this type. Despite progress in the management of Wiskott–Aldrich syndrome, the median survival is still only 6.5 years for patients born after 1964[2]. Bleeding, especially into the central nervous system, and infections are the causes of death in most instances, but malignancies account for more than 10% of fatalities. The vast majority of these malignancies are lymphoreticular tumours and leukaemias.

Pathology

Platelets are not only defective in number, but also display abnormal morphology – being less than half the normal size – as well as abnormal function. No quantitative anomaly of megakaryocytes can be demonstrated, but inefficient thrombopoiesis contributes, along with hypersplenism, to the platelet defects. An impaired humoral immune response to polysaccharide antigens is typical of the Wiskott–Aldrich syndrome. This is demonstrated by the low titres of isohaemagglutinins and failure of immunizations with polysaccharide antigens. An increased turnover of IgA, IgM and IgG leads to highly variable serum concentrations of immunoglobulins. A defect in the coupling of surface immunoglobulins on B cells to signal transduction pathways is suspected. The usual pattern consists of normal IgG, low IgM and elevated IgA and IgE levels. This abnormal metabolism explains the occurrence of transient paraproteinaemia. There is also a defect of cellular immunity, with cutaneous anergy, low numbers of circulating T lymphocytes but no imbalance of the T4/T8 ratio. The defect of cellular immunity deepens with age. This is paralleled by a gradual loss of lymphoid elements in T-dependent areas of peripheral lymphoid organs.

Genetics

The syndrome is transmitted in an X-linked fashion. The gene has been located on Xp11.22–11.3 in the following locus order: *DXS7–TIMP–(OATL1, WAS DXS255)–DXS146*[4]. Referred to as *WASP* and encoding a 501-amino acid protein, the gene was isolated using the positional cloning strategy[5]. Numerous mutations, insertions, deletions have now been reported[6].

Differential diagnosis

In a male infant with atopic dermatitis, the presence of purpuric streaks due to scratching should alert the physician to the possibility of the Wiskott–Aldrich syndrome.

Treatment

Symptomatic treatment aims at controlling the haemorrhages by platelet transfusions and/or splenectomy, and controlling infections by prophylactic infusions of immunoglobulins and antibiotic administration during acute episodes. Bone marrow transplantation is the treatment of choice in severe cases; it corrects the eczema, the immunological abnormality and the platelet defect.

References

1 Saurat JH. Eczema in primary immunodeficiencies: clues to the pathogenesis of atopic dermatitis with special reference to the Wiskott-Aldrich syndrome. *Acta Derm Venereol* 1985; **114** (suppl.): 125–8.

2 Perry GS, Spector BD, Schuman LM et al. The Wiskott–Aldrich syndrome in the United States and Canada (1892–1979). *J Pediatr* 1980; **97**: 72–8.

3 Simon HV, Mills GB, Hashimoto S et al. Evidence for defective transmembrane signalling in B cells from patients with Wiskott-Aldrich syndrome. *J Clin Invest* 1992; **90**: 1396–405.

4 Greer WL, Peacoke M, Siminovitch KA. The Wiskott-Aldrich syndrome: refinement of the localisation on Xp and identification of another closely linked marker locus, OATL-1. *Hum Genet* 1992; **88**: 453–6.

5 Derry JMJ, Ochs HD, Francke U. Isolation of novel gene mutated in Wiskott-Aldrich syndrome. *Cell* 1994; **78**: 635–44.

6 Kwan SP, Hagemann TL, Radtke BE et al. Identification of mutations in the Wiskott-Aldrich syndrome gene and characterization of a polymorphic dinucleotide repeat at DXS6940, adjacent to the disease gene. *Proc Nat Acad Sci* 1995; **92**: 4706–10.

Chronic mucocutaneous candidiasis

Definition

Chronic mucocutaneous candidiasis can be defined as a group of syndromes in which patients have an ineffective defence mechanism against *Candida*.

Clinical features

Usually the disease begins in infancy and persists into adulthood. In some cases, the onset may be delayed until after the age of 10 years. Candidiasis always affects the mouth, which assumes a chronic hyperplastic appearance. Cheilitis and painful, deeply fissured perlèche ensue. Other affected areas include the genital mucosae and the nails, with typical perionyxis. The cutaneous lesions extend in a centrifugal fashion and often display a 'glove and stocking' distribution (Figure 18.4), but any cutaneous location may be involved, including the face and scalp. Sometimes the lesions appear papillomatous and hyperplastic: this is the so-called monilial granuloma. Severe oesophageal and airways candidal infections are frequent, but septicaemia or systemic involvement remains rare. The disease is slowly progressive and does not notably affect the patient's general health. Patients may be classified into six subgroups, depending on the age of onset, the presence of associated disorders and the immunological profile[1,2].

Pathology

Cutaneous delayed hypersensitivity to *Candida* antigens is nearly always absent, and there is often total T-cell anergy. Autoimmune mechanisms are frequently responsible for associated disorders such as polyendocrinopathies. Autoantibodies to melanocytes and vitiligo have been reported in association with chronic mucocutaneous candidiasis[3].

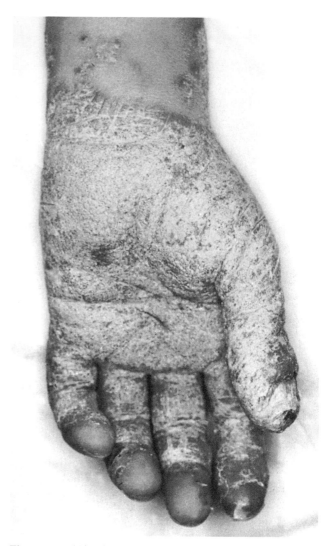

Figure 18.4 *'Glove' distribution of chronic mucocutaneous candidiasis*

Genetics

For practical purposes, chronic mucocutaneous candidiasis should be considered as an autosomal recessive disorder, although sporadic cases and even autosomal dominant inheritance have been described. This probably reflects the heterogeneity of the disorder[4].

Differential diagnosis

Potassium hydroxide examination of skin scrapings reveals mycelial elements, but cultures will ascertain the diagnosis and detect a possible superinfection with dermatophytes. Chronic candidal infection often appears as the initial manifestation in many forms of immunodeficiency with impaired T-cell function, so thorough studies of immunity should be carried out. In the same way, associated endocrinopathies, thymoma and iron deficiency should be ruled out.

Treatment

Topical and systemic administration of imidazole drugs is usually successful but the effect is transient. It does not influence the immune reactivity of the patients[5]. The newer triazoles, fluconazole and itraconazole, are also effective. Transfer factor, cimetidine and/or transfusions of intact peripheral blood leucocytes[1] are no longer used.

References

1 Kirkpatrick CH. Chronic mucocutaneous candidiasis. *Eur J Clin Microbiol Infect Dis* 1989; **8**: 448–56.
2 Mallory SB, Paller AS. Congenital immunodeficiency syndromes with cutaneous manifestations II. *J Am Acad Dermatol* 1991; **24**: 107–11.
3 Nordlung JJ, Howanitz N, Bystryn JC, Forget BM, Lerner AB. Anti-pigment-cell factors and mucocutaneous candidiasis. *Arch Dermatol* 1981; **117**: 210–12.
4 Byung IR. Chronic mucocutaneous candidiasis. *Int J Dermatol* 1988; **27**: 457–62.
5 Mobacken H, Lindholm L, Moberg S. Immunological studies in chronic mucocutaneous candidiasis before and after ketoconazole treatment. *Acta Derm Venereol* 1987; **67**: 257–60.

Hyperimmunoglobulinaemia E syndrome

Definition

The hyper-IgE syndrome is a group of specific immunodeficiency diseases of highly variable severity. The syndrome is defined by the association of recurrent bacterial infections of the skin and respiratory tract with an onset in infancy or early childhood, an extreme elevation of serum IgE levels and usually a defect of neutrophil chemotaxis. Controversy exists over the exact definition of the syndrome[1], and various clinical presentations – Job's syndrome[2], Buckley's syndrome[3] – can be united under the same heading (hyperimmunoglobulinaemia E syndrome), until the underlying defect or defects are better characterized.

Clinical features

The characteristic dermatologic abnormalities in these patients are represented by pyodermas and eczematous dermatitis, starting in infancy or early childhood. The pyodermas present as recurrent carbuncles or very deep staphylococcal 'cold' abcesses with little inflammation. They gave the name 'Job syndrome' to the disease, since affected patients resemble the biblical character who was afflicted with 'sore boils from the sole of his feet unto his crown'[2]. The eczematous dermatitis is essentially like that of atopic dermatitis; pruritic, affecting flexural surfaces, becoming lichenified, and characterized by a waxing and waning course, although superinfection may add a pustular element that modifies the clinical aspect. Other dermatological findings are chronic *Candida albicans* infections of the nails and mucosae, frequent urticaria and urticarial eruptions which often parallel episodes of active infections, and rarely ichthyosis of the ichthyosis vulgaris type. These patients also have coarse facial features and scrotal tongue.

Associated infections are common and often recurrent. They include staphylococcal pneumonia leading to pneumatoceles, otitis externa, chronic otitis media, gingivitis and sinusitis.

Pathology

Several immune abnormalities are usually found: increased levels of IgE, eosinophilia, increased levels of polyclonal IgG, IgA and IgM, decreased polymorphonuclear leucocyte function (chemotaxis), cutaneous anergy and presence of antistaphylococcal IgE. A speculative explanation of the excessive production of IgE is an imbalance of T-helper subsets (TH2) that regulate IgE production, possibly through the production of interleukin 4.

Genetics

The hyper-IgE syndrome occurs in a sporadic or autosomal dominant manner.

Differential diagnosis

There is no absolute frontier between severe atopic dermatitis and the hyper-IgE syndrome[4]. Parasitic infection, lymphocyte malignancy, T-cell disturbances and idiopathic hyperimmunoglobulinaemia E are distinguishable entities of hyper-IgE production[1].

Treatment

Currently the management of the hyper-IgE syndrome is limited to skin care (as for atopic dermatitis) and to the treatment of the infections and their complications. Treatment with H_2 antihistamines may be of help, but not on the grounds that the chemotaxis defect might be the result of elevated histamine levels[5]. An alternative in the future may be the administration of interferon gamma, since this drug has interesting effects in vitro on neutrophils from patients with Job syndrome[6].

References

1 Ring JD, Landthaler M. Hyper IgE syndromes. *Curr Probl Dermatol* 1989; **18**: 79–88.
2 Davis SD, Schaller J, Wedgewood RJ. Job's syndrome. Recurrent 'cold' staphylococcal abcesses. *Lancet* 1966; **i**: 1013–15.

3 Buckley RH, Becker WG. Abnormalities in the regulation of human IgE synthesis. *Immunol Rev* 1978; **41**: 288–314.
4 Donabedian H, Gallin JI. The hyperimmunoglobulin E recurrent infection (Job's) syndrome. A review of the NIH experience and the literature. *Medicine* 1983; **62**: 195–208.
5 Dreskin SC, Kaliner MA, Gallin JI. Elevated urinary histamine in the hyper-immunoglobulin E and recurrent infection (Job's) syndrome: association with eczematoid dermatitis and not with infection. *J Allerg Clin Immunol* 1987; **79**: 515–22.
6 Jeppson JD, Jaffe HS, Hill HR. Use of recombinant human interferon gamma to enhance neutrophil chemotactic responses in Job's syndrome of hyperimmunoglobulinemia E and recurrent infections. *J Pediatr* 1991; **118**: 383–7.

Griscelli–Prunieras syndrome

Definition

The Griscelli–Prunieras syndrome, so far described in four families, consists of a complex immunodeficiency associated with hypopigmentation.

Clinical features

Generalized hypopigmentation is present, and the hair, eyebrows and eyelashes have a peculiar silvery-grey hue. While T and B lymphocytes are present in normal numbers, both humoral and cellular immunities are profoundly disturbed, leading to various infectious complications.

Pathology

The two major features of this syndrome can be explained in terms of abnormal cell-to-cell interaction. The pigment dilution is secondary to an anomaly in the mechanism of melanosome transfer from melanocytes to keratinocytes. Similarly, a defect in the helper function of the T lymphocytes has been documented, and more generally T and B cell cooperation is impaired, thus explaining the immunodeficiency.

Genetics

Autosomal recessive transmission is postulated on the basis of the family histories of the few described cases.

Differential diagnosis

This peculiar association of anomalies resembles the Chédiak–Higashi syndrome, but the latter can easily be ruled out using a simple blood smear to demonstrate the absence of giant granules[1].

Treatment

Apart from non-specific measures, no treatment has proved satisfactory in the Griscelli–Prunieras syndrome[2].

References

1 Griscelli C, Durandy A, Guy-Grand D et al. A syndrome associating partial albinism and immunodeficiency. *Am J Med* 1978; **65**: 691–702.
2 Griscelli C. Anomalies héréditaires de l'immunité spécifiques. *Ann Nestlé* 1988; **46**: 146–59.

Phagocytic and granulocytic disorders

Chronic granulomatous disease

Definition

Neutrophils and monocytes activated during phagocytosis produce large amounts of microbicidal oxidants (e.g. superoxide, hydrogen peroxide). This process is called the phagocytic cells respiratory burst, which is catalysed by NADPH oxidase. This enzyme consists of at least four subunits. Chronic granulomatous disease is caused by defects in any of these four subunits. These defects have been extensively characterized and associated with different modes of inheritance, thus allowing a recent classification[1].

Clinical features

Clinical manifestations usually appear within the first year of life, but may be delayed until the second decade. There is increased frequency and severity of infections with catalase-positive bacteria and fungi. After the infection has been eliminated, inflammatory foci form granulomas. Skin, lung and bone are the most common infectious sites. Hepatic abscesses are a feature of chronic granulomatous disease. Chronic diarrhoea with abdominal pain can develop. Sepsis, meningitis and brain abscesses are rare[2]. Skin manifestations occur in over 70% of cases; eczematous lesions, distributed around the orifices, nose, ears or the scalp, thus resembling seborrhoeic dermatitis, are the earliest signs of the disease. Lymphadenopathies with draining sinuses (scrofulous lesions) are common in the inguinal and cervical areas. Children with this disease develop marked inflammatory and necrotic reactions in response to minor trauma, out of proportion to the initiating event. A hypodermic needle injection can induce necrotic lesions at the injection site. Granulomatous reactions can lead to the formation of firm papules around the nose, eyes and lips, and 'apple jelly' nodules of the cheeks, mimicking lupus vulgaris and sarcoidosis (see CVID, page 287).

Pathology

Histological examination of the lesions shows an infiltrate of histiocytes, neutrophils and giant cells, with areas of necrosis. These granulomas give the disease its name; however, especially in scrofulous lesions, they raise the possibility of tuberculosis or BCG infection[3].

Genetics

Four components of NADPH oxidase have now been identified, sequenced, cloned and characterized. They are respectively named gp91-phox, p22-phox, p47-phox and gp67-phox (phox – *ph*agocyte *ox*idase). The components gp91-phox and p22-phox form the two subunits of cytochrome B. Sixty per cent of affected patients show an abnormality of gp91-phox, inherited as an X-linked disorder. Transmission of the other defects (mutations in p22-phox, p47-phox and gp67-phox) are transmitted in an autosomal recessive fashion[1].

The carrier state can be detected with the nitroblue tetrazolium (NBT) dye test (granulocytes show an intermediate ability to reduce nitroblue tetrazolium) and with more complicated molecular biological techniques. Although this state is usually asymptomatic, carriers may suffer from a lupus erythematosus-like disease and recurrent aphthous ulcerations of mucosae[4].

Differential diagnosis

The various phagocytic disorders share many clinical features. If such a disorder is suspected, the initial assessment should include a peripheral white blood cell count and bone marrow aspirates. Reduction of NBT is typically pathologic in chronic granulomatous disease.

Rebuck skin windows allow testing of the motility and chemotaxis of phagocytes. The IgE level should be assessed.

Treatment

The usual treatment of patients with phagocyte defects is based on aggressive medical therapy (antibiotics) and surgical management. Like neutropenic patients, these patients may have severe infections with minimal clinical manifestations[5]. Interferon gamma therapy has proved to be very beneficial in a multicentre study[6], although its mechanism of action is not known.

References

1 Curnutte JT. Molecular basis of the autosomal recessive forms of chronic granulomatous disease. *Immunodef Rev* 1992; **3**: 149–72.
2 Tauber AL, Borregard N, Simons E, Wright J. Chronic granulomatous disease: a syndrome of phagocyte oxydase deficiencies. *Medicine* 1983; **62**: 286–309.
3 Windhorst DB, Good RA. Dermatologic manifestations of fatal granulomatosis disease of childhood. *Arch Dermatol* 1971; **103**: 351–7.
4 Garioch JJ, Sampson JR, Seywright M, Thompson J. Dermatoses in five related female carriers of X-linked chronic granulomatous disease. *Br J Dermatol* 1989; **121**: 391–6.
5 White CJ, Gallin JI. Phagocytes defects. *Clin Immunol Immunopath* 1986; **40**: 50–61.
6 Gallin JI, Malech HL, Weening RS et al. A controlled trial of interferon gamma to prevent infection in chronic granulomatous disease. *New Engl J Med* 1991; **324**: 509–16.

Myeloperoxidase deficiency

Definition

In affected patients, defective myeloperoxidase disrupts the mechanism responsible for the killing of micro-organisms inside the lysosomes of phagocytes.

Clinical features

Although myeloperoxidase-deficient phagocytes express a mild defect in bacterial killing and a marked defect in fungal killing in vitro, it is now accepted that severe infections with *Candida albicans* and bacteraemias occur only when an underlying illness, especially diabetes, coexists[1].

Pathology

In the presence of hydrogen peroxide and halide, myeloperoxidase produces hypochlorous acid and chloride which permits halogenation and destruction of phagocytosed bacteria. In myeloperoxidase deficiency, this mechanism is impaired.

Genetics

Total and partial congenital myeloperoxidase deficiencies have been described, both transmitted in an autosomal recessive mode. The molecular genetic mechanism involves a defect of post-translational processing of an abnormal precursor protein.

Treatment

The treatment is that of candidal infections, bacteraemias and the associated disorder[2,3].

References

1 Malech HL, Gallin JI. Neutrophils in human disease. *New Engl J Med* 1987; **317**: 687–94.
2 Nauseef WM, Root RK, Malech HL. Biochemical and immunologic analysis of hereditary myeloperoxidase deficiency. *J Clin Invest* 1983; **71**: 1297–307.
3 Parry MF, Root RK, Metcalf JA et al. Myeloperoxidase deficiency: prevalence and clinical significance. *Ann Int Med* 1981; **95**: 293–301.

Chédiak–Higashi syndrome

Definition

The characteristic abnormality in Chédiak–Higashi syndrome is the presence of giant granules in the cytoplasm of all lysosome-containing cells, including white blood cells, platelets, renal tubular epithelial cells, neural tissue, gastric mucosa, pancreatic cells, thyroid cells and melanocytes. Functionally, there is abnormal chemotaxis and a prolonged killing time of micro-organisms within phagocytes. The oxidative metabolism seems to be unaltered.

Clinical features

Patients have recurrent bacterial infections of the skin and other organs, and neurologic deterioration. The specific skin marker of the disease, partial albinism, would be better termed 'pigment dilution'[1]. The skin, hair and eyes are simultaneously involved in about 75% of cases. Hair has a silvery sheen and shows clumped pigment granules on microscopic examination. As in albinism, photophobia and nystagmus can be observed. In some cases, the depigmentation is confined to the nipples and genitalia, and the only hair abnormality is the particular metallic sheen. The disease may be fatal before the age of 10 years, following the so-called accelerated phase of the disorder, characterized by fever, jaundice, hepatosplenomegaly, lymphadenopathy, pancytopenia, tendency to bleed and infiltration of all organs by reactive mononuclear cells[2].

Pathology

The nature of the giant cytoplasmic inclusions of involved cells has been extensively studied[3]. In melanocytes, abnormally large melanosomes are produced, and the transfer mechanism of melanosomes to keratinocytes is altered. In phagocytes, the abnormalities of the bactericidal mechanisms explain the formation of huge secondary lysosomes. A peculiar immunologic defect in affected patients is a profound decrease in natural killer activity in peripheral lymphocytes. The underlying defect is still unknown.

Genetics

The Chédiak–Higashi syndrome is an autosomal recessive disease.

Differential diagnosis

The pigment dilution of Chédiak–Higashi syndrome is similar to that of Griscelli–Prunieras syndrome. In the latter syndrome, no giant granules are seen.

Treatment

Bone marrow transplantation is the treatment of choice of the immunologic and haematologic aspects. It does not influence the pigment dilution[4].

References

1 Windhorst DB, Zeligson A, Good RA. A human pigmentary dilution based on a heritable subcellular structural defect. The Chediak–Higashi syndrome. *J Invest Dermatol* 1968; **50**: 9–18.
2 Stolz W, Graubner V, Gerstmeier J, Burg G, Belohradsky BH. Chediak–Higashi syndrome: approaches in diagnosis and treatment. *Curr Probl Dermat* 1989; **18**: 93–100.
3 White JG, Clawson CC. The Chediak–Higashi syndrome: the nature of the giant neutrophil granules and their interactions with cytoplasm and foreign particulates. *Am J Pathol* 1980; **98**: 151–96.
4 Virelizier JL, Lagrue A, Durandy A et al. Reversal of natural killer defect in a patient with Chediak–Higashi syndrome after bone marrow transplantation. *New Engl J Med* 1982; **306**: 1055–7.

Leucocyte adhesion disorder

Definition

Formerly called 'delayed separation of the umbilical cord', 'lazy leucocyte syndrome' or 'CR3 deficiency', leucocyte adhesion disorder is characterized by the absence of a family of surface glycoproteins, called the CD11/CD18 complex. Patients with this deficiency show a defect in neutrophilic adhesion-related functions such as chemotaxis, adhesion to endothelial cells, antibody-dependent cell-mediated cytotoxicity, C3b-mediated phagocytosis and response to opsonized particles[1].

Clinical features

Affected children present with delayed separation of the umbilical cord, frequent skin infections, ecthyma gangrenosum, recurrent fever, perirectal abscesses, upper respiratory tract infections, gingivitis and stomatitis, and they are susceptible to staphylococcal and Gram-negative bacteria[2]. Leucocytosis with prominent neutrophil counts is common, due to the constant stimulation of granulocytes, resulting from the permanent presence of infectious micro-organisms and from the inability of granulocytes lacking adhesion function to exit the circulation. Healing is impaired and surgery should therefore be performed cautiously. Skin grafts are better avoided.

Pathology

There is a deficiency in the synthesis of the CD18 molecule, resulting in the absence of three main heterodimeric surface glycoproteins that share the CD18 beta-chain associated with one of the three CD11 alpha-chains. These glycoproteins are adhesion molecules called LFA-1 (CD18–CD11a), MAC-1 (CD18–CD11b) and p150–95 (CD18–CD11c). They are normally present on leucocytes, and their deficiency results in impairment of lymphocyte adhesion, natural killing, antibody-dependent cell cytotoxicity and most phagocyte adhesion-related functions[2,3].

Genetics

The disorder is inherited in an autosomal recessive fashion. The gene coding for CD18 has been localized on chromosome 21.

Differential diagnosis

Flow cytometric analysis with monoclonal antibodies to cell surface glycoproteins, showing normal HLA and CR1 expression but nearly absent levels of CD18/CD11 glycoproteins, allows a definite diagnosis.

Treatment

Only non-specific management of the complications of the disease could be offered until recently. Bone marrow transplantation can cure the defect. Gene therapy may be a good alternative in the future.

References

1 Yang KD, Hill HR. Neutrophil function disorders: pathophysiology, prevention, and therapy. *J Pediatr* 1991; **119**: 343–54.
2 Schmalstieg FC. Leukocyte adherence defect. *Ped Infect Dis J* 1988; **7**: 867–72.
3 Kishimoto TK, Springer TA. Human leukocyte adhesion deficiency: molecular basis for a defective immune response to infections of the skin. *Curr Probl Dermatol* 1989; **18**: 106–15.

Primary neutropenias

Definition

The neutropenias of childhood are a poorly defined group of disorders that share the common features of low polymorphonuclear leucocyte counts and frequent bacterial infections.

Clinical features

The range of the bacterial infections include infectious cellulitis, stomatitis, gingivitis and perirectal abscesses.

Genetics

There are two forms of the disease: a severe autosomal recessive form, and a relatively milder autosomal dominant form.

Differential diagnosis

Serial white blood cell counts and an accurate history are diagnostic[1].

The rare autosomal dominant cyclic neutropenia also belongs to this group of diseases: recurrent mouth ulcerations and skin pyodermas recurring in 3-week cycles should alert the clinician.

Neutropenia can be a feature of Schwachman's syndrome. Affected infants have diarrhoea due to pancreatic failure, neutropenia and thrombocytopenia in relation to bone marrow dysfunction. A defect in polymorphonuclear leucocytes may exist in these children. Interestingly, severe eczematoid dermatitis has been observed in these patients[2].

Treatment

Symptomatic management is usually sufficient in very mild disorders. Recombinant granulocyte colony-stimulating factor (G-CSF) has greatly improved the management of more severe neutropenias. Bone marrow transplantation is now rarely necessary in the severe form of cyclic neutropenia.

References

1 Pincus SH, Boxer LA, Stossel TT. Chronic neutropenia in childhood: analysis of 16 cases and a review of the literature. *Am J Med* 1976; **61**: 849–61.
2 Schwachman H, Diamond LK, Oski FA, Khaw KT. The syndrome of pancreatic insufficiency and bone marrow dysfunction. *J Pediatr* 1964; **65**: 645–63.

Tuftsin deficiency

It must be emphasized that there is no general agreement about the very existence of this disorder.

Definition

Tuftsin is a tetrapeptide that stimulates macrophages and polymorphonuclear leucocytes. The biologically active peptide Thr-Lys-Pro-Arg is enzymatically cleaved from a circulating precursor known as leucokinin. Tuftsin deficiency leads to recurrent bacterial infections.

Clinical features

Congenital familial tuftsin deficiency leads to severe recurrent infections in the neonatal period and early childhood. As the child grows up, infections become milder. Upper respiratory tract infections, pneumonitis and septicaemia are common. Skin infections consist of boils, furuncles and draining lymphadenitis. Seborrhoeic dermatitis may occur.

Pathology

To cleave the active tetrapeptide from its precursor molecule, two enzymes are needed, one located in the spleen and the other on the surface of phagocytes. These enzymes seem normal in familial tuftsin deficiency. The disease appears to be caused by the replacement of normal tuftsin by a mutant peptide that is strongly inhibitory to the normal molecule.

Genetics

The most common form of tuftsin deficiency is acquired, following loss of splenic function (e.g. splenectomy, leukaemia, infarction), but congenital familial forms exist. In two cases, one of the parents of the affected child had tuftsin deficiency, although asymptomatic. This points to a autosomal dominant trait, with variable penetrance. Thus, tuftsin activity should be assessed in other family members, as well as C5 activity, since tuftsin deficiency associated with C5 deficiency has been described[1].

Differential diagnosis

This awaits additional information about the real physiological role of tuftsin.

Treatment

Until the synthetic tetrapeptide is available, treatment consists of therapy with antibiotics and immunoglobulins[2].

References

1 Constantinopoulos A, Najjar VA, Smith JW. Tuftsin deficiency: a new syndrome with defective phagocytosis. *J Pediatr* 1972; **80**: 564–72.
2 Najjar VA. Biochemical aspects of tuftsin deficiency syndrome. *Med Biol* 1981; **59**: 134–8.

Complement deficiencies

Definition

The complement system comprises more than 20 glycoproteins, which interact in a manner reminiscent of the coagulation system: factors activate each other in a cascade of tightly regulated enzymatic reactions.

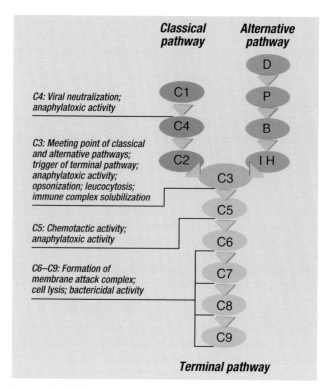

Figure 18.5 *The complement system*

The complement system can be conveniently divided into three subunits: the classical pathway, activated by immune complexes; the alternative pathway, which does not require antibodies for its activation, but instead is activated by contact with surfaces such as certain bacterial walls; and finally the terminal pathway, a common effector of both the classical and alternative pathway, whose function is to lyse target cells, especially Gram-negative bacteria.

Figure 18.5 schematically describes the organization of the complement system and shows the most important functions of the activated forms of major complement components. Detailed biochemical descriptions of the complement system are available elsewhere[1,2].

Deficiencies of all complement components have been described. Although it is not uncommon for these deficiencies to remain asymptomatic, when they do result in disease, the skin is likely to be involved.

Clinical features

The clinical features are summarized in Table 18.2. For practical purposes, it is convenient to distinguish five major groups of complement deficiencies, each having a different clinical expression.

Deficiency of C1 inhibitor

Deficiency of C1 inhibitor produces hereditary angioedema. This non-pruritic oedema has a subcutaneous

Table 18.2 *Diseases associated with complement deficiencies*

Complement component	Associated disease
C1q	SLE, GN
C1r	DLE, SLE, GN
C1r and C1s	SLE
C1 esterase inhibitor	Hereditary angioedema, SLE
C4	SLE, vasculitis, GN, Sjögren's syndrome
C2	DLE, SLE, GN, dermatomyositis, vasculitis, recurrent pneumonia, bacteraemia, meningitis
P (properdin)	Cellulitis, candidiasis, recurrent pneumonia, acute *Neisseria* infections
C3	SLE, annular rashes, GN, recurrent skin infections, pneumonia, bacteraemia, meningitis
I (C3 inactivator)	Similar to C3 deficiency
C5	*Neisseria* infections, SLE
C5 dysfunction	Leiner's disease
C6	*Neisseria* infections, toxoplasmosis
C7	*Neisseria* infections, scleroderma, SLE
C8	*Neisseria* infections, SLE, xeroderma pigmentosum
C9	*Neisseria* infections

DLE, SLE, discoid, systemic lupus erythematosus; GN, glomerulonephritis.

or submucous localization. As well as the skin and mucous membranes (with the possibility of life-threatening airways obstruction), the abdominal viscera may be affected, producing colicky pains. Hereditary angioedema patients are also at risk of developing connective tissue diseases.

Classical pathway deficiencies

Deficiencies of early components of the classical pathway are typically associated with collagen-vascular disease, the frequency of the association varying between 57% and 85% of cases. The severity of the associated disease is greatest with C1q deficiency, closely followed by total C4 deficiency. Systemic lupus erythematosus, associated with C4 and C2 deficiencies, is characterized by an early onset in childhood, extreme sensitivity to sun exposure, and absent or low-titre antinuclear antibodies.

Alternative pathway deficiencies

The most frequent alternative pathway deficiency is properdin (P) deficiency; this leads to fulminant meningococcal infections, to which female carriers also have an increased liability. This contrasts with terminal pathway deficiencies, in which neisserial infections curiously begin in the second decade of life and are recurrent but not especially severe. In alternative pathway deficiencies, there is no evidence for increased susceptibility to immune complex disease or to infections with other organisms than the Neisseriaceae[3].

Deficiency of C3

The most severe of all the complement deficiency states is C3 deficiency. All homozygous C3-deficient patients suffer from both infectious and connective tissue diseases. The central position of C3 in the complement system and the numerous biologic activities of C3 fragments account for the severity of this condition. Recurrent meningitis, bacteraemia, pneumonia, urinary tract infection and peritonitis are the most common infectious complications. Prominent pathogens include *Streptococcus pneumoniae*, *Haemophilus influenzae* and *Neisseria meningitidis*. Deficiency of C3 inactivator (factor I) produces a similar clinical syndrome: in the absence of the regulatory protein, unchecked consumption of C3 takes place, resulting in depletion of this factor.

Terminal pathway deficiencies

Terminal pathway deficiencies are characterized by recurrent neisserial infections or infections with uncommon serogroups. There is very little susceptibility to autoimmune diseases or to non-neisserial infections. Two types of deficiencies occur (at least for C6, C7 and C8), one with low but detectable amounts of the component, and one with total deficiency. Low amounts of functional terminal complement activity may be sufficient to protect against neisserial infections, and such affected patients may remain free of any symptoms[4].

Leiner's syndrome and its association with C5 dysfunction. In 1908, Leiner described 43 breast-fed infants with generalized seborrhoeic dermatitis, severe diarrhoea, failure to thrive and recurrent infections, and he concluded that nutritional factors might be responsible for the disorder[5]. In 1972, Jacobs and Miller described 2 infants with a similar syndrome, in whom a yeast opsonization defect caused by a functional abnormality of C5 was identified[6]. Since then, it has been determined that such a defect occurs in 5% of the general population, and that defective yeast opsonization is rather a consequence of impaired deposition of C3b/C3bi as a result of a cofactor deficiency. Moreover, it has been shown that the association of erythroderma, diarrhoea and failure to thrive in infancy, depicted as Leiner's disease, is not the result of a single disease but is the manifestation of various underlying immunologic defects[7]. Therefore, it seems best to abandon the term Leiner's syndrome or to consider it as a phenotype, highly suggestive of immunodeficiency, although not of a specific kind.

Pathology

Recurrent infections are expected features in a deficiency of an important effector of the organism's defence system, but the occurrence of hypersensitivity or autoimmune syndromes might seem paradoxical at first. Different theories have been proposed to explain this phenomenon: triggering of autoimmune diseases by uncontrolled viral infection in C2 deficiency, linkage of terminal pathway components deficiency with HLA-DR genotypes associated with autoimmune disorders, and diminished clearance of circulating immune complexes, especially in C3 deficiency[8]. These theories are not mutually exclusive, but increasing knowledge about the role played in immune complex clearance by red blood cell C3 receptors and receptors for other complement components makes the last explanation very likely[9].

Genetics

Most of the complement system proteins show autosomal codominant inheritance. The two exceptions to this rule are properdin (P) deficiency, which shows an X-linked mode of inheritance, and deficiency of C1 inhibitor, transmitted as an autosomal dominant trait. Proteins C4, C2 and factor B are coded for by genes situated on chromosome 6 within the major histocompatibility complex and especially linked to the HLA-DR region.

Differential diagnosis

When disorders compatible with a complement deficiency are present, the following steps should be taken. A careful personal and familial history must be obtained. The total haemolytic complement (CH_{50}) should be tested: it is low if any of the classical or terminal pathway protein is deficient. An alternative pathway deficiency can only be demonstrated using a specific test (APH_{50}), available in specialized laboratories only. Next, individual components should be assayed. Low values for multiple complement components suggest a consumption pathology rather than a hereditary defect, except in the case of genetic deficiencies of the regulatory proteins of the classical pathway (inhibitor of C1) and the alternative pathway (factors I and H). In 15% of patients with hereditary angioedema, normal levels of C1 inhibitor antigen are found, because these patients produce an antigenically normal but functionally inactive protein; a function test must therefore also be performed. In addition, an acquired form of deficiency of C1 inhibitor exists, usually associated with lymphoma.

Treatment

Hereditary angioedema can be handled with long-term prophylactic administration of androgenic steroids (e.g. danazol). The management of the other complement deficiencies has not so far been satisfactory. Except in the setting of acute infections, replacement therapy by plasma infusion is not warranted, because of the short half-life of complement proteins. Vaccination with polyvalent meningococcal and pneumococcal vaccines is recommended, but prophylactic antibiotics have limited usefulness[2].

References

1 Kinishita T. Biology of complement: the overture. *Immunol Today* 1991; **12**: 291–5.
2 Fries LF, O'Shea JJ, Frank MM. Inherited deficiencies of complement and complement-related proteins. *Clin Immunol Immunopath* 1986; **40**: 37–49.
3 Morgan BP, Walport MJ. Complement deficiency and disease. *Immunol Today* 1991; **12**: 301–6.
4 Würzner R, Orren A, Lachmann PJ. Inherited deficiencies of the terminal components of human complement. *Immunodef Rev* 1992; **3**: 123–47.
5 Leiner C. Uber Erythrodermia desquamativa, eine eigenartige universelle Dermatose der Brustkinder. *Arch Dermatol Syphilol* 1908; **89**: 163–89.
6 Jacobs JC, Miller ME. Fatal familial Leiner's disease: a deficiency of the opsonic activity of serum. *Pediatrics* 1972; **49**: 225–32.
7 Glover MT, Atherton DJ, Levinsky RJ. Syndrome of erythroderma, failure to thrive, and diarrhea in infancy: a manifestation of immunodeficiency. *Pediatrics* 1988; **81**: 66–72.
8 Ross SC, Densen P. Complement deficiency states and infection: epidemiology, pathogenesis and consequences of Neisserial and other infections in immune deficiency. *Medicine* 1984; **63**: 243–73.
9 Fearon DT. Complement, C receptors, and immune complex disease. *Hosp Pract* 1988; **23**: 63–7

Chapter 19

Genetic diseases predisposing to malignancy

J. I. Harper

Introduction

Genetic diseases that predispose to malignancy fall into several groups:

1. Disorders with a predisposition to specific skin cancers, in which there are premalignant skin lesions.
2. Disorders with a predisposition to skin and systemic malignancies.
3. Disorders with a predisposition to systemic malignancies but with cutaneous stigmata.

Table 19.1 details those genetic diseases relevant to dermatology that predispose to malignancy. Selected genetic diseases are discussed in this chapter; others are discussed elsewhere in the book, for example xeroderma pigmentosum (Figure 19.1) in Chapter 17.

Bazex syndrome

Definition

Bazex syndrome is characterized by the association of follicular atrophoderma and basal cell carcinomas.

Clinical features

First described by Bazex in 1964[1], the essential features are follicular atrophoderma, present from birth, and the development of multiple basal cell carcinomas of the face from adolescence onwards. The follicular atrophoderma typically affects the dorsa of

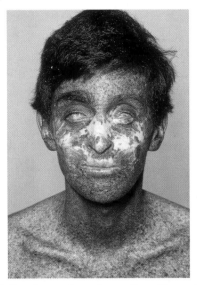

Figure 19.1 *Xeroderma pigmentosum (from Harper J. Handbook of Paediatric Dermatology.* Butterworth-Heinemann, Oxford, 1990)

the hands and feet, and sometimes the extensor limbs and lower back. The exaggerated follicular funnels ('ice-pick' marks) are caused by deep, lax follicular ostia rather than by true atrophy. The basal cell carcinomas present as lightly pigmented papules which resemble melanocytic naevi. Inconstant features include facial hypohidrosis with or without generalized hypohidrosis[2]. In some cases the hair has been notably sparse[3,4]. The hair shafts are defective and may show pili torti[5].

Table 19.1 *Genetic diseases predisposing to malignancy*

Genetic skin diseases	Tumour susceptibility	Inheritance	Gene localization
Albinism, several forms (Chapter 13)	Squamous cell carcinoma Basal cell carcinoma Malignant melanoma	Mainly AR	Tyrosinase gene, chromosome 11
Ataxia-telangiectasia (Chapter 18)	Lymphoma; leukaemia Epithelial carcinomas	AR	11q22–23
Bazex syndrome*	Basal cell carcinoma	AD	
Beckwith–Wiedemann syndrome (Chapter 11)	Wilms' tumour Adrenal carcinoma Hepatoblastomas	AD	11p15
Bloom's syndrome (Chapter 17)	Leukaemia; lymphoma Carcinoma of the gastrointestinal tract, cervix and larynx Wilms' tumour	AR	
Cowden syndrome*	Carcinoma of the breast, uterus and thyroid	AD	
Dyskeratosis congenita (Chapter 13)	Leucoplakia Squamous cell carcinoma	XLR	Xq28
Epidermolysis bullosa dystrophica (Chapter 4)	Squamous cell carcinoma	AR	Collagen VII gene, chromosome 3p21
Familial atypical mole–melanoma (FAMM) (dysplastic naevus syndrome) [1]	Cutaneous malignant melanoma	AD	? 1p36
Epidermodysplasia verruciformis*	Squamous cell carcinoma	?AR	
Fanconi's anaemia (Chapter 17)	Leukaemia Hepatic carcinoma	AR	20q12–13.3
Ferguson-Smith's self-healing epithelioma*	Self-healing 'squamous cell carcinomas'	AD	9q31–32
Gardner's syndrome*	Adenocarcinoma of the colon	AD	5q21–22
Gorlin's syndrome* (naevoid basal cell carcinoma syndrome)	Basal cell carcinomas Other internal malignancies	AD	9q22.3–31
Keratitis–ichthyosis–deafness (KID) syndrome (Chapter 5)	Squamous cell carcinoma	AD	
Maffucci's syndrome (Chapter 11)	Chondrosarcoma Ovarian tumours Gliomas	? AD	
Muir–Torre syndrome [2, 3]	Sebaceous tumours Keratoacanthomas Adenocarcinoma of the colon and other internal malignancies	AD	
Neurofibromatosis types I and II (Chapter 9)	CNS tumours Neurofibrosarcoma	AD	Type I: 17q11.2 Type II: 22q12
Peutz–Jeghers syndrome (Chapter 13)	Adenocarcinoma of the bowel Tumours at other sites including breast, ovary and testis	AD	

Table 19.1 *Continued*

Genetic skin diseases	Tumour susceptibility	Inheritance	Gene localization
Porokeratosis of Mibelli (Chapter 6)	Squamous cell carcinoma Basal cell carcinoma	AD	
Rothmund–Thomson syndrome (Chapter 12)	Squamous cell carcinoma Osteosarcoma	AR	
Sclerotylosis [4]	Squamous cell carcinoma of the skin, tongue and tonsil Bowel carcinoma	AD	4q28
Tuberous sclerosis (Chapter 9)	CNS, renal and cardiac tumours	AD	? 9q34; ? 16p
Turcot's syndrome [5]	Adenocarcinoma of the colon CNS tumours	AR	
Tylosis (Chapter 6)[6]	Oesophageal carcinoma	AD	17q23–ter
Von Hippel–Lindau disease (Chapter 11)	Renal cell carcinoma	AD	3p25–26
Werner's syndrome (Chapter 14)	Tumours of connective tissue or mesenchymal origin	AR	8p
Wiskott–Aldrich syndrome (Chapter 18)	Lymphoma Leukaemia	XLR	Xp11.4–11.21
Xeroderma pigmentosum, forms A–G (Chapter 17)	Squamous cell carcinoma Basal cell carcinoma Malignant melanoma Other internal malignancies	AR	Group A: 9q34.1 Group B: 2q21 Group D: 19

* Denotes genetic disorders discussed more fully in this chapter.
AD, autosomal dominant; AR, autosomal recessive; CNS, central nervous system; XLR, X-linked recessive.

References

1 Tucker MA. Individuals at high risk of melanoma. *Pigment Cell* 1988; **9**: 95–109.
2 Muir EG, Yates-Bell AJ, Barlow KA. Multiple primary carcinomata of colon, duodenum and larynx associated with keratoacanthoma of the face. *Br J Surg* 1967; **54**: 191–5.
3 Grignon DJ, Shum DT, Bruckschwaiger O. Transitional cell carcinoma in the Muir–Torre syndrome. *J Urol* 1987; **38**: 406–8.
4 Fischer S. La genodermatose scleroatrophiante et keratodermique des extremities. *Ann Derm Venereol* 1978; **105**: 1079–82.
5 Turcot J, Despres JP, St Pierre F. Malignant tumours of the central nervous system associated with familial polyposis of the colon: report of two cases. *Dis Colon Rectum* 1959; **2**: 465–8
6 Risk JM, Whittaker J, Fryer A et al. Tylosis oesophageal cancer mapped. *Nature Genet* 1994; **8**: 319–21.

Genetics

Bazex syndrome is determined by an autosomal dominant gene[6]. Gene localization is as yet unknown.

Differential diagnosis

The condition should be distinguished from Gorlin's syndrome. It must not be confused with a completely different disorder, acrokeratosis paraneoplastica, a cutaneous marker of malignancy which has also been labelled as Bazex syndrome[7].

References

1 Bazex A, Dupre A, Christol B. Genodermatose complexe de type indetermine associant une hypotrichose, un etat atrophodermique generalisé et des degenerescences cutanées multiples (epitheliomas-basocellulaires). *Bull Soc Fr Dermat Syphil* 1964; **71**: 206.
2 Viksnins P, Berlin A. Follicular atrophoderma and basal cell carcinomas. The Bazex syndrome. *Arch Dermatol* 1977; **113**: 948–51.
3 Gould DJ, Barker DJ. Follicular atrophoderma with multiple basal cell carcinomas (Bazex). *Br J Dermatol* 1978; **99**: 431–5.
4 Plosila M, Kiistala R, Niemi KM. The Bazex syndrome:

follicular atrophoderma with multiple basal cell carcinomas, hypotrichosis and hypohidrosis. *Clin Exp Dermatol* 1981; **6**: 31–41.

5 Meynadier J, Guilhou J-J, Barneon G, Malbros S, Guillot B. Atrophodermie folliculaire, hypotrichose, grains de milium multiples associés à des dystrophies ostéo-cartilagineuses minimes. Etude familiale de 3 cas. *Ann Dermatol Syphil Venereol* 1979; **106**: 497–501.

6 Mehta VR, Potdar R. Bazex syndrome: follicular atrophoderma and basal cell epitheliomas. *Int J Dermatol* 1985; **24**: 444–6.

7 Pecora AL, Landsman L, Imgrund SP, Lambert WC. Acrokeratosis paraneoplastica (Bazex syndrome). *Arch Dermatol* 1983; **119**: 820–6.

Cowden syndrome

Synonym: *Multiple hamartoma syndrome*

Definition

Cowden syndrome is a rare disorder in which multiple hamartomatous lesions of skin, mucous membranes, breast and thyroid are associated with a predisposition to malignant tumours, in particular of the breast. Cowden was the name of the family in whom the disease was first described[1].

Clinical features

The clinical features of Cowden syndrome [2–7] include skin-coloured papules up to 4 mm in diameter, tending to coalesce to give a 'cobblestone' appearance, which are distributed on and around the eyes and the mouth. On the dorsa of hands and wrists are lesions like those of acrokeratosis verruciformis. On the palms, soles, fingers and toes, there are small, translucent keratoses. Multiple angiomas and lipomas have been found in several cases. Malignant melanoma has occurred[8].

Verrucous and papillomatous lesions are seen in some patients on the labial and buccal mucosa, fauces and oropharynx, and may extend to the larynx.

In a series of patients[7], craniomegaly was noted to be the most frequent extracutaneous finding, affecting 70% of patients.

Of the many other abnormalities that have been reported in this syndrome, the most frequent involve thyroid and breasts. Approximately 30% of reported female cases developed breast cancer[7]. Fibrocystic disease of the breast sometimes leads to massive hyperplasia. Goitre or thyroid adenoma are present in many cases and thyroid carcinoma has been reported[2,9]. Adenocarcinoma of the uterus has been reported in 6% of women with multiple hamartoma syndrome[7]. Less frequent associations include adenoid facies, high-arched palate, vitiligo, *café au lait* spots, skeletal abnormalities, retinal glioma, pseudo-

tumour cerebri, gastrointestinal polyposis and various gynaecological disorders (menstrual irregularity, uterine fibroids).

Ruschak et al[10] described a patient with this syndrome who had a deficiency of T-lymphocyte function, with recurrent cellulitis and abscess formation and the eventual development of acute myeloid leukaemia.

Pathology

The skin lesions[11,12] around the mouth, eyes and chin are tricholemmomas[13]. The breast lesions are fibroadenomas which are liable to undergo malignant degeneration. A unique fibroma on the face and other sites has been described[9,12], composed of broad, acellular collagen bundles in a lamellar or whorl-like pattern with occasional giant cells. This has been referred to as 'Cowden's fibroma'[14]. There is a report of amyloid in association with multiple hamartoma syndrome[14].

Genetics

Inheritance of the disease appears to be determined by an autosomal dominant gene of variable expression. Carlson et al could demonstrate no linkage with any of a battery of markers in a family with 4 members affected in three generations[15].

Differential diagnosis

The skin lesions may be confused with Darier's disease or tuberous sclerosis.

Treatment

Cosmetic surgery may be helpful. The possibility of carcinoma of breast or thyroid must be borne in mind. Female patients with this syndrome should avoid oestrogen therapy and should have frequent breast checks, including mammography, or even prophylactic mastectomy[16].

References

1 Lloyd KM, Dennis M. Cowden's disease: a possible new symptom complex with multiple system involvement. *Ann Intern Med* 1963; **58**: 136–42.

2 Burnett JW, Goldner R, Calton GJ. Cowden disease. Report of two additional cases. *Br J Dermatol* 1975; **93**: 329–36.

3 Gentry WC, Eskitt NR, Gorlin RJ. Multiple hamartoma syndrome (Cowden disease). *Arch Dermatol* 1974; **109**: 521–5.

4 Nuss DD, Aeling JL, Clemons DE, Weber WN. Multiple hamartoma syndrome (Cowden's disease). *Arch Dermatol* 1978; **114**: 743–6.

5 Ocana Sierra J. Cowden's syndrome. *Actas Dermosifiliogr* 1974; **65**: 117–28.

6 Starink TM. Cowden's disease: analysis of fourteen new cases. *J Am Acad Dermatol* 1984; **11**: 1127–41.

7 Starink TM, Van der Veen JPW, Arwert F et al. The Cowden syndrome: a clinical and genetic study in 21 patients. *Clin Genet* 1986; **29**: 222–33.

8 Siegel JM. Cowden's disease: report of a case with malignant melanoma. *Cutis* 1975; **16**: 255–8.

9 Weary PE, Gorlin RJ, Gentry WC, Comer JE, Greer KE. Multiple hamartoma syndrome (Cowden's disease). *Arch Dermatol* 1972; **106**: 682–90.

10 Ruschak PJ, Kauh YC, Luscombe HA. Cowden's disease associated with immunodeficiency. *Arch Dermatol* 1981; **117**: 573–5.

11 Brownstein MH, Mehregan AM, Bikowski B, Lupulescu A, Patterson J. The dermatopathology of Cowden's syndrome. *Br J Dermatol* 1979; **100**: 667–73.

12 Starink TM, Meijer CJLM, Brownstein MH. The cutaneous pathology of Cowden's disease: new findings. *J Cutan Pathol* 1985; **12**: 83–93.

13 Salem OS, Steck WD. Cowden's disease (multiple hamartoma and neoplasia syndrome). *J Am Acad Dermatol* 1983; **8**: 686–96.

14 Barax CN, Lebwohl M, Phelps RG. Multiple hamartoma syndrome. *J Am Acad Dermatol* 1987; **17**: 342–6.

15 Carlson HE, Burns TW, Davenport SL et al. Cowden disease: gene marker studies and measurements of epidermal growth factor. *Am J Hum Genet* 1986; **38**: 908–17.

16 Walton BJ, Morain WD, Baughman RD, Jordan A, Crichlow RW. Cowden's disease: a further indication for prophylactic mastectomy. *Surgery* 1986; **99**: 82–6.

Epidermodysplasia verruciformis

Definition

Epidermodysplasia verruciformis[1] is due to a genetic susceptibility to human papillomavirus, with a risk of malignant transformation.

Clinical features

Lesions on the face and neck are indistinguishable from plane warts. Those on the trunk and extremities are larger and may coalesce to form plaques. They usually develop in childhood though they may arise at any age. Intraepidermal carcinoma and squamous cell carcinoma frequently develop, usually in light-exposed areas, often during the third decade but occasionally before the age of 20 years.

Pathology

The histology is that of a viral wart, intraepidermal carcinoma or squamous cell carcinoma, depending on the lesion examined. The cutaneous neoplasms are associated with the human papillomaviruses HPV-5, HPV-8 or HPV-14, suggesting that these viruses are potentially oncogenic.

Genetics

The condition is autosomal recessive and seems to represent a specific susceptibility to infection with certain human papillomaviruses.

Differential diagnosis

Immunosuppressed patients, particularly those with renal transplants, commonly have extensive viral warts and other keratotic skin lesions. Acrokeratosis verruciformis may be similar but is normally confined to the hands, feet, knees and elbows.

Treatment

Treatment with retinoids and interferon may be considered. Any lesion suggestive of squamous cell carcinoma should be excised.

Reference

1 Lutzner MA, Blanchet-Bardon C, Orth G. Clinical observations, virologic studies and treatment trials in patients with epidermodysplasia verruciformis, a disease induced by specific human papilloma-viruses. *J Invest Dermatol* 1984; **83**: 18–25.

Ferguson-Smith's self-healing epithelioma

Definition

Ferguson-Smith's self-healing epitheliomas are found in people of Scottish descent. Multiple squamous cell carcinomas develop mainly in light-exposed sites.

Clinical features

Skin lesions appear in early adult life, often on the face and scalp, and may arise in clusters[1,2]. The epitheliomas are dome-shaped and evolve to measure up to 1 cm in diameter (Figure 19.2). If left untreated they resolve over a period of about 4 months to leave unpleasant, ragged scars. Epitheliomas have developed in the nasal vestibule.

Pathology

Histologically the lesions show the changes of early invasive squamous cell carcinomas, but are distinct in most cases from multiple keratoacanthomas.

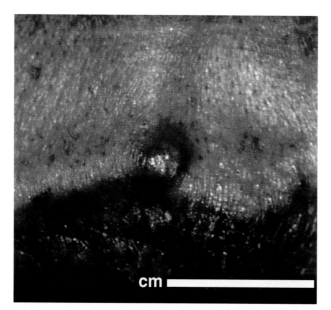

Figure 19.2 *Self-healing epithelioma of Ferguson-Smith: a dome-shaped epithelioma on the border of the lip (courtesy of Dr D Gawkrodger)*

Genetics

Family pedigrees have been established and an autosomal dominant inheritance seems likely. Linkage analysis has mapped the gene to chromosome 9q31–32[3].

Differential diagnosis

Squamous cell carcinomas associated with excessive sun exposure appear in older patients who have concomitant signs of actinic damage.

Treatment

Small lesions can be satisfactorily treated by cryosurgery. Larger epitheliomas are best treated by excision, otherwise unpleasant scarring results. The prognosis seems to be good.

References

1 Ferguson-Smith J. Multiple primary self-healing squamous epithelioma of the skin. *Br J Dermatol* 1948; **60**: 315–18.
2 Wright AL, Gawkrodger DJ, Branford WA, McLaren KM, Hunter JAA. Self-healing epitheliomata of Ferguson-Smith: clinical, cytogenetic and histological studies. *Dermatologica* 1988; **176**: 22–8.
3 Goudie DR, Yuille MAR, Affra NA et al. Localisation of the gene for multiple self-healing epithelioma (Ferguson-Smith type) to the long arm of chromosome 9. *Cytogenet Cell Genet* 1991; **58**: 1939.

Gardner's syndrome

Definition

Gardner's syndrome comprises multiple epidermoid cysts, fibrous tissue tumours, osteomas and polyposis of the colon. This syndrome was described in 1953 by Gardner and Richards[1].

Clinical features

The clinical features of Gardner's syndrome [1–5] (Figure 19.3) include polyposis of the colon or rectum, which usually arises during the second decade, but may occur in early childhood. It is present in about 50% of cases by the age of 20 years. There are few symptoms, and intussusception is not a feature. Malignant change develops some 15–20 years later in over 40% of reported cases. Sebaceous or epidermoid cysts, which may be numerous, are usually irregularly distributed on the face, scalp and extremities, and are less frequent on the trunk. They may first appear between the ages of 4 years and 10 years, but often considerably later, and are ultimately present in almost all cases. Osteomas develop mainly in the maxilla, mandible and sphenoid bones, but also in other bones of the skull and (less frequently) in the long bones. They are usually small, multiple and are present in some 50% of cases. The age of onset is often not accurately known, but the osteomas may be present at puberty. Fibromas or desmoid tumours are

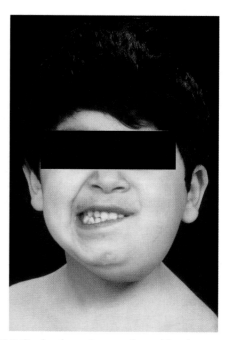

Figure 19.3 *Gardner's syndrome: a boy with a large submandibular tumour*

less frequently present. They are usually poorly localized tumours in incisional scars of the abdomen, but may occur at other sites. Fibrosarcomas have also been associated with the syndrome. Fibromatous growths of the mesentery may be discovered at operation, and severe peritoneal scarring may follow surgery. Lipomas in the subcutaneous tissues, and in other organs, have frequently been noted. Leiomyomas, of the stomach or ileum, or retroperitoneal, are sometimes present. The variable expression of the gene must be remembered when a family is investigated[6]. Cutaneous and skeletal changes may be present without polyposis, and polyposis may be present when one or more of the other features of the syndrome is lacking[7]. Congenital hypertrophy of the retinal pigment epithelium is a frequent finding in Gardner's syndrome and is a valuable clue to the presence of the gene in persons who have not yet developed other manifestations[8,9].

Pathology

The pathology and natural history of the polyposis are essentially similar to familial polyposis coli. Several groups have reported the association of hepatoblastoma with polyposis coli[10,11].

Genetics

Inheritance is determined by an autosomal dominant gene of variable expression. Gardner's syndrome is located on chromosome 5q, near bands 5q21–22 [12,13]. It is now thought that Gardner's syndrome and familial polyposis coli are allelic disorders.

Differential diagnosis

Multiple epidermoid or sebaceous cysts may be inherited as an isolated abnormality and may thus have no sinister significance. Their discovery is an indication for a detailed family history and a careful examination for osteomas, including radiological examination of the skull, and for other dermal tumours. The cutaneous lesions are an important indicator of possible asymptomatic polyposis.

References

1 Gardner EJ, Richards RC. Multiple cutaneous and subcutaneous lesions occurring simultaneously with hereditary polyposis and osteomatosis. *Am J Hum Genet* 1953; **5**: 139–47.
2 Danes BS. The Gardner syndrome. *Cancer* 1975; **36**: 2327–33.
3 Hornstein OP, Knickenberg M. Perifollicular fibromatosis cutis with polyps of the colon – a cutaneo-intestinal syndrome sui generis. *Arch Dermatol Res* 1975; **253**: 161–75.
4 McKusick VA. Genetic factors in intestinal polyposis. *J Am Med Assoc* 1962; **182**: 271–7.
5 Weary PE, Linthicum A, Cawley EP, Coleman CC, Graham GF. Gardner's syndrome: a family group study and review. *Arch Dermatol* 1964; **90**: 20–30.
6 Danes BS. The Gardner's syndrome: increased tetraploidy in cultured skin fibroblasts. *J Med Genet* 1976; **13**: 52–6.
7 Thomas KE, Watne AL, Johnson JG, Roth E, Zimmermann B. Natural history of Gardner's syndrome. *Am J Surg* 1968; **115**: 218–26.
8 Blair NP, Trempe CL. Hypertrophy of the retinal pigment epithelium associated with Gardner's syndrome. *Am J Ophthalmol* 1980; **90**: 661–7.
9 Traboulsi EI, Krush AJ, Gardner EJ et al. Prevalence and importance of pigmented ocular fundus lesions in Gardner's syndrome. *New Engl J Med* 1987; **316**: 661–7.
10 Kingston JE, Draper GJ, Mann JR. Hepatoblastoma and polyposis coli. *Lancet* 1982; **i**: 475.
11 Li FP, Thurber WA, Seddon J, Holmes GE. Hepatoblastoma in families with polyposis coli. *J Am Med Assoc* 1987; **257**: 2475–7.
12 Bodmer WF, Bailey CJ, Bodmer J et al. Localisation of the gene for familial adenomatous polyposis on chromosome 5. *Nature* 1987; **328**: 614–16.
13 Leppert M, Dobbs M, Scambler P et al. The gene for familial polyposis coli maps to the long arm of chromosome 5. *Science* 1987; **238**: 1411–13.

Gorlin's syndrome

Synonym: *Naevoid basal cell carcinoma syndrome*

Definition

Gorlin's syndrome[1,2] is characterized by multiple basal cell carcinomas, jaw cysts and skeletal malformations.

Clinical features

The basal cell skin lesions usually develop from puberty onwards, rarely in childhood[1,2]. They mainly affect the face, neck and trunk (Figure 19.4), and can number from a few to several hundred. The majority of the tumours behave in a benign fashion, but invasive basal cell carcinomas can develop and are particularly a problem around the eyelids, nose and nasolabial folds. Other skin lesions are epidermoid cysts, milia and distinctive pits on the palms and soles, which are a helpful pointer to the diagnosis (Figure 19.5).

Variable skeletal abnormalities include bone cysts, which are the most common and affect the mandible and maxilla, frontal bossing of the skull, hypertelorism, prognathism, bifid ribs, syndactyly, spina bifida occulta and kyphoscoliosis. Intracranial calcification also occurs. Ocular abnormalities, including congenital blindness, have been reported.

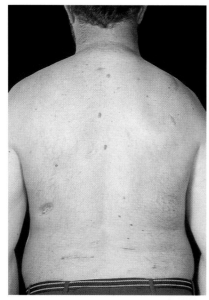

Figure 19.4 *Gorlin's syndrome: excision of multiple basal cell carcinomas*

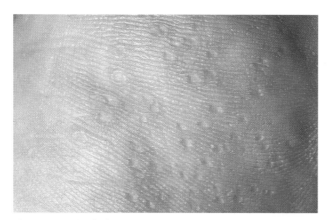

Figure 19.5 *Gorlin's syndrome: typical palmar pits*

There is a definite increase in incidence of non-dermatological malignancies, including squamous cell carcinoma and fibrosarcoma of the jaw cysts, and nasopharyngeal carcinoma. Other tumours that have been described in association with Gorlin's syndrome are medulloblastoma in childhood; ovarian and testicular tumours; cardiac and renal fibromas; melanoma; neurofibroma; leiomyoma; and rhabdomyoma/sarcoma. Mesenteric lymphatic or chylous cysts may occur.

Genetics

Inheritance is autosomal dominant. The gene for Gorlin's syndrome has been localized to chromosome 9q22.3–31 [3].

Differential diagnosis

The association of palmar pits and skeletal anomalies is normally sufficient to distinguish this syndrome from the case of an individual who has one or more basal cell carcinomas due to sun-damaged skin.

Treatment

All lesions around the eyelids, nose and nasolabial folds should be removed because of their destructive potential. Surgical excision is probably the best form of treatment; however, some have used curettage with cautery or diathermy, and cryosurgery. Radiotherapy should not be used. The prognosis should be good, provided no invasive tumours or other complications develop.

References

1 Howell JB, Caro MR. Basal-cell nevus: its relationship to multiple cutaneous cancers and associated anomalies of development. *Arch Dermatol* 1959; **79**: 67–80.
2 Gorlin RJ, Goltz RW. Multiple nevoid basal-cell epithelioma, jaw cysts and bifid rib. A syndrome. *New Engl J Med* 1960; **262**: 908–12.
3 Farndon PA, Del Mastro RG, Evans DGR et al. Location of gene for Gorlin syndrome. *Lancet* 1992; **339**: 581–2

Part Three

General Principles of Diagnosis and Management

Chapter 20

Genetic counselling in skin disorders

M. Baraitser

Introduction

At its most basic, genetic counselling is concerned with the calculation of risks of recurrence of conditions that are known to exist in the family, or that have occurred previously in a single member of that family. This counselling can be given by the dermatologist, by the clinical geneticist, or at a combined clinic. One of the advantages of separate counselling clinics, as opposed to genetic counselling in a busy dermatological department, is that genetic clinics are organized in such a way that rough pedigrees can often be drawn up before the patient is seen, from the information provided by families or their doctors, and a diagnosis or differential diagnoses can be formulated from reports from many sources, so that the clinical geneticist can be prepared to answer relevant questions. Counselling becomes increasingly difficult in the absence of a clear diagnosis, and every effort should be made to achieve the correct clinical designation. All counselling sessions begin with a diagrammatic representation of the pedigree, to establish who is affected and the relationship of the patient to others in the pedigree.

The risks are calculated and expressed as odds (for instance, the recurrence risk of having another affected child in an autosomal recessive condition is 1 in 4) or as a percentage (i.e. 25%). The risks can be viewed in many ways, and most counsellors will, when appropriate, express the risk figure in different terms to the two examples cited above. For instance, there would be 3 chances out of 4 for a good result in a situation in which there is a 1 in 4 chance of recurrence. The risk figure should be put into perspective by using as a background figure the general population risk that any couple would run of having a newborn child with a major malformation noted at birth. This background figure is of the order of 1 in 50 (2%); taking note of this, most people would agree that only risks greater than 1 in 10 (10%) should be considered as high, whereas risks that are less than 5% – i.e. less than 1 in 20 – should be considered as low. A risk between 5% and 10% is neither very high nor very low, and as the figure of 10% is approached it is difficult to make confident judgements and decisions. It has also become the practice in genetics not to specify very low risks, i.e. risks of less than 1 in 1000, as there are often published reports of very unusual and unexpected recurrences which cannot be easily predicted; so it is prudent to say in low-risk situations that the chances are less than 1% without quoting exact figures, unless they can be precisely calculated.

In many situations mendelian risk figures are not appropriate as the condition may be multifactorial. For instance, spina bifida and psoriasis, which are relatively common in the population, are weakly inherited and need more than one gene, or an additional environmental influence, before they are manifested. Risk figures in such conditions are derived from family studies and by studying the pedigree. Provided that the patients understand how the risk is calculated and can see that it is not a random estimate, they will usually accept that the advice is based on available evidence and could form the basis of a reasonable decision.

After advising the patient of the risk and putting it into perspective, the counsellor may follow with a few exploratory questions to make sure that the risk has been understood, such as, 'How do you feel about the risk?'; this might receive the response, 'I am not prepared to take any risk' or 'I don't want further children'. Provided that the geneticist is sure that the response indicates that the parents have understood the risk, and are not basing their immediate decision on a false assumption, no further enquiry which could challenge the patients' decision is appropriate. Even where the reasoning is controversial, the counsellor will be quick to say that we all see risks differently and that all actions within legal constraints are acceptable. The counselling process is always dynamic and should be used to allow parents to explore their own immediate thoughts. For instance, in autosomal recessive disorders, where both parents are carriers and may feel a stigma attached to being a carrier, the geneticist should take care to point out that there are good grounds to believe that all members of the population are likely to be gene carriers for at least one mutant – and therefore potentially harmful – gene. In single dose this would not cause problems, but in double dose, i.e. when both parents are carriers for the same mutant allele (or gene) and a child receives both mutant alleles, then an autosomal recessive condition manifests. An awareness of the anxiety which many people will feel, given genetic implications, is necessary, and hints of underlying turmoil need to be attended to and at all times put into perspective. It is also a frequent occurrence during counselling for parents to point out that very low risk figures are meaningless, because they have already been caught out despite the risks being greatly in their favour. For instance, the prior probability of any couple having a child with tuberous sclerosis is 1 in 30 000; parents who have such a child may be quick to point out that a recurrence risk of, say, 2% (the risk if neither parent shows any signs of the disease) may be small, but they have already been unlucky with a risk far smaller than that. It is this type of interaction that is time-consuming and yet very relevant in terms of counselling, and must be seen as part of the dynamics of genetic counselling. It should also be noted and pointed out to patients that in many situations risk figures are going to be 'the best that are available' and 'as accurate as possible', and every attempt should be made to convey this. It is also important in high-risk cases to discuss the possibility of prenatal diagnosis and artificial insemination by donor or even ovum transplantation (see below).

Who needs genetic counselling?

Genetic counselling is valuable in the following situations:

1. Where there is a positive family history of the condition. This should be seen in its fullest perspective, in that reassurance about a relative whose problem is not relevant to the condition under consideration is as important as confirmation of a relevant family history.
2. A previous child is diagnosed as having a genetic disorder.
3. A previous child has a multisystem involvement, i.e. multiple congenital abnormalities including a skin disorder.
4. A skin disorder exists which may have genetic implications.
5. There is a known genetic disorder and advice is needed about prenatal diagnosis.
6. Anxiety exists about an event that happened during pregnancy.
7. There is concern about age and its relationship to abnormality.
8. Blame – 'It must be something on your side of the family'.
9. Guilt – especially in X-linked disorders when the mother feels that she has passed on the problem.
10. Misconceptions – there is often a mistaken belief that if a disorder is genetic, it must have 'come from somewhere'. This is followed by endless delving into the family tree, mostly without success, to find another family member who might have the same condition.
11. The search for a diagnosis. There is often a strong desire for parents to be able to call their child's condition by a specific name. This enables them to communicate with other parents of children with the same condition; failing this, the geneticists who have become especially skilled in the diagnosis of rare syndromes may know of other patients seen previously. Most units will use one of the computerized databases of all the published syndromes and can simply ask for a differential diagnosis of any combination of features.
12. Information is needed about consanguinity. If there is nothing of note in the family tree, then the chance that first cousins would produce a child with a recessive disorder, which is their main risk, is of the order of 3%. This is a tenfold increase, but still well within the low order of risks. If the first-cousin parents have a previous child with an unrecognizable condition and they come from a population in which cousin marriage is infrequent, then it is highly likely that the condition could be recessively inherited. The same situation in populations in which first-cousin marriage is frequent will be more difficult to assess, and may result in intermediate risk figures based on the type of malformation under consideration.
13. Carrier detection. The detection of carriers in families who have had a child or adult with genetic disease may be appropriate, using biochemical, cytogenetic or DNA techniques. This requires a detailed explanation and the arrangement for blood samples to be taken.

It can be seen from the above that the counselling procedure is more than just a statement of risks, and that even those who do not want further children may benefit from a discussion of a number of the points above. In essence there are no exclusion criteria that make genetic counselling undesirable, and referral should be considered if any of the above is raised by the family.

In the past some doctors have shown a certain reluctance to refer people for counselling. The worry has been that by making a rare syndrome diagnosis doctors are doing nothing more than being clever without benefit to the patient. This is no longer the case, as without a diagnosis the assessment of risk is extremely difficult, and most people want accurate recurrence risks not vague reassurance. Medicolegal considerations have also persuaded doctors that precise labels and accurate recurrence risks are advisable. Parents not only want to read about the condition diagnosed in their child, but also want to meet other parents who have children with similar problems. As evidence for this there are now a number of patient groups dedicated to individual rare syndromes.

Genetic counselling identifies those who transmit genetic disease, and this occasionally creates difficulties. The act of taking a family pedigree not only elucidates the mechanism of inheritance, but may also identify members who were previously unaware that they were gene carriers or mildly affected. Countering the argument that unpleasant information may come to the surface by drawing up a family tree or by needing to take blood from a distant family member, is the view that if the situation is well handled, serious handicap can be prevented. There are certainly those who would argue that they would have preferred not to have known, but this is outweighed in most cases by the benefits of knowing.

Counselling in high-risk situations

All risks greater than 1 in 10 are high, although the counsellor may avoid the emotive word 'high' in favour of an indication that such a risk 'is one that may need serious thought'. It is part of the art of genetic counselling not to make value judgements (unless specifically asked), a technique incorporated in the concept of non-directive counselling, and there are good reasons for this approach. People may view a 1 in 4 (25%) risk in different ways; one extreme is where a couple arrive for counselling with the woman already pregnant, a situation in which the words 'high' and 'serious' are inappropriate, especially if the couple have strong views against termination of pregnancy. If the pregnancy has already progressed beyond 24 weeks, the counsellor, faced with limited options having given the correct recurrence risk, may emphasize the 3 chances out of 4 that the couple are

going to be lucky. It is in such situations that health visitors and social workers in attendance at the clinic can offer more long-term support than is possible during one counselling session.

There are other reasons why a high risk may be acceptable to a couple:

1. The availability of prenatal diagnosis (see below).
2. The high-risk condition may be viewed by the couple as being mild. The problem here is that the couple whose first child is affected may not realize that the condition could be manifested to a more serious degree; but provided that this is fully discussed – and the medical view of seriousness should not take precedence – even conditions involving mental retardation are, to some parents, acceptable.
3. High risks may be accepted by parents who have no healthy children and will accept the risk in order to have at least one healthy child. This is often seen soon after the death of a first-born affected child, when some parents will desperately want to replace the loss – perhaps being emotionally driven rather than being able to make an objective decision. It is one of the reasons why it is always appropriate to delay genetic counselling for 2–3 months after such an event.
4. Whether the condition is rapidly lethal, or chronic and debilitating. In some situations parents find it easier to accept a high risk for a condition which, if they were to be unlucky, would result in death within the first months of life. They would argue that it is less fair to the child and to themselves if the condition were to have a slowly progressive course over many years.

One way round a high-risk situation, especially in autosomal recessive disease but also in autosomal dominant conditions where the father is the affected parent, is to consider artificial insemination by donor (AID). Most counsellors would raise this as a possibility and wait to see how it is accepted by the parents. If it is acceptable, then recurrence risks should drop to that of the general population. Ovum donation, which is often more acceptable, and is especially applicable in X-linked recessive disorders where the mother is a carrier, has a success rate which is currently only 20–30%, and the technique is not readily available in most countries. The technical problems and organization of this latter procedure are still major drawbacks, and the procedure should not be offered unless the counsellor knows that it can be easily obtained.

Counselling in low-risk situations

Low risks are those that are less than 5%; risks that are very low, say less than 1 in 1000, are seldom a reality at genetic clinics. There are few situations which have never been known to recur within families, so it would be unwise for counsellors to use terms such as 'incredibly rare' or 'remote'. It is best to say that the risks are small, and quote a figure of less than 1%, followed by an explanation, where possible, of how this figure is derived. In general, the geneticist should be able to estimate how many cases have been reported and on how many occasions there have been rare, unexpected recurrences.

Some parents will be unexpectedly deterred by very low risks. Many come with the expectation of being told that there are no risks, and some will even want to consider prenatal diagnosis in situations where the chances of being unlucky are less than 1%. In essence, the experience of having had a child with a serious disorder (and sometimes even one that is not medically very serious) is, for some, so overwhelming that emotionally they could not go through it again. Low risks will be easier to cope with for both the counsellor and the parents, but care must be exercised not to prejudge the situation.

Counselling medium-order risks

Medium risks are those in the vicinity of 10%, and because it is neither very high nor very low, this risk figure is often a difficult one on which to make a decision. This order of risk is often the estimate in conditions determined by both genetic and environmental influences, after its occurrence in two first-degree relatives (for example spina bifida). It is also the order of risk where, say, half of all cases are known to be genetically determined (autosomal recessive) whereas the rest are known to have a solely environmental causation. Medium-order risks are often counselled where the exact nature of the condition cannot be determined, but the genetic counsellor has been something similar before in affected sibs, or is suspicious about a particular combination of signs, and is clearly worried about the situation. Provided that it can be shown how these risks are derived and that they are based on careful consideration of reported cases and experience, risk calculations of this nature can be justified.

Whether people accept middle-order risks and plan further children depends largely on the severity of the condition, the family structure and the availability of prenatal tests.

Risk calculation in autosomal recessive conditions

Individuals with an autosomal recessive disorder are homozygous for the mutant gene and therefore manifest the condition. Recurrence risks for the carrier parents (for practical purposes they must be carriers,

and fresh mutations need not really be considered) are 1 in 4, but offspring risks for those who are affected are generally small, as most recessive conditions are rare, and it is unlikely that the affected person will marry another carrier in the population. When the disease frequency is known, as in oculocutaneous albinism, then the following calculations apply. The disease frequency is about 1 in 10 000, and the gene frequency is the square root of this. The carrier frequency is twice the gene frequency:

$$\text{gene frequency} = \frac{1}{\sqrt{10\,000}}$$

$$= \frac{1}{100}$$

$$\text{carrier frequency} = \frac{1}{100} \times 2 = \frac{1}{50}$$

The chance that an affected person will have an affected child is calculated as follows. The affected person must pass on one of the mutant genes (i.e. the chance is 1); this is multiplied by 1/50 (the chance that an unrelated spouse is a gene carrier) and multiplied by 1/2 as there is a 1 in 2 chance of passing on the mutant gene:

$$1 \times \frac{1}{50} \times \frac{1}{2} = \frac{1}{100}$$

There is therefore a chance of 1 in 100 of having an affected child, i.e. the risk is low.

Sibs of those who are affected have a two-thirds chance of being gene carriers (Figure 20.1), but again are not at risk of having affected children, because carriers in the population are relatively few in number; the calculation is

$$\frac{2}{3} \times \frac{1}{50} \times \frac{1}{4} = \frac{1}{300}$$

In both the above situations it would be better if inbreeding (i.e. cousin marriage) were not contemplated.

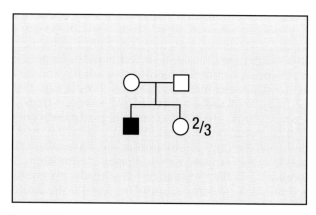

Figure 20.1

In summary, in autosomal recessive disease it is only the parents of the affected child who have a high risk of recurrence.

Risk calculation in autosomal dominant conditions

People who have an autosomal dominant condition are heterozygous for a mutant gene which expresses itself in single dose. Offspring risks for those who are affected are 50% (1 in 2), but in the case of an affected child where neither parent manifests any sign of the condition, recurrence risks for a further child are likely to be small, as the child would have the genetic disorder as a fresh mutation. Even in this situation there are small recurrence risks, either because in some genetic disorders expression is variable and penetrance may not be 100%, or, as is possibly more common, there are occasional unexpected recurrences because of gonadal mosaicism. This latter term implies that one or other parent is a genetic mosaic and carries the mutant gene only in a gonad or part thereof and therefore has no clinical manifestations. This mechanism possibly explains the sib recurrences in tuberous sclerosis where neither parent, on extensive investigation, manifests any signs of the disease. Recurrence risks of 1–2% are appropriate.

A knowledge of the likelihood of non-penetrance in individual diseases is necessary for accurate counselling. For instance, in neurofibromatosis penetrance by the age of 20 years is nearly always complete, so that if normal parents have an affected child, a fresh mutation can be diagnosed with relative confidence. Likewise, if an affected person has a child who, at the age of 20 years, wants to have children, and there are no skin lesions (or fewer than five *café au lait* patches) then risks to offspring are small (less than 1%).

The concept of 'fresh mutation' is difficult for parents. It is always worth pointing out that in simple terms, their genes are normal, and that they are in no way responsible for the gene change. The best way to explain this change is that it was a miscopy of a normal parental gene. This inevitably leads to enquiries about the cause of the miscopy, producing feelings in the parents that it was because they did something wrong, and this must be countered.

The most common cause of error in counselling about autosomal dominant diseases is to miss minimal manifestations by not examining both parents. Thorough examination is essential.

Another potential error in counselling is encapsulated in the term 'genetic heterogeneity'. For instance, epidermolysis bullosa can be inherited as either a dominant or a recessive condition, and within each of these groups there are many subtypes. Before counselling, a family tree, a history of the onset and course of the illness, and careful histological investigation may be needed before a decision is made on recurrence risks. This necessitates close collaboration between the dermatologist and geneticist.

In the unlikely event of a couple both having the same autosomal dominant disease, the ratio of 3 affected to 1 unaffected should be advised, and for many conditions it will not be possible to say whether the homozygous affected offspring (one of the three) will have the condition to a more serious degree than the two heterozygotes, although this is often the case.

Risk calculation in X-linked recessive conditions

If on pedigree evidence the mother is a carrier of a known X-linked recessive disorder, then theoretically half her sons would be affected and half her daughters would be carriers. This assessment of risk is often misunderstood by parents and it is easier to use the 'spinning coin' explanation to augment the concept. It should be pointed out that if a coin is thrown four times, theoretically two 'heads' and two 'tails' could be expected; however, any other combination may occur – three 'heads' and one 'tail', for example.

Pedigree evidence sufficient to diagnose an obligate carrier (arrowed) is shown in Figure 20.2.

The sister (arrowed) of an obligate carrier could herself be a carrier if their mother is a carrier (Figure 20.3). Alternatively, the mother of the affected boys in Figure 20.3 may be a carrier because of a fresh mutation, in which case the risk that the sister is a carrier may be small. An analysis of the pedigree may provide a clue as to which of the alternative possibilities is correct: for instance, if there are many normal men in the same generation as the two women under consideration (Figure 20.4), then it is unlikely that their mother is a carrier. It is seldom in practice

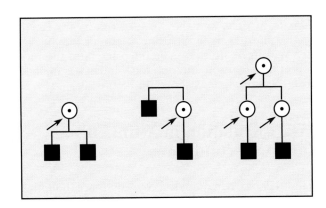

Figure 20.2

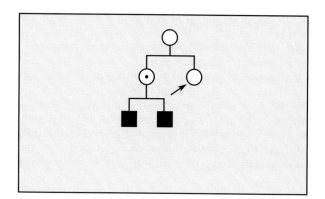

Figure 20.3

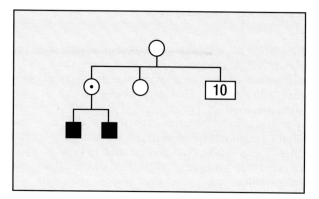

Figure 20.4

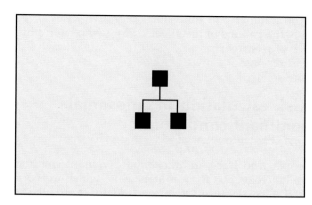

Figure 20.5 *Male-to-male transmission must suggest dominant inheritance*

pigmenti. Females manifest the condition and half of their female offspring could be affected. If an affected woman has two male offspring, then theoretically one would be severely affected and possibly aborted, whereas the other would be normal. In this way the 1:1 male to female sex ratio of the offspring of affected women would be altered to 2:1 in favour of females, and one of these females would be affected. In practice, in both of the conditions mentioned above, large pedigrees with many affected members are unusual, and the majority of cases seem to be fresh mutations. This should not, however, mean that minimal manifestations in the mother should not be sought.

possible to be sure, but Bayesian calculations will give a statistical likelihood of the possibilities by taking normal males into consideration. In some conditions it is now also possible to use DNA probes to determine whether females in an X-linked pedigree are carriers. For instance, in anhidrotic ectodermal dysplasia linkage has been established, and gene tracking within a family may provide data on carrier status. It is, however, necessary to examine possible carriers carefully, looking for clinical manifestations of heterozygosity.

All the female offspring of affected men will be obligate carriers, and they in turn run a 50% risk of having affected male offspring. None of the affected men will have affected male offspring, and the most important exclusion criterion for X-linkage is male-to-male transmission, as shown in Figure 20.5.

Risk calculation in X-linked dominant conditions

A number of dermatological conditions are thought to be inherited in an X-linked dominant manner. The best-known are Goltz's syndrome and incontinentia

Counselling in multifactorial inheritance

For practical purposes it matters not whether we speak of multifactorial or polygenic inheritance. The pedigree pattern produced will be the same, irrespective of whether we are dealing with many genes without environmental influence causing a disorder, or whether there is a harmful gene of major importance which needs a non-genetic contribution in order to have a deleterious effect. It should also be stated that the differentiation between multifactorial inheritance and a single mutant gene with reduced penetrance is equally difficult, but when it comes to risk calculation at the genetic clinic the difference is not important. The reason for this is that most recurrence risks in these situations are based on family studies, and provided that these are correctly done and are without bias, these figures can be used. A good example is atopy. Recent work has suggested that the condition might not arise from multifactorial inheritance, as has always been thought, but from a single gene of major effect which has variable expression. Recurrence risks will not be based on the mechanism

Other studies

Fetal skin obtained in utero has been used for the assessment of DNA repair in the prenatal diagnosis of trichothiodystrophy[46] and of collagenase expression by cultured dermal fibroblasts in the prenatal diagnosis of recessive dystrophic epidermolysis bullosa[47].

Complications

There were no sampling failures or known incorrect diagnoses in a series of over 150 cases (authors' unpublished observations). Fetal skin biopsy is likely to increase the risk of fetal loss by at least 1% over the background incidence of spontaneous abortions[48].

Scarring may result from the biopsy procedure[11], but the risk is reduced when a small 20-gauge cupped forceps is used. In the authors' experience scarring has not been a major problem, and the biopsy scars are often inconspicuous.

Conclusion

Prenatal diagnosis by middle trimester fetal skin biopsy at 15–22 weeks' gestation is generally a safe and rapid procedure. It is also reliable, especially for epidermolysis bullosa. However, its accuracy for certain forms of ichthyosis has been questioned[20,49].

Tests using DNA-based techniques have now been used for the diagnosis and prenatal diagnosis of some of the disorders mentioned in this chapter[50], including X-linked hypohidrotic ectodermal dysplasia[51], recessive dystrophic epidermolysis bullosa[52, 53] junctional epidermolysis bullosa[54, 55] and bullous congenital ichthyosiform erythroderma[56]. The DNA can be obtained from different sources including chorionic villus samples and amniotic fluid cells. A major advance over fetal skin biopsy is that the sampling (of chorionic villi) can be done earlier in pregnancy, i.e. at 10–11 weeks' gestation. However, the method is still invasive and not without complications[57]. Although these newer methods have considerable potential, fetal skin biopsy is likely to continue to be used for prenatal diagnosis until the alternative methods are better established and more widely available, and will remain as the only possibility for certain disorders in the absence of effective DNA markers.

Acknowledgements

The authors would like to thank Dr Adrian Heagerty for providing immunofluorescence micrographs, Mr David Gunner and Ms Trish Dopping-Hepenstal for excellent technical assistance, and Professors Charles Rodeck and Kypros Nicolaides for fruitful and enjoyable collaboration over the past 15 years.

References

1 Royal College of Physicians of London. *Prenatal Diagnosis and Genetic Screening*. Royal College of Physicians of London, 1989; 1–10.
2 Eady RAJ. Genodermatoses. In: Brock DJH, Rodeck CH, Ferguson-Smith, MA, eds. *Prenatal Diagnosis and Screening*. Churchill Livingstone, Edinburgh, 1992; 503–13.
3 Eady RAJ, Holbrook KA, Blanchet-Bardon C, Anton-Lamprecht I. Chair's summary: prenatal diagnosis of skin diseases. In: Burgdorf WHC, Katz SI, eds. *Dermatology, Progress and Perspectives*. Parthenon, New York, 1993; 1159–65.
4 Holbrook KA, Smith LT, Elias S. Prenatal diagnosis of genetic skin disease using fetal skin biopsy samples. *Arch Dermatol* 1993; **129**: 1437–54.
5 Davison BCC. Epidermolysis bullosa. *J Med Genet* 1965; **2**: 233–42.
6 Golbus MS, Sagebiel RW, Filly RA, Gindhart TD, Hall JG. Prenatal diagnosis of congenital bullous ichthyosiform erythroderma (epidermolytic hyperkeratosis) by fetal skin biopsy. *New Engl J Med* 1980; **302**: 93–5.
7 Rodeck CH, Eady RAJ, Gosden CM. Prenatal diagnosis of epidermolysis bullosa letalis. *Lancet* 1980; **i**: 949–52.
8 Anton-Lamprecht I, Rauskolb R, Jovanovic V et al. Prenatal diagnosis of epidermolysis bullosa dystrophica Hallopeau–Siemens with electron microscopy of fetal skin. *Lancet* 1981; **ii**: 1077–9.
9 Rodeck CH, Nicolaides KH. Fetoscopy and fetal tissue sampling. *Br Med Bull* 1983; **39**: 332–7.
10 Perry TB. Clinical procedures for prenatal diagnosis of inherited skin disease: amniocentesis, ultrasound, fetoscopy and fetal skin biopsy and blood sampling. *Sem Dermatol* 1984; **3**: 155–66.
11 Elias S. Use of fetoscopy for the prenatal diagnosis of hereditary skin disorders. In: Gedde-Dahl T, Wuepper KD, eds. *Prenatal Diagnosis of Heritable Skin Disease*. Karger, Basel; 1987; 1–13.
12 Eady RAJ. Fetoscopy and fetal skin biopsy for prenatal diagnosis of genetic skin disorders. *Sem Dermatol* 1988; **7**: 2–8.
13 Campbell S, Pearce J. Ultrasound visualization of congenital malformations. *Br Med Bull* 1983; **39**: 322–31.
14 Heagerty AHM, Kennedy AR, Gunner DB, Eady RAJ Rapid prenatal diagnosis and exclusion of epidermolysis bullosa using novel antibody probes. *J Invest Dermatol* 1986; **86**: 603–5.
15 Holbrook KA, Wapner R, Jackson L. Diagnosis and prenatal diagnosis of epidermolysis bullosa herpetiformis (Dowling-Meara) in a mother, two affected children and an affected fetus. *Prenat Diag* 1992; **12**: 725–39.
16 Anton-Lamprecht I. Prenatal diagnosis of genetic disorders of the skin by means of electron microscopy. *Hum Genet* 1981; **59**: 392–405.

17 Holbrook KA, Dale BA, Sybert VP, Sagebiel RW. Epidermolytic hyperkeratosis: ultrastructure and biochemistry of skin and amniotic fluid cells from two affected fetuses and a newborn infant. *J Invest Dermatol* 1983; **80**: 222–7.

18 Eady RAJ, Gunner DB, Doria Lamba-Carbone L et al. Prenatal diagnosis of bullous ichthyosiform erythroderma: detection of tonofilament clumps in fetal epidermal and amniotic fluid cells. *J Med Genet* 1986; **23**: 46–51.

19 Perry TB, Holbrook KA, Hoff MS. Prenatal diagnosis of congenital non-bullous ichthyosiform erythroderma (lamellar ichthyosis). *Prenat Diag* 1987; **70**: 145–55.

20 Holbrook KA, Dale BA, Williams ML et al. The expression of congenital ichthyosiform erythroderma in second trimester fetuses of the same family: morphologic and biochemical studies. *J Invest Dermatol* 1988; **91**: 521–31.

21 Blanchet-Bardon C, Dumez Y. Prenatal diagnosis of harlequin fetus. *Sem Dermatol* 1984; **3**: 224–8.

22 Suzumori K, Kanzaki T. Prenatal diagnosis of harlequin ichthyosis by fetal skin biopsy: report of two cases. *Prenat Diag* 1991; **11**: 451–7.

23 Eady RAJ, Blanchet-Bardon C, Gunner DB, Schofield OMV, Rodeck CH. Atypical intraepidermal vesicles serve as a marker for prenatal diagnosis of harlequin ichthyosis (abstract). *J Invest Dermatol* 1990; **95**: 468.

24 Kousseff BG, Matsouka LY, Stenn KS et al. Prenatal diagnosis of Sjögren–Larsson syndrome. *J Pediatr* 1982; **101**: 998–1001.

25 Eady RAJ, Gunner DB, Garner A, Rodeck CH. Prenatal diagnosis of oculocutaneous albinism by electron microscopy of fetal skin. *J Invest Dermatol* 1983; **80**: 210–12.

26 Eady RAJ. Prenatal diagnosis of oculocutaneous albinism: implications for other hereditary disorders of pigmentation. *Sem Dermatol* 1984; **3**: 241–6.

27 Shimizu H, Ishiko A, Kikuchi A. Prenatal diagnosis of tyrosinase-negative oculocutaneous albinism. *Lancet* 1992; **340**: 739–40.

28 Anton-Lamprecht I, Arnold ML, Rauskolb R. et al. Letter to the Editor. *Hum Genet* 1982; **62**: 18.

29 Holbrook KA. The biology of human fetal skin at ages related to prenatal diagnosis. *Pediatr Dermatol* 1983; **1**: 97–111.

30 Eady RAJ, Gunner DB, Tidman MJ, Nicolaides KH, Rodeck CH. Rapid processing of fetal skin for prenatal diagnosis by light and electron microscopy. *J Clin Pathol* 1984; **37**: 633–8.

31 Haynes ME, Robertson E. Can oculocutaneous albinism be diagnosed prenatally? *Prenat Diag* 1981; **1**: 85–9.

32 Gershoni-Baruch R, Benderly A, Brandes JM, Gilhar A. DOPA reaction test in hair bulbs of fetuses and its application to the prenatal diagnosis of albinism. *J Am Acad Dermatol* 1991; **24**: 220–7.

33 Fine J-D. Basement membrane related antigens: their significance in epidermolysis bullosa. In: Priestley JB, Tidman MJ, Weiss J, Eady RAJ, eds. *Epidermolysis Bullosa: A Comprehensive Review of Classification, Therapy and Laboratory Studies.* DEBRA Publications, Crowthorne, 1990; 40–9.

34 Katz SI. The epidermal basement membrane zone: structure, antigens and role in disease. *J Am Acad Dermatol* 1984; **11**: 1025–37.

35 Eady RAJ. Babes, blisters and basement membranes: from sticky molecules to epidermolysis bullosa. *Clin Exp Dermatol* 1987; **12**: 161–70.

36 Heagerty AHM, Kennedy AR, Eady RAJ et al. GB3 monoclonal antibody for the diagnosis of junctional epidermolysis bullosa. *Lancet* 1986; **i**: 860.

37 Verrando P, Pisani A, Ortonne J-P. The new basement membrane antigen recognized by the monoclonal antibody GB3 is a large size glycoprotein; modulation of its expression by retinoic acid. *Biochim Biophys Acta* 1988; **942**: 45–56.

38 Schofield OMV, Fine J-D, Verrando P et al. GB3 monoclonal antibody for the diagnosis of junctional epidermolysis bullosa: results of a multicenter study. *J Am Acad Dermatol* 1990; **23**: 1078–83.

39 Fine J-D, Horiguchi Y, Couchman JR. 19-DEJ-1, a hemidesmosome anchoring filament complex-associated monoclonal antibody. *Arch Dermatol* 1989; **125**: 520–5.

40 Heagerty AHM, Kennedy AR, Leigh IM, Purkis P, Eady RAJ. Identification of an epidermal basement membrane defect in recessive forms of dystrophic epidermolysis bullosa by LH7:2 monoclonal antibody: use in diagnosis. *Br J Dermatol* 1986; **115**: 125–131.

41 Leigh IM, Eady RAJ, Heagerty, AHM et al. Type VII collagen is a normal component of epidermal basement membrane which shows altered expression in recessive dystrophic epidermolysis bullosa. *J Invest Dermatol* 1988; **90**: 639–42.

42 Heagerty AHM, Eady RAJ, Kennedy AR et al. Rapid prenatal diagnosis of epidermolysis bullosa letalis using GB3 monoclonal antibody. *Br J Dermatol* 1987; **117**: 271–5.

43 Nazzaro V, Nicolini U, De Luca L, Berti E, Caputo R. Prenatal diagnosis of junctional epidermolysis bullosa associated with pyloric atresia. *J Med Genet* 1990; **27**: 244–8.

44 Fine J-D, Eady RAJ, Levy ML et al. Prenatal diagnosis of dominant and recessive dystrophic epidermolysis bullosa: application and limitations in the use of KF1 and LH 7.2 monoclonal antibodies and immunofluorescence mapping technique. *J Invest Dermatol* 1988; **91**: 465–71.

45 Fine J-D, Holbrook KA, Elias S, Anton-Lamprecht I, Rauskolb R. Applicability of 19-DEJ-1 monoclonal antibody for the prenatal diagnosis and exclusion of junctional epidermolysis bullosa. *Prenat Diag* 1990; **10**: 219–29.

46 Blanchet-Bardon C, Sarrasin A, Renault G, Dumez Y, Civatte J. Prenatal diagnosis of BIDS and IBIDS syndromes: trichothiodystrophies with DNA repair defect. *Br J Dermatol* 1989; **121** (suppl. 34): 18.

47 Bauer EA, Lindman MD, Goldberg JD, Berkowitz RL, Holbrook KA. Antenatal diagnosis of recessive dystrophic epidermolysis bullosa: collagenase expression in cultured fibroblasts as a biochemical marker. *J Invest Dermatol* 1986; **87**: 597–601.

48 Rodeck CH. Prenatal diagnosis of epidermolysis bullosa. In: Priestley JB, Tidman MJ, Weiss JA, Eady RAJ, eds. *Epidermolysis Bullosa: A Comprehensive Review of Classification/Therapy and Laboratory Studies.* DEBRA Publications, Crowthorne, 1990; 10–12.

49 Arnold ML, Anton-Lamprecht I. Problems in prenatal diagnosis of the ichthyosis congenita group. *Hum Genet* 1985; **71**: 301–11.

50 Christiano AM, Uitto J. DNA-based prenatal diagnosis of heritable skin diseases. *Arch Dermatol* 1993; **129**: 1455–9.

51 Zonana JH, Schinzel A, Upadhaya M et al. Prenatal diagnosis of X-linked hypohidrotic ectodermal dysplasia by linkage analysis. *Am J Hum Genet* 1990; **35**: 132–5.

52 Hovnanian A, Hilal L, Blanchet-Bardon C et al. DNA-based prenatal diagnosis of generalised recessive dystrophic epidermolysis bullosa in six pregnancies at risk for recurrence. *J Invest Dermatol* 1995; **104**: 456–61.

53 Dunnill MGS, Rodeck CH, Richards AJ et al. Use of type VII collagen gene (COL7A1) markers in prenatal diagnosis of recessive dystrophic epidermolysis bullosa. *J Med Genet* 1995; **32**: 749–50.

54 Vailly J, Pulkinen L, Miguel C et al. Identification of a homozygous one base-pair deletion in exon 14 of LAMB3 gene in a patient with Herlitz junctional epidermolysis bullosa and prenatal diagnosis in a family at risk for recurrence. *J Invest Dermatol* 1995; **104**: 462–6.

55 McGrath JA, Kiviriko S, Ciatti S et al. A homozygous nonsense mutation in the α3 chain gene of laminin 5 (LAMA3) in Herlitz junctional epidermolysis bullosa: prenatal exclusion in a fetus at risk. *Genomics* 1995; **29**: 282–4.

56 Rothnagel JA, Longley MA, Holder RA, Kuster W, Roop DR. Prenatal diagnosis of epidermolytic hyperkeratosis by direct gene sequencing. *J Invest Dermatol* 1994; **102**: 13–16.

57 Silverman NS, Wapner RJ. Chorionic villus sampling. In: Brock DJH, Rodeck CH, Ferguson-Smith MA, eds. *Prenatal Diagnosis and Screening*. Churchill Livingstone, Edinburgh, 1992; 25–38.

Chapter 22

Preimplantation diagnosis

R. J. A. Penketh

Introduction

The period following fertilization of the human oocyte until the blastocyst implants into the endometrium some 6–7 days later is known as the preimplantation period. During this time, the conceptus is a free-living organism in the genital tract of the mother, and until the recent development of human in vitro fertilization[1], these early stages of human life were extremely difficult to study.

Since the 1970s there have been enormous advances in the prenatal diagnosis of genetic disease. The availability of genetic typing by DNA analysis has allowed diagnoses to be made on any tissue of the pregnancy, and thus enabled the introduction of first-trimester diagnosis by chorionic villus sampling[2]. Samples of placental villi are removed under ultrasound guidance, either following the passage of an instrument through the cervix, or by transabdominal needling. The range of genodermatoses that can be diagnosed in the first trimester will increase with knowledge of the molecular basis of each condition. In essence, if the causative mutation in a mendelian disorder is known for the particular family then prenatal diagnosis by DNA is possible. Such a disorder can also become a candidate for preimplantation diagnosis.

Advances in the technologies of both in vitro fertilization and the diagnosis of single gene disorders by DNA methods allowed serious consideration of the possibility of diagnosis before implantation[3,4]. The first clinical trial of preimplantation sexing in the context of avoiding serious X-linked disease was reported in 1990[5] and preimplantation

exclusion of cystic fibrosis after in vitro fertilization 2 years later[6]. The success of superovulation, in vitro fertilization and embryo transfer has steadily improved since the 1980s. Developments such as ultrasound guided vaginal oocyte retrieval[7], improved superovulation with luteinizing hormone releasing hormone (LHRH) analogues[8] and delayed administration of human chorionic gonadotrophin (HCG)[9] have improved not only the success but also the acceptability of the technique for infertile patients.

Prenatal diagnosis of sickle cell disease using Southern blotting techniques required the DNA from perhaps a million cells, but introduction of the polymerase chain reaction[10] enabled the diagnosis to be made using the DNA from only 75 cells in the first instance, and more recently using only single cells. The technique has been applied to single copy gene sequences in spermatozoa[11], single oocytes[12] and cells removed from the early embryo.

In addition, those closely involved in prenatal diagnosis have realized a need among some of their patients to be able to begin a pregnancy in the knowledge that it will not be affected by the disorder for which their families are at risk. This would avoid the distressing period of pregnancy before genetic diagnosis is completed, and the parents can be reassured that the pregnancy is unaffected by the disorder and begin to get to know their baby without the fear of possible termination of an affected fetus after prenatal diagnosis.

This chapter outlines the strategies for preimplantation diagnosis, the range of patients who might benefit from the application of such technology, and current progress.

In vitro fertilization and early human development

In vitro fertilization (IVF) follows the hormonal stimulation of multiple follicular development by one of a variety of stimulation regimens. Each patient's response to hormonal stimulation is closely monitored by ultrasound examination of follicular development, and measurement of the hormone output (serum oestradiol) from the ovaries. When the response is judged to be appropriate, maturation of the oocytes is induced by administration of HCG which mimics a luteinizing hormone surge.

Oocytes are collected approximately 34 hours later by either transvaginal ultrasonographically controlled [7, 13, 14] or laparoscopically guided needle aspiration of the follicles[15,16]. After a short period of pre-incubation the oocyte cumulus complex is transferred to medium containing motile spermatozoa which have been separated from the ejaculate. Approximately 18 hours later, the oocytes are examined for the presence of pronuclei which indicate that fertilization has occurred. The following day embryos are examined for cleavage, and up to three with the best morphology are transferred to the patient's uterus between the two-cell and eight-cell stages. The concentration of serum beta subunit of HCG is measured 14 days after oocyte recovery in order to detect pregnancy, and ultrasound examination after 28 days confirms that intrauterine implantation has occurred.

Figure 22.1 demonstrates the appearances of human embryos during cleavage, through to the formation of a blastocele cavity and eventually to the hatching of the blastocyst from the zona pellucida. The individual cells during early cleavage are called blastomeres. By the blastocyst stage, two distinct cell types have evolved: those on the outside, known as trophecto-derm, which are destined to form placental tissues; and those of the inner cell mass, which form the yolk sac, umbilical cord and eventually the fetus itself. All stages up to the hatching blastocyst have been successfully cultured in vitro, but only 22–59% of spare embryos after human IVF reach the blastocyst stage. Unfortunately, as yet there has been little success in obtaining pregnancies after transfer of blastocysts to the uterus after IVF, possibly due to developmental delay during culture in vitro[17], but 35% of women established a pregnancy after transfer of a thawed blastocyst[18].

There is potential for preimplantation genetic diagnosis at three stages:

1. Preconception, using the first polar body to infer the genotype of the oocyte.
2. Biopsy during the cleavage stage of the embryo, typically at the six-cell to eight-cell stage (Figure 22.1).
3. Trophectoderm biopsy at the blastocyst stage.

Preimplantation diagnosis at the blastocyst stage offers an alternative method of obtaining embryos, namely uterine lavage. Lavage was first performed in humans for the treatment of infertile couples by insemination of a donor female with the husband's sperm[19]. Lavage of the uterine cavity 5–8 days following insemination yielded a low recovery of healthy blastocysts which following transfer to the recipients resulted in healthy pregnancies. Subsequently this approach has been investigated by Buster's group and two further groups in Italy[20]. Unfortunately, despite the development of new systems for flushing the uterine cavity, employing ultrasound control to ensure no flushing medium passes up the fallopian tubes and into the peritoneal cavity, several blastocysts have not been recovered from the

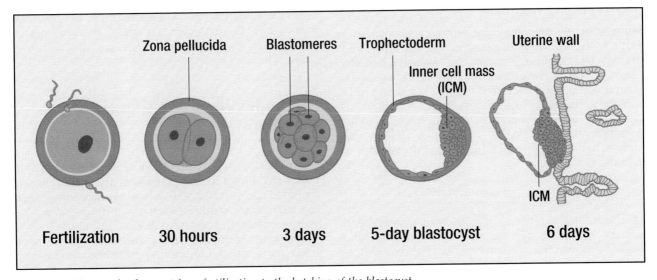

Figure 22.1 *Human development from fertilization to the hatching of the blastocyst*

same woman in one collection cycle despite super-ovulation[21]. A major anxiety with uterine lavage is the possibility of leaving the patient pregnant, particularly with an ectopic gestation if all the embryos are not recovered. The ultrasonographically controlled approach to flushing minimizes the possibility of retrograde lavage up the fallopian tubes, and hormonal manipulation can prevent pregnancy in the cycle of embryo collection. This is fine during research, but would necessitate cryopreservation of the biopsied blastocysts for transfer in a subsequent cycle.

Despite these difficulties, the approach of uterine lavage followed by blastocysts biopsy is extremely attractive. Firstly the ordeal and cost of IVF are removed and the couple can conceive by the normal route, which would be of emotional benefit to some couples. In addition, biopsy of the trophectoderm does not involve interference with the cells destined to become the embryo proper and may therefore be viewed as an early chorionic villus biopsy from the ethical point of view. Thus trophectoderm biopsy following uterine lavage may be more acceptable in ethical terms than cleavage biopsy following IVF, an important factor in some countries.

Which patients might benefit from preimplantation diagnosis?

In the context of the genodermatoses, the women likely to be considering preimplantation diagnosis in the future are those at risk of having a baby with an X-linked disorder (embryo sexing) or a mendelian disorder in which the mutation is known. Certain groups may particularly benefit.

Women already sterilized

Before effective prenatal diagnosis became available, couples who were at high risk of giving birth to a child affected with a serious monogenic disorder had the choice of taking the chance that the child would be normal, accepting gamete donation, or refraining from further pregnancies and considering adoption. It would therefore be entirely appropriate to offer preimplantation diagnosis to couples where the woman had undergone tubal ligation, but was still of reproductive age.

Tragically unlucky families

All those who practise in the fields of genetics and prenatal diagnosis become aware of families who despite (for example) the probability of three chances out of four that they will conceive a healthy child, are unlucky time and time again. They often have no

difficulty conceiving, and as is often the case with couples at genetic risk, they fall pregnant 'by accident'. This is perhaps because planning a pregnancy is associated with the stress and possible disappointment of prenatal diagnostic testing. When prenatal testing fails to result in the news of an unaffected child, the couple experience an enormous drive to replace the pregnancy, and may present for prenatal diagnosis again and again despite repeated failure. Those of us who have never had reproductive or genetic problems cannot begin to appreciate their determination, and suggest adoption or gamete donation. For these tragic families such suggestions are unacceptable, as the pregnancies that have been lost are genetically their own, they feel that they must provide the solution themselves.

Infertile couples and those at genetic risk

The infertile population will contain a similar proportion of sufferers or carriers of genetic disease to their fertile counterparts. It is therefore important to identify those at genetic risk by a careful family history or examination. For example, individuals affected by neurofibromatosis type I may well be overlooked if mildly affected. With large IVF centres treating 2000 infertile couples each year a few couples may present at risk of transmitting one of the genodermatoses.

Patients with moral objections to termination of pregnancy

Objections to termination of pregnancy may not preclude selection of unfertilized oocytes, or preimplantation diagnosis and selective transfer of embryos. However, it is likely to be unacceptable until the reliability is well established, because this group can be expected to reject a confirmatory prenatal test in pregnancy.

Strategies for preimplantation diagnosis

The methodology of preimplantation diagnosis falls under two broad headings, namely the embryological methods necessary to achieve a diagnostic sample and the technology required to make a diagnosis on the sample obtained. The embryological approaches cover three areas including non-invasive diagnosis, preconception removal of the first polar body, and biopsy of cells from the embryo either during cleavage or at the blastocyst stage.

Non-invasive diagnosis

Culture of human embryos in microdrops under oil after fertilization in vitro has allowed serial measurements of their production of lactate and consumption of pyruvate and glucose from the medium[22]. Diagnosis based on this type of approach is very attractive in that the embryo itself is not damaged in any way, but is likely to be limited to a few rare metabolic disorders which may be expressed at such an early stage.

Preconception diagnosis

Preconception diagnosis has many advantages, the greatest of which is an ethical one, as the procedure does not involve interference with the preimplantation embryo. For single gene disorders that are inherited in an autosomal recessive fashion, if the genetic contribution of the oocyte can be typed to be normal, then whether a normal or abnormal gene is inherited via the sperm the baby will be unaffected. The same is true of X-linked disorders which, although the sex of the embryo is determined by the sperm, the defective gene is inherited via the oocyte. If a dominant disorder is present in the mother, again typing of the oocyte will be effective in determining whether the offspring is affected. Thus the majority of single gene disorders could benefit from this approach.

Genetic analysis of the oocyte itself would of course destroy the very cell needed for fertilization. However, during the reduction division or meiosis to produce the oocyte, degenerative microcells (polar bodies) containing one of the two products of chromosome segregation are formed – but can the genetic make-up of the oocyte be inferred from the polar bodies?

The first meiotic division is completed just before ovulation, and the first polar body is extruded. This contains a single set of chromosomes that have already divided, each into two chromatids; one of the two chromatids may have exchanged genetic material by crossing over with a chromatid that remains in the oocyte. After removing the cumulus cells, a small slit can be made in the zona pellucida and the polar body removed by micromanipulation. The polymerase chain reaction can then be used to examine the gene locus in question, on the assumption that the oocyte will have the opposite genotype to that of the first polar body. This approach has been attempted using human oocytes tested for the presence of the unaffected allele of the alpha-1-antitrypsin gene, deficiency of which may cause severe liver disease in the neonate[23]. Amplified polar body DNA was hybridized with both the normal (M) and the abnormal (Z) allele-specific oligonucleotide probes, and two fertilized oocytes whose polar body contained only the abnormal allele were transferred to the uterus as six-cell embryos. Pregnancy did not result.

The major anxiety with this approach is crossing-over during female meiosis, the frequency of which is dependent on the chromosome involved and the distance of the gene from the centromere. Extensive preliminary studies to examine this issue for each disease system tested must be undertaken before such diagnosis is offered to patients.

Embryo biopsy

During cleavage

In humans the retention of the zona pellucida is desirable in order to prevent spontaneous loss of blastomeres and to protect the embryo during transfer. Micromanipulative removal of single human blastomeres at the eight-cell stage after drilling a small hole in the zona pellucida with an acidic solution[24] has confirmed the ability of an eight-cell human embryo to adjust for the loss of a blastomere at this stage, because healthy infants have been born following the transfer of biopsied embryos. Alternative approaches to biopsy at this stage involve slitting the zona or pushing a hole in the zona thus allowing entry of the biopsy pipette. At the eight-cell stage one or two cells may be removed without a significant decrease in viability[25], but it is thought that this is the latest stage at which the blastomeres remain totipotent and thereafter biopsy is best left to the trophectoderm at the blastocyst stage on day 6 or 7 following fertilization. Eight-cell embryos are observed early on day 3, and rapid diagnosis has allowed transfer of sexed embryos later on the same day.

Blastocyst biopsy

The above approaches to obtaining samples rely on obtaining oocytes and fertilizing them in vitro. An alternative, biopsy at the blastocyst stage, may allow collection of embryos after natural conception by uterine lavage, therefore avoiding many of the disadvantages of fertilization in vitro.

At the blastocyst stage, days 5–7 in the human, the cells of the embryo have segregated into an outer layer of trophectoderm destined to form placental tissue, and an inner cell mass of cells which remain totipotent, of which a small proportion give rise to the fetus itself. Biopsy at this stage offers the possibility of removing cells that are not destined to become the embryo itself, and may in fact eventually degenerate, because in the human the placenta forms adjacent to the inner cell mass and the trophectoderm opposite the inner cell mass will form the chorion laeve.

Blastocyst biopsy of human embryos following IVF has been achieved[26–28], and as several cells are removed, multiple diagnoses would be possible. Such techniques have not yet been applied in clinical preimplantation diagnosis.

Genetic diagnosis

In future practice the method actually used to make the genetic diagnosis, with respect to embryos at risk of inheriting a genodermatosis, will almost always be DNA analysis exploiting the exquisite sensitivity of the polymerase chain reaction (PCR). It may be that it will become routine to check the karyotype of embryos selected for transfer, but the primary diagnosis will be detection of the mutant DNA sequence. In situ hybridization of molecular DNA probes directly on to metaphase chromosomes may well play a role in sexing embryos where an X-linked genodermatosis is concerned. The technique of using fluorescent markers for Y and X specific sequences has improved steadily since the first attempts, and has been reviewed by Handyside and Delhauty[29].

Advantages of fluorescent in situ hybridization (FISH) include the fact that the cell is observed and therefore shown to be present during analysis, both X and Y signals are detected, and an assessment of the number of X chromosomes can be made[32–35]. The technique can be extended to assess the number of copies of specific autosomes, raising the possibility of interphase karyotyping on single cells[36, 37].

To date, diagnosis at the protein level has not looked too helpful. In particular, using hypoxanthine phosphoribosyl transferase deficiency as a model of the Lesch–Nyhan syndrome, promising results in mouse embryos[30] have not been replicated in human embryos[31], emphasizing the importance of species differences in gene expression in the early embryo.

The greatest success so far has been the use of the polymerase chain reaction (Chapter 1) to detect specific changes in DNA sequence following biopsy of the six-cell to eight-cell embryo. The sensitivity of PCR means that contamination, even by a single skin cell from the operator, is the greatest potential problem. There have already been clinical trials of embryo sexing in families at risk of X-linked disease[5]. Follow-up of the pregnancies with chorionic villus sampling revealed one error in eight such pregnancies[29], and this group now favours FISH for pre-implantation sexing. The methods are now considerably improved and further clinical trials are under way. The same team[6] has developed pre-implantation diagnosis for couples at risk of cystic fibrosis, and several healthy children have already been born following this procedure. A number of

other mutations have already been diagnosed using PCR, including Lesch–Nyhan syndrome, Duchenne muscular dystrophy (A. Handyside, personal communication) and Tay–Sachs disease[38]. The introduction of whole genome amplification will allow the possibility of multiple diagnoses on a single cell and it has been possible to amplify six loci from a single human blastomere[39, 40]. Preimplantation diagnosis promises to offer a further choice to couples facing genetic risks, and many more healthy babies will be born as a result of these developments.

References

1 Steptoe P, Edwards RG. Birth after reimplantation of a human embryo. *Lancet* 1978; **ii**: 336.
2 Old JM, Ward RHT, Petrou M et al. First trimester diagnosis for haemoglobinopathies: three cases. *Lancet* 1982; **ii**: 1413–16.
3 McLaren A. Prenatal diagnosis before implantation: opportunities and problems. *Prenat Diag* 1984; **5**: 85–90.
4 Penketh R, McLaren A. Prospects for prenatal diagnosis during preimplantation human development. *Balliere's Clin Obstet Gynaecol* 1987; **1**: 747–64.
5 Handyside AH, Kontogianni EH, Hardy K, Winston RML. Pregnancies from biopsied human embryos sexed by Y-specific DNA amplification. *Nature* 1990; **334**: 768–70.
6 Handyside AH, Lesko JG, Tarin JJ, Winston RMI, Hughes MR. Birth of a normal girl after in vitro fertilisation and preimplantation diagnostic testing for cystic fibrosis. *New Engl J Med* 1992; **327**: 905–9.
7 Feichtinger W, Kemeter P. Transvaginal sector scan sonography for needle guided transvaginal follicle aspiration and other applications in gynacologic routine and research. *Fertil Steril* 1986; **45**: 722–5.
8 Rutherford AJ, Subak-Sharpe R, Dawson K et al. Dramatic improvement in IVF success following treatment with LHRH agonist. *Br Med J* 1988; **296**: 1765–8.
9 Conaghan J, Dimitry ES, Mills M, Margara RA, Winston RML. Delayed human chorionic gonadotrophin administration for in vitro fertilisation. *Lancet* 1989; **i**: 1323–4.
10 Saiki RK, Scharf S, Faloona F et al. Enzymatic amplification of beta globin genomic sequences and restriction site analysis for diagnosis of sickle cell anaemia. *Science* 1985; **230**: 1350–4.
11 Li H, Gyllensten UB, Cui X et al. Amplification and analysis of DNA sequences in single human sperm and diploid cells. *Nature* 1988; **335**: 414–17.
12 Coutelle C, Williams C, Handyside A et al. Genetic analysis of DNA from single human oocytes – a model for preimplantation diagnosis of cystic fibrosis. *Br Med J* 1989; **299**: 22–4.
13 Dellenbach P, Nisand L, Moreau L et al. Transvaginal, sonographically controlled ovarian follicle puncture for egg retrieval. *Lancet* 1984; **6**: 1647.
14 Dellenbach P, Nisand L, Moreau L et al. Transvaginal, sonographically controlled follicle puncture for oocyte retrieval. *Fertil Steril* 1985; **44**: 656–62.
15 Renou P, Trounson AO, Wood C, Leeton JF. The collection of human oocytes for in vitro fertilisation. An instrument for maximising oocyte recovery rate. *Fertil Steril* 1981; **35**: 409.

16 Wood C, Leeton J, McTalbot J, Trounson AO. Technique for collecting mature human oocytes for in vitro fertilisation. *Br J Obstet Gynaecol* 1981; **88**: 756.

17 Dawson K-J, Rutherford AJ, Winston NJ, Subak-Sharpe R, Winston RML. Human blastocyst transfer, is it a feasible proposition? Abstracts of the fourth meeting of the ESHRE. *Hum Reprod* 1988; **14** (suppl.): 44–5.

18 Fehilly CB, Cohen J, Simons R-F, Fishel SB, Edwards RG. Cryopreservation of cleaving embryos and expanded blastocysts in the human: a comparative study. *Fertil Steril* 1985; **45**: 638–44.

19 Buster JE. Embryo donation by uterine flushing and embryo transfer. *Clin Obstet Gynaecol* 1985; **12**: 815–24.

20 Brambati B, Tuli L. Preimplantation genetic diagnosis: a new simple uterine washing system. *Hum Reprod* 1990; **5**: 448–50.

21 Carson SA, Smith A, Scoggan J, Buster JE. Super-ovulation fails to increase human blastocyst yield after uterine lavage. *Prenat Diag* 1991; **11**: 513–22.

22 Hardy K, Hooper MAK, Handyside AH et al. Non-invasive measurement of glucose and pyruvate uptake by individual human oocytes and preimplantation embryos. *Hum Reprod* 1989; **4**: 188–91.

23 Verlinsky Y, Rechitsky S, Evsikov S et al. Preconception and preimplantation diagnosis for cystic fibrosis. *Prenat Diag* 1992; **12**: 103–10.

24 Handyside AH, Pattinson JK, Penketh RJA et al. Biopsy of human preimplantation embryos and sexing by DNA amplification. *Lancet* 1989; **1**: 347–9.

25 Hardy K, Martin KL, Leese HJ, Winston RML, Handyside AH. Human preimplantation development in vitro is not adversely affected by biopsy at the 8cell stage. *Hum Reprod* 1990; **5**: 708–14.

26 Dokras A, Sargent IL, Ross C et al. Trophectoderm biopsy in human blastocysts. *Hum Reprod* 1990; **5**: 821–5.

27 Dokras A, Sargent IL, Gardner RL et al. Human trophectoderm biopsy and secretion of chorionic gonadotrophin. *Hum Reprod* 1991; **6**: 1453–9.

28 Muggleton-Harris AL, Glazier AM, Pickering S et al. Genetic diagnosis using polymerase chain reaction and fluorescent in situ hybridisation analysis from both the cleavage and blastocyst stages of individual cultured human preimplantation embryos. *Hum Reprod* 1995; **10**: 183–92.

29 Handyside AH, Delhauty JDA. Cleavage stage biopsy of human embryos and diagnosis of X-linked recessive disease. In: Edwards RG, ed. *Preimplantation Diagnosis of Human Genetic Disease*. Cambridge University Press, 1993.

30 Monk M, Handyside A, Hardy K, Whittingham DG. Preimplantation diagnosis of deficiency of hypoxanthine phosphoribosyl transferase in a mouse model for Lesch–Nyhan syndrome. *Lancet* 1987; **ii**: 423–5.

31 Braude PR, Monk M, Pickering SJ et al. Measurement of HPRT activity in the human unfertilized oocyte and pre-embryo. *Prenat Diag* 1989; **9**: 839–50.

32 Griffin DK, Handyside AH, Penketh RJ et al. Fluorescent in situ hybridisation to interphase nuclei of human preimplantation embryos with X and Y-chromosome specific probes. *Hum Reprod* 1991; **6**: 101–5.

33 Harper JC, Coonen E, Ramaekers FC et al. Identification of the sex of human embryos in two hours using an improved spreading method and fluorescent in-situ hybridisation (FISH) using directly labelled probes. *Hum Reprod* 1994; **9**: 721–4.

34 Griffin DK, Handyside AH, Harper JC et al. Clinical experience of preimplantion diagnosis of sex by dual fluorescent in situ hybridisation. *J Assist Reprod Genet* 1994; **11**: 132–43.

35 Delhanty JD, Griffin DK, Handyside AH et al. Detection of aneuploidy and chromosomal mosaicism in human embryos during preimplantation sex determination by fluorescent in situ hybridisation (FISH). *Hum Mol Genet* 1993; **3**: 1183–5.

36 Harper JC, Coonen E, Handyside AH et al. Mosaicism of autosomes and sex chromosomes in morphologically normal, monospermic preimplantation human embryos. *Prenat Diag* 1995; **15**: 41–9.

37 Munne S, Sultan KM, Weier HU et al. Assessment of numeric abnormalities of X, Y,18 and 16 chromosomes in human preimplantation embryos before transfer. *Am J Obstet Gynecol* 1994; **172**: 1191–9.

38 Gibbons WE, Giltin SA, Lanzendorf SE et al. Pre-implantation genetic diagnosis for Tay Sachs disease: successful pregnancy after pre-embryo biopsy and gene amplification by polymerase chain reaction. *Fertil Steril* 1995; **63**: 723–8.

39 Griffo JA, Tang YX, Munne S et al. Healthy deliveries from biopsied human embryos. *Hum Reprod* 1994; **9**: 912–16.

40 Snabes MC, Chong SS, Subramanian SB et al. Pre-implantation single cell analysis of multiple genetic loci by whole genome amplification. *Proc Nat Acad Sci* 1994; **91**: 6181–5.

Chapter 23

What future is there in gene therapy?

C. Kinnon and M.E. Pembrey

Introduction

With the advent of recombinant DNA technology many advances in the diagnosis and treatment of human genetic diseases have been postulated. These advances have already been translated into improved methods for the prenatal diagnosis of many diseases and the use of recombinant gene products in treatment regimens. It is envisaged, however, that with further developments it will soon be possible to correct the genetic defects themselves in affected individuals, through the use of somatic gene therapy techniques. The potential of this form of treatment has generated much interest and the possible applications of somatic gene therapy have been much discussed [1–3]. In this chapter the applications of somatic gene therapy in the treatment of diseases that affect the skin are discussed, as well as the possibility of genetically modifying the skin itself and using it as a drug delivery system.

Somatic gene therapy can be defined as the introduction of a functioning exogenous gene into a cell that either does not express its own copy of the gene or has a defective copy of that gene. In most cases the introduced gene would be in addition to the copy of the gene already present in the cell, which would technically result in gene augmentation. A more difficult technique would be gene replacement, whereby a defective gene would be removed and replaced with a functional gene in the correct orientation and chromosomal location. Such gene replacement would be technically difficult, although a model for gene targeting involving homologous recombination is being developed [4]. This, however, currently involves introducing the gene into the germ line,

which means that it could be passed on to subsequent generations. With somatic gene therapy techniques the gene is introduced only into the somatic cells of the patient and not into the germ line, and therefore the gene cannot be passed on to subsequent generations.

Methods of gene insertion

There are two approaches to the problem of introducing cloned genes into cells: namely, physical and viral [5]. Physical methods include coprecipitation of DNA with calcium phosphate; the use of polycations or lipids to complex the DNA; cell fusion techniques utilizing liposomes, erythrocyte ghosts or protoplasts; microinjection; and electroporation techniques. While large numbers of cells can be treated at once (except by microinjection), these techniques have the disadvantage that the efficiency of integration is low and multiple copies of the DNA are usually integrated.

Viruses have often been used to introduce DNA into cells in culture; the first expression vectors utilized the DNA tumour viruses, SV40 and polyoma [6]. More recent work in this area has focused on the murine retroviruses, including Moloney leukaemia virus (MLV) and myeloproliferative sarcoma virus (MPSV), and on adenoviruses and adenoassociated viruses. In essence, a viral vector replaces the viral protein genes with the DNA to be transferred (Figure 23.1).

Retroviruses have a number of features which make them suitable for use as vectors for gene therapy. The production of progeny virus is non-lytic, leading to the establishment of permanent, viral producer cell lines which give high-titre virus for infection of target

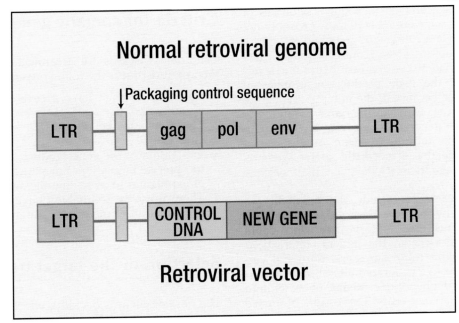

Figure 23.1 *How the new DNA replaces the* gag, pol *and* env *envelope genes in the retrovirus genome*

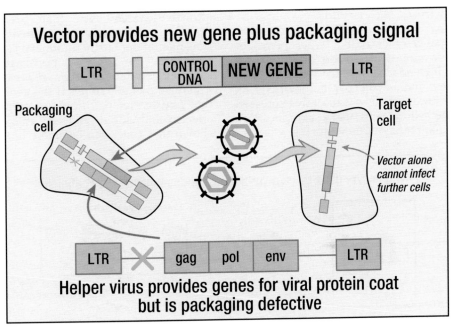

Figure 23.2 *The use of cells containing a packaging-defective virus to supply viral coat proteins and therefore allow one round of infection of the target cell by the vector carrying the new DNA*

cells. The *gag, pol* and *env* genes, required for viral encapsidation, can be supplied *in trans*, which means that replication-defective retroviruses can be produced that are capable of only one round of infection, technically eliminating the problem of constant reinfection of cells (Figure 23.2). Any infective retroviruses that did arise in the patient should, however, be efficiently neutralized by complement present in the patient's own sera. Retroviral vectors can infect up to 100% of target cells and the DNA is usually integrated as a single copy. Once integrated into the host genome the provirus acts as a cellular gene in that it is faithfully passed onto progeny cells.

However, there are several disadvantages to using retroviruses as vectors for gene therapy. Perhaps the most obvious drawback is the fact that retroviral vectors can only encode up to about 7 kilobases of introduced DNA, which in most cases is probably not sufficient to encode a full-length gene and its appropriate control sequences. Loss of control sequences may lead to inappropriate tissue expression and low levels of expression of the gene product. A number of problems can arise because of the non-specific nature of the integration event where the gene is randomly inserted into the genome. These can include non-expression of the introduced gene or insertional mutagenesis, whereby a normally active gene is silenced or a silent deleterious gene may become activated.

Further disadvantages include the possibility of recombination between the exogenous retroviral vector and endogenous human retroviruses which could produce infective virus in the patient. Interactions between endogenous retroviruses and retroviral vectors can give rise to phenotypic alterations such as pseudotyping and phenotypic mixing even without genetic recombination events. Expression of mixed exogenous proviruses could give rise to the production of replication-competent viruses. These potential problems have suggested the need to develop new packaging cell lines from species that have fewer endogenous retroviruses, such as birds.

It is possible that safer, more efficient, higher-titre viral vectors, capable of encoding larger pieces of DNA, may be developed based on other viruses including adenovirus, adenoassociated virus, vaccinia and herpesviruses, and bovine papillomavirus[5,6]. Indeed, the cystic fibrosis gene was recently expressed in rat airway epithelium cells using a replication-deficient recombinant adenovirus vector[7].

Criteria for somatic gene therapy

Candidate diseases for treatment by this type of therapy must meet the following criteria:

1. The disease must have a severe and predictable phenotype.
2. The gene to be introduced must have been cloned.
3. Expression of the gene product should not require too precise regulation, nor particularly high levels of expression to overcome the defect.
4. There must be a suitable delivery system for the implantation of the genetically modified cells.

Selection of the target tissue

The next problem is deciding which target tissue the gene should be delivered to. Currently, the most suitable target tissues are those of the haematopoietic system, in particular the bone marrow and the lymphoid system. The bone marrow is a particularly attractive system since there are many candidate disorders which are now treated by bone marrow transplantation. Furthermore, the search is under way to identify the human bone marrow multipotential stem cell population. If these cells can be infected, then it may be possible to insert the gene once and correct the genetic defect throughout the lifetime of the affected individual. Indeed, studies in mice have shown that genes can be stably introduced into bone

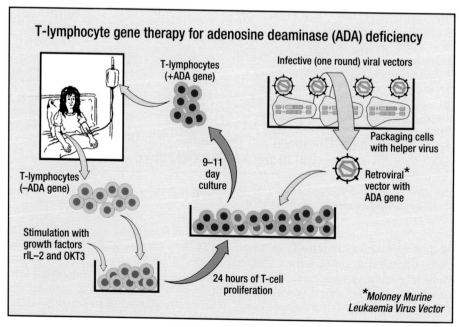

Figure 23.3 *The approach used in the first clinical study of gene therapy for adenosine deaminase (ADA) deficiency, exploiting the long-lived nature of some peripheral blood lymphoctyes*

marrow stem cells by retroviral vectors and expression in differentiated progeny cells has been detected for some time afterwards. The lymphoid system has been utilized as a delivery system for the adenosine deaminase (ADA) gene (R.M. Blaese, personal communication), which is defective in a form of severe combined immunodeficiency (Figure 23.3). These approaches may prove useful for skin diseases which are caused by an absence or insufficiency of a humoral product such as a hormone, growth factor, enzyme or other diffusible protein. In diseases where this is found to be the case, once the defective gene has been identified and cloned, a functional copy of the gene may be introduced into the patient's own bone marrow stem cells or lymphoid cells and the normal gene product may be secreted from the modified cells and/or their descendants into the blood stream to circulate to the affected sites in the skin. The effectiveness of such an approach would presumably depend on sufficient quantities of these proteins reaching their target cells. This may necessitate high levels of gene expression and/or the prerequisite for specific uptake or receptor systems being present in the targeted cells.

Skin cells such as fibroblasts and keratinocytes are also attractive as target tissues for gene transfer. Such cells are readily accessible by skin biopsy and can easily be cultured and manipulated in vitro. They are relatively easy to transform with vectors and can be reintroduced by autografting. Skin fibroblasts have an additional advantage in that they reside in a highly vascularized compartment of the dermis and so transduced cells would have direct access to the circulatory system. Thus, this approach could be manipulated to deliver other secreted gene products into the circulation, such as factor IX for haemophilia[8], and adenosine deaminase[9] or purine nucleoside phosphorylase[10] for certain forms of severe combined immunodeficiency. Similarly, cultured epidermal keratinocytes could provide another potential target tissue but would not have the advantage of such a highly vascularized compartment. Some promising results in the development of gene therapy for haemophilia B using primary human keratinocytes have been reported[11].

A patch of genetically altered skin producing a growth factor or other gene product could be easily controlled since the graft could be removed or varied in size according to need. Furthermore, by use of suitable promoter or other regulatory sequences it may ultimately be possible to regulate levels of gene product by external stimuli such as light or temperature.

Conclusion

It is clear that the potential for genetic manipulation in the treatment of skin diseases is vast. This chapter merely outlines a few of the potential applications; much of this work is still at the level of basic research and, indeed, is dependent on the elucidation of the basic molecular defects in the majority of these conditions. In recent years, there have been significant advances in our understanding of a number of important genetic skin diseases (for example, epidermolysis bullosa). Many of the major problems of gene therapy, such as gene transfer and targeting, are now being investigated and in time will be solved. Once these problems are resolved, treatment of skin diseases by the technique of somatic gene therapy may become practicable.

References

1 Anderson FW. Prospects for human gene therapy. *Science* 1984; **226**: 401–9.
2 Kantoff PW, Freeman SM, Anderson FW. Prospects for gene therapy for immunodeficiency diseases. *Ann Rev Immunol* 1988; **6**: 581–94.
3 Friedmann T. Progress toward human gene therapy. *Science* 1989; **244**: 1275–81.
4 Capecchi MR. Altering the genome by homologous recombination. *Science* 1989; **244**: 1288–92.
5 Sambrook J, Fritsch EF, Maniatis T. In: *Molecular Cloning: A Laboratory Manual*. 2nd ed. Cold Spring Harbor Press, 1989.
6 Rigby PWJ. In: Williamson R, ed. *Genetic Engineering*, vol 3. Academic Press, New York, 1982; 84–134.
7 Rosenfeld MA, Yoshimura K, Trapnell BC et al. In vivo transfer of the human cystic fibrosis transmembrane conductance regulator gene to the airway epithelium. *Cell* 1992; **68**: 143–55.
8 St Louis D, Verma IM. An alternative approach to somatic cell gene therapy. *Proc Nat Acad Sci USA* 1988; **85**: 3150–4.
9 Palmer TD, Hock RA, Osborne WRA, Miller AD. Efficient retrovirus-mediated transfer and expression of a human adenosine deaminase gene in diploid skin fibroblasts from an adenosine deaminase-deficient human. *Proc Nat Acad Sci USA* 1987; **84**: 1055–9.
10 Osborne WRA, Miller AD. Design of vectors for efficient expression of human purine nucleoside phosphorylase in skin fibroblasts from enzyme-deficient humans. *Proc Nat Acad Sci USA* 1988; **85**: 6851–5.
11 Gerrard AJ, Hudson DL, Brownlee GG et al. Towards gene therapy for haemophilia B using primary human keratinocytes. *Nature Gen* 1993; **3**: 180–3.

Index